Family-Centered Maternity/Newborn Care

A BASIC TEXT

Family-Centered Maternity/Newborn Care

A BASIC TEXT

Celeste R. Phillips, R.N., Ed.D.

Maternity Instructor,
Cabrillo College, Aptos, California;
Director of Professional Relations,
the Borning Corporation,
Spokane, Washington

with 163 *illustrations*

new line drawings by

Jeffrey A. Nagel

contributor

J. Duncan Phillips, M.D.

University of California,
Los Angeles, California

The C. V. Mosby Company

ST. LOUIS • WASHINGTON, D.C. • TORONTO 1987

MOSBY

A TRADITION OF PUBLISHING EXCELLENCE

Project editor: Sylvia Kluth
Production editor: John A. Rogers
Manuscript editor: Editing, Design & Production, Inc.
Book design: Liz Fett
Production: Editing, Design & Production, Inc.

Printed in the United States of America

The C.V. Mosby Company
11830 Westline Industrial Drive, St. Louis, Missouri 63146

Library of Congress Cataloging-in-Publication Data

Phillips, Celeste R., 1933-
Family-centered maternity/newborn care.

Includes bibliographies and index.
1. Obstetrical nursing. 2. Neonatology. I. Phillips, J. Duncan. II. Title. [DNLM: 1. Family—nurses' instruction. 2. Obstetrical Nursing. 3. Pediatric Nursing. WY 157 P558f]
RG951.P63 1987 610.73'678 86-23828
ISBN 0-8016-3918-2

C/VH/VH 9 8 7 6 5 4 3 2 01/D/011

To my first teachers, my parents
Catherine M. Nagel and **Erwin W. Nagel**
and my new teachers, my children
J. Duncan Phillips, M.D., and
Catherine Rose Phillips, R.N., B.S.N.
who will teach me so much

Preface

This second edition of Family-Centered Maternity/Newborn Care has been revised, expanded, and updated to include the latest information on care of childbearing families. Although longer and more detailed, this edition has remained a basic text for use by beginning students with no previous maternity experience. The book format remains the same, with goals and objectives identified adjacent to the appropriate text material in each unit. Self-assessment exercises follow each unit so that the student can have immediate feedback on attainment of objectives. Also at the end of each unit, learning activities, audiovisual materials, and in-depth study activities are suggested. These exercises are offered only as recommended ways in which the learning could be expanded upon and enriched. Answers for the self-assessment exercises are given at the end of the book.

To individualize the manner in which this text might be used, it has been printed so that pages may be removed easily to be used as assignments, work sheets, or clinical tools. Clinical learning objectives and learning tools are included for students and instructors to use where and when appropriate. The clinical applications at the back of the text provide suggestions for creating nursing care plans. However, to keep this text a reasonable size and price, and also to make it useful to all entry level health care providers, nursing care plans were not included. When needed, an excellent supplemental reference for writing and using nursing care plans for childbearing families is *Nursing Care Plans for the Childbearing Family*, by Virginia Aukamp, R.N., M.S. This 1984 reference is published by Appleton-Century-Crofts, 25 Van Zant Street, East Norwalk, Connecticut, 06855.

The updated references used and listed in the bibliography at the end of each unit still are mainly from nursing journals and books to which beginning students can refer. Extremely detailed and complex references were purposely avoided so that the student might not be discouraged when reading source material.

This second edition is accurate and current with added information on preterm labor, vaginal birth after cesarean (VBAC), mother-baby nursing, ambulation and a variety of positions for labor and birth, and nipple stimulation as a technique for antepartum stress testing. Expanded sections on high-risk pregnancy and newborn care, fetal monitoring, breastfeeding, and education for birth and parenting contribute to the comprehensiveness of this new edition.

It is assumed that the student who uses this book has had a basic preparation in anatomy and physiology, medical terminology, medical and surgical nursing, and fundamental nursing skills.

Whatever terms are finally used, it is important to remember that 85% to 90% of all births in the United States occur without major dangers or complications. However, in our culture the majority of pregnant women are hospitalized for birth in institutions for the care of the sick. Hospital maternity units are adjacent to areas where people may have terminal illnesses; visiting times for family and friends often are scheduled and regimented to accommodate the regulations necessary to manage a large, multifaceted institution caring for medical and surgical patients. In this context, childbirth often is treated as an illness and the woman's hospital experience is regimented and compartmentalized into the prenatal unit, labor and delivery unit, postpartum unit, and newborn nursery. As a result, the childbearing woman and her family may have to interact with numerous health care providers on these separate units; frequently they must repeat answers to the same questions again and again. Although this book was organized for clarity into time periods in the childbearing cycle (prenatal, intrapartum, postpartum, and newborn), the theme of family care was threaded throughout, and an attempt has been made not to compartmentalize the childbearing experience. Family-centered maternity/newborn care providers offer individualized care for the entire family unit, thus providing continuity to the childbearing cycle and reducing fragmentation of care.

Just like the original text, this edition is also a family project, with my own family and friends helping in every way they could. However, this time my son, Dr. J. Duncan Phillips, contributed significantly by writing the anatomy and physiology content, reviewing all of the units, and offering suggestions.

Important suggestions also were contributed by my daughter, Catherine Rose Phillips, R.N. I will never be able to thank her enough for her love and support.

Appreciation goes to my mother, Catherine Nagel, and to my father, Erwin Nagel, for their patience and support for a daughter who undertakes projects they don't always understand. This can be a very difficult thing to do and requires a great deal of caring.

To the couples, families, nurses, and hospitals who shared their special photographs go special thanks.

I would also like to give special recognition to my nephew, Jeffrey A. Nagel, who prepared the new illustrations to supplement the originals drawn by Sharon J. Leibolt, and to Dr. Loel Fenwick and Charles Pomeroy of Borning Corporation for the use of their illustrations and photographs.

For manuscript typing, much appreciation goes to Ann Bennett, who read my writing and interpreted my symbols.

Last but not least, extra special thanks go to my husband, Roger Phillips, for his faith in me. As the years of our lives together continue, he remains consistently excellent in every way.

Celeste R. Phillips

Contents

UNIT I
Introduction and overview

GOALS

This unit is designed to provide the reader with information that will:

□ provide a background for the study of family-centered maternity/newborn care.
□ develop an awareness of parenting processes: mothering and fathering.
□ develop an appreciation for variations influencing the parenting process.

STUDENT OBJECTIVES

After studying this unit, you should be able to:

1. List two developments in maternity care for each of the following historical periods.
   a. Ancient
   b. Renaissance
   c. Seventeenth century to nineteenth century
   d. Twentieth century
2. Identify the numerical position of the U.S. infant mortality rate in the world.
3. Discuss the concept of family and explain how pregnancy and birth can affect other family members.
4. Differentiate between the key components of conventional and family-centered models of maternity care.
5. Indicate several ways in which fathers may be helped to face the reality of pregnancy.
6. With your classmates or family discuss at least two basic differences in attitudes toward childbearing and birth.
7. Identify three emotional phases for men and three for women to experience during pregnancy to begin bonding with their unborn baby.
8. Identify four experiences that could interfere with the parent-infant relationship and result in bonding difficulty.

Events in recent years have brought tremendous change into the world of childbearing families. As a result, the health care requirements of these families in pregnancy and birth and childbearing can be expected to change. As this study of the childbearing family begins, it is appropriate to look briefly at where we have been to better understand where we are and where we are going.

Obstetrics is that branch of medicine defined as the art and science of caring for the childbearing woman and her unborn baby. Actually, the term *obstetrics* was derived from the Latin verb *obstare*, "to stand before." From this point, or whenever possible, we will purposely omit the terms *obstetrics* and *obstetric nurse and personnel* because this old terminology pertains to standing before the mother and concentrating on adapting care around her medical treatment. For effective and meaningful change to occur in childbearing in this decade, *family-centered maternity and newborn care* should become the norm, in which health care personnel offer support during the whole childbearing cycle and emphasize the individual needs of the mother and family. Family-centered maternity and newborn care involves caring for not one but for all family members: mother, father, infant, siblings, grandparents, and significant other people. At no time during the childbearing experience should any person in this multisided unit be neglected, for exclusion of one member of the family can have serious consequences for all members.

HISTORICAL BACKGROUND

Ancient

DEVELOPMENTS IN MATERNITY CARE

Until the nineteenth century, few people, including physicians, were concerned with providing women in childbirth with other than untrained women attendants. In fact, the first services provided to women at childbirth really were maternal, with mothers helping their own daughters give birth. However, even in these early times, women with special skills were recognized as midwives who would assist at deliveries outside their own families. The midwives concentrated on the labor and delivery; physicians were called only when there were complicating medical problems. Even in these problem cases, however, the physician would usually only supervise or give advice while the midwife assisted the delivery.

In ancient Greece, the writings of Hippocrates marked the beginning of the scientific study and practice of medicine, including the practice of obstetrics. Soranus of Ephesus, the "Father of Obstetrics," wrote the oldest known textbook for midwives (AD 120). In the Roman Empire, according to the *lex caesarea* (law of Caesar's land), cesarean sections were performed to save the baby of a dying mother.

Medieval period

During the medieval period there was no progress in obstetrics; medical practice regressed into mysticism.

Renaissance

During the Renaissance, establishment of Italian medical schools advanced obstetric education. Although the Church opposed dissection, persistent physicians robbed graves to obtain bodies on which to study. During this period, Ambrose Paré helped establish the first midwifery school in France and also helped establish obstetric practice as part of medicine.

Seventeenth century to nineteenth century

Milestones in obstetric care occurred in this period: discovery of fetal heart tones and fetal circulation in the seventeenth century, release of the Chamberlen family secret of obstetric forceps in 1813, calculation of expected date of confinement (EDC) in the early nineteenth century, and measurement of the female pelvis to determine the eventual course of labor. Also, in the eighteenth century the use of male physicians as obstetricians came into vogue. When many of these physicians chose to deliver babies in hospitals, a new scourge, known as puerperal sepsis, or "childbed fever," claimed the lives of many previously healthy mothers. Dr. Oliver Wendell Holmes in the United States and Dr. Ignaz Semmelweis in Vienna published papers warning of the contagiousness of puerperal fever and outlining the steps necessary (e.g., careful handwashing) to reduce the mortality rate of the disease. Although many physicians laughed at the simple practice of handwashing by those attending a birth, maternal mortality declined significantly when this act was enforced. In 1860, Louis Pasteur discovered the organism causing puerperal fever—*Streptococcus*—and thus provided the scientific rationale for the theories of Holmes and Semmelweis.

In 1853 Simpson introduced chloroform as an anesthetic in obstetrics. Although anesthetics had been used for surgery prior to this time, they were not used in obstetrics because it was believed that God meant for women to bring forth children in pain and suffering.

Twentieth century

Antepartal and postpartal care were finally seen as important parts of the care of pregnant women when the U.S. Congress established a Children's Bureau in 1912 to educate the public on the need for prenatal care. Advances in general medicine and surgical knowledge, discovery and use of antibiotics, and advances in anesthesia and analgesia all have served to make giant strides in improving maternity care in the 20th century. The "circle" of maternity care today begins in the preteen years with good nutrition and education for parenthood and continues during and after pregnancy from generation to generation.

DEFINITIONS

At the end of each unit is a vocabulary list for the major terms in that unit. However, a few key terms will be defined here because they are basic to understanding today's maternity care.

neonatal period The period extending from birth through the first 28 days of life. During this period the infant is referred to as a *neonate,* also called a *newborn.*

perinatal period The period extending from the 28th week of gestation through the 28th day after birth.

neonatologist A pediatrician with special training in the care of the infant in the neonatal period (neonate).

perinatologist An obstetrician with special interest in the perinatal period and particular interest in high-risk mothers and infants.

infant mortality rate (IMR) The number of deaths in the first year of life per 1000 live births.

maternal mortality rate The number of maternal deaths per 100,000 live births.

neonatal mortality rate The number of deaths before 28 days of life per 1000 live births.

Note that infant mortality is listed in rates per 1000, whereas maternal mortality is listed in rates per 100,000. This higher base for reporting maternal mortality denotes the significant improvements in these rates.

CURRENT PROBLEMS AND TRENDS

Infant mortality rate

NUMERICAL POSITION OF U.S. INFANT MORTALITY RATE

In 1983 there were 3.61 million live births in the United States.

According to data gathered by the National Center for Health Statistics and by the Statistical Office of the United Nations for 1983, the United States placed 17th lowest in infant mortality rates among 25 countries listed. Even though 16 other countries had lower rates, infant mortality in the United States fell to its lowest level in history in 1983. The estimated infant mortality rate (IMR) of 10.9 per 1000 live births was down from 11.2 in 1982 and 18.5 in 1972. Most of this dramatic decline in infant mortality occurred in the neonatal period as a result of improved intensive intrapartum and neonatal care (Fig. 1-1).

FACTORS CONTRIBUTING TO IMR

IDENTIFY FOUR MAJOR CAUSES OF INFANT MORTALITY

Causes for these figures are:

1. Premature births and low birth weight
2. Asphyxia
3. Birth injuries
4. Intrauterine hypoxia
5. Respiratory distress syndrome
6. Congenital malformation

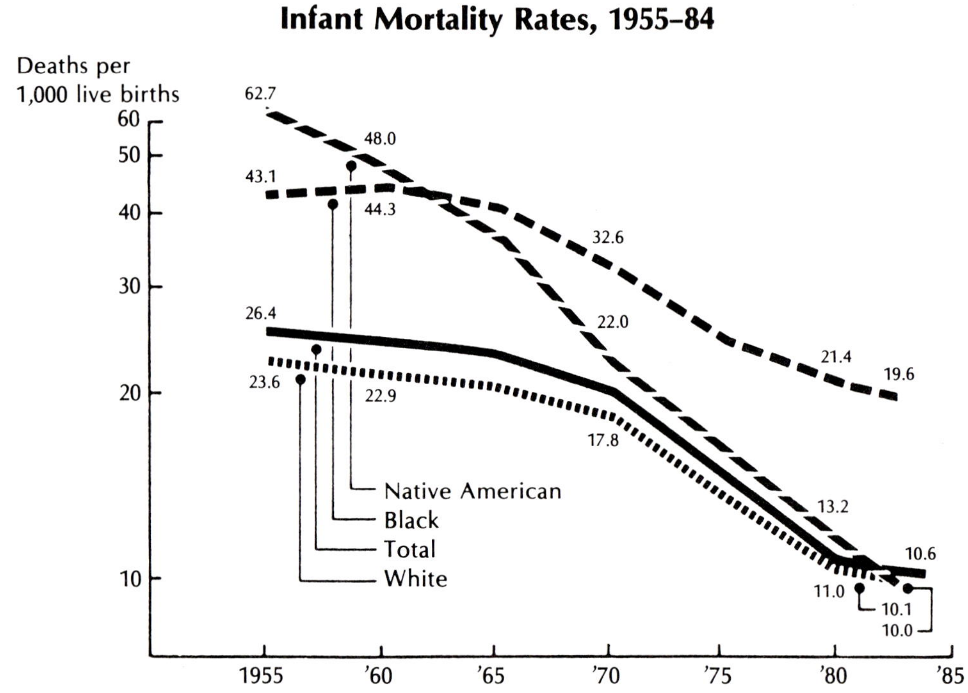

Fig. 1-1. Neonatal and postnatal mortality rates, according to race: United States, 1950 to 1979. (From Health Resources and Services Administration *Chronicle*, Vol. 12, No. 2 (August 1985).

DESCRIBE THE FACTORS CONTRIBUTING TO DIFFERENCES IN INFANT AND MATERNAL DEATH RATES AMONG WHITE AND NONWHITE FAMILIES

However, in the United States the infant mortality rate for blacks remained two to three times that for whites. A lack of prenatal care has been demonstrated to bear a direct relationship to the rate of prematurity and low birth weight. In the United States, where a baby is born, what color he or she is, and how much money the parents make affect the infant's chances of surviving the first year of life. Infant mortality rates are highest in rural nonmetropolitan counties and in inner city areas of large cities.

It is very apparent when viewing the alarmingly higher rate of infant mortality among blacks and other minorities that something is radically wrong. The people most in need of instruction regarding preconception and conception health actually receive the least amount of education. While women attending tax-supported prenatal clinics are receiving a minimal amount of instruction, the opposite is occurring for women obtaining private medical care, since classes in prepared childbirth are proliferating throughout the United States for families who can afford private care.

Maternal mortality

Maternal death rates in the United States have declined more than 30-fold since 1940. In 1935 there were 582.1 maternal deaths per 100,000 live births. However, in 1982 in the United States there were 8.9 maternal deaths per 100,000 live births. Greater use of prenatal care, improved intrapartum care, technical advances in medical care, lower parity, fewer unwanted births, and a decrease in the number of illegal abortions have all contributed to these lower rates of maternal mortality. However, as with infant mortality, the rate of maternal mortality for women of black and other races is three times higher than for white women. Increased efforts to provide access to family planning and prenatal services for women of black and other races could probably significantly reduce the differential between their mortality rate and that of white women.

IMPROVING MATERNITY CARE

In view of the overwhelming effects of social influences on infant and maternal mortality rates, it would seem that we should seriously re-examine our priorities. A step in the right direction may be to change our goal from discovering a new substance in the amniotic fluid or developing a new and better electronic monitoring system to alleviating prematurity and low birth weight.

PROPOSE THREE STEPS THAT COULD BE TAKEN BY SOCIETY TO IMPROVE MATERNITY CARE FOR ALL PEOPLE IN THE U.S.

Since 80% to 95% of women experience normal childbirth, a new maternity model may be appropriate, designating two levels of care:

1. Normal—a simple, humanistic model for healthy women
2. High risk—a more complex but still humanistic model for women with medical complications or complications of pregnancy

In keeping with the concept of levels of care, many states have regionalized maternity and newborn care. Basically, this involves dividing a state into regions according to population distribution and geography and then providing levels of care ranging from routine care for the uncomplicated births to the most complicated birth and newborn care. These levels include:

Level III ("tertiary" care): A teaching and research hospital providing care for high-risk maternal-fetal and neonatal patients with complications. This regional center has a minimum of 2000 births a year, many of these being normal deliveries.

Level II ("intermediate" care): A hospital providing care for the normal mother and newborn and limited care for the high-risk mother and newborn. This district center has 1000 to 2000 births per year and special care nurseries for stabilization of newborns prior to transfer to the level III center. This hospital also has 24-hour laboratory, radiology, ultrasound, and in-house anesthesia services.

Level I ("primary" care): A hospital providing primarily routine maternity and newborn care. This is usually a small community hospital with at least 1000 births a year. The goal of these hospitals is to detect high-risk mothers and babies and transfer them early to the regional center.

Although there is still considerable debate surrounding regionalization, we cannot ignore the reduction in infant deaths that has occurred in areas where regionalization has been implemented. The proponents of regionalization stress that it also avoids needless and costly duplication of services. However, although the concept of three levels will continue to be useful, the actual program development is a dynamic process. As regionalization continues, consumer input in planning is vital to assure inclusion of both preventive care and the humanistic care of low-risk families.

THE FAMILY

The family is the oldest human institution, and in many ways it is the most important. Families have existed since earliest times and will continue to exist in *some form* as long as human beings live on earth. Families began and have survived as the basic unit of society because they serve vital human needs (Fig. 1-2).

There are five models of the family, each with its own definition. The two most frequently considered when hospital maternity policies are written are the legal family model and the family structure model. Three other models are (1) the normative or moral model, (2) the social-psychological model, and (3) the functional model. Each of these five models of the family is defined in Table 1-1.

According to Duvall, the new image is that of a family functioning as a nurturing center for human development (Fig. 1-3). In this contemporary family the following functions are emerging: (1) affection, (2) personal security and acceptance, (3) satisfaction and a sense of purpose, (4) continuity of companionship and association, (5) socialization, and (6) establishment of limits. These new and modified functions of a family can be met by

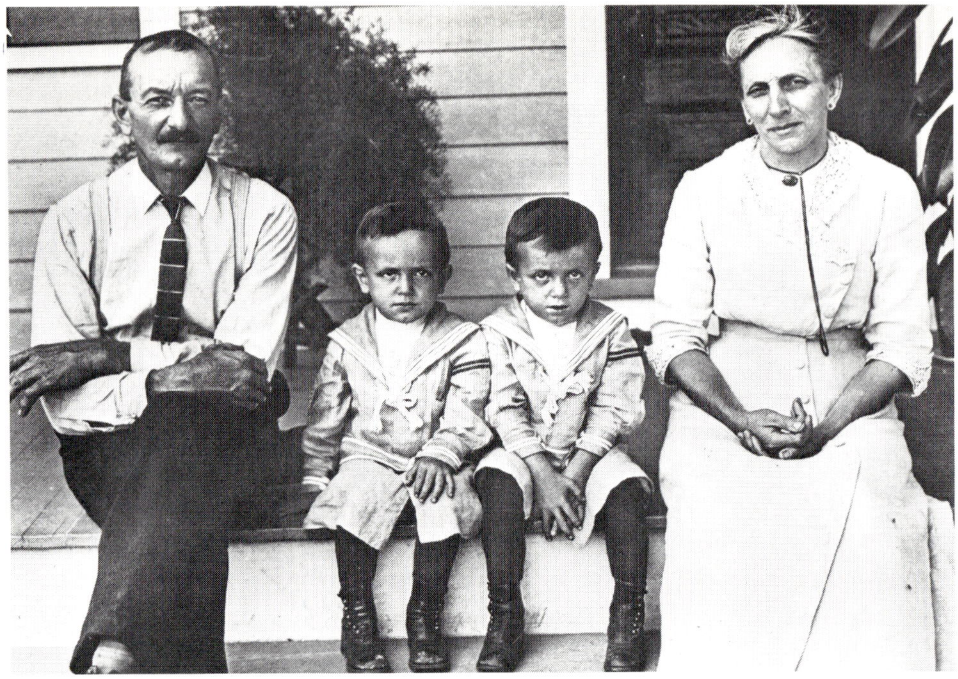

Fig. 1-2. Turn-of-the-century American family.

Table 1-1. Family definitions

Model	Definition
Legal family model	Defined by law and varies from one state to another but commonly consists of married heterosexuals and their legitimate children. (There were 2,444,000 marriages reported in 1983.)
Family structure model	Defined by the U.S. Census Bureau for statistical purposes as two or more persons, residing together, who are related by blood, marriage, or adoption.
Normative or moral model	Defined by most religions as the nuclear family for the purpose of determining biological links, legal recognition, and patriarchal hierarchy. Families headed by women are excluded.
Social-psychological model	Defined as a group in which parents and children interact, live in residence, or have significant and frequent contact. The phrase "significant other" identifies them.
Functional model	Defined by linking family and society. The family is viewed as passive, whose purpose is sharing of consumption of material goals.

Modified from Snyder, D.P.: *The family in post-industrial America,* Boulder, Colo., 1979, pp. 25-33, Westview Press.

changing family forms that include:

Communal settlements. Groups of persons not all of one family, sharing living accommodations and goods.

Social contract marriages. Couples "living together" without a marriage ceremony.

Single parents. It is estimated that by 1990 25% of all children in the United States (or 16.2 million children) will be in single-parent families. Single parenting can be the result of separation, divorce, or death of a partner or can simply be a matter of individual choice. Although many single parents worry about being an effective mother or father to their children, they can fill the dual role successfully. An understanding of what forces (other than parental) contribute to childhood development, how these forces interact, and how to find and use them is essential for single parents.

Blended families. Blended families are defined as one adult and one or more children

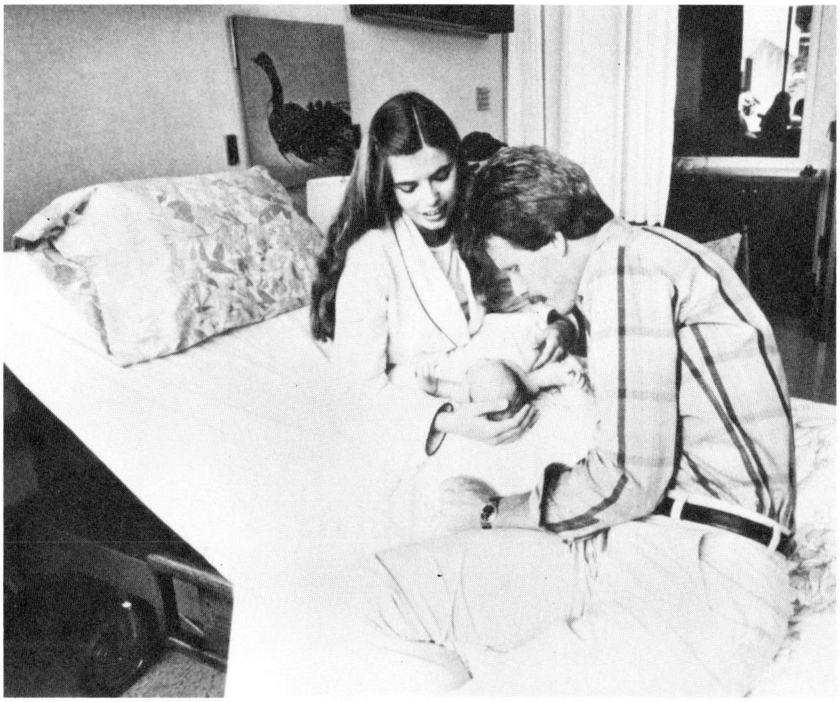

Fig. 1-3. American family in the late 1900s.

from one family and one adult and one or more children from another family. Blended families constitute 15% of all families with children under 18 years of age.

Divorced families. In 1983 there were three times as many divorces as there were in 1955 and two times as many as in 1965. The median duration of marriage prior to divorce was 7 years.

BIRTH RATE FOR UNMARRIED ADOLESCENTS AND MARRIED PERSONS DURING THE LAST 10 YEARS

Adolescent parents. While the birth rate for married persons has consistently dropped in the United States in the last 10 years, the rate of birth to unmarried adolescents has almost doubled. Adolescence is a time of turmoil in which the person must achieve many developmental tasks. Perhaps the most difficult task an adolescent must accomplish is to develop a personal identity. This can be very difficult for a young woman who has to recognize the growing fetus inside her as being a person also.

LIST THREE REASONS WHY ADOLESCENT PREGNANCY IS CLASSIFIED AS HIGH RISK

Complicating adolescent pregnancy is the fact that this is a high-risk population for medical and social complications because of such factors as late prenatal care, inadequate nutrition, and inconsistency in following instructions about health care. Also, teenage anatomy is often not as well developed as it should be for childbirth. In the general population, teenage pregnancies present an elevated rate of perinatal mortality compared with pregnancies of women in their twenties (30% higher in some studies).

Although the motivations for pregnancy in adolescence are as numerous as those for any pregnancy, pregnancy during adolescence is frequently unwanted and therefore a crisis. The key to reducing complications in adolescent pregnancy is the quality and quantity of prenatal care.

Many adolescent girls decide to keep their babies instead of placing them for adoption or considering an abortion. With an adequate support system, some young mothers are very capable of child care, whereas others have a very difficult time with mothering. The adolescent needs a great deal of help in decision-making from a support person who can be trusted for honesty, consistency, and stability. The crisis of adolescent pregnancy can be a time of responsible planning, difficult decision-making, and ultimately becoming mature and assuming increased responsibility.

WAYS IN WHICH A SINGLE FATHER MAY BE HELPED TO FACE THE REALITY OF THE PREGNANCY

In the process of providing support and counseling for the adolescent mother, the single father is often forgotten. It is wrongly assumed that he is unconcerned about the pregnant girl, her safety, or the well-being of his child. If he wants to be involved, it is important to include the single father to help in planning alternative solutions regarding the child's future. Many young single fathers have difficulty believing that they are about to become fathers. Being involved in the prenatal care, pregnancy outcome planning, and even the labor and birth helps them face the reality of the situation and the responsibilities involved.

Because we live in a time of transition and rapid change, we cannot understand families without recognizing the economic factors, life-styles, and values that influence them. Unemployment, inflation, the shrinking dollar, and increased costs of raising children often cause family stress. A smaller proportion of women today fill the traditional full-time housekeeping role. It is predicted that by 1990 three fourths of all American women 20 to 54 years of age will be in the labor force. And with social change, pregnancy no longer need end a woman's career. The Pregnancy Discrimination Act of 1978 mandates that employers can no longer force a pregnant woman, who can still do her job, to quit working. Nor can a woman be denied a job or passed over for a promotion because she is pregnant.

Many children of the World War II baby boom are now in their thirties. Having delayed pregnancy, many of these women at ages 35 to 50 are now responding to their biological clocks. A report from the National Center for Health Statistics says women aged 30 to 40 averaged 14.6 first births per 1000 women in 1982, which is more than double the 7.0 rate of 1972. And for those aged 35 to 39, the increase was 83% from 1.8 to 3.3 first births per 1000. By contrast, in the same period the birth rate for younger women decreased.

These changing economic factors, life-styles, values, and childbirth practices affect children and their families in many ways. How family members see their roles may vary significantly within different cultural groups; nevertheless, in every family the action of one individual affects all other members. A birth in the family affects each family member according to that person's own needs and expectations (Fig. 1-4). A new baby in the family can mean competition for a sibling, more work for grandparents, financial worry for the father or mother, less physical space in the house for all family members, loss of privacy for some family members, and change in life-styles for all family members. As pregnancy and the idea of a new baby are introduced to the family, the relationship of the family to the physical and emotional changes of the mother must also be considered.

As families changed in this country, so did the way in which birth happened in these families. Most births in the early 1900s occurred at home because of lack of money or lack of access to a hospital or simply because of family tradition. However, as society became more complex and industrialized, the role of institutions in people's lives became

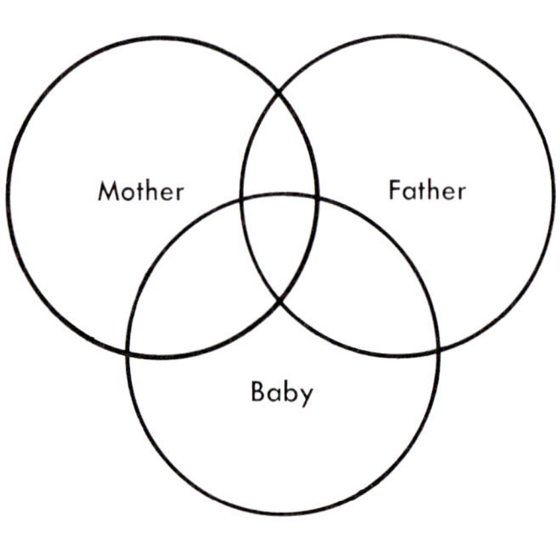

Fig. 1-4. The family nucleus.

more important and the setting for childbirth moved to the hospitals. By 1935 approximately 96% of births were occurring in hospitals. Maternal and infant mortality statistics improved significantly in these years, and proponents of hospital birth attributed this reduction to advances in hospital care. There is no doubt that modern hospital care and techniques have improved statistics, particularly for complicated labor and birth.

However, these great improvements were not without a price. As hospitals became larger, more complex, and more sophisticated in using technology, they often became impersonal, mechanistic institutions in which the human needs of families were disregarded. Disenchantment with the impersonal treatment in many hospitals has led more and more couples to seek alternatives to traditional hospital birth. Attempts are being made by many hospitals to look at the traditional multitransfer surgical system for birth and at outdated policies and procedures and then to change to meet the needs of today's families and still offer safe maternity care. The move to family-centered maternity and new-born care is evidence that changes are happening.

FAMILY-CENTERED MATERNITY AND NEWBORN CARE

DISCUSS CURRENT CONCEPTS IN FAMILY-CENTERED MATERNITY CARE

Family-centered maternity and newborn care focuses on the physical, social, psychological, and economic needs of the total family unit, however the family may be defined. The family is included in decision-making and planning, and its individual needs and responsibilities are recognized. Whenever possible, the birth process is made accessible to as many family members as desire to share in the process.

A joint position statement published on "The Development of Family-Centered Maternity/Newborn Care in Hospitals" was approved by the American College of Obstetricians and Gynecologists, the American Academy of Pediatrics, the American College of Nurse-Midwives, the American Nurses' Association, and the Nurses Association of the American College of Obstetricians and Gynecologists. In this position paper, the following family-centered childbirth policies were recommended:

1. Hospitals offer preparation for birth classes for both mothers and fathers, including instruction on the role of men at birth.
2. Fathers be permitted to accompany women giving birth during the entire process, including being present in the delivery room and helping at the birth itself.
3. Hospitals offer the option of using a homelike "birthing room" rather than a standard delivery room. The birthing room would contain informal furnishings and bear little resemblance to a surgical facility, as delivery rooms now do.
4. Hospitals consider an end to restrictions (some spelled out by state law or health department regulation) on young children visiting their mothers and newborn siblings in the hospital.
5. Hospitals develop programs for early discharge of mothers after birth so that the family can quickly move back into the more psychologically secure atmosphere of the home. (To do this, hospitals would probably have to develop programs in which health professionals make home visits.)

INDICATE THE MAJOR CHANGE IN MATERNITY CARE NEEDED TO MAKE FAMILY-CENTERED CARE WORK

Before listing these possible physical and functional changes, the position statement emphasized that the major change in maternity care needed to make family-centered care work was *attitudinal*.

Table 1-2 provides a comparison of conventional and family-centered models of maternity care.

Cultures

Family-centered maternity care deals not only with members of the white, middle-class majority, but also with people from various cultures, social classes, and ethnic groupings. Although it is beyond the scope of this book to go into detail on the care of

Table 1-2. Comparison of conventional and family-centered models of maternity care

Conventional medical model	Family-centered model
No childbirth education.	Prepared childbirth education required.
Pregnancy, labor, and delivery considered an illness.	Pregnancy, labor, and delivery considered a time of emotional, social, and physical change/stress.
Care is task oriented, routinized.	Care is individualized.
Staff, in position of authority, makes treatment decisions. Family is dependent.	Staff uses expertise to inform family of options; family makes decision; family and staff create team for treatment.
Staff is rigid.	Staff is flexible.
Mother and infant considered separate patients.	Mother and infant served as a unit.
Labor, delivery, recovery, and postpartum and neonatal care take place in different locations.	Labor, delivery, recovery, and postpartum and neonatal care occur in one location.
Infant cared for primarily in nursery.	Infant remains with mother.
Visiting hours prescribed.	Family and friends encouraged to be present at any time mother wishes.
Father or supportive person informed of labor progress and birth.	Father or supportive person present and actively involved in labor, delivery, postpartum, and neonatal care.

culturally diverse people, it must be emphasized that a goal of family-centered maternity care is to treat each family with dignity, as individuals.

STATE A GOAL THAT IS USEFUL WHEN GIVING CARE TO FAMILIES WHOSE CULTURE IS DIFFERENT FROM YOUR OWN

When values differ from our own, we should listen, be nonjudgmental, reach out, be sensitive to the differences, and understand any reluctance the family may have in accepting new and foreign ideas. There is certainly no simple formula in working with a culturally different family, but there is one rule that always holds true: We *never* have the right to impose our own personal convictions on anyone.

Rights

As providers of care for the childbearing family, we have a responsibility to ask ourselves again and again: Whose birth is this? To whom does the baby belong?

EXPLAIN THE FAMILY'S RIGHTS FOR MEANINGFUL HUMANISTIC CARE DURING THE CHILDBEARING CYCLE

People are beginning to realize that they do not give up rights when they enter a health care institution. They do not gain any rights either, but they have the same rights as any other human beings in our society. A great many patients' rights are derived from the necessity to obtain informed consent. Informed consent simply means that patients have a right to participate in the decisions that determine what may or may not be done with their bodies and their minds. . . . They need to be sufficiently aware of what is going to happen so that they can appropriately make those decisions.

In 1972 the American Hospital Association adopted a "Patient's Bill of Rights" as a national policy statement and distributed it to its member hospitals throughout the country. This statement intended to give the consumer something to go by in understanding what to expect in more effective patient care.

The Committee on Patients' Rights, headed by Doris and John Haire, published the "Pregnant Patient's Bill of Rights." "The Pregnant Patient's Responsibilities" was prepared by members of the International Childbirth Education Association. Both of these papers are reproduced here so that you can study and discuss them.

Attitudes

BASIC DIFFERENCES IN ATTITUDES TOWARD CHILDBEARING AND BIRTH

Take a few minutes to complete the attitude survey that follows, expressing your true feelings as you complete each sentence. When you have satisfied yourself that your answers express your true feelings, exchange your answers with another classmate or with a member of your family for discussion and sharing.

THE PREGNANT PATIENT'S BILL OF RIGHTS*

1. *The Pregnant Patient has the right,* prior to the administration of any drug or procedure, to be informed by the health professional caring for her of any potential direct or indirect effects, risks or hazards to herself or her unborn or newborn infant which may result from the use of a drug or procedure prescribed for or administered to her during pregnancy, labor, birth or lactation.
2. *The Pregnant Patient has the right,* prior to the proposed therapy, to be informed, not only of the benefits, risks and hazards of the proposed therapy but also of known alternative therapy, such as available childbirth education classes which could help to prepare the Pregnant Patient physically and mentally to cope with the discomfort or stress of pregnancy and the experience of childbirth, thereby reducing or eliminating her need for drugs and obstetric intervention. She should be offered such information early in her pregnancy in order that she may make a reasoned decision.
3. *The Pregnant Patient has the right,* prior to the administration of any drug, to be informed by the health professional who is prescribing or administering the drug to her that any drug which she receives during pregnancy, labor and birth, no matter how or when the drug is taken or administered, may adversely affect her unborn baby, directly or indirectly, and that there is no drug or chemical which has been proven safe for the unborn child.
4. *The Pregnant Patient has the right* if Cesarean section is anticipated, to be informed prior to the administration of any drug, and preferably prior to her hospitalization, that minimizing her and, in turn, her baby's intake of nonessential pre-operative medicine will benefit her baby.
5. *The Pregnant Patient has the right,* prior to the administration of a drug or procedure, to be informed if there is NO properly controlled follow-up research which has established the safety of the drug or procedure with regard to its direct and/or indirect effects on the physiological, mental and neurological development of the child exposed, via the mother, to the drug or procedure during pregnancy, labor, birth, or lactation—(this would apply to virtually all drugs and the vast majority of obstetric procedures).
6. *The Pregnant Patient has the right,* prior to the administration of any drug, to be informed of the brand name and generic name of the drug in order that she may advise the health professional of any past adverse reaction to the drug.
7. *The Pregnant Patient has the right* to determine for herself, without pressure from her attendant, whether she will accept the risks inherent in the proposed therapy or refuse a drug or procedure.
8. *The Pregnant Patient has the right* to know the name and qualifications of the individual administering a medication or procedure to her during labor or birth.
9. *The Pregnant Patient has the right* to be informed, prior to the administration of any procedure, whether that procedure is being administered to her for her or her baby's benefit (medically indicated) or as an elective procedure (for convenience or teaching purposes).
10. *The Pregnant Patient has the right* to be accompanied during the stress of labor and birth by someone she cares for, and to whom she looks for emotional comfort and encouragement.
11. *The Pregnant Patient has the right* after appropriate medical consultation to choose a position for labor and for birth which is least stressful to her baby and to herself.
12. *The Obstetric Patient has the right* to have her baby cared for at her bedside if her baby is normal, and to feed her baby according to her baby's needs rather than according to the hospital regimen.
13. *The Obstetric Patient has the right* to be informed in writing of the name of the person who actually delivered her baby and the professional qualifications of that person. This information should also be on the birth certificate.
14. *The Obstetric Patient has the right* to be informed if there is any known or indicated aspect of her baby's care or condition which may cause her or her baby later difficulty or problems.
15. *The Obstetric Patient has the right* to have her and her baby's hospital medical records complete, accurate, and legible and to have these records, including Nurses' Notes, retained by the hospital until the child reaches at least the age of majority, or, alternatively, to have the records offered to her before they are destroyed.
16. *The Obstetric Patient,* both during and after her hospital stay, *has the right* to have access to her complete medical records, including Nurses' Notes, and to receive a copy upon payment of a reasonable fee and without incurring the expense of retaining an attorney.

It is the obstetric patient and her baby, not the health professional, who must sustain any trauma or injury resulting from the use of a drug or obstetric procedure. The observation of the rights listed above will not only permit the obstetric patient to participate in the decisions involving her and her baby's health care, but will help to protect the health professional and the hospital against litigation arising from resentment or misunderstanding on the part of the mother.

*Prepared by Doris Haire, Chair., Committee on Health Law and Regulation, International Childbirth Education Association.

THE PREGNANT PATIENT'S RESPONSIBILITIES*

In addition to understanding her rights the Pregnant Patient should also understand that she too has certain responsibilities. The Pregnant Patient's responsibilities include the following:

1. The Pregnant Patient is responsible for learning about the physical and psychological process of labor, birth and postpartum recovery. The better informed expectant parents are the better they will be able to participate in decisions concerning the planning of their care.
2. The Pregnant Patient is responsible for learning what comprises good prenatal and intranatal care and for making an effort to obtain the best care possible.
3. Expectant parents are responsible for knowing about those hospital policies and regulations which will affect their birth and postpartum experience.
4. The Pregnant Patient is responsible for arranging for a companion or support person (husband, mother, sister, friend, etc.) who will share in her plans for birth and who will accompany her during her labor and birth experience.
5. The Pregnant Patient is responsible for making her preferences known clearly to the health professionals involved in her case in a courteous and cooperative manner and for making mutually agreed-upon arrangements regarding maternity care alternatives with her physician and hospital in advance of labor.
6. Expectant parents are responsible for listening to their chosen physician or midwife with an open mind, just as they expect him or her to listen openly to them.
7. Once they have agreed to a course of health care, expectant parents are responsible, to the best of their ability, for seeing that the program is carried out in consultation with others with whom they have made the agreement.
8. The Pregnant Patient is responsible for obtaining information in advance regarding the approximate cost of her obstetric and hospital care.
9. The Pregnant Patient who intends to change her physician or hospital is responsible for notifying all concerned, well in advance of the birth if possible, and for informing both of her reasons for changing.
10. In all their interactions with medical and nursing personnel, the expectant parents should behave towards those caring for them with the same respect and consideration they themselves would like.
11. During the mother's hospital stay the mother is responsible for learning about her and her baby's continuing care after discharge from the hospital.
12. After birth, the parents should put into writing constructive comments and feelings of satisfaction and/or dissatisfaction with the care (nursing, medical and personal) they received. Good service to families in the future will be facilitated by those parents who take the time and responsibility to write letters expressing their feelings about the maternity care they received.

All the previous statements assume a normal birth and postpartum experience. Expectant parents should realize that, if complications develop in their cases, there will be an increased need to trust the expertise of the physician and hospital staff they have chosen. However, if problems occur, the childbearing woman still retains her responsibility for making informed decisions about her care or treatment and that of her baby. If she is incapable of assuming that responsibility because of her physical condition, her previously authorized companion or support person should assume responsibility for making informed decisions on her behalf.

*By members of the International Childbirth Education Association.

EXPLORE YOUR ATTITUDES AND FEELINGS ABOUT CHILDBEARING AND BIRTH

1. Pregnancy is ____________________
2. Babies are ____________________
3. Childbirth is ____________________
4. I think that childbirth makes a woman more ____________________
5. I think that childbirth makes a man more ____________________
6. When I gave birth, it was ____________________
7. A pregnant woman should be treated ____________________
8. As a result of pregnancy, a woman looks ____________________
9. Expectant fathers are ____________________
10. A pregnant woman should work until ____________________
11. Expectant fathers worry about ____________________
12. Expectant mothers worry about ____________________

Our own background, culture, religion, and value system influence the care we give to childbearing families in both positive and negative ways. We are often caught in a conflict between our own values and those of the people we are trying to help. Although our attitudes can interfere with our objectivity, it is vital that we attempt to be nonjudgmental as we work with childbearing families whose attitudes differ from our own or from what we have experienced.

Attitudes toward childbearing and birth differ depending on each person's past experiences. A woman or a couple who experienced a painful and very difficult birth may have very negative attitudes about birth, and a woman or a couple who experienced a pain-free and joyous birth may have very positive attitudes. Also, people who have never given birth may have extremely positive or negative attitudes formulated by family stories of births or family and cultural myths.

FATHERING: PATERNAL INVOLVEMENT IN LABOR AND BIRTH

In our culture, literature relating to the father's involvement in pregnancy and birth has been sparse until recently. On reviewing the psychologic literature, it would seem that the American male's parental role is limited to impregnation, paying the bills 9 months later, and then magically appearing again as a role model for adolescent boys.

This very lack of information on fathers and fathering has reinforced the idea that fathers in our culture are not interested in birth and babies. Nothing could be farther from the truth. Most men who are invited and encouraged to participate in the pregnancy, labor, and birth are very happy to be involved. In fact, most participating fathers think of their help in labor and delivery as essential to their experience as expectant fathers. For a well-prepared father, being at the side of the mother when their baby is born can be a satisfying and moving experience, as well as a tremendous help to the woman.

MEN'S INVOLVEMENT IN BIRTH IN OUR CULTURE DURING THE PAST CENTURY

In our culture, the father's role in childbearing has changed greatly in the past 100 years. In the nineteenth century childbirth was accepted as a natural part of the life cycle, usually occurring at home, with the assistance of a midwife, a woman relative, a family physician, or the father if he was the only one available to assist. But whether the father had to assist in the delivery or not, he was close at hand, proudly interested in the labor and birth.

As society became more complex, more women gave birth in hospitals if they could afford it. Now instead of actively participating at the birth, the father found himself waiting in a hospital fathers' waiting room, designed just for him.

Our culture's stereotyped sex roles also had a great deal to do with moving childbirth to women's wards in hospitals and keeping it there. A man in our culture has had to repress his feelings of tenderness and gentleness, causing him to downplay his role as father, thus making fatherhood a social obligation, while motherhood has always meant nurturing and meeting the physical and emotional needs of the family.

A man in our culture is expected to be "manly" and provide financially for his family, while a woman is expected to be "motherly"—nurturing.

The irony of all this is that the role of the father is tremendously important for the mental health of the family. Study after study indicates that emotional disturbances in children can be traced to the detachment or lack of involvement of a father with his children.

IDENTIFY SOME FEELINGS AN EXPECTANT FATHER HAS TOWARD (1) HIS ROLE AS A FATHER, (2) HIS PARTNER, AND (3) THE BABY, AS HE ADAPTS TO FATHERHOOD

Men's reactions to fatherhood are many and diverse. Many expectant fathers have a joyful reaction to impending fatherhood, whereas others may react with depression, fear, anger, or jealousy. How a man reacts may depend on his childhood memories of his own father, his mother's pregnancies, his own childhood, financial status, and number of children he already has.

During pregnancy a man must deal with the role change of his partner to mother at the same time that he is becoming a father. In addition, he may further be confused by the woman beginning to evaluate him in terms of what kind of a father he will be, even as he may be wondering himself. Pregnancy may be a time when the man also needs mothering and feels strongly dependent.

Pregnancy may be a real testing ground for a man-woman relationship as well as a training ground for parenthood. Pregnancy can be a crisis time for men as well as women.

During pregnancy men are often worried about the increasing financial responsibilities they will have. Also, it is not unusual for some men in pregnancy to unintentionally acquire the symptoms presented by the pregnant women, such as nausea and vomiting in the first trimester.

The labor and birth, as the culmination of pregnancy, and the beginning of the relationship between father and child can have a marked influence on the father, both positive and negative. The more fathers are encouraged to become involved in pregnancy through prenatal classes and visits to the physician, the more likely they are to welcome the opportunity to be with their wives in labor.

Benefits of the father's participation

LIST FOUR BENEFITS OF THE FATHER'S PARTICIPATION IN LABOR AND/OR BIRTH

From the fathers who are participating and speaking out, data are coming in to support their new role as a vital introduction to fatherhood. Studies have shown that the father's presence in the labor room results in decreased need for pain relief medication and that his presence can make labor a supportive and valuable interpersonal experience for the couple.

In investigating the role of husbands in labor and birth, Tanzer compared groups in which the husband was and was not present at birth. The results of this study indicate that the wives experienced a positive and highly desirable effect when their husbands were present during birth. All women who reported a rapturous or peak experience during birth had their husband present in the delivery room.

A survey published in *American Baby* (June 1972) reported that 80% of the 2796 couples who responded were positive about the childbirth experience. Not all couples thought the husband was useful in the delivery room, but all felt positive about labor. The conclusions were that "something significant is happening" and that there is a need to further explore attitudes about childbearing in this country.

Cogan studied two groups of couples, all enrolled in childbirth education classes. In one group the fathers attended labor and birth; in the second group the fathers attended only the first stage of labor. Women in the total participation group reported less pain and received less medication. This group also reported more positive feelings about the total birth experience.

Cronewett and colleagues questioned 158 fathers concerning their feelings about their infants and wives during labor and delivery. Those who attended labor and delivery rated their overall experiences during childbirth significantly more positively than the fathers who did not have these experiences. According to this study, even without preparation, attendance at delivery positively influenced the couple's relationship.

A doctoral dissertation by Hott showed that there was similarity of self-concept and concept of wife among participating fathers and those who chose not to participate in labor and delivery. This study would seem to dispel the theories often put forth by professionals and lay people that men who want to be present at birth are morbidly curious or zealots of "natural childbirth" or want to experience an "ego trip."

When fathers interact with their newborns from the moment of birth, the fathering role is a natural extension of the pregnancy and birth process. Most men who share such an experience relate that they seemed to develop a continuing relationship with their child—a natural relationship right from the start. Interrupted relationships are often more difficult to hold together when stressful events occur in a family.

Expectant fathers may experience a type of "culture shock" when entering a hospital labor and delivery area. An unfamiliar physical environment can be disorienting and cause the father to feel as if he were a visitor instead of a participant. Many fathers begin labor physically tired after weeks of sleep that was interrupted by dreams. Also, their needs for food and for elimination do not stop as their mates labor. The question is: What is meaningful participation for a father in the birth process? What are his needs? Merely allowing fathers to enter labor and delivery areas does not mean that their needs are being met. It is also important to recognize that some fathers may be perfectly content to wait in a separate room during the labor and birth. When fathers choose *not* to participate, nurses need to respect and support that choice.

PSYCHOLOGICAL ASPECTS

Psychological aspects for siblings

Once again, it is important to individualize care. Some parents want their children present at the birth of their new sibling; others do not. There is a diversity of opinions on the issue of sibling presence, as present theories on sibling participation are still quite primitive. Parents have a right to make their own decisions, while medicine and nursing provide education, guidance, and sensitive care. If the parents choose sibling participation at birth, preparation for the experience is essential. Issues to cover during preparation include the wetness, smells, and sounds of birth; the basic anatomy and physiology of labor and birth; the hard work, intensity, and pain of labor and birth; plus the procedures involved. Another essential for the sibling is a supportive person, in addition to the father, to help the child during labor and birth.

Whether or not siblings participate in the labor and birth, it is very important for them to visit their mother and their new brother or sister after birth. Our goal should be to *minimize* separation anxiety (from parents) and jealousy toward the new baby. When meeting the new baby, the sibling should be told to examine the baby and discover his or her unique traits, thus bridging the gap between reality and fantasy (Fig. 1-5). Sibling-to-sibling relationships endure beyond parent-child relationships and are longer than husband-wife relationships. In our society, sibling relationships are often characterized bv life-long struggle, rivalry, and competitiveness. Could this be changed?

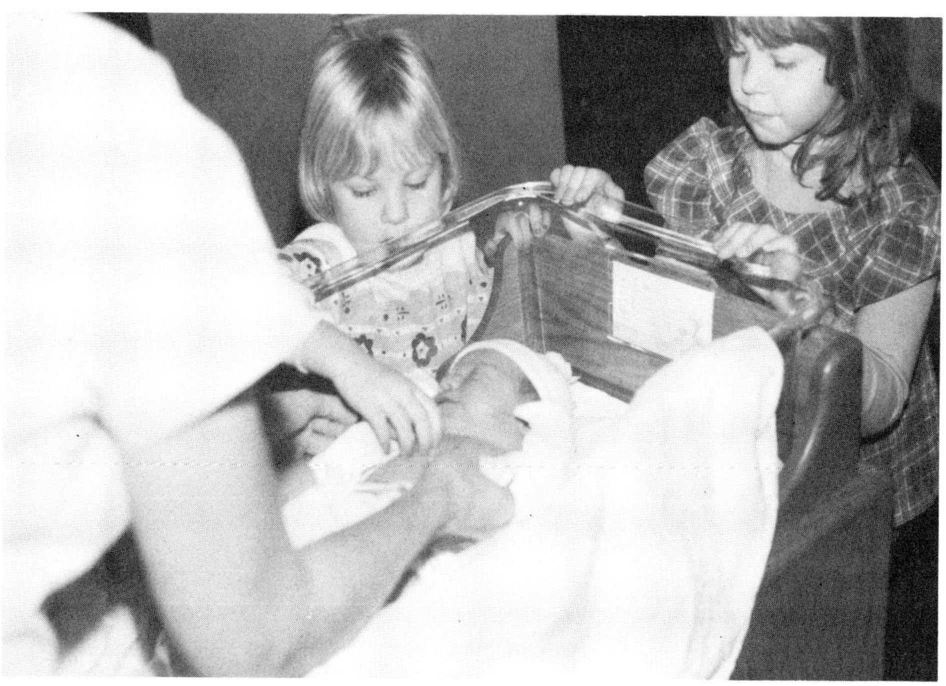

Fig. 1-5. Big sisters with baby brother. (Courtesy Holy Family Hospital, Spokane, Wash.)

Psychological involvement of grandparents

Biological links and generational ties are profound. Grandparents want to see and hold the new baby but often feel left out, especially when hospitals limit visitors to one person besides the father.

Many grandparents do not understand new trends in childbirth preparation classes and father participation. Often, women who had scopolamine for their own births relive their suppressed birth experience when they see their daughters' labor. These women need nursing support so they resolve their long-buried feelings.

Psychological aspects of postpartum period

During the postpartum period new parents have to balance their own, partner's, and infant's needs. They also have to cope with changes in self, relationships, and routines while redefining relationships with parents and friends.

Men become fathers and grandfathers. Women become mothers and grandmothers (Fig. 1-6). Children become brothers and sisters, and numerous other roles change for family members and friends through the birth experience. Although all of these changes began months earlier, the result of 8 to 16 hours of an average labor brings the reality of a new life and all that means to everyone in the family.

BONDING: PARENT-INFANT ATTACHMENT

Bonding is the early attachment that takes place between parents and infants within the first hours and days after birth. It can be facilitated and reinforced by physical contact

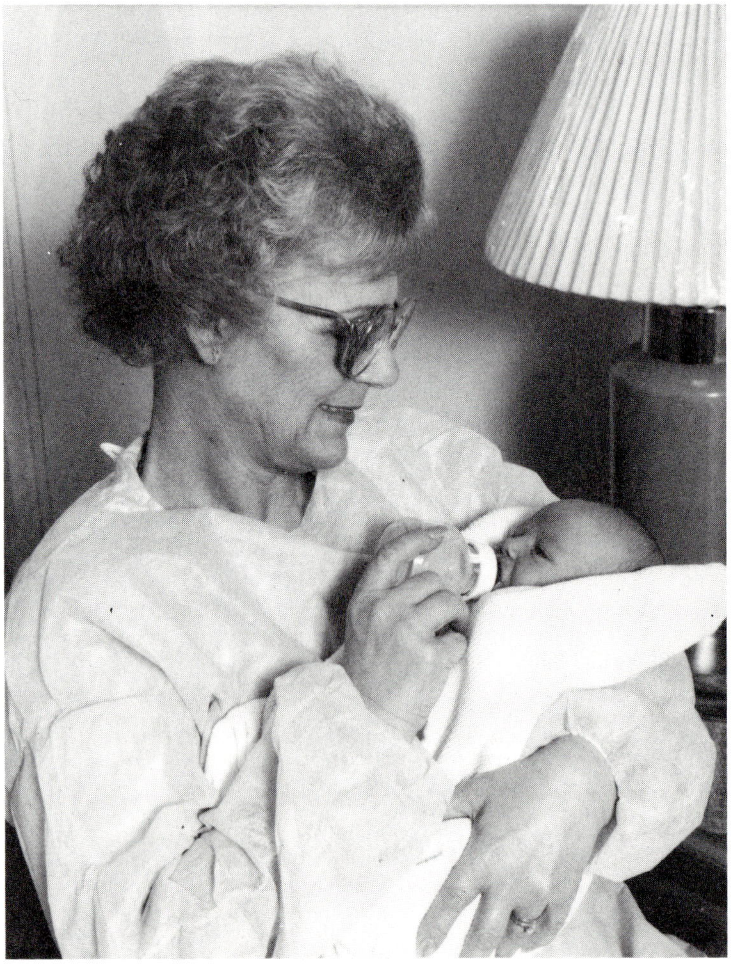

Fig. 1-6. Grandma and the new baby. (Courtesy Valley Hospital and Medical Center, Spokane, Wash.)

and is primarily unidirectional from parent to infant. When there is bonding difficulty, the infant may be at risk of being abused. All health care providers who work with childbearing families should be able to recognize behavior that indicates successful bonding or bonding difficulty or delay.

Attachment is an affectional tie between infants and parents that begins during pregnancy, continues through birth, and flourishes over a lifetime. Attachment is reciprocal both to and from mother to infant and to father. Many variables influence attachment.

Bonding during pregnancy

EMOTIONAL PHASES FOR MEN AND FOR WOMEN TO EXPERIENCE DURING PREGNANCY IN ORDER TO BEGIN BONDING WITH THEIR UNBORN BABY

Bonding does not occur magically at the time of birth but progresses throughout pregnancy, beginning when the mother confirms the pregnancy. With any pregnancy, whether planned or unplanned, a woman has many new and different feelings, including ambivalence toward the pregnancy. Rubin describes the first trimester for women as the "who, me? now?" stage. We will describe the first trimester for men as the "why me? why now?" stage. When learning of the woman's pregnancy, the man is often ambivalent, sometimes both pleased that he can "father" biologically but worried about what kind of father he will be. The lack of obvious physical evidence of the pregnancy permeates this stage, and both the mother and father focus on themselves and their own needs.

As the pregnancy progresses and fetal movement is felt and the woman blossoms out into maternity clothes, Rubin identifies the period as that of "radiant health." Uncertainty about the pregnancy is removed by the positive presence of the fetal movement. If they have accepted the pregnancy and moved through the ambivalence of the first trimester, the couples' focus is now on the baby. During the second trimester many men go through a period of creative, warm feelings. Feeling the baby move for the first time is a profound experience, and they begin thinking seriously about becoming fathers.

Rubin describes the last trimester as a period of "watchful waiting" for women; this time we will term a period of anxious concern and waiting for the father. He is often very concerned about his mate's physical safety as the time for birth approaches. Bonding with their unborn baby begins as both the man and woman move through these emotional phases of pregnancy on their way to successful role changes (Table 1-3).

All family members of a pregnant woman, as well as the woman herself, should be offered prenatal classes or prenatal counseling and teaching to prepare for the birth and to help them work through the emotional phases and preparatory tasks of pregnancy.

Bonding behavior

Marshall Klaus and colleagues have been actively studying whether or not human mothers have a "sensitive period" immediately after birth, as has been reported among animal mothers. In many animals, if mother and baby are separated immediately after birth, the mother will reject the baby when they are reunited, even after a separation of only 1 or 2 hours. Conversely, if animal mother and baby are together in the first few days, then separated and reunited, the mother quickly accepts her baby. Dr. Klaus and associates have also found that human mothers who have close contact with their babies immediately after birth are more responsive and sensitive to their babies' needs. Their other studies suggest that extra contact, even if not immediately after birth, may strikingly improve both subsequent mothering and child health.

Table 1-3. Emotional phases of pregnancy

	Women (mother)	Men (father)
First trimester	Who, me? Now?	Why me? Why now?
Second trimester	Radiant health	Creative, warm feelings
Third trimester	Watchful waiting	Anxious concern and waiting

Table 1-4. Stages of attachment

Parent	Infant/child
Assessing own parenting . . . actual and remembered: nurturing received, relationship with own parents	**Before pregnancy**
Pregnancy (planned, accepted, unwanted)	**9 months**
	Intrauterine experience: maternal heart rate, voice; light and dark environment, sounds; maternal emotions and health; placental transfer
Couple relationship . . . age, marital status, work, other family members Fantasies: mother-father role perception Experiencing stresses/developing support system: having energy to be ready to attach Cultural definition of parenting Preparation for experience of birth	
	Birth
Length and type of labor and birth: control/awareness, support, fatigue, pain, medication Resolution of labor and birth experience Acceptance of real versus mythical infant; for example, sex, appearance Caregiving in supportive environment: verbal, visual, tactile interaction; positive or negative perception of infant	Period of increased alertness: first reactive phase Adjustment to new world, response to caregiver contact . . . phases and states of awareness Simple differential response to mother's odor, voice, face
	Approximately 3 months after birth
Feeling of love for infant	Complex differential response to mother, father, strangers

Unfortunately, Klaus and Kennel's work has often been misinterpreted by some people to mean that there is a one-chance critical period for bonding to occur immediately after birth. Developmental stages in the process of attachment seem more theoretically defensible than critical periods. Table 1-4 outlines the stages of attachment.

In studying parent-infant behavior immediately after birth, it has been demonstrated that parents want to make eye contact with their babies. Very early after delivery, mothers have been heard to say, "Open your eyes," "What color are your eyes?," and "Oh, she's looking at me!" The parents and baby need to have eye contact to respond to each other. Since babies can focus on an object at 12 to 16 inches, breast feeding immediately after birth is an ideal opportunity to have eye contact. The initial position that facilitates eye contact has been given the term "en face." It has been reported that immediately following birth the baby is most alert and can make eye contact with the mother, visually following her for 180 degrees.

Another behavior that has been noted with infants is the manner in which parents first touch their babies. The initial touching is very lightly with fingertips to the baby's extremities and then gradually increasing to palm and then to full hand touching, encompassing the trunk and head with the hand.

EXPERIENCES THAT COULD INTERFERE WITH THE PARENT-INFANT RELATIONSHIP AND RESULT IN BONDING DIFFICULTY

A variety of experiences may interfere with the parent-infant relationship to the point that bonding does not occur. These happen throughout pregnancy and immediately after birth. Some of the more common are:

1. Unplanned pregnancy
2. Poor relationship between partners
3. Lack of education about what is happening both physically and emotionally
4. Attitude of health care providers toward parents
5. Separation at time of birth
6. Lack of money
7. Previous negative experiences in childbirth

8. Disappointment about birth outcome (need for anesthesia, unexpected cesarean, infant with congenital anomalies, etc.)

Factors that could be described as bonding difficulty are:

LIST SEVERAL INDICATIONS OF BONDING DIFFICULTY

1. Parents not touching infant; holding infant at arm's length
2. Disinterest in infant; perceiving infant to be ugly
3. Anger and noncommunication between parents
4. Expectations for baby—wanting a female or male *only*

Factors that could be described as indicating bonding are:

LIST SEVERAL INDICATIONS OF BONDING

1. Eye contact (parent-infant-parent)
2. Touching baby and holding it close to body
3. Talking, cooing, smiling, seeing infant as pretty or cute
4. Undivided attention toward baby
5. Calling baby by name

Klaus and Kennel have developed the following specific recommendations for maternity care to enhance the father-mother-infant bond:

1. Identify specific needs for a mother that would influence the birth and ability to adapt to mothering (also true for fathers).
2. Encourage all parents to attend prenatal education classes to ensure their role as active participants in childbirth (does not mean natural birth only).
3. Encourage that a significant person be present with the mother during labor and delivery to offer support and reassurance.
4. Enhance attachment by allowing privacy (long periods of father-mother-infant contact and the opportunity for the parents to assume all care for their infant with a nurse available to assist when needed).
5. Avoid putting silver nitrate in the infant's eyes until the parents have been able to have close contact with the baby during the first hour of life.
6. Allow the mother, infant, and father to interact as a new family without interruptions.
7. Encourage rooming-in to assist the parents in recognizing the normal behavior of their infant before going home.
8. Allow families, including children, to make hospital visits to provide emotional support for all the family members and to prevent possible trauma from the separation.

These recommendations are made as an attempt to improve the childbirth and parenting experience for the total family. Parent-infant attachment is a complex process involving all biological, psychological and social influences surrounding the pregnancy and birth of the baby. Health care providers must be aware of the attachment process and its impact on the development of a baby as an integral member of the family unit.

SUMMARY

The first unit was designed to provide a brief look at obstetric care yesterday and family-centered maternity and newborn care today, with both their problems and their joys. It was also intended to provide a stimulus for you to examine your own feelings and attitudes about pregnancy and birth as you embark on this study of the childbearing family. What you have learned to this point will set the tone and influence the quality of care you provide. As you progress through all the other units in this text, remember that the major change in maternity care needed to make family-centered care work is *attitudinal.*

BIBLIOGRAPHY

Anisfeld, E., and Lipper, E.: Early contact, social support, and mother-infant bonding, Pediatrics, **72**(1): 79-83, 1983.

Clark, A.L., editor: Culture, childbearing health professionals, Philadelphia, 1978, F.A. Davis Co.

Cox, F.: American marriage: A changing

scene, Dubuque, Iowa, 1972, William C. Brown Co., Publishers.

Curtis, F.L.S.: Observations of unwed pregnant adolescents, Am. J. Nurs. **74**:100-102, Jan. 1974.

Devitt, N.: The transition from home to hospital birth in the United States, 1930-1960, Birth Fam. J. **4**:2, Summer 1977.

Duvall, E.M.: Family development, ed. 4, Philadelphia, 1971, J.B. Lippincott Co.

Harrison, L.K.: Making a good thing better: The regionalization of neonatal intensive care units, J.O.G.N. Nurs. **4**:49-52, May/June, 1975.

Horn, M., and Manion, J.: Creative grandparenting, bonding the generations, J.O.G.N. Nurs. **3**:233-236, May/June 1984.

Interprofessional Task Force on Health Care of Women and Children: A joint position statement on the development of family-centered maternity/newborn care in hospitals, June 1978.

Israel, S.L.: Teaching the art of caring for women, J. Am. Med. Assoc. **191**:393-396, 1965.

Klaus, M.H., and Kennell, J.H.: Parent-infant bonding, ed. 2, St. Louis, 1982, The C.V. Mosby Co.

Lipkin, G.B.: Parent-child nursing: Psychosocial aspects, ed. 2, St. Louis, 1978, The C.V. Mosby Co.

Lytle, L.A., editor: Nursing of women in the age of liberation, Dubuque, Iowa, 1977, William C. Brown Co., Publishers.

McKay, S., and Phillips, C.: Family-centered maternity care implementation strategies, Rockville, Md., 1984, Aspen Systems Corp.

McRae, M.: An approach to the single parent dilemma, MCN **2**:164–167, May/June 1977.

Mead, M., and Heyman, K.: Family, New York, 1965, Macmillan, Inc.

Mercer, R.: Relationship of the birth experience to later mothering behaviors, Journal of Nurse-Midwifery **30**:204-211, July/August 1985.

Pannor, R.: The unmarried father: The forgotten man, Nurs. Outlook, **18**:36-37, Nov. 1970.

Petrella, J.M.: The unwed pregnant adolescent: Implications for the professional nurse, J.O.G.N. Nurs. **7**:22-26, July/August 1978.

Phillips, C.: Interviews with fathers, 1974-1976, unpublished manuscript.

Phillips, C.R., and Anzalone, J.T.: Fathering: Participation in labor and birth, St. Louis, 1978, The C.V. Mosby Co.

Rubin, R.: Cognitive style in pregnancy, Am. J. Nurs. **70**:508-520, March 1970.

Shearer, M.H.: The effects of regionalization of perinatal care on hospital services for normal childbirth, Birth Fam. J. **4**:4, Winter 1977.

Snyder, O.P.: The family in post-industrial America, Boulder, Colo., 1979, Westview Press.

Speert, H.: Iconographic gynitrica. A pictorial history of gynecology and obstetrics, Philadelphia, 1973, F.A. Davis Co.

Sugarman, M.: U.S. Health care regionalization and the consumer. In Kaleidoscope of childbearing: Preparation, birth and nurturing, Seattle, 1978, Pennypress.

Tankson, E.A.: The adolescent parent: One approach to teaching child care and giving support, J.O.G.N. Nurs. **5**:9-15, May/June 1976.

Taylor, D.: A new way to teach teens about contraceptives, MCN **1**:378-383, Nov./Dec. 1976.

Wegman, M.E.: Annual summary of vital statistics, Pediatrics **73**(6):981, 1984.

DEFINITIONS

Define the following terms:

adolescent
antepartal
asphyxia
atelectasis
attachment
attitudes
bonding
commune
congenital malformations
culture
ethnic
family-centered maternity/newborn care
fetal
infant mortality rate
low birth weight
maternal mortality rate
morbidity
mortality
myths
neonatal mortality rate
nonjudgmental
nuclear family
obstetrics
postpartal
prenatal
puerperal sepsis
regionalization
ruptured membranes
Semmelweis
urban
values

LEARNING ACTIVITIES AND EXPERIENCES

1. Group discussions.
2. Guest speakers: Childbearing couples of different ages, races, cultures.
3. Visit a regionalized perinatal center and report on its goals and activities.
4. View audiovisual aids and discuss.

ENRICHMENT/IN-DEPTH STUDY

1. Read and report on "A Joint Position Statement on The Development of Family-Centered Maternity/Newborn Care in Hospitals," June 1978, Interprofessional Task Force on Health Care of Women and Children.
2. Design a plan for improving maternity care

in your community. Use only current local resources and resources available within a 250-mile radius.

3. Write a paper on the therapeutic use of self in maternity care. Describe how you can best use yourself in a helping way while providing care to childbearing families.
4. Read and report on "Guidelines for Perinatal Care," American Academy of Pediatrics and American College of Obstetricians and Gynecologists, 1983.
5. Read and report on "Standards for Obstetric-Gynecologic Services," American College of Obstetricians and Gynecologists, 1985.
6. Read and report on "Standards for Obstetric, Gynecologic, and Neonatal Nursing," 3rd ed., the Nurses Association of the American College of Obstetricians and Gynecologists, 1986.

SELF-ASSESSMENT

For questions 1 through 12, determine if each statement is true or false. Fill in the space to the left of the statement by indicating T for true and F for false.

_____ 1. During the ancient historical period, obstetricians provided care for all childbearing women.

_____ 2. The oldest known textbook for midwives was written in the nineteenth century.

_____ 3. Obstetric practice was established as part of medicine during the twentieth century.

_____ 4. During the Renaissance, establishment of Italian medical schools advanced obstetric education.

_____ 5. In the twentieth century male physicians as obstetricians came into vogue.

_____ 6. "Childbed fever" (puerperal fever) claimed the lives of many women giving birth before Pasteur discovered the organism causing puerperal fever in 1860.

_____ 7. In the twentieth century postpartal and antepartal care were recognized as being important when caring for childbearing women.

_____ 8. The U.S. Congress established a Children's Bureau in 1912 to educate the public in the need for prenatal care.

_____ 9. The United States ranked second in the world in infant mortality between 1955 and 1984.

_____10. Infant mortality rates are highest in rural nonmetropolitan counties and inner cities among blacks and other minorities.

_____11. Sometimes people experience childbirth as a warm, giving experience.

_____12. Men in our culture had never been actively involved in the birth process.

For questions 13 through 16, choose the best answers and indicate your choice by circling the answer.

13. A new baby in the family can mean:
    a. competition for a sibling
    b. more work for grandparents
    c. financial worry for the family
    d. no noticeable change in lifestyle
    e. diminished privacy for all

    Answer (circle one): 1. a and c
    2. a, b, c, and e
    3. all of the above

14. The pregnant couple during the first trimester often feels that the pregnancy is:
    a. a welcome, wanted responsibility
    b. a threat to their own freedom
    c. both a and b

15. The progression parents use in first touching their baby is:
    a. whole hand to body
    b. fingertip to palm to increased body contact
    c. palm to fingertip

16. The unwed father may be helped to face the reality of pregnancy by:
    a. involving him in prenatal care
    b. informing him that he has no rights if he does not provide child support

c. encouraging him to go on "about his business"
d. involving him in the pregnancy planning

Answer (circle one): 1. a and d
2. b
3. c

Supply the correct answer(s) for items 17 through 22.

17. What are some of the rights of a childbearing family?
    a.
    b.
    c.
    d.
    e.
18. List three factors that could be described as bonding delay.
    a.
    b.
    c.
19. Describe three steps that could be taken by this society to improve maternity care for all people in the United States.
    a.
    b.
    c.
20. List four major causes of infant mortality.
    a.
    b.
    c.
    d.
21. List three reasons why adolescent pregnancy is classified as high risk.
    a.
    b.
    c.
22. List three hospital policies that would be considered family-centered.
    a.
    b.
    c.

Fill in the blanks for items 23 through 27.

23. The major change in maternity care needed to make family-centered care work is ________________________________.
24. Family-centered maternity care includes all family members in ____________ for the birth experience.
25. A goal of family-centered maternity care is to treat each family with ________, as individuals, no matter what makes them seem "different."
26. "Rights" always bring with them ________________________.
27. The birth rate for married persons has consistently dropped in the United States in the last 10 years; the rate of birth to unmarried adolescents has ____________.

UNIT II

Basic anatomy and physiology of the reproductive system

GOALS

This unit is designed to provide the reader with information that will:

□ form a basis for understanding the primary parts and functions of the female and male reproductive systems.

□ facilitate explaining basic reproductive system anatomy and physiology to future parents and family members.

STUDENT OBJECTIVES

After studying this unit, you should be able to:

1. Correctly label diagrams of the male and female internal and external reproductive systems.
2. Briefly diagram the blood supply of the uterus.
3. Trace the passage of spermatozoa from their origin until they are ejaculated.
4. Given a diagram of a mammary gland, label the following structures: chest wall, nipple, areola, lactiferous duct, lobule.
5. Demonstrate a basic understanding of the anatomy of the uterus by identifying three distinct areas of uterine demarcation.
6. Demonstrate a basic understanding of the anatomy of the female bony pelvis by:
   a. Listing the four bones of the pelvis
   b. Identifying the three bones that unite to form the innominate bone
   c. Identifying the four joints of the bony pelvis
   d. Identifying the anatomic landmark separating the false from the true pelvis
   e. Identifying the three planes of the pelvis that have obstetric significance
   f. Identifying the axis of the true pelvis
7. Explain the processes of menstruation, ovulation, and fertilization by naming the hormones responsible for these processes and describing their functions.
8. Define premenstrual syndrome (PMS).
9. Name the three phases of the menstrual cycle and state what changes take place during each phase.

FUNCTIONS OF THE FEMALE REPRODUCTIVE SYSTEM

Human life begins with the union of two different cells, one from the female, called the ovum, and one from the male, called the spermatozoon. This beginning of life, known as fertilization or conception, begins inside the female, whose body then nurtures the fertilized ovum until it grows and develops into a new and separate human being.

LIST THE PRIMARY FUNCTIONS OF THE FEMALE REPRODUCTIVE SYSTEM

The female reproductive system has three very basic functions:

1. To reproduce (to give life)
2. To produce the hormones responsible for female sexual characteristics and reproductive functions
3. To provide sexual gratification

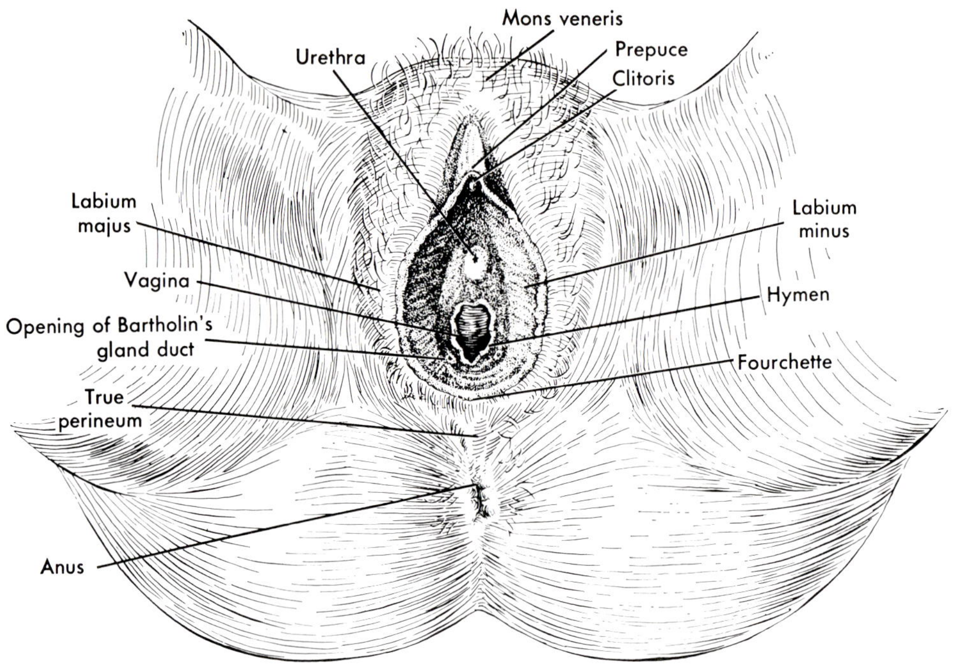

Fig. 2-1. External female genitalia.

EXTERNAL FEMALE GENITALIA

EXTERNAL FEMALE GENITALIA

The external parts of the female reproductive system (Fig. 2-1) form the *vulva* (from the Latin word meaning covering). These include two pair of lips, or *labia.* The outermost, heavy lips, called the *labia majora,* are composed of skin and fat and covered with pubic hair. These outer lips are continuous with, and extend down from, the mons pubis (or mons veneris), which is a skin-covered mound of fat covering the pubic bone, to the perineum. Although the entire pelvic floor is usually called the *perineum* in both the male and female, in the pregnant woman the area between the vaginal opening and the anus is called the perineum.

The two smaller lips, called the *labia minora,* are folds of skin that lie within the labia majora and meet at the top to form a hood, which covers the clitoris. The *clitoris* is a small, cylindrical, erectile organ covered with mucous membrane. It is like the male organ, the penis, in that it responds to sexual excitation by becoming erect. Toward the anus, the labia minora blend together with the labia majora to form a ridge of tissue called the *frenulum of the labia,* or *fourchette.*

The triangular or almond-shaped area between the labia minora is called the *vestibule.* The vaginal opening and the urethral orifice through which urine is voided are found within this space. Just above and to each side of the vaginal opening are mucus-producing *Bartholin's glands* (also called *greater vestibular glands*). These glands may become infected and swollen. The vaginal opening is surrounded by a fold of mucous membrane called the *hymen.* On each side of the urethral orifice are *Skene's glands* (also called *paraurethral glands*), which discharge lubricating secretions.

The *anus* lies below the perineum and serves as an outlet for the rectum.

FEMALE INTERNAL REPRODUCTIVE ORGANS

FEMALE INTERNAL REPRODUCTIVE ORGANS

The internal reproductive organs are found within the pelvis (Fig. 2-2).

The two *ovaries* are the primary sex glands of the female. These almond-shaped bodies lie just above and behind the uterus and are located on each side of it. Each ovary is about an inch long, half an inch thick, and three quarters of an inch wide. They contain

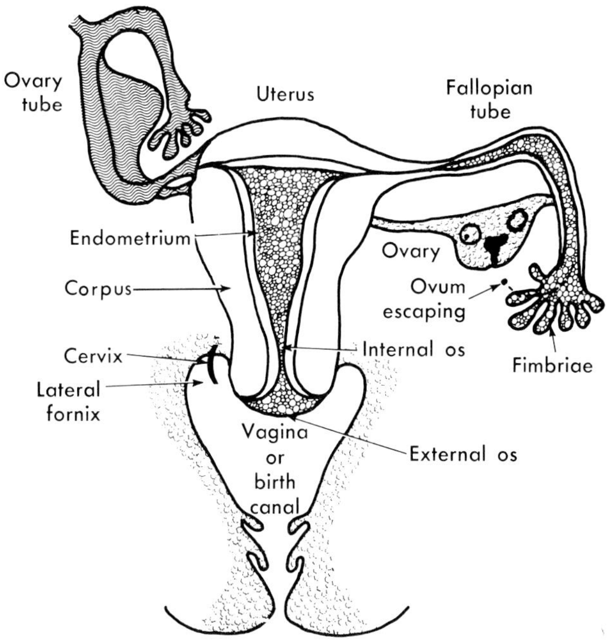

Fig. 2-2. Internal female reproductive organs.

small secretory sacs, or *follicles*, each of which contains an *ovum* that matures and is discharged from the ovary into the pelvic cavity by the process of *ovulation*. In addition to maturing and discharging ova, the ovaries produce the two major hormones necessary for reproduction to occur: *estrogen* and *progesterone*.

The two *fallopian tubes* (also called *oviducts* or *uterine tubes*), attached to each side of the upper body of the uterus, are small, muscular structures, nearly 5 inches long. These tubes carry the egg from the ovaries to the uterus by the action of the cilia in the lining of the tubes and by peristaltic action. It is important to understand that there is no direct connection between the ovaries and the fallopian tubes. Extending from the ends of the tubes are small, finger-like projections called *fimbriae*. Their movements cause a current in the peritoneal fluid, which sweeps the ovum into the tube. It takes about 5 days for the ovum to travel the 5 inches from the ovary to the uterus. Fertilization occurs in the end of the fallopian tube (farthest from the uterus), and the fertilized egg usually continues down into the uterus where it implants itself. Sometimes a fertilized egg implants itself in the lining of the tube, and this is called a *tubal pregnancy*. Rarely, a fertilized egg does not find its way into the tube at all and attaches itself to the peritoneal cavity, causing an *abdominal pregnancy*. Any pregnancy outside of the uterus is known as *ectopic* or *extrauterine*.

The *vagina* is a muscular, membranous tube about 3 inches (7.5 centimeters) long connecting the uterus with the vulva. Directly in front of the vagina are the urethra and urinary bladder, and in back of it is the rectum. The walls of the vagina contain many folds, or *rugae*, which allow the vagina to stretch during childbirth and sexual intercourse. The vagina receives the penis during sexual intercourse, receives the semen, discharges menstrual flow in nonpregnant women, and is the passage through which the birth occurs.

The cervix, or lowermost part of the uterus, dips down into the upper vagina so that a circular space is formed around the cervix and between the walls of the vagina. The areas of this circular space are known as *fornices*, with the deepest of these spaces behind the cervix called the *posterior fornix*. A needle can be introduced into the vaginal canal and then poked through the thin tissue of the posterior fornix and into the abdominal cavity to withdraw samples of any fluid that might have accumulated there. Because this

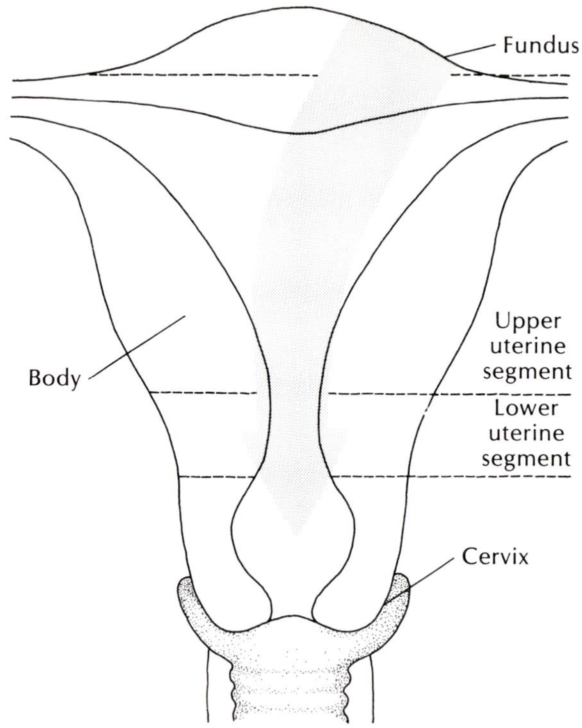

Fig. 2-3. Areas of the uterus.

lowermost portion of the abdominal cavity is called the *cul-de-sac,* this procedure is known as *culdocentesis.*

DISTINCT AREAS OF UTERINE DEMARCATION

The *uterus* is a hollow, pear-shaped muscular organ, which in the nonpregnant female is about the size of a closed fist. The uterus contains three distinct areas (Fig. 2-3): (1) the uppermost, rounded top portion, above the level where the fallopian tubes enter, called the fundus, (2) the middle portion, called the *body,* or *corpus,* and (3) the lower, smaller portion, called the *cervix,* or *neck.* The prolongations of the uterus into which the fallopian tubes fit are termed the *cornu (horns).* In about 80% of women, the uterus is tipped forward, or *anteverted.* If the uterus is tipped backward, it is *retroverted.*

The uterus is located in the middle of the pelvic cavity between the bladder and the rectum. It is held in place by ligaments that stretch to allow the uterus to expand and rise up out of the pelvis into the abdominal cavity during pregnancy.

LIST THE THREE DIVISIONS OF THE CERVIX

The cervix is divided into three parts (Fig. 2-2): (1) the *internal os,* opening into the uterus, (2) the *external os,* opening into the vagina, and (3) the *cervical canal,* the area between the internal and external osea.

LIST THE THREE LAYERS OF TISSUE COMPOSING THE UTERUS

IDENTIFY THE ARRANGEMENT OF THE UTERINE MUSCULATURE

The interior surface of the uterus, the *endometrium,* is composed of secretive tissue containing blood vessels and glands. This is the layer of the uterus that sloughs each month during menstruation. The walls of the uterus are made of a smooth muscle called *myometrium.* The outside of the uterus is covered by connective tissue called *perimetrium.* The myometrium is the thickest of the three layers. Its walls contain a network of muscle fibers that can grow and stretch as the uterus grows in pregnancy (Fig. 2-4). The outer layer of the myometrium is made up mainly of lengthwise fibers that extend into various supporting ligaments. The fibers of the inner layer run in a circular direction, while the fibers of the thick middle layer form an interlacing network and are arranged in figure-eight patterns. Because blood vessels run through these interlacing patterns, when these fibers contract after the birth, the blood vessels are kinked and constricted, thus controlling uterine bleeding.

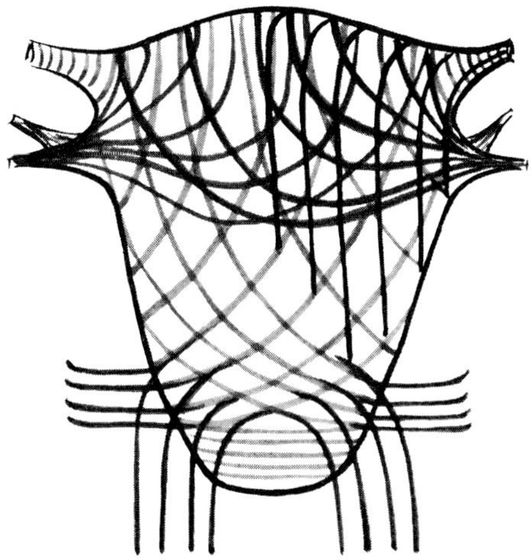

Fig. 2-4. Muscle fibers of the uterus. (From Lerch, C., and Bliss, V.J.: Maternity nursing, ed. 3, St. Louis, 1978, The C.V. Mosby Co.)

Blood supply

Although the nonpregnant uterus receives only 50 to 60 milliliters of blood per minute, the pregnant uterus at term can receive up to 700 to 800 milliliters per minute. This is equal to 10% of all blood pumped by the maternal heart at term. About 70% of the abundant blood supply of the uterus is provided by the uterine artery and 30% by the ovarian arteries (Fig. 2-5, **A**). To understand where these arteries arise, trace them back to the aorta. As you can see, to get to the uterus, either a red blood cell could travel from the aorta through a common iliac artery, then through an internal iliac (hypogastric) artery, then through the uterine artery, *or* the red cell could travel directly off the aorta, through an ovarian artery, to the uterus. The uterine artery also supplies blood for the cervix, upper vagina, fallopian tubes, and round ligament.

Once the uterine and ovarian arteries reach the uterus, they penetrate the uterine wall to reach the myometrium, the thick middle muscular layer. There they branch into arteries that run parallel to the surface. From these arteries arise the *radial arteries*, which point inward toward the uterine cavity like the spokes of a bicycle wheel. Where the radial arteries terminate, they are very tortuous and convoluted and thus are called *spiral arteries*. Because the spiral arteries are so coiled and twisted, they can easily stretch out to supply the placenta as it and the uterus change in size and position during pregnancy (Fig. 2-5, **B**).

The ovaries are supplied by the ovarian artery.

Veins follow essentially the same paths as the arteries. They penetrate all the layers of the uterus and are especially plentiful in the myometrium.

Nerve supply

The innervation of the female reproductive organs can be divided into efferent (motor) and afferent (sensory) components. Motor fibers to the uterus are primarily sympathetic nervous system fibers, which originate in the lower thoracic and upper lumbar portions of the spinal cord. After leaving the cord and traveling down toward the pelvis, these fibers eventually form large, intertwining tangles called *plexi* (singular: *plexus*). The *hypogastric plexus* is the large plexus formed above the sacral promontory. This plexus sends sympathetic fibers to the uterus, fallopian tubes, vagina, and ovaries. The ovaries and fallopian tubes also receive sympathetic fibers via the *ovarian plexus*. The pelvic organs receive a lesser amount of innervation from the parasympathetic nervous system via the *pelvic splanchnic nerves (nervi erigentes)*, which originate from spinal cord seg-

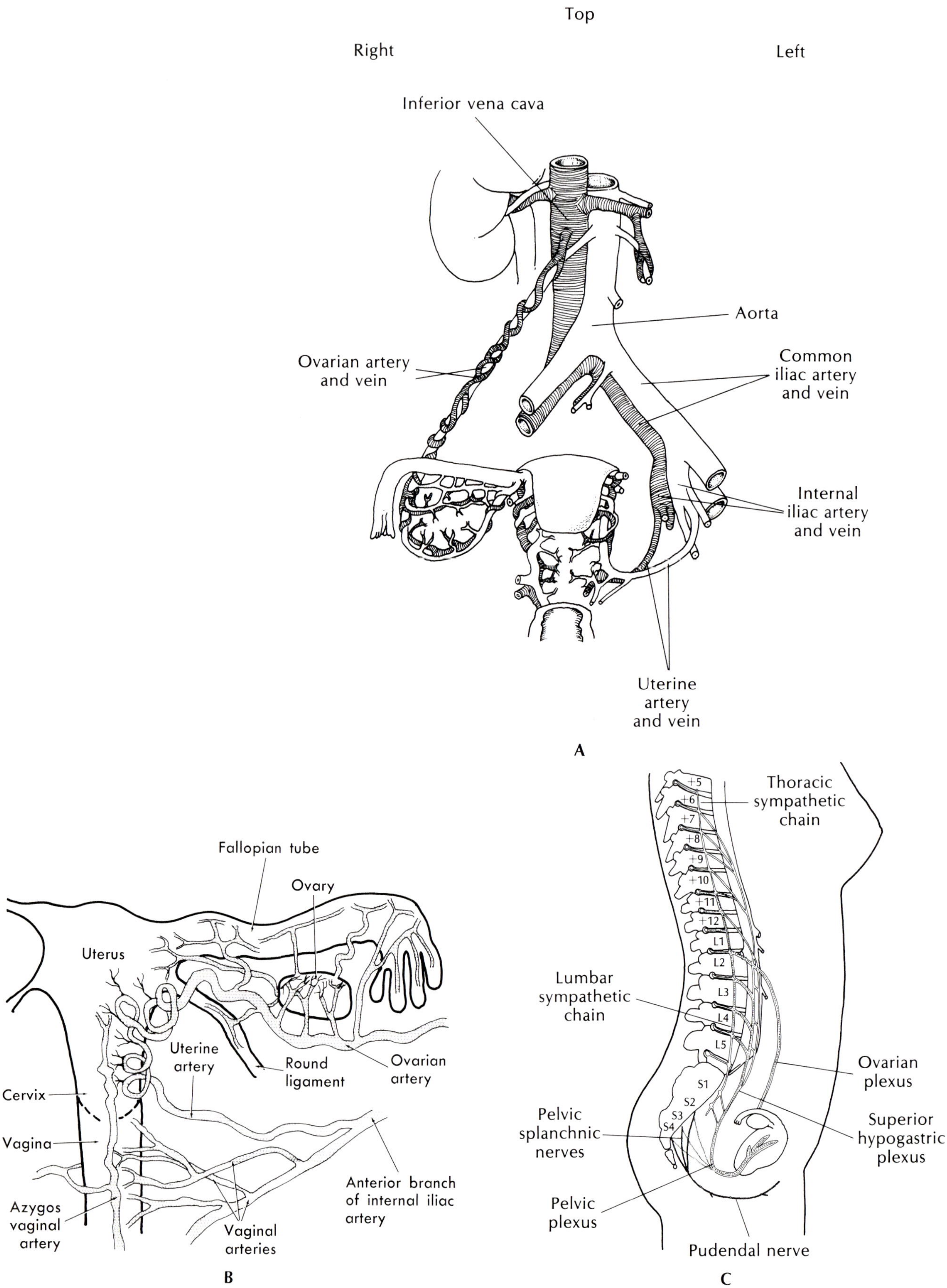

Fig. 2-5. A, Blood supply to pelvis. **B,** Blood supply to uterus. **C,** Nerve supply to uterus.

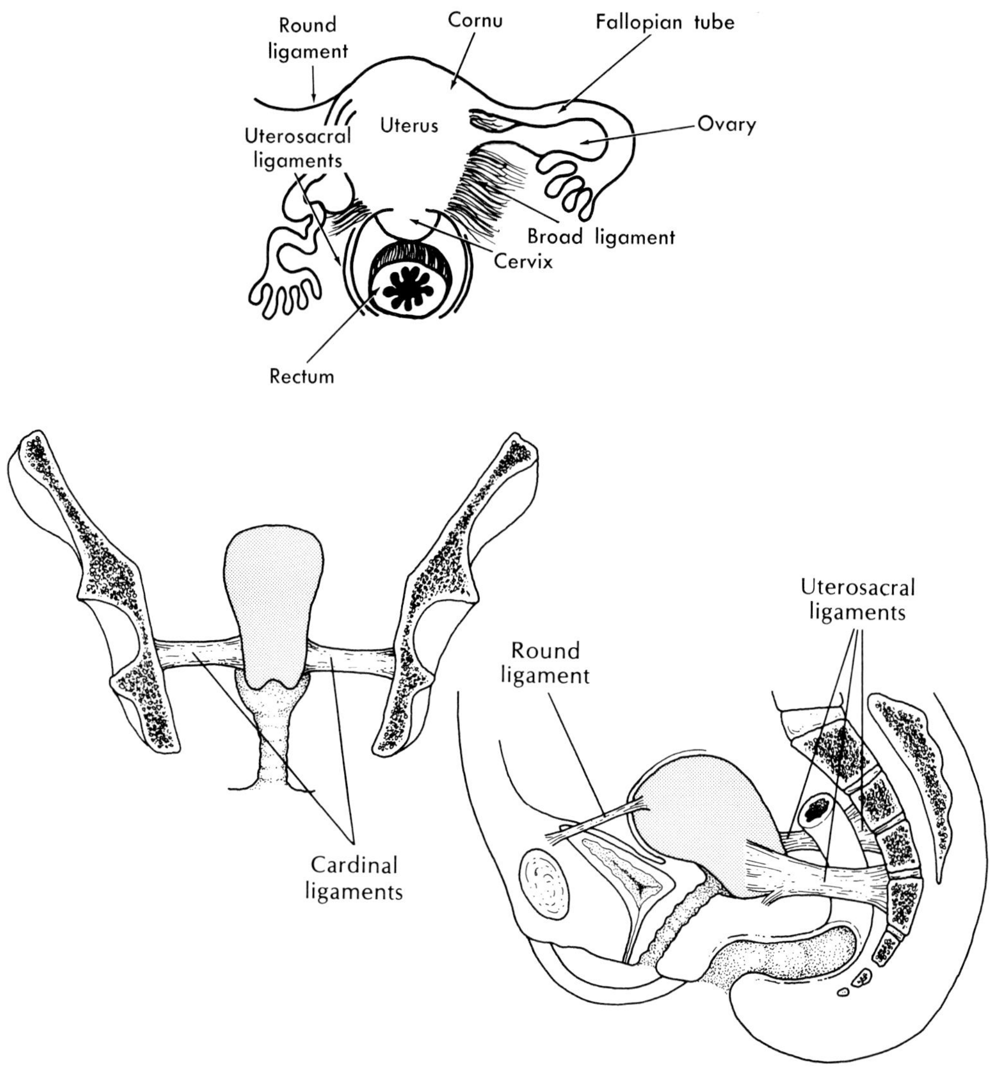

Fig. 2-6. Uterine support.

ments S2, S3, and possibly S4. The pelvic splanchnics enter the pelvic plexus before reaching the pelvic organs.

Sensory fibers from the uterus, as well as pain fibers from the vagina and cervix, are found in the nervi erigentes (S2-S4). However, it is currently thought that sensory fibers also accompany the sympathetic component.

It is currently believed that the sensation of "pain" in labor is transmitted as follows:

1. First stage of labor: dilation and effacement of the cervix sends impulses along with the sympathetic nerves to T11, T12, and L1.
2. Second stage: distention of the vagina and perineum sends impulses along branches of the *pudendal* nerve to S2, S3, and S4.
3. Third stage: dilation of the cervix sends impulses along with the sympathetic nerves to T11, T12, and L1. (See Fig. 2-5, **C,** nerve supply to uterus.)

Uterine support

The uterus is supported in its position in the pelvic cavity by ligaments (Fig. 2-6). The paired *broad ligaments* attach the uterus to each side of the pelvic cavity. Uterine blood vessels and nerves pass through the broad ligaments. They serve to anchor the ovaries and tubes in place. The *uterosacral ligaments* connect the sacrum to the uterus,

IDENTIFY THE FOUR LIGAMENTS THAT SUPPORT THE UTERUS AND ITS PORTIONS

one on each side of the rectum. The *cardinal ligament* extends laterally from the vagina and cervix and runs within the lowest part of the broad ligament to the pelvic sidewall. The cardinal ligament is the chief ligament that keeps the uterus from dropping down into the vagina. The *round ligaments* extend from a point on the uterus just below the fallopian tubes through the inguinal canal to the labia majora. Because the uterus is suspended from ligaments (which can be pulled, stretched, and distorted), it can rise up out of the pelvic cavity as it enlarges during pregnancy.

Pelvic floor

DESCRIBE THE LAYERS OF THE PELVIC FLOOR MUSCLES

The pelvic floor muscles are composed of three layers. The outermost two layers are made up mainly of sphincters (Fig. 2-7, *A*). These ring-like muscles, which are relatively weak, close the outer openings of the urinary meatus, rectum, and vagina. The outermost layer contains the ischiocavernosus muscle, the bulbocavernosus muscle, and the superficial transverse perineal muscle. The bulbocavernosus muscle, with the external anal sphincter muscle, forms a figure-eight around the vagina and rectum. The middle layer, not visible in the diagram, contains the sphincter urethrae (which surrounds the urethra) and the deep transverse perineal muscle. Lying inside these outer muscle layers are deeper, stronger muscles that run from the pubis to the coccyx and form the base of the abdominal cavity (Fig. 2-7, *B*). These most powerful muscles are the *levator ani* and the *coccygeus*. The levator ani has three portions: (1) pubococcygeal, (2) iliococcygeal, and (3) puborectalis muscles. These muscles form a hammock, or sling, above which the vagina, rectum, bladder, and uterus are suspended by ligaments and fasciae. These fascial sheaths surround and embrace each pelvic organ and are subject to tearing during birth.

EXPLAIN TWO FUNCTIONS OF THE PELVIC FLOOR

Breasts

MAMMARY GLANDS

The mammary glands, or breasts, are also considered part of the femal reproductive system (Fig. 2-8). The breasts are two glands situated over the pectoralis muscles on the anterior chest. Each breast is composed of fatty tissue containing 15 to 20 lobes, each lobe containing many lobules. Breast size has no effect on the number of lobes. The lobules contain *acini cells*, which begin to secrete colostrum in midpregnancy and milk after birth. Closed lactiferous ducts connect all lobes and lobules and join under the areola to make sinuses (ampullae), which can enlarge to serve as a reservoir for colostrum and milk. The pigmented area of smooth skin around the nipple is the *areola*. In the areola sebaceous glands form *Montgomery's tubercles*, which secrete oil to lubricate and protect the nipples. The tubercles appear as small, white, elevated patches on the pigmented areola. The nipple, located in the center of the areola, is the outlet for the ducts. The nipple is made of sturdy, pigmented skin tissue. Although the breasts are complex in their structure and function, it is very easy for women to become familiar with how their breasts feel. In fact, women and their partners can become so sensitive to the normal texture of the breasts that breast lumps often are first detected by them.

Female bony pelvis

ANATOMY OF THE FEMALE BONY PELVIS

The pelvis is a bony, basket-like structure that carries the weight of the upper part of the body and transfers this weight to the lower limbs. It is the cavity that contains the reproductive organs and through which the baby must pass.

BONES OF THE PELVIS

Bones. The *female bony pelvis* is made up of four bones: the coccyx, the sacrum, and the two innominate bones (Fig. 2-9). The sacrum is the wedge-shaped bone at the back of the pelvis. Attached to the bottom of the sacrum is the coccyx. The sacrum and coccyx can be thought of as lowermost extensions of the spinal column. The innominate, or hip, bones make up the sides and front of the pelvis. Each innominate bone is composed of three fused bones: the ilium, the ischium, and the pubis (Fig. 2-9). Fusion of these three bones begins at about the twelfth year and is usually complete by the eighteenth. The

THREE BONES THAT UNITE TO FORM THE INNOMINATE BONE

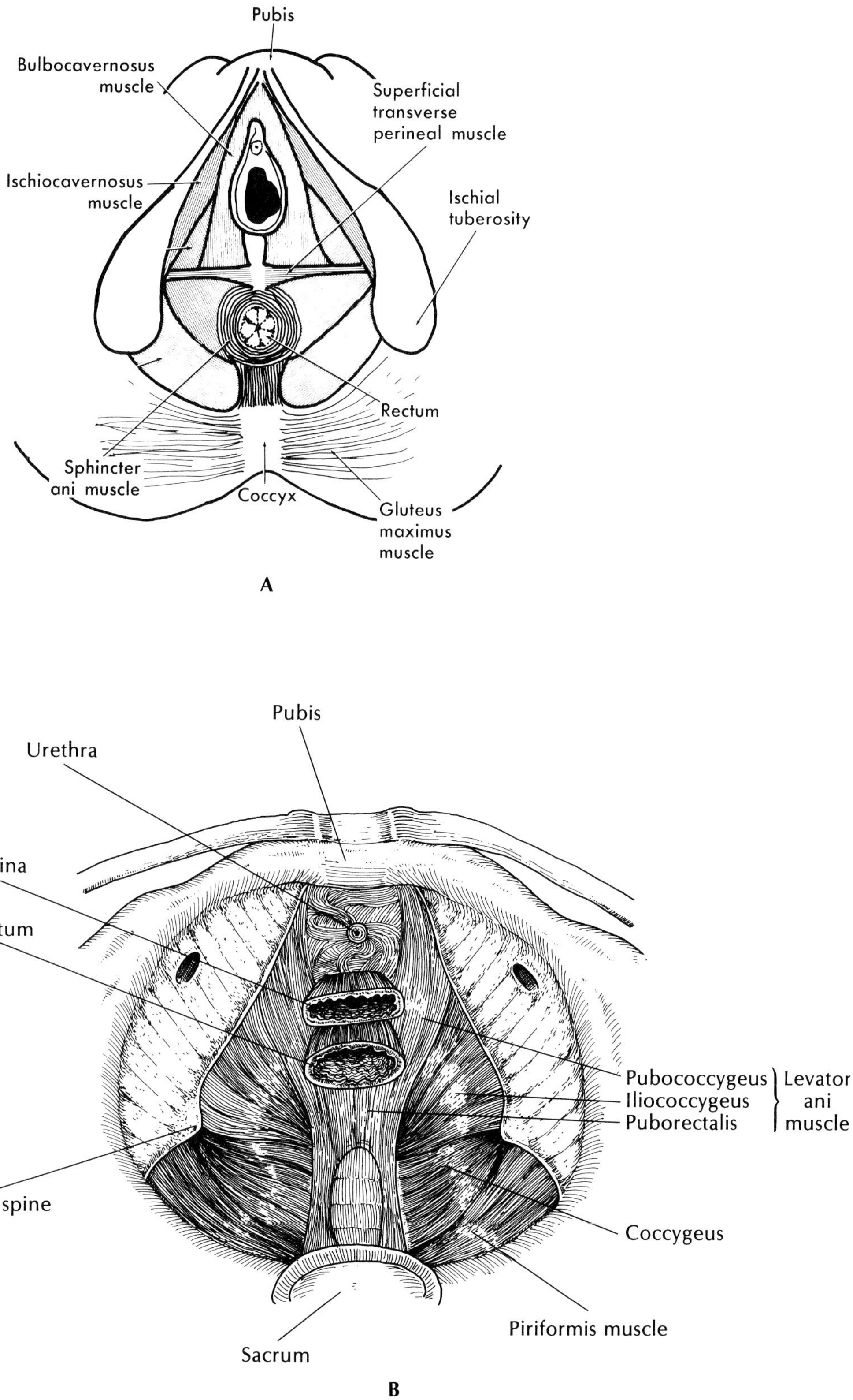

Fig. 2-7. A, Muscles of perineum. **B,** Muscles of pelvic floor from above.

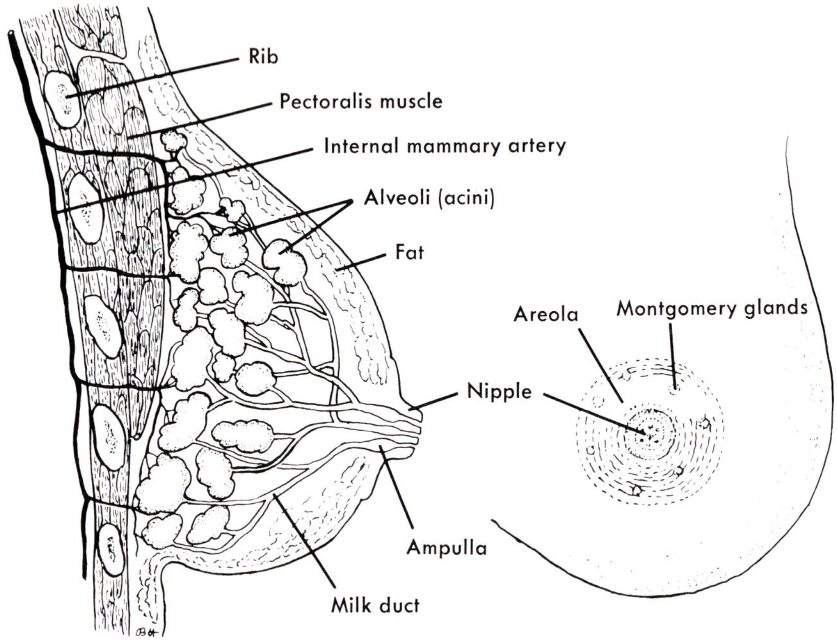

Fig. 2-8. Breasts. (From Hamilton, P.M.: Basic maternity nursing, ed. 5, St. Louis, 1985, The C.V. Mosby Co.)

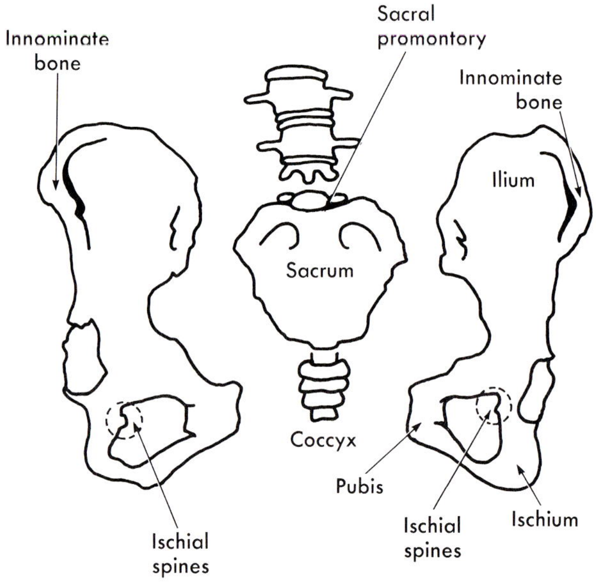

Fig. 2-9. Female bony pelvis.

top anterior portion of the sacrum tilts forward, forming a bony ridge known as the *sacral promontory.* The two pubes join in front to form the *symphysis pubis.*

JOINTS OF THE BONY PELVIS

Joints. In the bony pelvis there are four joints of importance: the two *sacroiliac* joints, between the sacrum and the ilia on each side, the *symphysis pubis,* in the front between the two pubic bones, and the *sacrococcygeal,* between the sacrum and the coccyx (Fig. 2-10). These joints are lined with fibrocartilage, which becomes thickened and softened during pregnancy, thus allowing greater mobility of the pelvic bones.

ANATOMICAL LANDMARKS SEPARATING THE FALSE FROM THE TRUE PELVIS

Division. The pelvis is divided into two parts by the *linea terminalis;* these parts are named the false pelvis (upper part) and the true pelvis (lower part) (Fig. 2-11). The false pelvis is less important for labor. It can be thought of as a large funnel that supports the uterus during late pregnancy and directs the fetus into the true pelvis when labor begins.

THREE PLANES OF THE PELVIS

The true pelvis has three planes: an inlet, a tunnel-like cavity, and an outlet (Fig. 2-12). The *inlet,* or the entryway to the true pelvis, is the brim that separates the false from

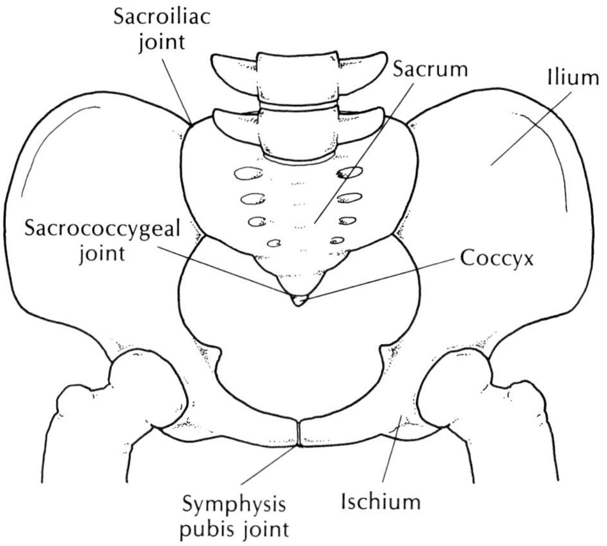

Fig. 2-10. Bony pelvis and joints.

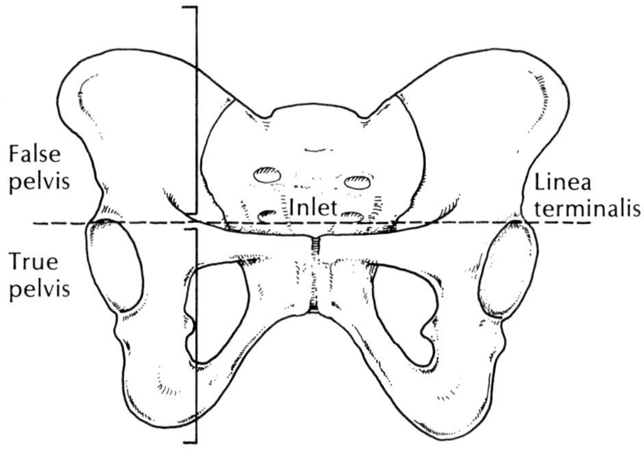

Fig. 2-11. False and true pelvis.

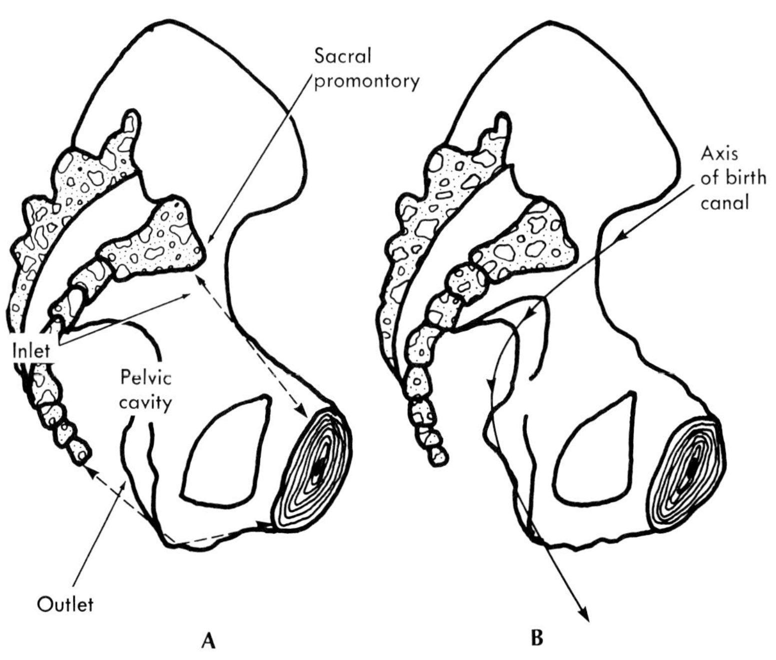

Fig. 2-12. Pelvic planes and axis. **A,** Cavity of true pelvis. **B,** Axis of birth canal.

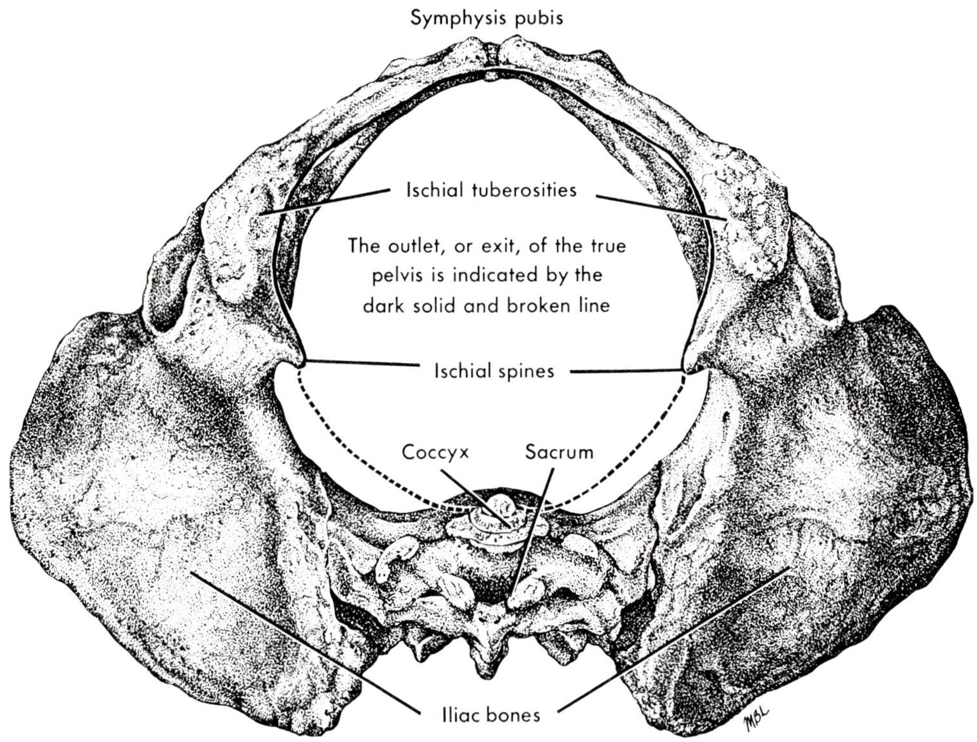

Fig. 2-13. Pelvic outlet.

the true pelvis. It is heart-shaped, with the promontory of the sacrum forming a slight projection into it from behind. It extends forward to the uppermost part of the symphysis pubis. It is widest from side to side and narrowest from front to back.

The pelvic *outlet* is the space between the ischial tuberosities (the sit-upon bones) on the sides, the coccyx in the back, and the symphysis pubis in the front. Note that the outlet is diamond shaped (Fig. 2-13). The greatest diameter of the outlet is the anteroposterior (A-P) (from front to back).

AXIS OF THE TRUE PELVIS

Axis. The pelvic cavity is the space between the inlet above and the outlet below and the walls of the pelvis. Note the *axis* of the cavity is curved (Fig. 2-12) so that the baby must accommodate itself to the curved path when coming through the canal. The curve is similar to that of a sliding board, and the baby in a favorable position can slide on out, head first.

On both sides of the inner part of the ischium are bony knobs of significance called the *ischial spines* (Figs. 2-9 and 2-13), which can be palpated during manual pelvic examination. These are landmarks for determining how high the baby is in the pelvis by measuring the height of the baby's presenting part in relationship to the level of these bony ischial spines. The prominence of these ischial spines and the distance between them are important measurements of the adequacy of the pelvis.

The size of the true pelvis is very important because the baby must pass through it to be born.

DISTINGUISH FOUR PELVIC TYPES ACCORDING TO THEIR SHAPE

Pelvic types. There are four main classifications of pelves: (1) gynecoid (female), (2) android (male), (3) anthropoid (oval), and (4) platypelloid (flat) (Fig. 2-14). Most women have pelves that do not fit into a single category but incorporate features of two varieties. Thus, the preceding classification is based on the shape of the *inlet.* It is generally believed that the gynecoid pelvis is the most favorable for normal delivery.

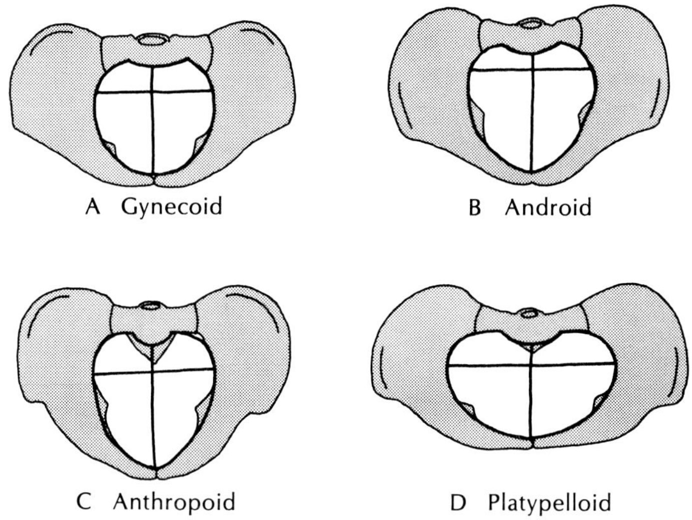

Fig. 2-14. Four types of pelves: **A,** Gynecoid. **B,** Android. **C,** Anthropoid. **D,** Platypelloid.

MALE EXTERNAL REPRODUCTIVE ORGANS

LIST THE PRIMARY FUNCTIONS OF THE MALE REPRODUCTIVE SYSTEM

The scrotum and penis are the external reproductive organs of the male (Fig. 2-15). The male reproductive system has three basic functions:

1. To reproduce (to give life)
2. To produce the hormones responsible for male sexual characteristics and reproductive functions
3. To provide sexual gratification

Penis

MALE EXTERNAL REPRODUCTIVE SYSTEM

The penis is a cylindrical organ made of three chambers of a sponge-like tissue containing many blood-filled spaces. These spaces are relatively empty when the penis is in a relaxed state but fill with blood and distend when sexual excitation occurs, making the penis erect. The male urethra passes through one of the three chambers. It is through the urethra that the urine empties from the bladder and the reproductive cells and secretions are carried to the outside.

The head of the penis is composed of an enlarged portion called the glans; covering the glans is the loosely fitting skin, called the *prepuce,* or *foreskin,* which is removed if a circumcision is done.

Scrotum

The scrotum is the pouch suspended between the thighs that holds the male gonads (testes). The scrotum is divided into two sacs by a septum down the middle. Each sac contains a testis (testicle), an epididymis, and a portion of the spermatic cord. Spermatozoa require a temperature lower than body temperature for their development and maintenance, thus the temperature of the scrotum is a few degrees cooler than that of the body. Muscle fibers in the tissue of the scrotum can move the testes closer to the abdomen when very cold or lower the testes away from the abdomen when very hot.

MALE INTERNAL REPRODUCTIVE ORGANS

The internal organs include two testes, two epididymides, two seminal ducts and vesicles, two ejaculatory ducts, two spermatic cords, the urethra, the prostate, and the bulbourethral (Cowper's) glands. As these internal reproductive organs are described, refer to Figure 2-15 to locate each part.

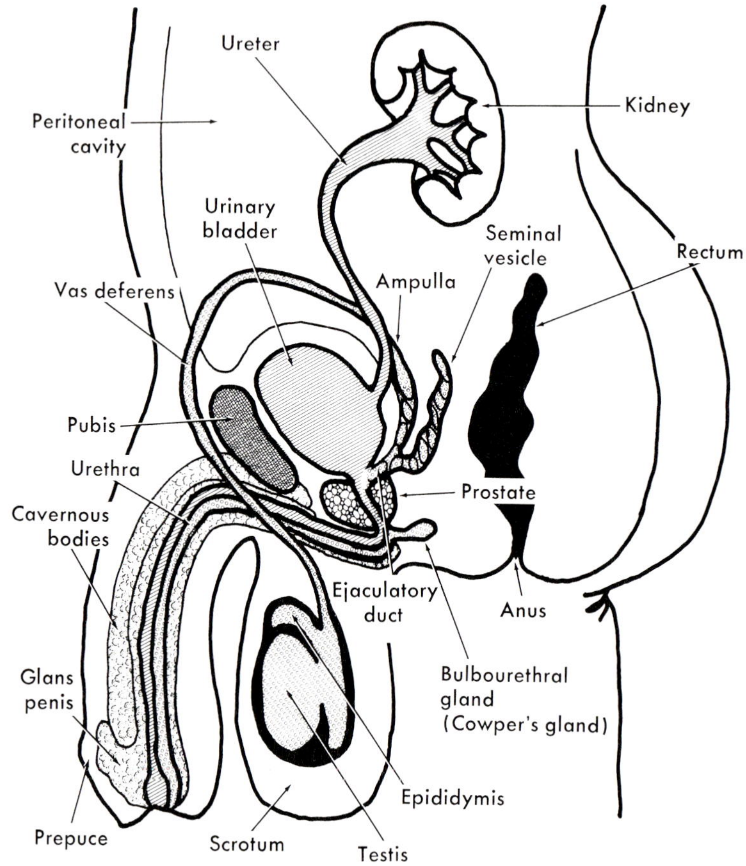

Fig. 2-15. Male genitourinary system.

Testes

The testes are paired, oval-shaped glands about 2 inches long and 1 inch wide. Each testis contains specialized tissue arranged in tubules *(seminiferous tubules)* where the spermatozoa are produced. Between the tiny tubes are small groups of cells that produce the male sex hormone *testosterone,* responsible for the masculine characteristics of the male body. Part of the seminal fluid, or *semen,* in which the spermatozoa are transported is also produced in the tubules in the testes.

PASSAGE OF SPERMATOZOA FROM THEIR ORGIN UNTIL THEY ARE EJACULATED

The tubes for carrying the spermatozoa begin with the tubules inside the testis itself. From these tubes the spermatozoa are collected by a coiled tube, 20 feet long if stretched to its full extent, called the *epididymis,* situated above and behind the testis. The mature spermatozoa enter the epididymis from the testis, become motile there, and pass through it to the *vas deferens* when ejaculated.

Vas deferens

The vas deferens is a duct about 18 inches long that continues through a small canal in the abdominal wall and then curves back behind the urinary bladder where it joins the duct of the seminal vesicle to form the *ejaculatory duct.* The vas deferens carries the semen to the urethra. Traveling with the vas deferens are the testicular artery, autonomic nerves, veins, lymphatics, and a small muscle. These structures collectively make up the *spermatic cord.*

Seminal vesicles

The seminal vesicles are two small muscular glands at the base and rear of the urinary bladder. They are somewhat irregularly shaped and consist of many small sacs, or pock-

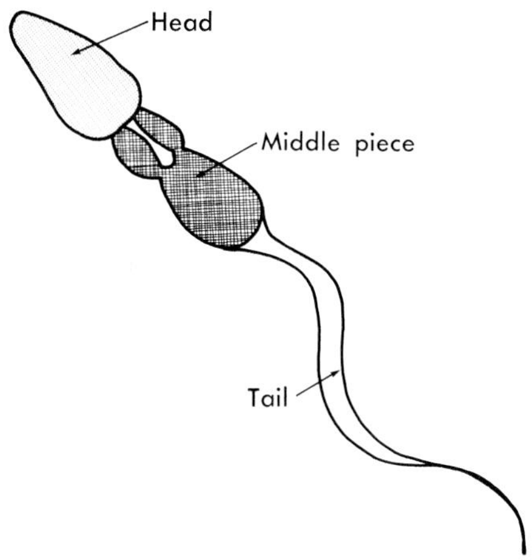

Fig. 2-16. Spermatozoon.

ets. Their glandular lining produces a thick, milky secretion that forms much of the ejaculated semen. The ducts of the seminal vesicles join the vas deferens to form the ejaculatory ducts, which empty into the urethra.

Prostate gland

The prostate gland is a single, fibromuscular, doughnut-shaped gland completely surrounding the urethra, just below the bladder. The prostate secretes a thin, clear fluid that becomes part of the ejaculate by entering the urethra by way of about 60 tiny *prostatic ductules*. The prostate is also composed of muscular tissue that contracts to aid in the ejaculation of semen into the urethra.

Bulbourethral glands (Cowper's glands)

The bulbourethral glands are a pair of pea-sized organs located below the prostate gland. These glands secrete mucus into the urethra to serve as a lubricant.

Spermatozoa

Spermatozoa are very tiny detached cells that look like tadpoles with oval heads and long tails. Over 200 million spermatozoa are deposited in the vagina in the average ejaculation. Once ejaculated, spermatozoa have a life expectancy of 24 to 72 hours. Roughly one in a million will actually make the entire journey to the egg. The head of a spermatozoon contains chemicals that help it to penetrate the ovum, and the tail propels it as it swims to meet the ovum (Fig. 2-16).

The spermatozoa are produced in the testes, stored in the epididymis, and travel through the vas deferens to the ejaculatory duct to the urethra and out the penis. In sexual intercourse the spermatozoa are deposited in the vagina by the erect penis through the process of ejaculation.

REPRODUCTION

Puberty is the term given to the period of time (11 to 17 years of age) when the reproductive organs of both the male and female reach maturity. The childbearing years begin for a female when she produces mature ova *(ovulation)* several months after her first menstrual period *(menarche)* and end when she experiences a permanent cessation of menses *(menopause)*. The ability to father a child begins for the male when he produces functional spermatozoa, usually during his early teens. Although the female's ovaries contain over one million immature ova at birth, males constantly produce new spermatozoa after each ejaculation. Thus, the male is capable of remaining fertile until well advanced in years.

Hormones

LIST THE TWO FEMALE HORMONES

The two main female sex hormones are (1) *estrogen*, responsible for the development of female characteristics, and (2) *progesterone*, which prepares the endometrium for pregnancy, maintains the endometrium during pregnancy, and suppresses ovulation during pregnancy.

Ovarian cycle: ovulation

PROCESS OF OVULATION

Although the ovarian cycle may vary in length from female to female, the average cycle is 28 days, the first day of the menstrual period being day 1. The anterior lobe of the pituitary, a small endocrine gland at the base of the brain, secretes gonadotropic hormones that control the ovarian cycle in women. These hormones are the *follicle-stimulating hormone* (FSH) and the *luteinizing hormone* (LH). In turn, release of LH and FSH is controlled by *luteinizing hormone-releasing hormone* (LHRH), a chemical compound secreted by the hypothalamus (a part of the brain) to act on the anterior pituitary gland.

Beginning at puberty, one of the ovaries is stimulated to prepare an egg (ovum) for release, and possible fertilization, about once a month. Each egg, and its surrounding specialized mass of supporting and nutrient-supplying cells, is called a *follicle*. At the

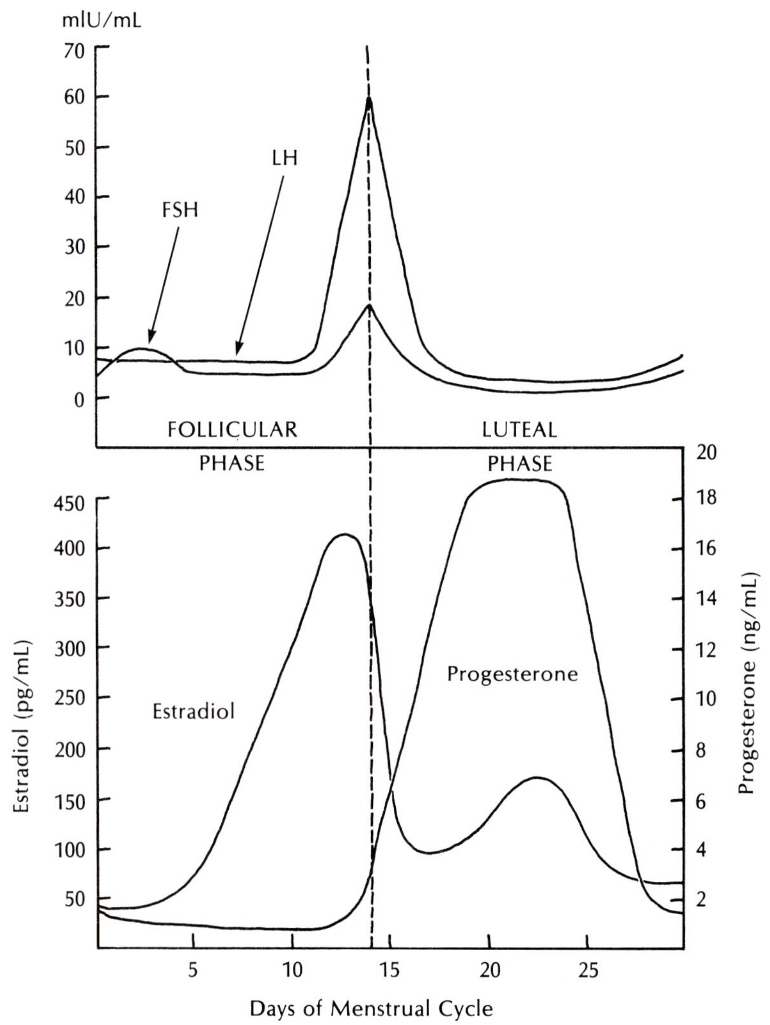

Fig. 2-17. A, Luteinizing hormone (LH), follicle-stimulating hormone (FSH), estradiol, and progesterone levels in the peripheral circulation.

onset of each ovarian cycle, FSH released by the anterior pituitary travels through the bloodstream to stimulate the growth and maturation of several follicles (Fig. 2-17, **A**). One follicle outgrows the others to form a prominent, mature *graafian follicle*, which becomes large enough to stick out above the surface of the ovary. Thus, the first half of the ovarian cycle is termed the *follicular phase*. (Although FSH is generally thought to be the most important anterior pituitary hormone to stimulate follicle growth, *both* FSH and LH are necessary.)

As the graafian follicle matures, some of its cells secrete increasing amounts of estrogen (primarily in the form of estradiol). It has been shown that if estradiol levels in blood are *high enough* for *long enough* periods of time, the anterior pituitary will release LH. Thus, approximately 14 days into the average ovarian cycle, the anterior pituitary releases a "surge" of LH, which triggers a small area of the graafian follicle to become thin and translucent, resembling a blister. It then bursts, and the ovum, covered by several cell layers, floats out of the follicle into the end of the fallopian tube. This "bursting" is termed ovulation.

After ovulation, the graafian follicle collapses and the mass of tissue forms a new structure termed the *corpus luteum* (Fig. 2-17, **B**). The cells of the corpus luteum (luteal cells) produce both estrogen and progesterone in large amounts for approximately 14 days. Thus the second half of the ovarian cycle is termed the *luteal phase*. About 9 days after ovulation, the corpus luteum begins to wither and die if fertilization does not occur. As the corpus luteum dies, its hormone-producing powers die with it, and thus estrogen and progesterone levels in the bloodstream fall to their lowest levels.

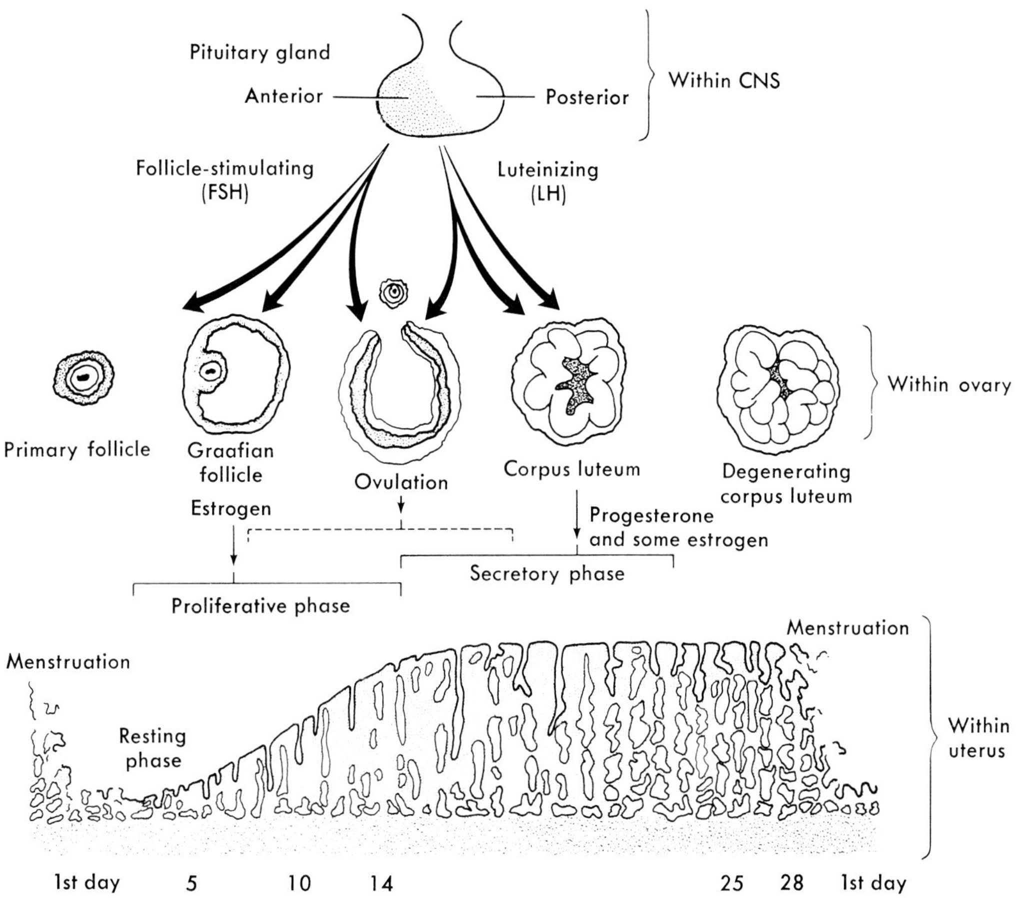

Fig. 2-17. B, Menstrual cycle. (From Jensen, M. and Bobak, I.M.: Maternity and gynecologic care: the nurse and the family, ed. 3, St. Louis, 1985, The C.V. Mosby Co.)

One might ask, if rising estrogen levels cause the anterior pituitary to release the LH "surge," why doesn't a second LH "surge" occur during the luteal phase as estrogen levels rise? The answer lies in progesterone's ability to inhibit this feedback mechanism. Thus, because the corpus luteum secretes large amounts of progesterone, a second ovulation, during the same ovarian cycle, is normally prevented.

If the ovum is fertilized by a spermatozoa in the fallopian tube, menstruation does not occur, and the corpus luteum continues to secrete progesterone during the first 3 months of pregnancy. The placenta gradually takes over the secretion of progesterones.

Uterine cycle: menstruation

PROCESS OF MENSTRUATION

The menstrual cycle prepares the endometrium for implantation of the ovum should fertilization occur. Once again, we are using a 28-day cycle for study. The four phases of the menstrual cycle are described as follows (Fig. 2-17, **B**).

PHASES OF THE MENSTRUAL CYCLE

1. Proliferative phase. This coincides with the last 8 to 12 days of the follicular phase of the ovarian cycle, depending on the duration of an individual woman's menstrual flow. During the proliferative phase, a period of endometrial repair is in progress. Cells from the uterine glands spread over the base of the endometrium as it regenerates and thickens. Endometrial glands become more and more tortuous. This growth is stimulated by the estrogen secreted from the developing ovarian follicle(s).

2. Ovulatory phase. Ovulation occurs on about the fourteenth or fifteenth day.

3. Secretory phase. Technically, this phase begins at ovulation and includes the ovulatory phase. The secretory phase coincides with the luteal phase of the ovarian cycle. In normal circumstances, the secretory phase is a constant 14 days in duration, no matter what the length of a woman's menstrual cycle (for example, 28 days, 31 days, 26 days). Progesterone, the hormone responsible for the secretory phase, prepares the already-thickened endometrium for possible implantation of the fertilized ovum. The endometrium becomes edematous and highly vascular. By the eighth day of the secretory phase (twenty-second day of the cycle), endometrial activity and gland secretory activity reach their peak, coinciding with maximal corpus luteum activity and highest progesterone levels. From the tenth to fourteenth days, edema subsides and the endometrium regresses. As the endometrium shrinks, the endometrium loses its blood supply and becomes ischemic. Tissue necrosis develops.

4. Menstrual phase. The tissue necrosis produced during the secretory phase causes blood vessels to open, producing scattered endometrial hemorrhages. These enlarge and form hematomas, which in turn cause shedding of the endometrium. The pattern of this shedding varies considerably in duration and amount of flow and is termed *menstruation.*

Normally, the cycle begins again and continues at regular intervals except during pregnancy and after menopause.

SUMMARY

Unit II was designed to provide you with a very basic understanding of the anatomy and physiology of the male and female reproductive systems, with an emphasis on the female.

BIBLIOGRAPHY

Anderson, J.E.: Grant's atlas of anatomy, ed. 8, Baltimore, 1983, Williams & Wilkins Co.

Benson, R.D., editor: Current obstetric and gyneologic diagnosis and treatment, ed. 4, Los Altos, Calif., 1982, Lange Medical Publications.

Benson, R.D.: Handbook of obstetrics and gynecology, ed. 8, Los Altos, Calif., 1983, Lange Medical Publications.

Cox, H.: Midwifery manual: A guide for auxiliary midwives, New York, 1971, McGraw-Hill Book Co.

Deutsch, R.M.: The key to feminine response in marriage, New York, 1968, Random House, Inc.

Hamilton, P.M.: Basic maternity nursing, ed. 5, St. Louis, 1984, The C.V. Mosby Co.

Memmler, R.L., and Wood, D.L.: The human body in health and disease, Philadelphia, 1977, J.B. Lippincott Co.

Oxorn, H., and Foote, W.R.: Human labor and birth, ed. 3, New York, 1975, Appleton-Century-Crofts.

Tortora, G.J., and Anagnostakos, N.P.: Principles of anatomy and physiology, San Francisco, 1975, Canfield Press.

DEFINITIONS

Define the following terms:

acini cells
anteverted
areola
Bartholin's glands
bulbourethral gland
cervix
cilia
clitoris
coccygeus
colostrum
convoluted
cornu
corpus luteum
cul-de-sac
culdocentesis
ejaculation
endometrium
estrogen
fallopian tubes
fibrocartilage
follicle
follicle-stimulating hormone (FSH)
follicular phase
fundus
gynecoid
hymen
hypogastric plexus
innominate bones
ischial spines
ischium
labia majora
labia minora
levator ani muscle
linea terminalis
lobes
lobules
luteal phase
menstruation
Montgomery's tubercles
myometrium
ovulation
pelvic floor
pelvic splanchnics
perimetrium
perineum
peristaltic action
prepuce
progesterone
secretory phase
Skene's glands
spermatozoa
spiral arteries
symphysis pubis
testes
urethra
uterus
vas deferens
vestibule
vulva

LEARNING ACTIVITIES AND EXPERIENCES

1. In an anatomy laboratory inspect a bony female pelvis and a male pelvis. Compare the general shape and curvature of the pubic arch.
2. View audiovisual aids and discuss.

SELF-ASSESSMENT

1. External female reproductive organs. Label the following structures: labium majus, labium minus, vagina, clitoris, anus, perineum.

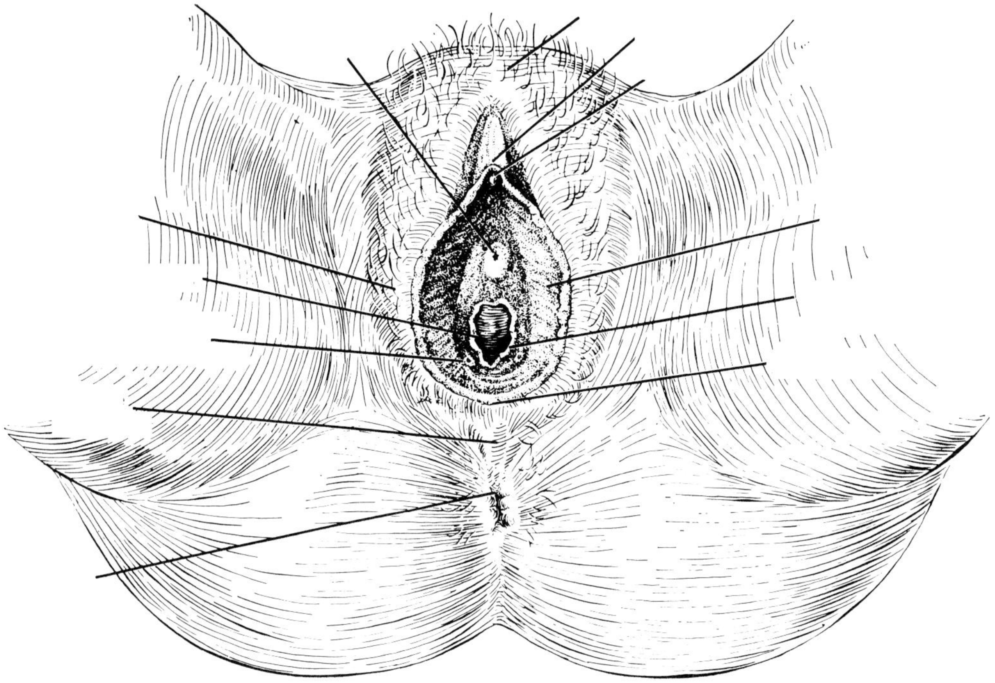

2. Male reproductive system. Label the following structures: bladder, urethra, pelvic bone, penis, scrotum, testis, vas deferens, prostate gland, epididymis, foreskin, glans penis, seminal vesicle.

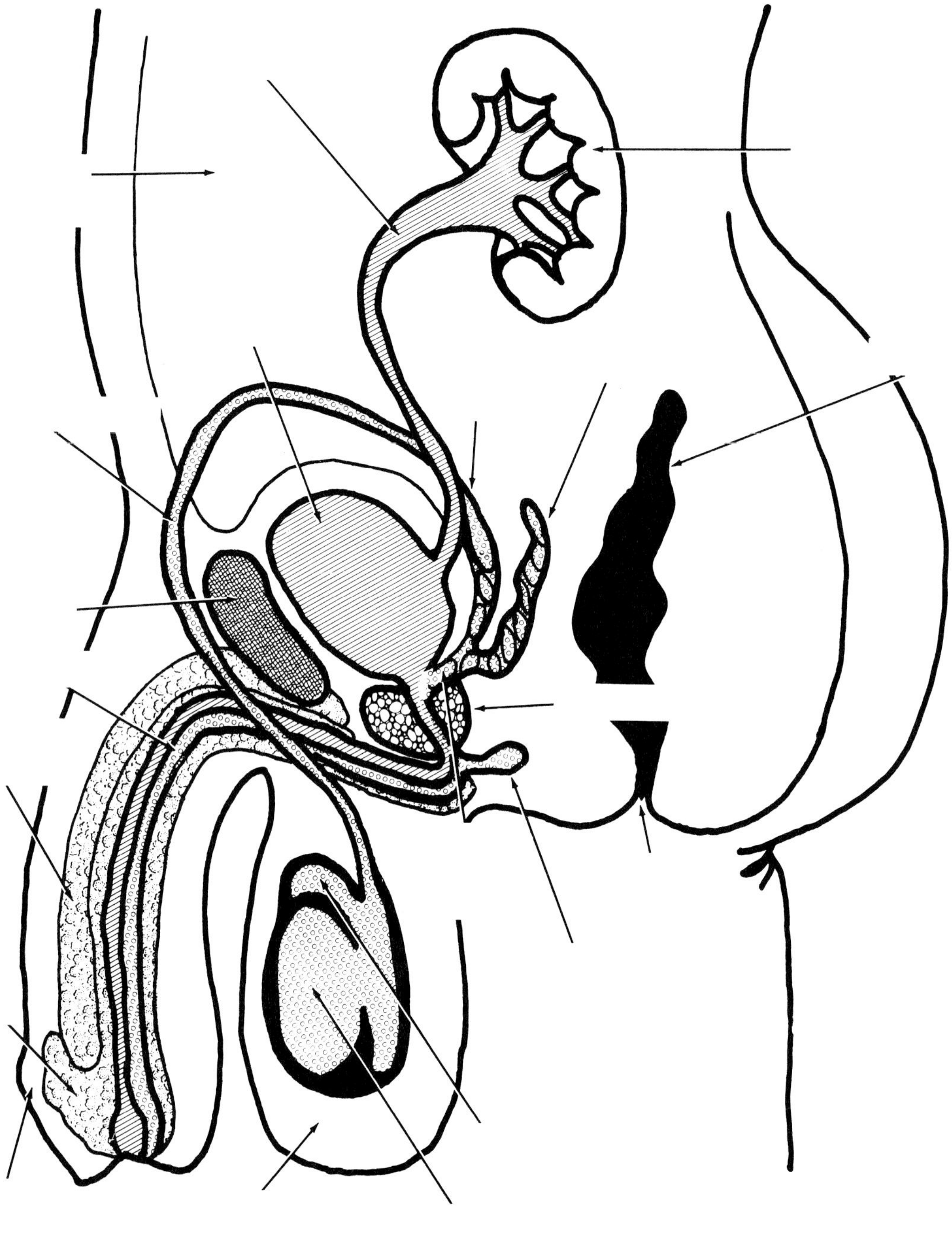

3. Internal female reproductive organs, front view. Label the following structures: fundus, cervix, corpus, fallopian tube, fimbriae, ovum, vagina, endometrium.

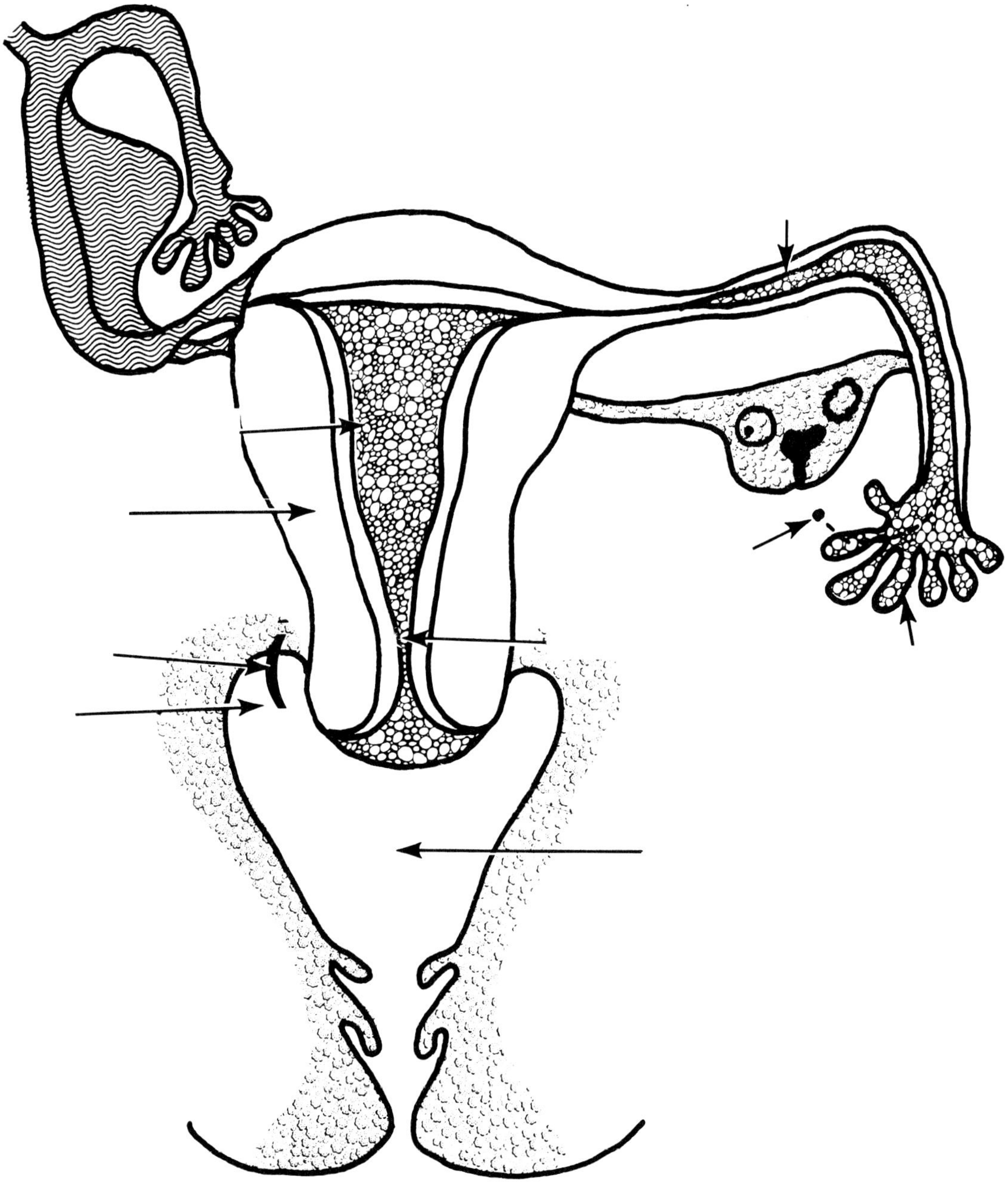

4. Label the following structures of the breast: nipple, areola, Montgomery glands, rib, pectoralis muscle, internal mammary artery, alveoli (acini), fat, milk duct, sinuses (ampullae).

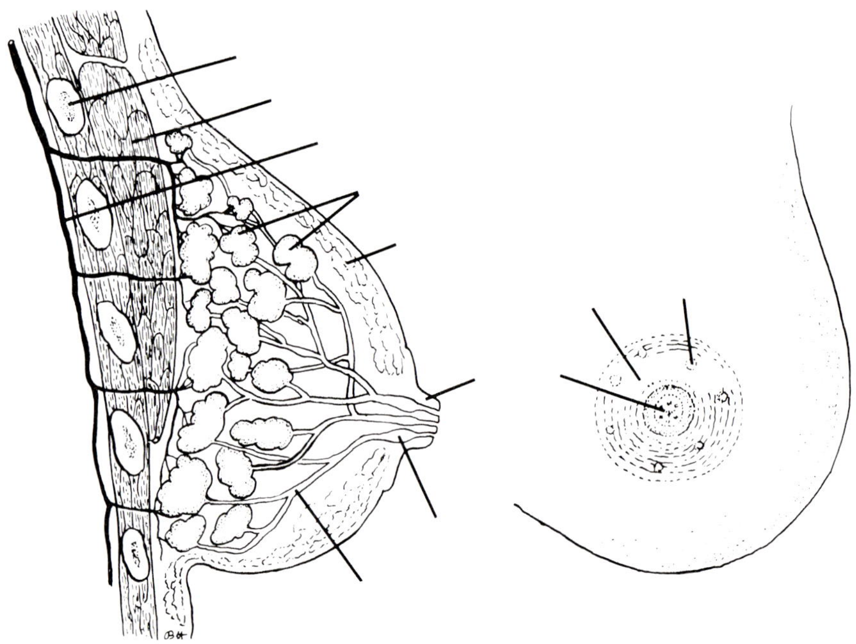

5. Female pelvic bones. Label the following: innominate bones, sacrum, coccyx, sacral promontory, ischial spines, pubis, ischium.

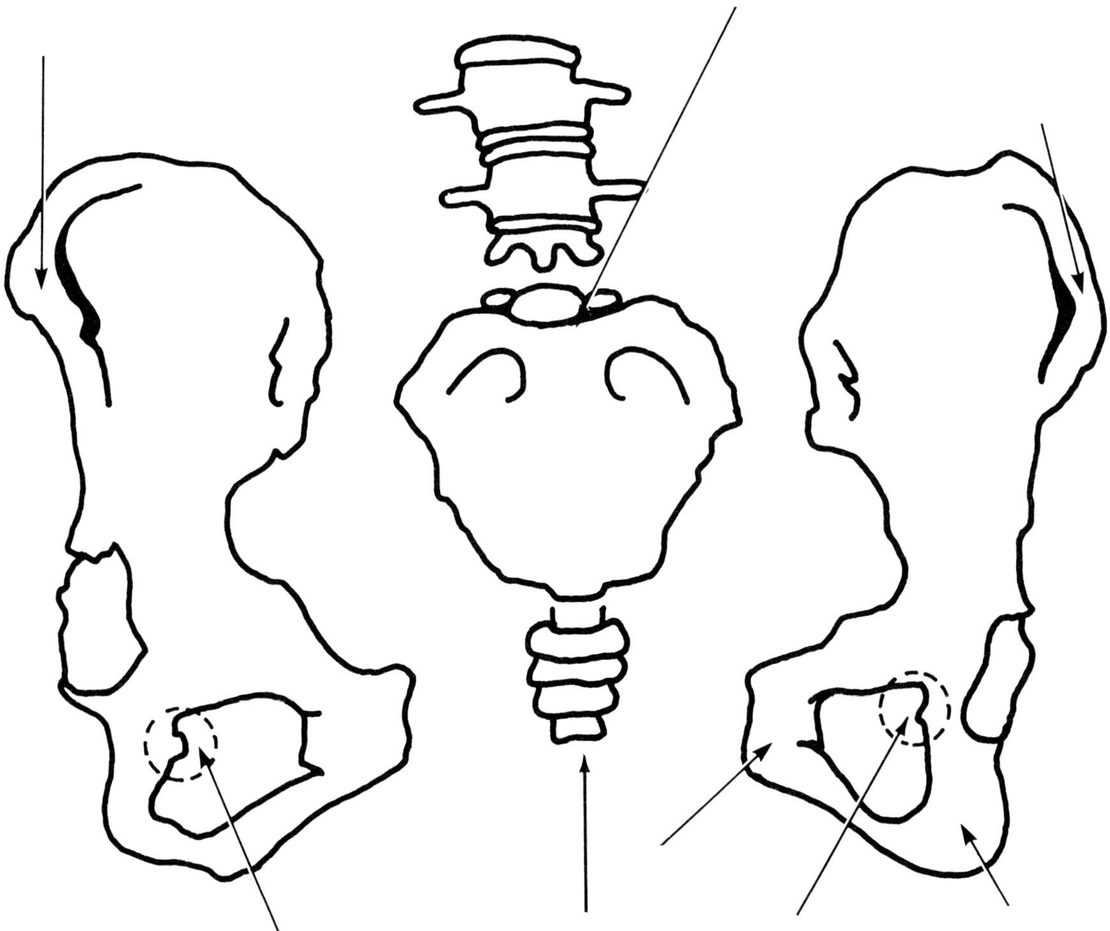

6. Identify the four pelvic types according to their shape:

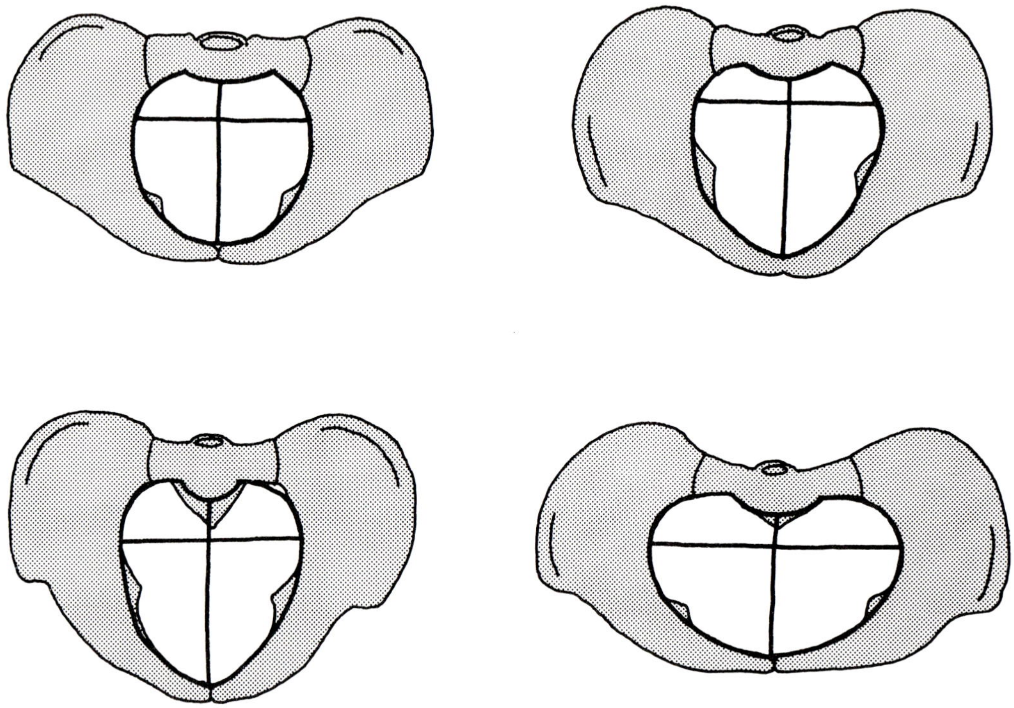

7. Explain two functions of the pelvic floor:
   a.
   b.

For questions 8 through 13, circle the best answers.

8. The three divisions or parts of the cervix are:
   a. meatus
   b. internal os
   c. corpus
   d. isthmus
   e. external os
9. Three of the bones listed below unite to form the innominate bone. Which one does *not?*
   a. pubis
   b. ilium
   c. coccyx
   d. ischium
10. The lowermost part of the uterus is called the:
    a. clitoris
    b. vagina
    c. endometrium
    d. cervix
11. The uppermost part of the uterus is called the:
    a. cervix
    b. corpus
    c. fundus
    d. myometrium

12. The three layers of tissue comprising the uterus include all of the following *except:*
    a. embriometrium
    b. endometrium
    c. perimetrium
    d. myometrium
13. The anatomic structure of the breasts that produces milk is:
    a. acini cell
    b. sinus
    c. areola
    d. Montgomery's tubercle

Supply the correct answer(s) for items 14 through 17.

14. Which layer of uterine muscle is the thickest and shaped like a figure-eight?
15. The three basic functions of the male and female reproductive systems are:
    a.
    b.
    c.
16. List the four bones of the pelvis.
    a.
    b.
    c.
    d.
17. The four phases of the menstrual cycle are:
    a.
    b.
    c.
    d.
18. The two phases of the ovulatory cycle are:
    a.
    b.
19. On the line to the left of each item in Column A match the appropriate hormones from Column B.

Column A

______1. stimulates development of the follicle
______2. initiates buildup of the lining of the uterus
______3. causes ovulation and develops the corpus luteum
______4. finishes preparation of uterus for pregnancy
______5. a drop in this hormone in particular precedes menstruation

Column B

a. LH (luteinizing hormone)
b. estrogen (estradiol)
c. FSH (follicle-stimulating hormone)
d. progesterone

20. Match the structures listed in column B with their proper characteristics in column A.

Column A

______1. a muscular hammock supporting the internal organs
______2. attaches the uterus to each side of the pelvic cavity
______3. extends from the uterus to the labia majora
______4. connects the sacrum to the uterus
______5. ligament that keeps the uterus from dropping down into the vagina
______6. a superficial muscle that makes a figure-eight around the vagina and rectum

Column B

a. uterosacral ligaments
b. broad ligaments
c. levator ani
d. round ligaments
e. cardinal ligament
f. bulbocavernosus muscle

For items 21 through 24, fill in the blanks:

21. Two female sex hormones are ____________________ and ____________________.
22. Ovulation occurs during the ____________________ phase of the menstrual cycle.
23. The lining of the uterus thickens to prepare for pregnancy during the ____________ phase of the menstrual cycle.
24. The anatomic landmark that separates the false pelvis from the true pelvis is ____________________.
25. Trace two possible pathways of blood from the aorta to the uterus, naming all intervening blood vessels.

26. Name the nerve pathways that transmit uterine pain.

27. Describe, in two sentences, the function of the corpus luteum.

28. Draw a rough sketch, indicating relative amounts of LH, FSH, estradiol, and progesterone during the menstrual cycle and ovarian cycle.

29. Name all of the structures that add fluid to semen.

UNIT III
Conception and prenatal development

GOALS

This unit is designed to provide the reader with information that will:

☐ promote an understanding of conception, implantation, and placental development.
☐ develop an awareness of the influence of environmental factors on embryonic and fetal development.
☐ develop an awareness of the problem of infertility.

STUDENT OBJECTIVES

After studying this unit, you should be able to:

1. Describe the process of implantation (transition from zygote to blastoderm).
2. Describe the umbilical cord (length and composition) and explain the significance of a single umbilical artery in the cord.
3. Characterize the significant changes in growth and development of the fetus in utero at 20 weeks of gestation, 28 weeks of gestation, and 32 weeks of gestation.
4. Describe the growth of the embryo from the first through third month.
5. Diagram the fetal circulatory structures.
6. Explain how common characteristics are inherited in terms of dominant and recessive traits and sex-linked traits.
7. Discuss the relationship between the incidence of Down's syndrome and maternal age.
8. Identify a chromosomal abnormality that can be detected by examination of amniotic fluid cells following amniocentesis.
9. Discuss known environmental agents associated with birth defects.

FERTILIZATION

DESCRIBE THE PROCESS OF FERTILIZATION

During sexual intercourse spermatozoa are ejaculated from the male penis into the female vagina. At the time of ejaculation over 200 million spermatozoa may be deposited in the vagina; moving by means of their long, thin tails, they travel up into the cervical canal. Contractions of the uterus and fallopian tubes are primarily responsible for propelling the sperm through these organs to the ovum. Three hundred to a thousand (roughly one in one million) survive to make it to the vicinity of the ovum. The spermatozoa live for an average of 24 to 48 hours, swimming about waiting for an ovum. If the female ovulates during this time, a single spermatozoa can enter the ovum, thus fertilizing it. A human ovum remains viable for about 12 to 24 hours and is capable of being fertilized for only a short period after ovulation (probably not more than 12 hours). Thus in each woman's menstrual cycle, there is a period of approximately 60 hours (48 plus 12), called the *fertile period*, during which fertilization can occur. This period occurs approximately 14 days into the ovarian cycle. The spermatozoon contains an enzyme that facilitates penetration of the outer covering of the ovum (the *zona pellucida*). *Fertilization* usually ocurs in the dilated portion of the fallopian tube called the ampulla (see Unit II).

The fertilized cell resulting from the union of sperm and ovum is called a *zygote*. The zygote is one cell in which the nucleus of the sperm and the nucleus of the ovum have met to form a single nucleus containing all the necessary components for the development of another human being.

CLEAVAGE

Soon after the zygote has formed, it divides into two daughter cells, called *blastomeres*, then four, eight, sixteen, and so forth by a process of cell division called *cleavage*. This cell division occurs while the fertilized ovum is being moved down the tube by the wave-like action of cilia and the peristaltic action of the tube itself. The trip to the uterus takes approximately 3 to 4 days, during which time the ovum becomes a round mass of cells called a *morula*, because of its resemblance to a mulberry. Although there are more than 16 cells by now, there has been no increase in the size of the developing cell cluster. It is still no larger than the point of a straight pin. As the cells continue to divide, fluid passes into the morula from the uterine cavity, and the cells regroup themselves into a hollow ball filled with fluid. The outer layer of cells, called the *trophoblast*, obtains food for the inner layer (or *embryoblast*) and eventually forms the placenta. The embryo develops from the inner layer of cells. At this stage the fertilized ovum is called a *blastocyst* (Fig. 3-1).

IMPLANTATION

As the blastocyst falls into the uterus, it sheds its outer membrane (the *zona pellucida*) and prepares to implant in the thick lining of the endometrium by day 6 or 7. By this time, the endometrial lining has been prepared by circulating progesterone during the secretory phase (see Unit II) and is now thick, edematous, and vascular. The endometrium is at its "ripest" stage. The blastocyst, by this time consisting of approximately 200 cells, usually implants in the front or back of the upper portion of the uterus. To burrow into the uterine lining, the trophoblastic cells secrete an enzyme that dissolves

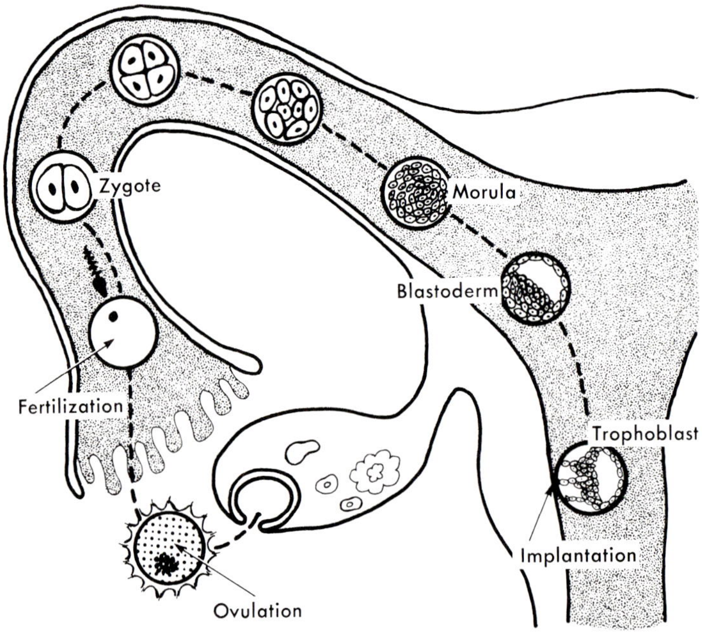

Fig. 3-1. Fertilization, cleavage, and implantation. The numbers indicate days after fertilization.

and absorbs some of the endometrium, literally eating its way into the endometrium. The endometrium is now called the *decidua*, and the area directly under the trophoblast is called the *decidua basalis*. As the trophoblastic cells invade, they differentiate into two types: those at the blastocyst-decidua interface blend together to from the *syncytiotrophoblast*, and those trophoblast cells next to the developing embryo remain separate as *cytotrophoblasts*.

TROPHOBLASTIC STAGE

Once implantation has occurred, the growing embryo can no longer survive only on nutrients from its own yolk sac; therefore the trophoblastic cells begin to form the *chorion*, or outermost sac. Covering the chorion are thousands of root-like projections called *villi*, which further dig into the decidua and lay the foundation for the *placenta*.

The yolk sac gradually disappears as the amniotic cavity encloses the embryo. The embryo develops from the body stalk within the amniotic cavity, and as development continues, the chorionic villi that are not attached to the decidua fall off, leaving a transparent sac called the fetal membranes, which are made up of the *amnion (inner)* and *chorion (outer)* membranes. These membranes help to protect the embryo (and later the fetus) by sealing it off from the outside (Fig. 3-2)

The syncytiotrophoblast cells produce the hormone *human chorionic gonadotropin* (hCG), which signals the corpus luteum in the ovary to continue to manufacture levels of progesterone and estrogen high enough to prevent menstruation and ovulation. After the first few weeks of gestation, the corpus luteum is no longer essential to maintain pregnancy, and thus hCG's function thereafter is unclear. The hormone hCG is excreted in the woman's urine and is the basis of pregnancy testing beginning 1 or 2 weeks following a missed menstrual period. Implantation is completed by about day 12 (Fig. 3-3).

AMNIOTIC FLUID

LIST THREE FUNCTIONS OF AMNIOTIC FLUID

The amnion secretes *amniotic fluid* in which the fetus floats and moves for the duration of the pregnancy. This fluid-filled space (often known as the "bag of waters") contains 500 to 1500 milliliters of clear fluid by the end of the pregnancy.

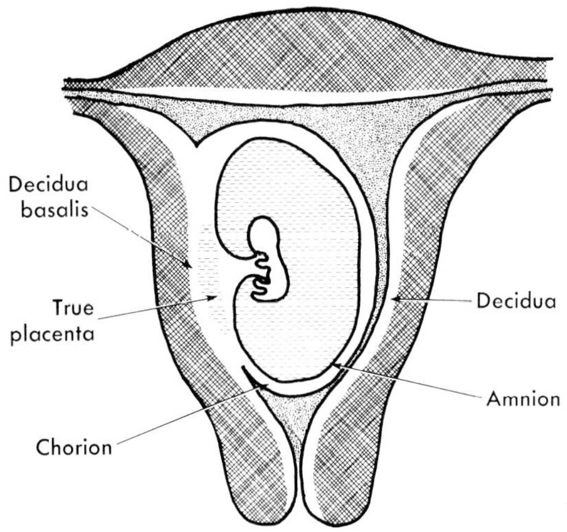

Fig. 3-2. Fetal membranes.

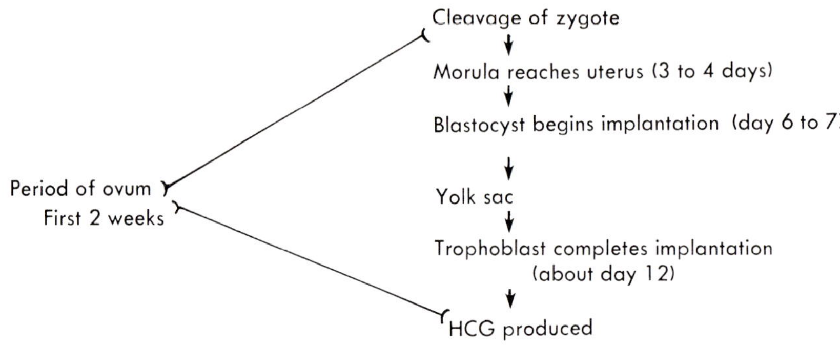

Fig. 3-3. Period of the ovum: first 2 weeks.

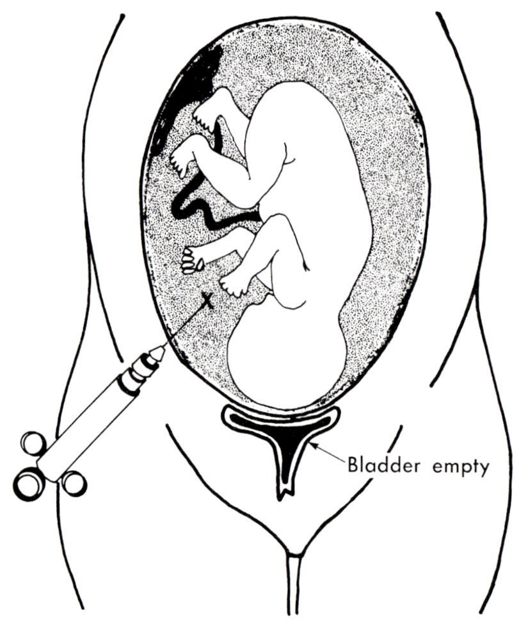

Fig. 3-4. Amniocentesis.

The functions of the amniotic fluid include keeping the fetus at an even temperature, serving as a protective cushion for the fetus, equalizing pressures, and allowing the fetus to move freely without adhering to the amnion. Also contributing to the formation of amniotic fluid are fluid from the maternal blood, the fetal lungs, and the fetal kidneys. The fetus near term drinks about 500 ml of amniotic fluid each day, which is about the same as the daily milk consumption of the newborn. Because the fetus drinks and inhales amniotic fluid, urinates into the amniotic fluid, and constantly sheds cells into it, studies of amniotic fluid obtained by *amniocentesis* (withdrawing some fluid from the amniotic sac for cell study) (Fig. 3-4) can reveal fetal maturity, sex, and general well-being. Too much *(polyhydramnios)* or too little *(oligohydramnios)* amniotic fluid often indicates fetal abnormalities. Certain genetic disorders can also be diagnosed by utilizing amniocentesis.

EMBRYO

DIFFERENTIATION BETWEEN EMBRYO AND FETUS

The product of conception is termed an *embryo* until the eighth week of growth and a *fetus* thereafter. As soon as the fetus is born, it is termed a *newborn* (infant).

The most striking advances in development occur during the first 7 weeks—often before the woman even realizes she is pregnant. This is especially important when one

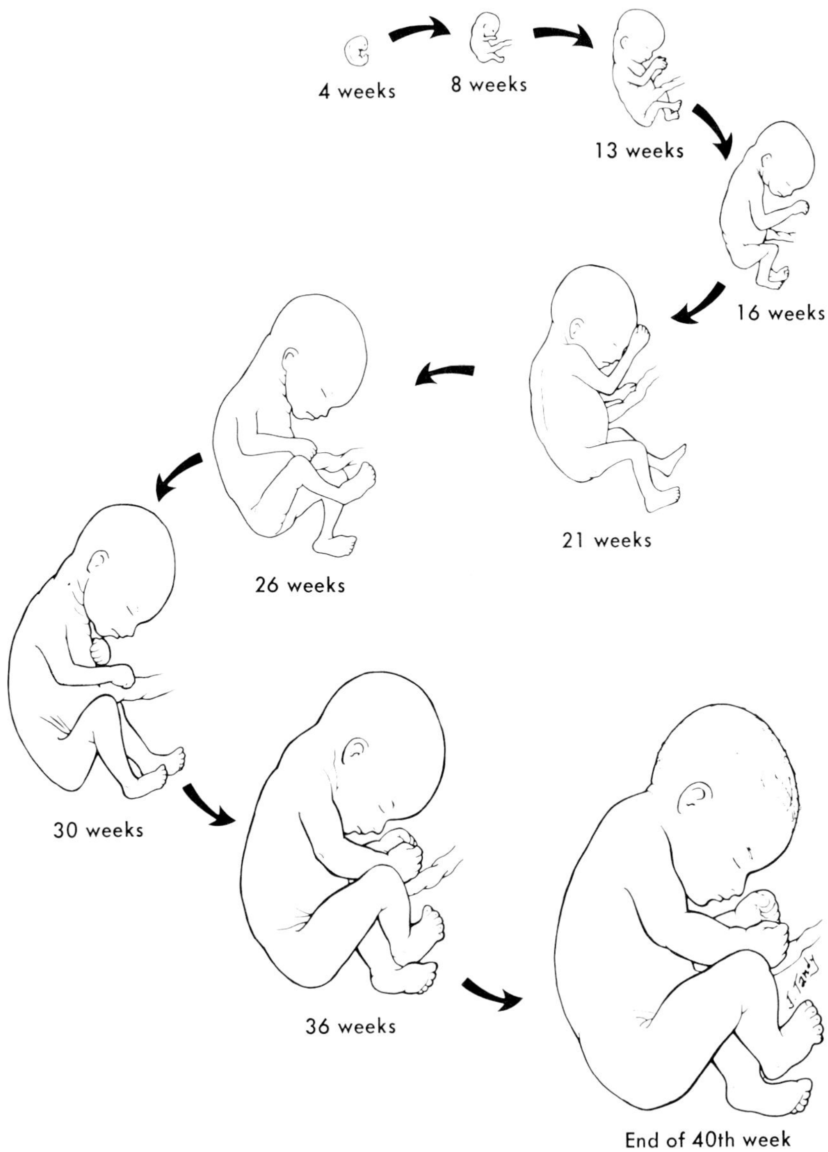

Fig. 3-5. Growth and development. (From Jensen, M., Benson, R.C., and Bobak, I.M.: Maternity care: the nurse and the family, St. Louis, 1977, The C.V. Mosby Co.)

considers the list of all potential environmental hazards that can cause birth defects. By the end of the seventh week (the embryonic period), the beginnings of *all* major structures are present.

Embryonic development

GROWTH OF THE EMBRYO FROM THE FIRST THROUGH THE THIRD MONTH

By the end of the first 3 weeks following conception, the heart and brain are beginning to be formed. One week later there is beginning formation of eyes, ears, and nose, and small buds that will eventually become arms and legs. Development of the embryo generally proceeds from the head to the tail *(cephalocaudal)*.

During the next 28 days, the embryo grows to be about 1⅛ inches long. Because of the rapid development of the brain, the head is very large in comparison to other parts of the embryo. External genitalia appear, but sex cannot be differentiated (Fig. 3-5).

Development of the growing embryo is most easily affected by harmful environmental agents—including drugs, chemicals, and certain viruses—during the *organogenetic period.* This is the time when the body's basic organ systems are being formed, usually

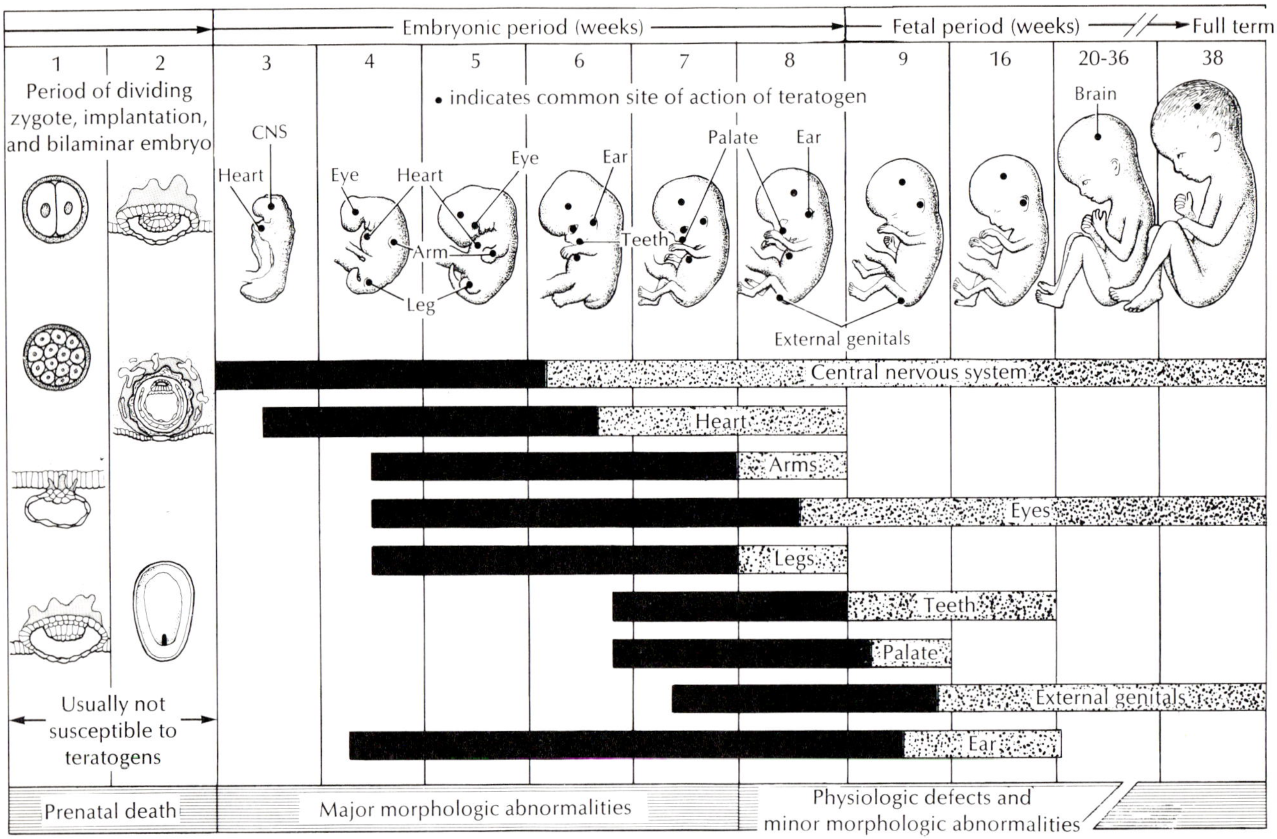

Fig. 3-6. Sensitive, or critical, periods in human development. (From Moore, K.L.: Before we were born, Philadelphia, 1974, W.B. Saunders Co.)

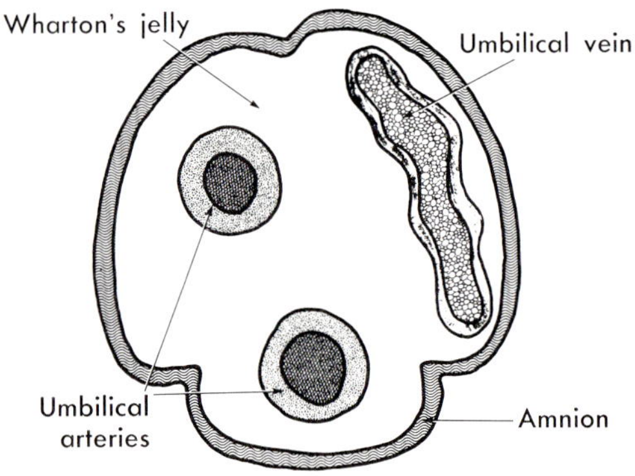

Fig. 3-7. Cross-section of the umbilical cord.

from week 3 through week 8 (see Fig. 3-6). It is at this time that the embryo is most sensitive to agents known to cause congenital malformations.

PLACENTA

As the developing embryo continues to grow, the chorionic villi (fetal side) embedded in the decidua basalis and the decidua basalis (maternal side) form the *placenta*. At the end of a full-term pregnancy, about 80% of the normal placenta is of fetal origin. The capillaries unite to form larger and larger veins until finally joining to form the umbilical vein in the body stalk. Blood is sent back to the placenta from the embryo through two umbilical arteries (Fig. 3-7). The umbilical vein and two arteries are enclosed in the

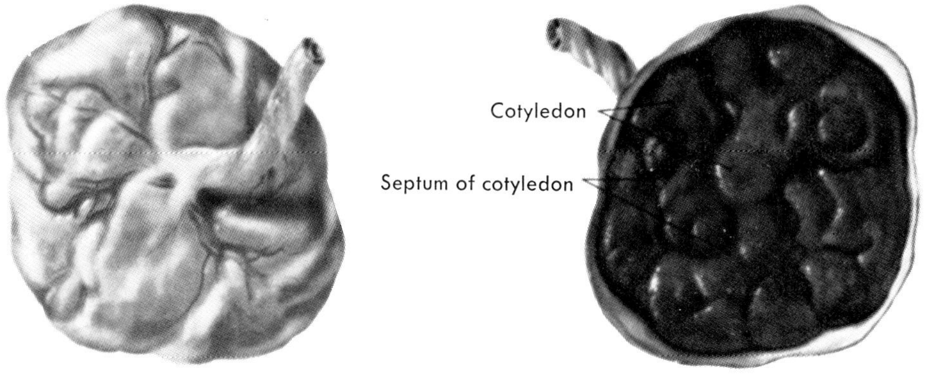

Fig. 3-8. A, Fetal surface of placenta. **B,** Maternal surface of placenta. (From Placental circulation, Nursing Education Aid No. 2, Ross Laboratories, Columbus, Ohio.)

umbilical cord, which is about 2 feet long at birth and filled with a whitish, gelatinous substance called *Wharton's jelly*. Wharton's jelly prevents kinking of the cord and interference with circulation.

SIGNIFICANCE OF A SINGLE UMBILICAL ARTERY IN THE CORD

The umbilical cord should always be inspected at the time of birth. In 1 out of every 500 deliveries, the umbilical cord contains only one artery instead of two. If this is the case, the baby should be examined carefully, because there is a higher risk of abnormalities in babies with a single umbilical artery.

The embryo is now floating in fluid and is anchored to the uterine wall by the umbilical cord and placenta. The placenta consists of maternal portions (decidua basalis) and fetal portions (chorionic villi) and acts as the organ of transfer between the mother and the fetus. The maternal surface is deep red and divided into sections, or *cotyledons*. The fetal surface (covered with amniotic membrane) is smooth and grayish with prominent blood vessels. The umbilical cord usually arises from the middle of the placenta (Fig. 3-8). At the end of pregnancy the placenta is about 8 inches in diameter, 1 inch thick, and weighs more than 1 pound.

Placental transfer

It is important to understand that the maternal and fetal blood are in separate systems and do not mix. There are three tissue layers between maternal and fetal blood in the human placenta. These are (1) fetal trophoblast, (2) the connective tissue core of the fetal villus, and (3) the endothelium of fetal capillaries. Any substance passing between mother and fetus must cross these three permeable tissue layers (often known as the *placental barrier*). Contrary to the old myth that this placental barrier stops all harmful substances and protects the fetus, we know now that the placenta is literally a bloody sieve, allowing almost all substances, if small enough, to cross it in varying degrees. Nourishment passes from the maternal side to the fetal side, and waste products pass from the fetal side to the maternal side as a result of several factors, both static and dynamic. Oxygen from the maternal side passes through the placenta to the fetal side, and CO_2 passes from the fetal side to the maternal side by *diffusion* (the passive passage of gases from an area of high concentration to one of low concentration). On the mother's side of the placental barrier, the uterine arteries bring blood into the intervillous space, and uterine veins drain that blood. On the fetal side, umbilical arteries bring blood into the fetal placental area, and the umbilical veins drain it. To remember this terminology, remember that the term *artery* always refers to a vessel that brings blood *away* from a heart (maternal or fetal), and vein always refers to a vessel that brings blood *to* a heart. As these two separate blood systems come close at the placental membrane site, the exchange of substances occurs (Fig. 3-9).

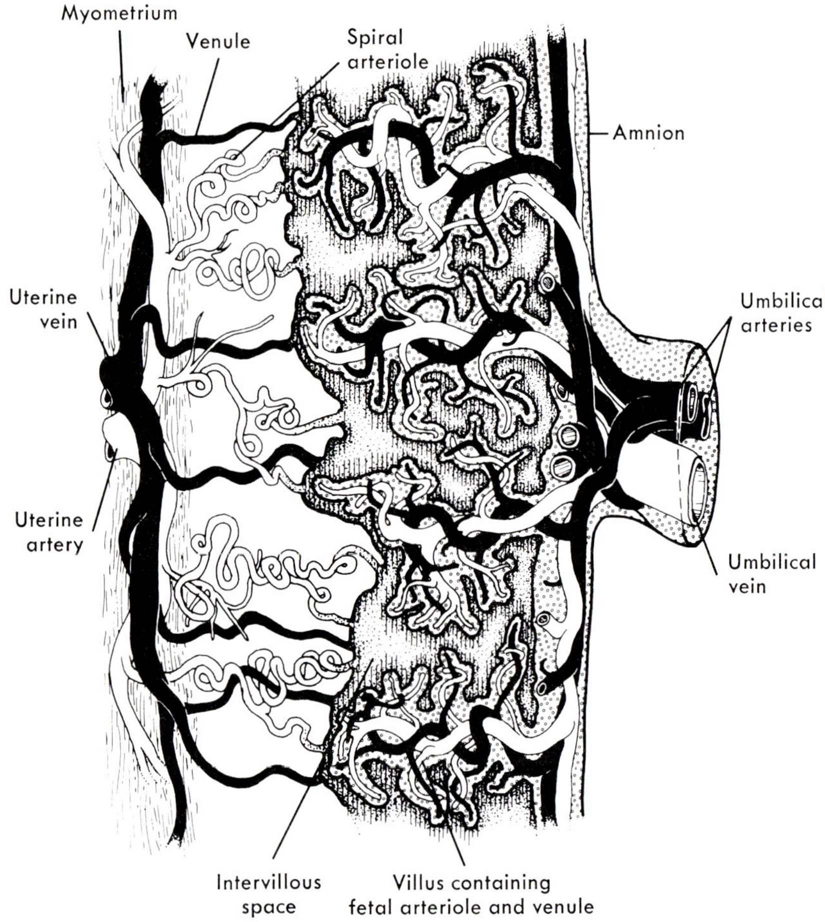

Fig. 3-9. Placental transfer. (From Tucker, S.M., and Bryant, S.: Fetal monitoring and fetal assessment in high-risk pregnancy, St. Louis, 1978, The C.V. Mosby Co.)

IDENTIFY THREE MAJOR FUNCTIONS OF THE PLACENTA

The placenta has three major functions: (1) transfer—O_2, CO_2, nutrients, electrolytes, some antibodies, and waste; (2) metabolism—the placenta manufactures fatty acids, glycogen, and cholesterol; and (3) endocrine secretion—hCG, human chorionic somatomamotropin (hCS), thyrotropin, estrogens, and progesterones. As stated earlier, during the first part of pregnancy the corpus luteum produces the progesterone, but after about 3 months of pregnancy, the placenta takes over the secretion of progesterone, which is essential for the maintenance of pregnancy. At this point the corpus luteum is no longer needed and degenerates.

FETAL DEVELOPMENT

Fertilization age is measured from the time the zygote is formed by the union of sperm and ovum. However, because this date is not usually known with certainty, a more useful term is *gestational age.* Gestational age is dated from the time of onset of the last menstrual period. From the first day of the last menstrual period, the length of an average pregnancy is 280 days, 10 lunar months (month by the moon), 9 calendar months, or 40 weeks. As you study fetal development, refer again to Fig. 3-5.

At the beginning of the *fourth lunar month (16 weeks gestation),* the fetus usually looks like a miniature baby with pink skin but a rather large head. It is 6 inches long (15.2 centimeters), weighs 6 ounces (170 grams), and has formed fingers and toes. The buds for "baby" teeth are present, and the kidneys are developing and secreting small amounts of urine. Brain configuration is nearly complete, and heart muscle is developed. *Meconium* (a thin, dark green to black sterile substance) begins to be present in the intestines.

SIGNIFICANT CHANGES IN THE GROWTH AND DEVELOPMENT OF THE FETUS IN UTERO

By the *fifth lunar month (20 weeks gestation)* the fetus has grown considerably and is approximately 8 inches long (20.3 centimeters), weighing 10 ounces (284 grams). A fine downy hair called *lanugo* covers the body. Fetal movements are felt by the mother *(quickening)*, and the heart beat can be heard with a fetoscope. (Actually the heart beat can be heard as early as the sixteenth week with the sensitive electronic instrument called an *ultrasonic fetoscope*, or Doppler.)

By the *sixth lunar month (24 weeks gestation)* the fetus is 12 inches long (30.4 centimeters) and weighs 24 ounces (680 grams). The skin of the fetus is red and wrinkled; if born, the infant may not survive.

By the *seventh lunar month (28 weeks gestation)* the fetus is about 14 inches long (35.4 centimeters), has a head circumference of approximately 26 centimeters and weighs 2½ pounds (1136 grams). A cheesy, greasy, white substance, called *vernix caseosa*, covers the wrinkled red skin to serve as a protective coating for the fetus floating in the amniotic fluid. Without this lubricating vernix, the fetus might shrivel like a prune. The eyes have lids that open and close now and eyebrows and lashes. If born, the fetus can survive with life support systems and expert intensive care.

By the *eighth lunar month (32 weeks gestation)* the fetus is about 16 inches long (40.6 centimeters), has a head circumference of about 30 centimeters and weighs about 3½ pounds (1590 grams). The fetus now has the appearance of a "little old man" and, if born, has a chance of surviving if given expert care.

By the *ninth lunar month (36 weeks gestation)* the fetus is about 18 inches long (45.6 centimeters), has a head circumference of about 32 centimeters and weighs about 5½ pounds (2500 grams). The fetus now has fingernails reaching to the fingertips and is able to survive outside of the uterus.

By the *tenth lunar month (40 weeks gestation)* the fetus is 20 inches long (50.8 centimeters), has a head circumference of about 35 centimeters and weighs about 7 pounds (3200 grams). The body has filled out because of subcutaneous fat deposits. The soft lanugo hair has almost disappeared except on the shoulders and upper back, and vernix caseosa is mainly in the folds and creases of the skin. The fetus is ready to be born.

The fetus of a pregnancy that goes past a 42-week gestation period is termed *postmature*. This can be a serious situation for the fetus because as the placenta ages, the mother deposits fibrin in the placenta. Extensive fibrin deposits can cut off the villi and cause a compromised placenta that becomes less and less efficient in supplying O_2 and nutrients. A postmature baby appears to have very dry, parchment-like skin with little subcutaneous fat and no vernix. This postmature baby is at risk of developing major problems such as meconium aspiration and hypoglycemia. There are biochemical and biophysical tests that can be performed to determine both the gestational age and the wellness of the fetoplacental unit. If the tests indicate that the fetus is being compromised, the pregnancy can be terminated and the baby born before serious life-threatening complications occur.

Fetal circulation

Because the source of oxygen for the fetus is the placenta, the fetus does not need its lungs to exchange oxygen; and because the source of nutrients for the fetus is the placenta, it does not need its own liver to serve as a nutrition factory. Consequently, there are three special shunts to route most of the fetal blood past the fetal lungs and liver. These shunts are the *ductus venosus*, which goes straight through the liver, and the foramen ovale and ductus arteriosus, which bypass the lungs (Fig. 3-10). These will be discussed subsequently.

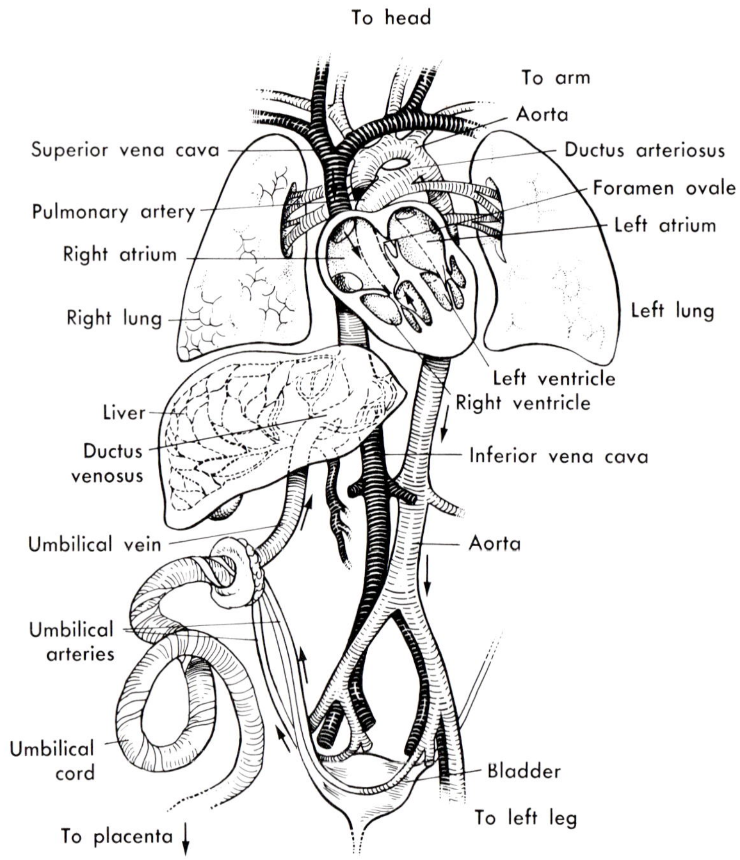

Fig. 3-10. Fetal circulation. (From Lerch, C., and Bliss, V.J.: Maternity nursing, ed. 3, St. Louis, 1978, The C.V. Mosby Co.)

Comparison of fetal and adult circulation

CONTRAST ADULT AND FETAL CIRCULATION

Adult circulation. In an adult the unoxygenated blood returns to the heart via the superior vena cava (SVC) and inferior vena cava (IVC). The blood enters the right atrium, travels next to the right ventricle, then leaves via the pulmonary artery for oxygenation in the lungs. In the capillary beds of the pulmonary circulation, the blood not only picks up O_2 but also gives off CO_2. The blood then returns to the left atrium by way of the pulmonary veins. From the left atrium it travels to the left ventricle and is then pumped out the aorta, under high pressure, to perfuse the rest of the body (trace the path just described in Fig. 3-11).

FETAL CIRCULATORY STRUCTURES

Fetal circulation. Because in the fetus the source of O_2 is the placenta and not the fetal lungs, blood rich with O_2 and nutrients flows through the umbilical vein (remember: blood returning from an oxygen source always travels through veins). Blood from the umbilical vein enters the *portal venous system* (which drains all blood from the intestines and other digestive organs), and then 20% to 80% of this mixed blood is shunted quickly through the liver, bypassing the normal liver by way of the special ductus venosus. It is not known what factors determine how much umbilical vein blood goes through the ductus venosus and how much traverses the liver.

Once fetal blood leaves the liver, it enters the IVC and continues its journey toward the heart. One would think that IVC and SVC blood would mix completely in the right atrium; however, this is not the case. Much of the blood from the IVC is directed preferentially through the right atrium to the left side of the heart via the *foramen ovale* (a small hole between the two atria). Thus this relatively oxygen-rich blood (remember: it has just recently returned from the placenta) flows from the left atrium to the left ventricle and out the ascending aorta to the oxygen-hungry fetal brain.

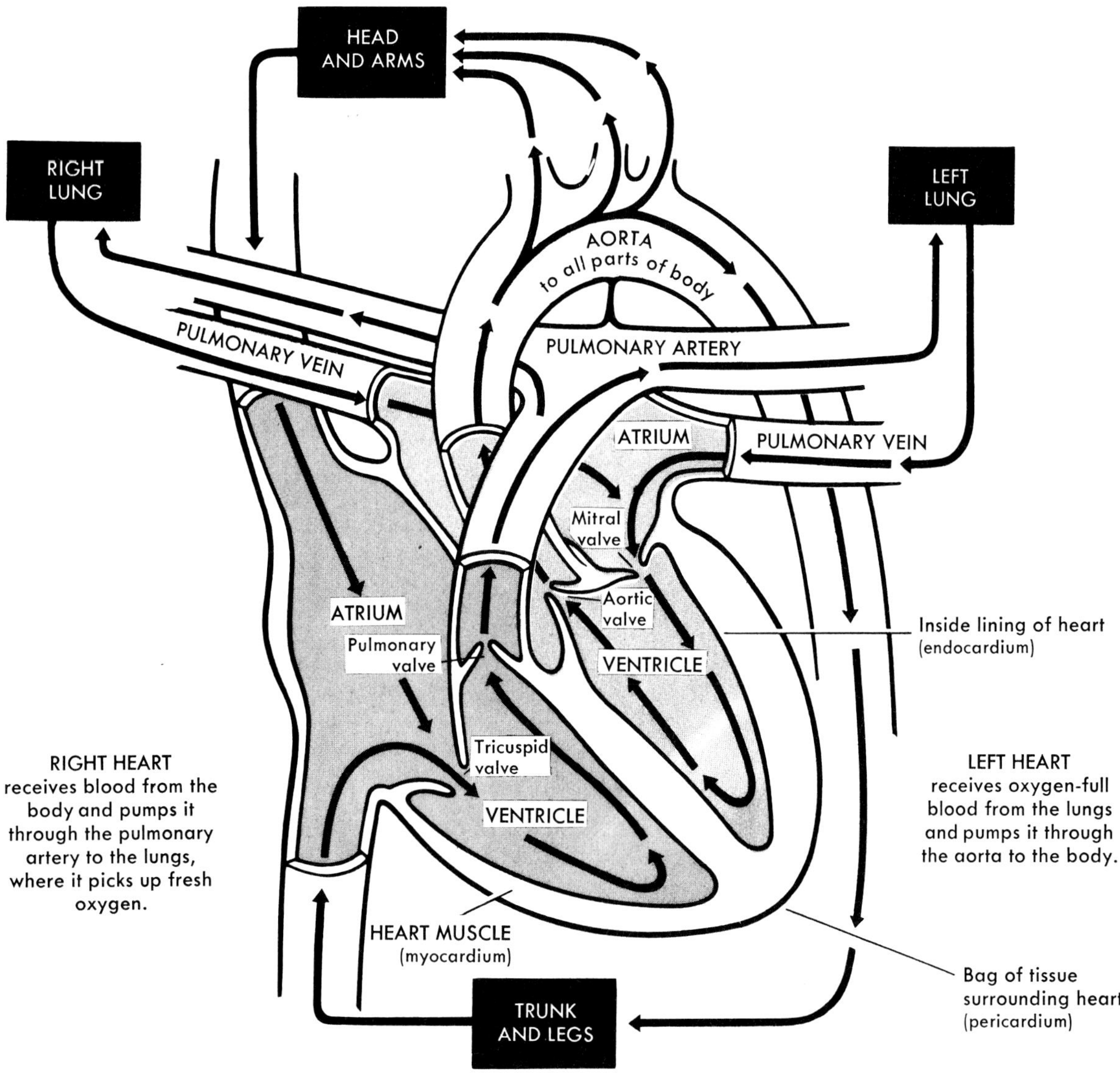

Fig. 3-11. Adult circulation. (Reprinted with permission © American Heart Association.)

On the other hand, blood returning from the fetal head is relatively oxygen-poor. Thus, most SVC blood is efficiently streamlined to pass through the right atrium into the right ventricle and out the pulmonary artery. However, blood traveling through non-breathing lungs serves little purpose (except to provide the small amount of blood necessary to keep the fetal lungs alive). Thus the third fetal shunt is the *ductus arteriosus*, a short artery between the pulmonary artery and the descending aorta. The ductus arteriosus allows 85% to 90% of pulmonary artery blood to bypass the lungs and thus begin its trip down the descending aorta toward the placenta to be reoxygenated. The fetal heart pumps the blood at a rate of 120 to 160 beats per minute to the body. (Trace the path of fetal circulation in Fig. 3-10).

Circulation changes at birth. With the first breath, the lungs expand and the pulmonary vessels open. This drop in pulmonary vascular resistance lowers the blood pressure on the right side of the heart, thereby reversing the blood flow through the shunts (foramen ovale and ductus arteriosus). The foramen ovale closes by a small flap of tissue sealing over the hole during the first 24 hours. The ductus venosus and arteriosus shrivel up and are converted to fibrous ligaments within 2 or 3 months. The umbilical arteries wither from disuse and are converted to fibrous cords. The umbilical vein becomes a round ligament of the liver (the ligamentum teres).

SEX DETERMINATION

DISTINGUISH BETWEEN GENES AND CHROMOSOMES

All human cells contain 23 paired *chromosomes* (total 46) in their cell nuclei except for the spermatozoon and the ovum. Each ovum carries 23 chromosomes, one of which is the x chromosome (sex chromosome). Each spermatozoon carries 23 chromosomes, one of which is the sex chromosome, which can be either x or y. If an x-carrying spermatozoon fertilizes an ovum, two x's are joined creating a female. However, if a y-carrying spermatozoon fertilizes an ovum, an x and y are joined, creating a male.

$$x + x = xx = \text{female}$$
$$x + y = xy = \text{male}$$

When the sperm and ovum unite at conception, the resulting zygote contains 46 chromosomes: 23 chromosomes, including a sex chromosome, from each parent (Fig. 3-12).

HEREDITY

The chromosomes contain many *genes*, which carry the factors responsible for transmitting the characteristics or traits of individuals. Thus each individual inherits characteristics from his or her mother and father by receiving their genes. The chromosomes are made up chemically of DNA (deoxyribonucleic acid) and protein. The genes are actually portions of the DNA molecule.

Dominant and recessive traits

DOMINANT AND RECESSIVE TRAITS AND SEX-LINKED TRAITS

Some physical traits passed on from generation to generation are said to be either *dominant* or *recessive*. If the genes the individual receives from each parent are different (*heterozygous*), the dominant gene will determine the characteristic more likely to appear. If there are like recessive genes present (*homozygous*), a recessive trait will appear. People may carry an abnormal trait without showing the trait themselves.

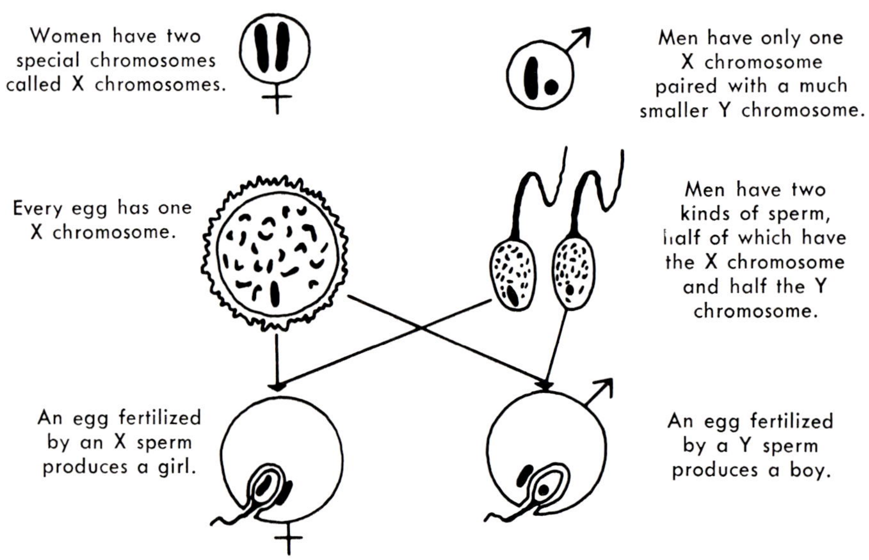

Fig. 3-12. Sex determination. (From Morgan, C: Introduction to psychology, ed. 2, New York, 1961, McGraw-Hill.)

Some dominant traits:

Dark hair
Brown eyes
Curly hair

Some recessive traits:

Blue or grey eyes
Light hair
Rh negative blood

Example: Gene for eye color

Father
Blue-eyed gene

Mother
Blue-eyed gene

Two blue-eyed genes
Baby has blue eyes

Father
Blue-eyed gene

Mother
Brown-eyed gene

One blue-eyed gene (recessive)
One brown-eyed gene (dominant)
Baby has brown eyes

Sex-linked characteristics

Still other physical traits are associated with the genes in the x and y, or sex, chromosomes and do not affect the two sexes equally. Rare sex-linked (x-linked) recessive disorders occur almost exclusively in males with the females being carriers. This occurs because very few genes are present on the y chromosome. Thus, a gene present on one x chromosome is easily "dominant" in a male who can offer no other x genes. More than 50 traits are known to be inherited in this manner, including color blindness and hemophilia.

Example: Hemophilia

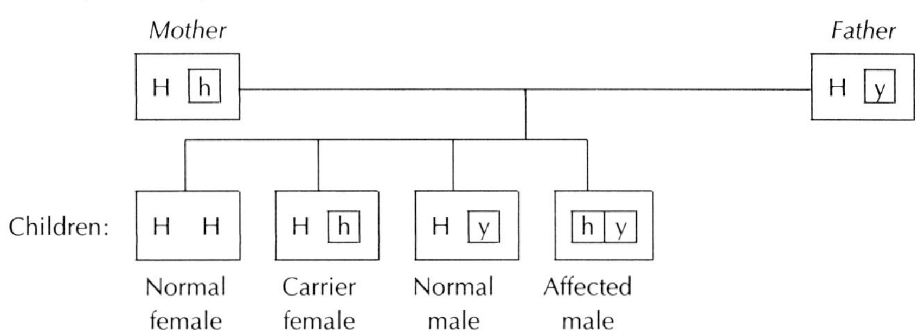

risk: 50% for female carrier
50% for male with hemophilia

H = normal gene

h = hemophilia gene

y – absence of hemophilia gene on y chromosome

It is possible as early as the third month of pregnancy to determine the sex of the fetus in utero by doing an amniocentesis. If a Barr body (sex chromatin found in female cells) is found in 20% to 40% of the nuclei of the fetal cells collected, the fetus in utero is probably a female. It could be important to predict fetal sex in the event of sex-linked diseases such as described previously. The parents may choose to abort a fetus who could be a carrier or may have a sex-linked disorder; or by simply knowing the probabilities, they may be better prepared to cope with potential problems.

BIRTH DEFECTS

Although traits and abnormalities can be passed on from generation to generation as just discussed, birth defects can result from three other major causes: (1) chromosomal abnormalities, (2) environmental agents, and (3) a combination of genetic and environmental factors.

Chromosomal abnormalities

CHROMOSOMAL ABNORMALITIES

As discussed previously, each spermatozoon and each ovum have 23 chromosomes, which unite at conception to form 46. Rarely, a sperm or ovum keeps one complete pair, thus giving it 24 chromosomes, or drops a pair, giving it 22 chromosomes. If an ovum with an extra chromosome is fertilized by a normal sperm, the resulting fetus is either aborted or a baby is born with *autosomal trisomy*. The most frequent chromosomal abnormality is trisomy 21 (Down's syndrome). The incidence of Down's syndrome increases as the mother's age increases. In women under 20 years of age, the incidence is 1:1500 to 2000. In women over 44 years of age, the incidence is 1:50. In this case, it is thought that the ova of the older woman, having been present in her ovaries since birth, may have begun to deteriorate. These women are also candidates for amniocentesis, since trisomies can be detected by a study of the amniotic fluid.

DOWN'S SYNDROME AND MATERNAL AGE

CHROMOSOMAL ABNORMALITY THAT CAN BE DETECTED BY EXAMINATION OF AMNIOTIC CELLS FOLLOWING AMNIOCENTESIS

If this problem arises in a sex chromosome, it is called a *sex-linked trisomy*. An example of this is Klinefelter's syndrome, in which the male has a xxy trisomy and usually has immature sexual organs, may be impotent, and is often mentally retarded.

In *monosomy*, only one of a particular pair of chromosomes is present. Turner's syndrome is an example of this, in which the female has a xo monosomy and usually has no ovaries, a webbed neck, and congenital heart disease. Fortunately, these aberrations are usually one-time occurrences and are not passed on to the next generation.

Environmental agents

EXPLAIN TERATOGEN

Exposure to toxic agents can cause prematurity, birth defects, spontaneous abortions, stillbirths, intrauterine growth retardation, and a decrease in fertility. Agents capable of causing birth defects are called *teratogens*. Even before a woman may realize that she is pregnant, the embryo is particularly vulnerable to the teratogenic effects of environmental agents. These agents include drugs and medicines, environmental pollutants, smoking, radiation, viral diseases and infections, and sexually transmissible diseases (STDs). A chart of potentially harmful medicines (see Appendix D) should be consulted whenever a pregnant (or possibly pregnant) woman gives a history of taking prescription medications or other drugs.

IDENTIFY FIVE POTENTIAL TERATOGENS FOR THE FETUS

More commonly encountered is the pregnant woman who smokes cigarettes or drinks alcohol. Heavy cigarette smoking has been correlated with an increased incidence of low-birth-weight babies. Even light smoking (less than 10 cigarettes per day) has been shown to increase the risk of fetal death, damage in utero, abruptio placentae, and placenta previa. Heavy alcohol consumption has been correlated not only with a high incidence of newborn mental retardation but also with the "fetal alcohol syndrome," in which a high percentage of infants born to alcoholic mothers have one or more of the following characteristics: growth retardation, microcephaly (small head size), central nervous system abnormalities, joint anomalies, and heart defects. It appears that there is a dose-effect relationship; that is, the more one drinks, the more likely one is to have a baby with the full-blown syndrome. However, no one knows whether drinking even a small amount of alcohol during pregnancy could have harmful effects on the fetus.

Many environmental agents are currently under investigation after reports of potentially harmful effects. A disproportionate amount of spontaneous abortions and birth defects have been reported in women who work in offices with video display terminals and computers. It is unclear whether this is a true correlation or merely statistical chance. Industrial solvents found at toxic waste dumps have been associated with a variety of birth defects and high rates of infant mortality. Exposure to dioxin, used by the U.S. government on forests, highways, and power lines, has been associated with birth defects and spontaneous abortions. Although environmental agents do not usually cause abnormalities during the fetal period, if exposure to them occurs during the fetal period, they can cause abnormalities of the external genitalia, teeth, brain, and palate because the development of these structures is not completed during the embryonic period. Because the brain is particularly susceptible, adverse environmental conditions may cause mental retardation.

The infections that have been convincingly shown to cause serious birth defects are known as the TORCH group:

T for toxoplasmosis
O for "other"(syphilis)
R for rubella
C for cytomegalovirus
H for herpes simplex

Women who contract these infections while pregnant have an increased risk of delivering malformed offspring.

Toxoplasmosis is caused by the parasite *Toxoplasma gondii.* Infectious organisms are transmitted primarily in the feces of cats who hunt rodents that harbor the parasite. However, the disease can also be spread by eating undercooked or raw meat from sheep, pigs, or cattle that feed from contaminated sources. Associated congenital anomalies include intrauterine growth retardation (IUGR), microcephaly or *hydrocephaly* (large, fluid-filled brain), *microphthalmia* (small eyes), *chorioretinitis* (an inflammation of the eyes), calcifications in skull radiographs, low platelet counts, and jaundice. An infected infant that survives the neonatal period is usually mentally retarded, affected by seizures, and has neuromuscular disease and poor vision. Pregnant women should avoid cats, litter boxes, and raw meats.

Syphilis is caused by the bacterium *Treponema pallidum* and is spread by direct contact with infectious lesions (usually sexually). The earlier in pregnancy the fetus is exposed to the organism, the more severe the fetal infection. If an infant is born with symptoms, these are likely to include a bullous rash *(syphilitic pemphigus);* enlarged liver, spleen, and lymph nodes; anemia; low platelet count; inflammation of the mouth and respiratory tract (producing the "syphilitic snuffles"); and the so-called Pseudoparalysis of Parrot due to pain caused by bone and joint infection. However, newborns with congenital syphilis are often asymptomatic when born and thus do not receive potentially curable treatment with antibiotics. They can thus develop tooth abnormalities ("Hutchinson's teeth" and "mulberry molars"), eye disease, deafness, facial anomalies (the "saddle nose"), and bowing of the legs ("saber shins"). These deformities are not reversible.

Rubella (German measles) is caused by a viral organism that can cross the placenta. If the mother becomes infected while pregnant, there is a 20% to 60% chance that the offspring will have major anomalies. These include low platelet count, hepatitis, microcephaly, congenital heart disease, low birth weight, cataracts, deafness, and mental retardation. Because there is no treatment, women should be vaccinated against the virus prior to becoming pregnant.

Cytomegalovirus (CMV), a member of the Herpes virus family, can cause a mononucleosis-type illness in adults or an asymptomatic infection. The general mode of transmission is sexual (either oral or genital contact). Congenital CMV infections vary from mild (jaundice, feeding difficulties, irritability, muscle weakness, spasticity) to severe (IUGR, microcephaly, mental retardation, and involvement of multiple organ systems). Infants may excrete the virus in saliva and urine for years; therefore, infected infants should be isolated in isolettes or incubators while in the hospital. Again, there is no specific treatment.

Herpes simplex virus type II (HSV-2) is the organism thought to be responsible for congenital herpes infection. Although there *are* cases of herpes simplex virus type I (typically present in the mouth as the cause of "cold sores") reported in the genital mucosa, it is usually HSV-2 that is reponsible for "herpes below the waist." HSV-2 lesions are typically fluid-filled vesicles and ulcers on the genitalia. In women they can involve the vagina, cervix, and bladder. There may be extreme pain and tenderness in the infected tissues until the lesions heal. Typically, the virus remains latent for a time, only to reappear with recurrent vesicles later. Congenital herpes is acquired during the passage down the birth canal as the newborn slides past active lesions. Thus infection of the infant can be prevented by cesarean delivery if maternal lesions are present. This is effective only if done within 4 hours after rupture of the membranes. Congenital herpes is associated with skin lesions (which can cover the entire body), psychomotor retardation, microcephaly, seizure disorders, optic atrophy, cataracts, and eye inflammation.

Infectious agents other than those of the TORCH group have been linked to harmful effects on the fetus and/or newborn. These include *hepatitis B, chlamydia, gonorrhea,* and the presumed *AIDS* virus.

Hepatitis B is caused by a virus and is spread by contact with contaminated blood, urine, saliva, feces, vaginal secretions, tears, and other bodily fluids. Offspring of infected mothers can be infected either transplacentally (in utero) or during delivery. Most infected infants are asymptomatic. However, 90% of infected newborns become chronic carriers of the virus, continually shedding the virus in their bodily fluids. Some sources have estimated that 25% of these infants who carry the hepatitis B virus will develop chronic active hepatitis in later life, with the potential consequences of liver cirrhosis and liver cancer. Infected fetuses have increased risks of prematurity and stillbirth. As a preventive measure, hepatitis B immune globulin or immune serum globulin can be given on the first day of life to all infants born to affected mothers. Although this will not prevent transplacental infection, it can prevent infection by contact with bodily fluids.

Chlamydia is caused by the intracellular microorganism *Chlamydia trachomatis.* This infection, not well recognized until recently, is probably the most prevalent sexually transmissible disease in the United States, with approximately three million new cases of genital chlamydia per year. Perhaps 5% of pregnant women are infected. Chlamydia can cause *pelvic inflammatory disease (PID),* an infection of the fallopian tubes, which can lead to tubal obstruction and ectopic pregnancies. Maternal chlamydia infection has been thought to cause IUGR, premature delivery, and stillbirths. However, the evidence for this correlation is still incomplete. What is known with certainty is that maternal chlamydia infection can cause newborn infection as the organism is transferred to the fetus during delivery. Newborn infections include *inclusion conjunctivitis* (eye), *pneumonitis* (lung), and *otitis media* (ear). Treatment is with antibiotics like erythromycin.

Gonorrhea is caused by the bacterium *Neisseria gonorrhoeae* and is spread by sexual contact. The infection can be transmitted to the newborn during delivery through the birth canal and can result in *ophthalmia neonatorum,* a congenital eye infection. Treatment is with penicillin or ampicillin.

The *acquired immune deficiency syndrome (AIDS)* is thought to be caused by the *human T-cell leukemia virus III (HTLV-III).* This disease, which usually effects intravenous drug abusers, homosexual men, and hemophiliacs, is thought to be spread by contact with virus-carrying blood or through sexual intercourse. Infected newborns are thought to have acquired the disease transplacentally (in utero).

GENETIC COUNSELING

EXPLAIN NURSING RESPONSIBILITIES IN GENETIC COUNSELING

Genetic counseling services are available to couples who suspect that their future children may be at risk for inheriting a disorder. There are now more than 100 counseling centers in the United States where people can go to gather the information necessary to obtain a probability estimate for genetic problems.

In these centers a family history is taken to develop a family *pedigree chart* (a form for recording data about a family tree). Next, extensive physical examinations are conducted, and special testing is done to give the couple a probability estimate. The final decision about what to do with all this information is one that only the couple can make; however, the nurse can be very helpful by encouraging them to talk about their decision, thus possibly finding areas of misunderstanding. If such misunderstandings exist, the nurse can clarify them by providing the correct information they need to make an informed decision. The well-informed nurse can also help with genetic counseling by case-finding, making referrals, and explaining the genetic counseling procedure to couples, thus preventing or alleviating anxiety.

INFERTILITY

Infertility affects approximately 10% to 15% of couples at some time during their reproductive life. The causes of infertility are diverse and range from inability to conceive to inability to carry pregnancy to term. Although causes may be multiple in any given couple, a general categorization of causes is as follows: male, 45%; trouble with ovulation, 20%; tubal problems, 20%; cervical problems, 5%; and unknown, 10%. Because infertility can be caused by an abnormality in either or both partners, both partners should be evaluated together in an infertility investigation. Evaluation may include a thorough history and physical of both partners, documentation of ovulation by basal body temperature, endometrial biopsy, examination of cervical mucus, determination of tubal patency, and analysis of the man's seminal fluid.

IDENTIFY MAJOR PHYSIOLOGIC CAUSES OF INFERTILITY

The major physiological causes of female infertility are tubal, hormonal, and cervical. Causes of blocked tubes include PID, postabortal sepsis, adhesions, and other pathology. The diagnosis can be made with either a hysterosalpingogram, in which an x-ray picture is taken of the uterus and fallopian tubes after contrast material is squirted into the uterus, or with laparoscopy, in which a viewing tube is inserted through a small abdominal incision for direct inspection of the tube. Tubes that have been closed can often be opened by tubal insufflations with carbon dioxide gas, sexual rest, antispasmodics, and tubal surgery *(tuboplasty)*.

Hormonal factors causing infertility usually involve lack of ovulation because of low levels of hormones or deficiencies in endocrine organs. Clomiphene (Clomid) therapy is used to stimulate ovulation in these women. The drug is relatively safe with few side effects. It works by stimulating the leutinizing hormone "surge" (see Unit II). For women who become pregnant after treatment with clomiphene, multiple births are possible. Indeed, the incidence of twins born to such women is 1 in 16 (versus 1 in 89 in the general population), and 1 in 200 will have three or more children born at the same time. Women who fail to respond to clomiphene will sometimes respond to gonadotropins. Pergonal HMG and Ortho HMG are two intramuscular preparations of gonadotropins available for clinical investigation. There is also a higher than normal rate for multiple births with Pergonal.

Cervical and uterine factors causing infertility include cervical "incompetence," which may be corrected by a *cerclage* procedure, or placement of a suture around the cervix to hold it closed. The cerclage may be done before conception or during pregnancy. The procedure of choice may be "permanent," in which subsequent delivery will have to be by cesarean birth, or "temporary," in which the suture can be removed prior to delivery. Congenital abnormalities of the uterus that can predispose to abortion are bicornuate, septate, and double uteri. The treatment for these uterine abnormalities is surgical. The possibility of endometriosis is also considered when evaluating infertility because it may be a causative factor.

Physiological causes of male infertility are lack or deficiency of sperm and impotence. Infertility diagnostic studies begin with semen analysis. Seminal fluid is analyzed for volume of fluid, sperm count, sperm shape, and sperm motility. Because of variability, at least two specimens should be examined. Normal is defined as volume, 3 to 5 cc; count greater than 20 million per cc; shape greater than two thirds normal; and motility greater than 50% at 1 to 2 hours. Excessive use of alcohol or tobacco affects sperm production, as do some genitourinary problems and/or surgery.

Psychological factors involving infertility are often more difficult to evaluate than the physiological factors. Some investigators feel that the physiological factors causing infertility sometimes have a psychological basis. Therapy as well as education and a supportive relationship with health care providers can be very helpful for these couples. In working with infertile couples, it is important to remember that infertility is a stressful situation for people who want to reproduce. They should be encouraged to express their feelings and understand that their emotional response is normal.

It is important to provide a supportive atmosphere while helping to dispel the myths about infertility with accurate information. An infertile couple may feel a loss of control over their own futures. Numerous diagnostic tests that require strict scheduling may add to the feeling of being externally controlled. Some control can be returned to the couple by allowing them choices for scheduling diagnostic and treatment regimes wherever possible. Mutual support and education are available through local support groups and the national self-help organization for infertile couples known as *RESOLVE*.

Adoption, donor insemination, and even embryo transplantation are possible alternatives for those couples who remain infertile after evaluation and treatment. Adoption is the legal placement of an infant or child with parents, to whom the state gives full legal responsibility for the child. For adoption to occur, the infant's biologic mother usually gives up her rights to her baby voluntarily. In some instances, the court terminates her rights; however, when this happens, it is usually on the basis of abandonment.

An alternative to adoption is donor insemination, in which donor semen or the husband's own sperm is deposited in the woman's vagina via syringe during her fertile period. When donor sperm is used, an attempt can be made to match the physical characteristics of the donor to those of the husband.

A potential new hope for the childless couple is embryo transplantation. This involves recovery of an ovum from the woman using the laparoscope, with subsequent fertilization in a laboratory medium and then implantation in her own uterus. Pregnancy rates of 20% to 25% have been achieved with this technique.

SUMMARY

Unit III briefly describes the fascinating trip of the fertilized ovum to its bed in the uterus as life begins. In this unit we traced the development of both the embryo and the fetus and became aware of some of the hazards along the way to healthy development. The next unit explores ways to assure optimal wellness for this new life.

BIBLIOGRAPHY

Bahr, J.E.: Herpesvirus hominis type 2 in women and newborns, MCN **3**:16-21, Jan./Feb. 1978.

Bernstein, J., and Mattox, J.H.: An overview of infertility, JOGN Nurs. **5**:309-314, Sept./Oct. 1982.

Bleyer, W.A., and Breckenridge, R.T.: Studies on the detection of adverse drug reactions in the newborn, J. Am. Med. Assoc. **213**:2049-2053, 1970.

Edwards, M.S.: Venereal herpes: a nursing overview, JOGN Nurs. **7**:7-15, Sept./Oct. 1978.

Eppink, H.: Genetic causes of abnormal fetal

development and inherited disease, JOGN Nurs. **6**:14-22, Sept./Oct. 1977.

Gaver, J.R.: Birth defects and your baby, New York, 1972, Lancer Books.

Golub, S.: Genetic counseling: Heading off birth tragedies, RN, pp. 38-47, Nov. 1969.

Hamilton, P.M.: Basic maternity nursing, ed. 4, St. Louis, 1979, The C.V. Mosby Co.

Iorio, J.: Childbirth: family-centered nursing, ed. 3, St. Louis, 1975, The C.V. Mosby Co.

Kistner, R.W.: The infertile woman, Am. J. Nurs. **73**:1937-1943, Nov. 1973.

Mocarski, V.: The nurse's role in helping infertile couples, MCN **2**:264-266, July/Aug. 1977.

Moore, K.L.: Human embryology, Philadelphia, 1975, W.B. Saunders Co.

Moore, M.L.: Realities in childbearing, ed. 2, Philadelphia, 1983, W. B. Saunders Co.

Palmisano, P.A., and Polhill, R.B.: Fetal pharmacology, Pediatr. Clin. North Am. **19**:3-20, 1972.

Sever, J.L., and Cleghorn, C.: Rubella diagnostic tests: What is a significant result?, Postgrad. Med. **71**:73-78, March 1982.

Unger, K.P.: Warning: environment hazardous to reproductive health, ICEA News **24**:2,8-9, Nov. 1985.

Wiehe, V.R.: Psychological reactions to infertility: Implications for nursing in resolving feelings of disappointment and inadequacy, JOGN Nurs. **5**:28-32, July/Aug. 1976.

DEFINITIONS

Define the following terms:

amniocentesis
amnion
Barr body
bicornuate
biochemical
biophysical
blastoderm
cerclage
chromosomes
chorion
cleavage
cytomegalovirus (CMV)
decidua
decidua basalis
dominant
double uteri
ductus arteriosus
ductus venosus
endometriosis
endothelium
embryo
fertilization age
fibrin
foramen ovale
genes
genetic counseling
gestational age
heterozygous
homozygous
human chorionic gonadotropin (hCG)
"incompetent" cervix
meconium
morula
ovulate
placenta
pulmonary
quickening
recessive
retroverted
rubella
septate
syphilis
toxoplasmosis
trisomy
trophoblast
tuboplasty
vernix caseosa
viable
villi
zygote

LEARNING ACTIVITIES AND EXPERIENCES

1. Group discussions.
2. Guest speakers: a genetic counselor, a couple who has experienced genetic counseling.
3. Visit a genetic counseling center and report on its method of developing family pedigrees.
4. View audiovisual aids and discuss.
5. Look at three-dimensional model of placental circulation.
6. Look at three-dimensional models of growth of embryo and fetus.
7. Write for information on services of RESOLVE, Inc., P.O. Box 474, Belmont Mass. 02178

ENRICHMENT/IN-DEPTH STUDY

1. Visit a biology laboratory to examine specimens of embryos. If there are embryos of animals present, compare their development with that of a human embryo.
2. Make a list of genetic counseling centers within a 150-mile radius of your home.
3. Obtain a placenta from a hospital maternity department and examine it. Check the number of vessels in the cord.

SELF-ASSESSMENT

For questions 1 through 15 determine if the statements are true or false. Fill in the space to the left of the statement by indicating T for true and F for false.

_____ 1. Human development begins when an ovum is fertilized by a sperm.

_____ 2. Fertilization takes place in the tube at the point where the tube enters the uterus.

_____ 3. The ovum lives 12 to 24 hours if not fertilized.

_____ 4. The genes carry the chromosomes.

_____ 5. The spermatozoon cell determines whether the baby will be a boy or a girl.

_____ 6. The sex of the embryo is determined at conception.

_____ 7. Each ovum and each sperm contain 23 chromosomes.

_____ 8. The fertilized cell resulting from the union of a sperm and ovum is called a gonadotropin.

_____ 9. During pregnancy the endometrium is termed the decidua.

_____10. The zygote moving through the fallopian tube is called an embryo.

_____11. The cells that provide nourishment for the developing zygote are the trophoblasts.

_____12. Implantation usually occurs near the cervix of the uterus.

_____13. The period of the ovum lasts 8 weeks.

_____14. The transparent sac in which the fetus floats is made up of two membranes: amnion and chorion.

_____15. Implantation is completed by the trophoblast.

For questions 16 through 22, circle the best answer.

16. Which of the following functional activities is **not** performed by amniotic fluid?
    a. protection
    b. fluid exchange
    c. temperature regulation
    d. gas exchange
17. The structures in fetal circulation that allow a detour of most blood past the fetal lungs and liver are:
    a. ductus venosus
    b. foramen ovale
    c. ductus arteriosus
    d. mitral valve
    Answer (circle one):
    1. a, b, and c
    2. a, b, and d
    3. all of these
18. Traits are passed on from parents to their offspring by:
    a. genes
    b. chromosomes
    c. hormones
19. The zygote contains the following number of chromosomes:
    a. 46 plus 2 sex chromosomes
    b. 44 plus 2 sex chromosomes
    c. 42 plus 2 sex chromosomes

20. The embryo can be affected by all *except* one of the following:
    a. viruses affecting the mother
    b. drugs taken by the mother
    c. nutritional deficiency of the father
    d. nutritional deficiency of the mother
21. An example of a recessive trait is:
    a. dark hair
    b. brown eyes
    c. diabetes mellitus
    d. curly hair
22. The umbilical cord ordinarily contains:
    a. two arteries and one vein
    b. two veins and one artery
    c. one vein and one artery
23. On the line to the left of each item in Column A match the appropriate time periods from Column B. Each item in Column B may used more than once.

Column A	Column B
______1. fetus weighs 3½ pounds	a. 28 weeks gestation
______2. lanugo covers fetus	b. 32 weeks gestation
______3. if born, fetus might survive	c. 20 weeks gestation
______4. fetal heartbeat can be heard through stethoscope	
______5. vernix caseosa covers fetus	

24. On the line to the left of each item in Column A match the appropriate time periods from Column B.

Column A	Column B
______1. rapid development of brain	a. end of first 3 weeks
______2. heart and brain formed	b. end of first 4 weeks
______3. formation of eyes, ears, and nose	c. end of first 7 weeks

25. Draw a sketch of adult circulation and of fetal circulation, tracing the flow of blood through the adult heart and the fetal heart. Label structures in the fetal heart that differ from adult circulation.

For questions 26 through 33, fill in the blanks:

26. The incidence of Down's syndrome increases as the mother's ______________ increases.
27. A chromosomal abnormality that can be detected by examination of amniotic fluid cells following amniocentesis is ______________.
28. What are the nursing responsibilities in genetic counseling?
29. There is a higher risk of ______________ in babies born with only one umbilical artery in the cord.
30. At the sixth week of pregnancy the product of conception is termed the ______________.
31. The fetal period extends from the eight week until ______________.
32. Development during the fetal period is primarily concerned with ______________ and ______________ of tissues and organs.
33. Three major functions of the placenta are ______________, ______________ and ______________.
34. Identify the infections known as the TORCH group:
    T for ______________
    O for ______________
    R for ______________
    C for ______________
    H for ______________
35. Infertility affects approximately ______% to ______% of couples at some time during their reproductive life.

UNIT IV
The antepartum family

GOALS

This unit is designed to provide the reader with information that will:

□ develop awareness of the psychological responses to pregnancy.
□ promote an understanding of the physiological changes resulting from pregnancy.
□ develop a basis for understanding recommended care during pregnancy.
□ explore the nursing role in antepartum care.

STUDENT OBJECTIVES

After studying this unit you should be able to:

1. Explain both the basic physiological and psychological factors affecting attitudes and feelings on love, sex, and intimate relations during pregnancy.
2. Indicate the time interval when intercourse can be resumed for most well couples following childbirth.
3. Describe the physiological changes resulting from pregnancy by identifying at least one change in each body system.
4. Differentiate among the presumptive, probable, and positive signs and symptoms of pregnancy and be able to explain when they occur, why they occur, and a possible other cause for each.
5. Identify the normal values for the following laboratory tests commonly done during the antepartum period: Hct (hematocrit), Hgb (hemoglobin), serology, Rh factor, rubella, urine content of sugar, and albumin.
6. Design a plan to cover a woman's basic nutritional needs during pregnancy.
7. Explain the cause of the following common discomforts of pregnancy and suggest ways to alleviate them:
   a. frequent urination
   b. nausea
   c. heartburn
   d. flatulence
   e. constipation
   f. backache
   g. dyspnea
   h. varicose veins
   i. hemorrhoids
   j. leg cramps
   k. edema
   l. vaginal discharge
8. List the danger signs that may indicate complications of pregnancy that should be reported to a physician.

MOTIVATIONS

DISTINGUISH BETWEEN POSITIVE AND NEGATIVE MOTIVATIONS FOR PREGNANCY

The decision to be pregnant may be conscious and thought out thoroughly or may be buried deep in the subconscious. Many times a couple decides to have a baby because they love one another and want to have a child to share their life. This is the beginning that each human being deserves but may not have when any of the following motives for pregnancy are present:

1. To have a child for a status symbol
2. To have a child to please others
3. To have a family heir
4. To escape a job or new responsibility
5. To prove femininity or masculinity
6. To save a relationship
7. To prove independence
8. To convey hostility toward a parent or the "system"

Being pregnant and alone or deciding to give the baby up for adoption does not necessarily mean that the woman or the couple were ignorant of contraception. One or more of the above motives may have precipitated the pregnancy, or a complex psychological mechanism revolving around feelings of guilt and punishment if contraceptives are used may have been involved. If one prepares for intercourse by obtaining contraceptives, then the act is planned. Some may fear that the fantasized "magic" and "hearing violins playing" may not happen if the act is not "spontaneous."

MYTHS

DISCUSS FOUR MYTHS ASSOCIATED WITH CHILDBEARING AND BIRTH

Just as there are numerous reasons why a woman becomes pregnant, there are also many myths or old wives' tales surrounding childbearing and birth. Some of these center around harm to the unborn child, such as: (1) "Don't reach above your head or the cord will strangle the baby," (2)"If you see a monkey, your baby will look like a monkey," (3) "If you walk in the moonlight, your baby will be a lunatic."

Other myths are concerned with the sex of the baby, such as: (1) "If you carry the baby low, it will be a boy," (2) "If you stick out in front, the baby will be a girl."

Still other myths involve the physical symptoms a woman may have, such as: (1) "If you have heartburn, your baby will have curly hair," (2) "If your baby is active, he or she will be a poor sleeper."

We could go on at great lengths about myths because each culture has its own. It is necessary to explore the attitudes, motivations, and myths each person brings to the childbearing experience; many times what one believes to be true is often as important as what is actually true.

SEXUALITY

BASIC PHYSIOLOGICAL AND PSYCHOLOGICAL FACTORS AFFECTING ATTITUDES AND FEELINGS OF LOVE, SEX, AND INTIMATE RELATIONS DURING PREGNANCY

Pregnancy, labor, and birth are all facts of female sexuality, closely related physiologically and psychologically. Consequently, because childbirth is a sexual experience, we need a basic understanding of the attitudes as well as the feelings couples may have on love, sex, and intimate relations during pregnancy.

Masters and Johnson have shown that sex habits vary widely among different couples and these habits may change throughout pregnancy. Therefore, it is important to individualize and not compare the needs of one couple with those of another. A couples' sexual interest before and during pregnancy may remain the same or differ, depending on their expectations.

The human sexual response cycle as observed by Masters and Johnson has shown women to be as sexually responsive as men, if not more so. In both men and women the two principal physiological responses to sexual stimulation are (1) vasocongestion of tissues in the pelvic region and (2) an increase in voluntary and involuntary muscle tension.

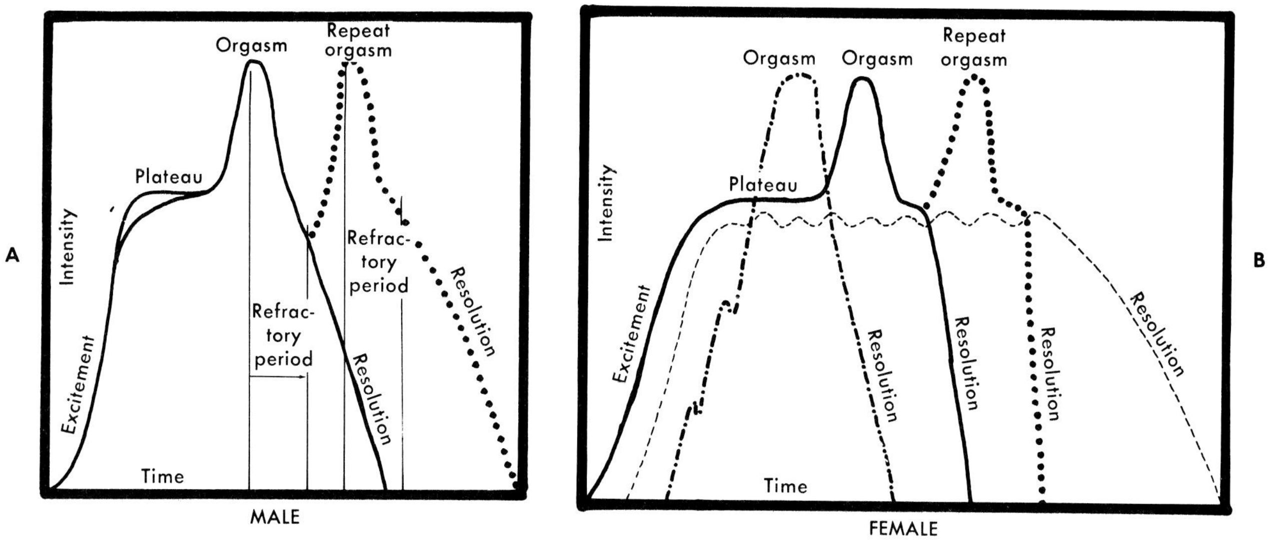

Fig. 4-1. A, Male; and **B,** Female sexual response cycle. (Modified from Masters, W., and Johnson, V.: Human sexual response, Boston, 1966, Little, Brown & Co.)

The phases of sexual arousal and stimulation are excitement, plateau, orgasm, and resolution. The excitement phase develops from sources of physical or psychological stimuli. In the plateau phase sexual tension becomes intensified and may lead to orgasm, the involuntary climax of sexual tension. In orgasm vasocongestion and muscle tension often intensify; and although the total body is involved, the sensations are concentrated in the pelvic region. During the resolution phase sexual tension subsides and the person returns to the pre-excitement state (Fig. 4-1). Some females have a multiorgasmic potential and, if adequately stimulated, may experience another sexual response cycle before resolution. The male experiences a refractory period following ejaculation during which he cannot be restimulated. This sexual response cycle is both highly individualistic and subjective in regard to what is sexually arousing and what is adequate physical stimulation.

To understand what is happening to the couple, we must look at the entire couple, not just their pregnancy. How childbearing couples integrate sexual expression into their lives during pregnancy and postpartum depends on many factors. These factors include their sexual value systems, religious beliefs, folklore, general health and specific pregnancy-related health concerns, and the quality of the couple relationship.

Numerous studies on sexuality during pregnancy indicate that, in general, there is a decline in sexual interest, activity, and satisfaction as pregnancy progresses. However, every study includes both men and women for whom this is not true. When sexuality is incorporated into counseling sessions or teaching plans, the approach and information shared should vary according to the individuals involved.

First trimester changes

For most women during the first trimester (first 3 months of pregnancy), there is a decrease in sexual desire and consequently in frequency of sexual intercourse. Normal physiological alterations of pregnancy that may cause this decrease in sexual desire are:

1. Nausea and perhaps vomiting
2. Breast tenderness
3. Fatigue
4. Feeling of fullness
5. Pelvic vasocongestion

Psychologically, a woman may feel that she is now a "mother" and should behave differently, or that she should protect her baby from possible trauma during intercourse.

Fathers often view the newly pregnant woman with awe, worrying that they may harm the baby during intercourse, thus causing uncertainty and reluctance to engage in sexual activity. On the other hand, some men, having impregnated their partners, feel more "manly" and desire sexual contact more often than before.

Second trimester changes

In the second 3 months of pregnancy most women experience a general feeling of well-being, with the fatigue gone and an increase in pelvic engorgement all contributing to easier and more frequent sexual arousal. If the woman is happy with her pregnancy and things are going well with the couple in other areas of their lives, the woman may have greatly increased desire for sexual encounter.

Fathers often feel very warm, loving, and protective toward their mates as they bloom in the second trimester. The initial fear of harming the fetus is put aside as physical evidence of the pregnancy in the form of the growing uterus reassures both partners that the pregnancy is a reality and seems to be going well.

The second trimester is often a time of loving caresses, expressions of appreciation for each other, and a fulfilling sex life.

Third trimester changes

During the last 3 months of pregnancy there is often again a decrease in sexual interest and reduced sexual activity.

Often the mother's loss of interest results from her increasing size and concentrating on her baby and mentally preparing herself for motherhood. As she "rests," the father's old fears of injury to the baby often return and he shows less interest in sexual intercourse to support his mate's increased needs and to protect the fetus from any harm.

Until recently it was traditional for physicians to prohibit sexual intercourse for all couples during the last 6 weeks of pregnancy and the first 6 weeks postpartum. This practice was recommended because it was believed that for 6 weeks before birth sexual intercourse could induce premature labor and for 6 weeks after birth could cause serious infection. Not only were these reasons invalid, but many couples continued to have intercourse in spite of the instructions and then had to deal with guilt feelings associated with what should be an act of love and giving.

Today it is recognized that sexual intercourse is contraindicated in pregnancy when the following complications are present:

1. Vaginal bleeding
2. Ruptured membranes
3. Incompetent cervix
4. Threatened premature labor
5. Prematurely ripe cervix
6. Vaginal infection
7. History of miscarriage (abortion)

TIME INTERVAL WHEN INTERCOURSE CAN BE RESUMED

No longer are all women instructed to refrain from intercourse during the last 6 weeks of pregnancy and the first 6 weeks postpartum. Advice is based on a realistic appraisal of each couple's individual needs, desires, and circumstances. Following childbirth sexual intercourse can usually be resumed when vaginal discharge has stopped, there is no perineal discomfort, and the couple is psychologically ready. For the first few months after delivery the vagina may not lubricate well and a water-soluble gel may be recommended for lubrication.

Pregnancy and the postpartum period need not be times of sexual frustration for the pregnant couple but can be a time to increase intimacy and strengthen their bonds.

AIMS OF PRENATAL CARE

The physical and psychological health care a family receives during pregnancy is termed antepartal (*ante*, before; *partal*, birth) care, or prenatal care.

IDENTIFY FOUR AIMS OF PRENATAL CARE

The aims of antepartal care for the family include:

1. To protect and promote the physical and emotional health and well-being of the expectant mother
2. To protect and support optimal health of the unborn baby
3. To assist the expectant father in adapting to his new role of father with a high degree of wellness
4. To assist siblings and other family members to adapt to the changing family structure resulting from a new baby in the family

DIFFERENTIATE BETWEEN GRAVIDA AND PARA

In beginning a study of the antepartum, there are several terms you should become familiar with because they will be used frequently. These are:

gravid the stage of being pregnant.

gravida the number of pregnancies a woman has had, regardless of outcome. It includes the present pregnancy. It is the pregnancy that is counted and not the number of babies in utero.

nulligravida a woman who has never been pregnant.

primigravida a woman pregnant for the first time.

multigravida a woman pregnant more than once.

para the pregnancy that terminates in the birth (live or dead) of a fetus or fetuses who reached the stage of viability (generally designated at 28 weeks of gestation).

primipara a woman who has given birth to a fetus or fetuses (live or dead) who reached the stage of viability.

multipara a woman who has given birth to more than one infant (live or dead) at the stage of viability. A woman who has delivered three children and is in labor now with her fourth pregnancy is gravida IV, para III. A woman who is pregnant for the first time is a primigravida. When she gives birth to her first child, she will be a primipara.

PHYSIOLOGICAL CHANGES

Reproductive system

PHYSIOLOGICAL CHANGES RESULTING FROM PREGNANCY

In the healthy, regularly menstruating woman, an absence of the menses beyond 2 weeks of the expected menstrual date is suggestive of pregnancy.

In the first 3 months of pregnancy, the uterus becomes enlarged and more anteflexed than normal. Uterine growth is due to stretching and enlargement of existing cells rather than growth of new cells. This results initially from estrogen's effects on the uterus and later from mechanical stretching. The blood supply to the uterus increases (see Unit II), and the blood vessels become larger. By the end of the pregnancy, the capacity of the uterus will increase to more than 500 times what it was before pregnancy. By the fourth month of pregnancy, the uterus has lost its nonpregnant "pear" shape and is more globular in shape. It emerges from the pelvis and can be palpated above the symphysis pubis. Uterine contractility increases, and after the first trimester, irregular infrequent painless contractions begin (the so-called *Braxton-Hicks' contractions*). As the pregnancy progresses, these contractions become more regular but are often unnoticed by the pregnant woman.

About 4 weeks after conception, the softening of the cervix *(Goodell's sign)* is detectable by pelvic examination. The endocervical glands become more active and secrete large amounts of cervical mucus. At about the 6th or 8th week of pregnancy, the lower segment of the uterus becomes softer and this softening *(Hegar's sign)* can be felt by the examiner during a bimanual examination (Fig. 4-2). This is one of the most reliable early signs of pregnancy. Also, during a vaginal examination at 8 to 10 weeks of pregnancy the examiner can see a violet tinge to the cervical and vaginal mucous membranes *(Chad-*

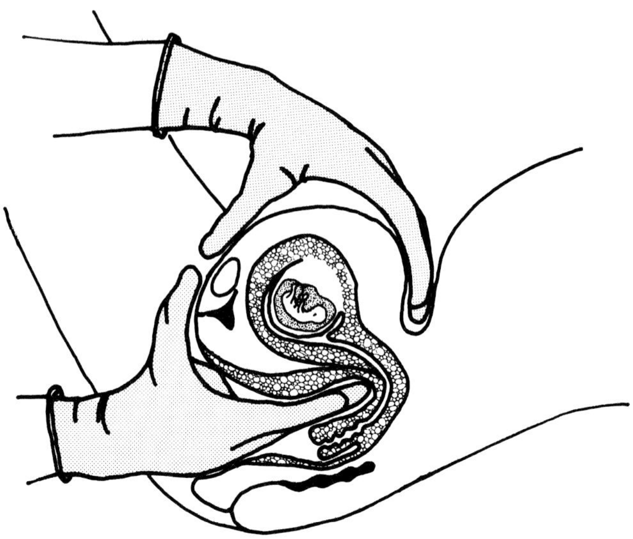

Fig. 4-2. Hegar's sign.

wick's sign). This is caused by the increased vascularity of the pelvic organs. The vagina also becomes softer and more congested.

In the first 3 to 4 months of pregnancy, the fetus is small compared to the amount of amniotic fluid; therefore it will rebound against the examiner's fingers *(ballottement)* when the examiner gently pushes against the uterus, through either the vagina or the abdomen.

Breast changes, the result of hormonal changes, cause the areolae to become dark, the nipples to become firmer, and the weight of the breasts to increase. The breasts also become tender, and light blue veins are visible beneath the skin. Visible striations may develop as the lobules enlarge and stretch the connective tissue and skin of the breasts. After the first few months of pregnancy, a thin, yellowish, clear fluid called *colostrum* may sometimes be expressed from the nipples. This is the substance that precedes the milk from the breasts when milk letdown occurs 3 to 4 days after delivery. The presence of colostrum does not indicate whether the woman will be able to breast feed.

Skeletal and muscular systems

The increase in both hormone supply and blood supply to the pelvis causes relaxation of the pelvic joints during pregnancy, which can cause a "waddling" walk. The pelvic bones actually spread out slightly, thus shifting some of the weight of the heavy uterus to surrounding muscles and ligaments. The normal lumbar curve of the spine becomes more pronounced as the weight of the uterus and its contents tilt the pelvis forward. This extra weight-supporting burden put on the muscles and ligaments may cause the backache many women experience toward the end of pregnancy.

Circulatory system

Because there is an increase in the amount of blood needed for the reproductive system in pregnancy, the blood volume in the body increases by approximately 30% to 50% so that the rest of the body will not be depleted. However, the increase in plasma volume is greater than the increase in red blood cell volume, so that there is a slight dilution of the hemoglobin content of the blood. This is normal and called, by some, the "physiological" anemia of pregnancy. The hemoglobin to hematocrit ratio in pregnancy is often 12 to 36, instead of 13.3 to 40 as seen in a nonpregnant menstruating woman. However, a hemoglobin of less than 11 or 12 is still indicative of "real" anemia.

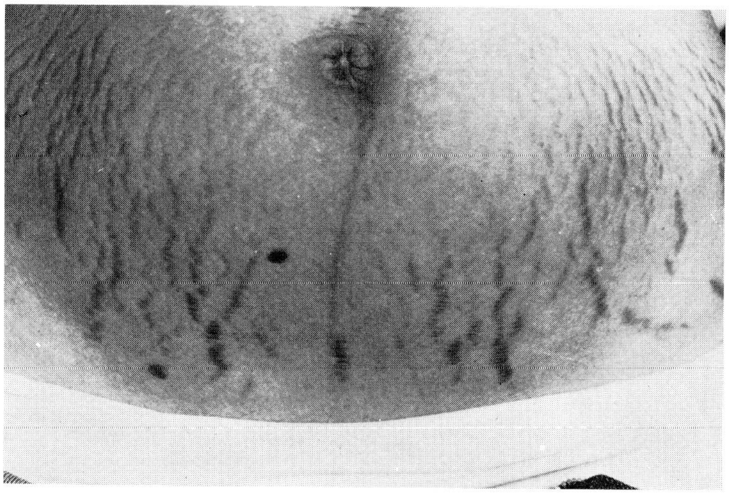

Fig. 4-3. Striae (stretch marks). (Courtesy Mercy Hospital and Medical Center, San Diego.) (From Ingalls, A.J., and Salerno, M.C.: Maternal and child health nursing, ed. 4, St. Louis, 1979, The C.V. Mosby Co.)

The heart is displaced upward and to the left by the enlarging uterus and the displaced abdominal organs. Cardiac output increases by approximately 30% early in pregnancy and remains elevated until delivery. During labor there is a further increase in cardiac output. Uterine contractions can increase output by up to 400 milliliters per minute. There is a marked positional effect: in the supine position the enlarged, heavy uterus frequently lies against the inferior vena cava and obstructs venous return to the heart, reducing cardiac output by as much as 1 liter per minute (see Unit III). This compression can lead to serious hypotension and even fetal compromise.

Heart rate increases early in gestation by approximately 20% (10 to 15 beats per minute). Although there is no significant change in systolic blood pressure, there is a slight decrease in diastolic blood pressure. A pressure of 90/70 is not unusual in the pregnant woman. The increased blood flow in pregnancy occurs mainly to the breasts, gut, skin, kidneys, and uterus.

As the pregnancy progresses, the pressure on the enlarged veins of the pelvis and lower extremities increases because of the pressure of the growing uterus. This makes the woman a good candidate for varicose veins in the legs, thighs, and vulva, as well as for phlebitis and hemorrhoids.

Integumentary system

Increases in hormone levels cause many skin changes in pregnancy. Some of these are *linea nigra*, a dark vertical line running from the umbilicus to the mons pubis (veneris), and *chloasma* ("mask of pregnancy"), irregular mottled brownish pigmentation of the face. The *linea nigra* and *chloasma* fade and sometimes disappear after pregnancy. It is thought that these skin changes may be the result of increased levels of melanocyte-stimulating hormone (MSH) during pregnancy, causing increased production of the pigment melanin. *Angiomas* or tiny capillary branches ("vascular spiders") frequently occur on the skin of the shoulders, arms, hands, or face and tend to disappear after birth. They are thought to be caused by estrogen. There are also silvery-blue stretch marks *(striae gravidarium)* on the sides of the abdomen, breasts, and thighs (Fig. 4-3). These may fade but never entirely disappear.

Respiratory system

The pregnant woman breathes deeper and more frequently than the nonpregnant woman to maintain optimal pressures of O_2 and CO_2 for herself and the fetus. Because respiratory rate is slightly increased, and tidal volume increases, the total amount of air exchanged is elevated approximately 40%. However, oxygen consumption increases only 15% to 20% (primarily accounted for by the uterus and its contents). Thus, the "hyperventilation of pregnancy" is probably a reserve mechanism for the fetus. The pregnant woman frequently experiences difficulty breathing *(dyspnea)* in the latter months of pregnancy as the large uterus displaces the diaphragm. Although the lungs are crowded, the ribs flare out so that lung capacity is not decreased.

Gastrointestinal system

Nausea and vomiting ("morning sickness") are common in early pregnancy. The high level of circulating hormones is probably one of the primary causes of nausea. By the third or fourth month of pregnancy, the placenta has assumed major responsibility for progesterone production, and circulating estrogen levels begin to exceed progesterone. At this time, nausea stops being a problem for most women.

During pregnancy there is relaxation of the sphincter between the esophagus and stomach causing a reflux of gastric juices into the esophagus. This reflux causes heartburn. Constipation and flatulence are very common, resulting from pressure of the growing fetus on the large intestines and a generalized reduction in gastric tone and motility. Because of uterine enlargement pushing the intestines aside, the pain of appendicitis may actually present in the upper abdomen (near the rib cage) rather than in its traditional position in the right lower abdomen.

Urinary system

Frequency of urination is common in both early and late pregnancy because of the pressure of the uterus on the bladder. This frequent urination is alleviated to some degree in the second trimester as the uterus rises out of the pelvis to the level of the symphysis. However, because the edema of pregnancy (swollen feet and ankles) is relieved when the pregnant woman lies down at night, this fluid is often mobilized. Thus, it is common for the pregnant woman to have to get up several times at night to urinate. The increased hormone level in pregnancy causes the walls of the ureters to soften and lose much of their muscular tone, thus causing them to dilate. As a result, urinary tract infections, such as cystitis (bladder infection) and pyelonephritis (kidney infection) frequently occur in pregnancy. There is also a change in the kidney filtration system in pregnancy, which may cause some spilling of sugar into the urine.

Endocrine system

The thyroid increases in size during pregnancy, and as it does, the basal metabolic rate increases. The posterior lobe of the pituitary secretes the oxytoxic hormone, which stimulates uterine muscle to contract. The anterior lobe of the pituitary secretes hormones necessary to the normal physiology of pregnancy and also the hormone *prolactin*, which causes milk secretion after birth.

WEIGHT GAIN

INDICATE THE NORMAL WEIGHT GAIN IN PREGNANCY

The recommended weight gain in pregnancy is 24 to 28 pounds for all women, usually even those who are obese. The normal weight gain can be plotted on a grid, reflecting a gradual and progressive increase in weight (Fig. 4-4). In the first trimester there is little weight gain—usually a total of 2 to 4 pounds (1 to 2 kilograms). During the second and third trimesters, there is a steady gain of 0.9 pounds (0.4 kilograms) per week. The weight gain of pregnancy is distributed as follows:

Fetus	7.7 pounds (3.5 kilograms)
Placenta	1.4 pounds (0.64 kilograms)
Amniotic fluid	1.8 pounds (0.82 kilograms)

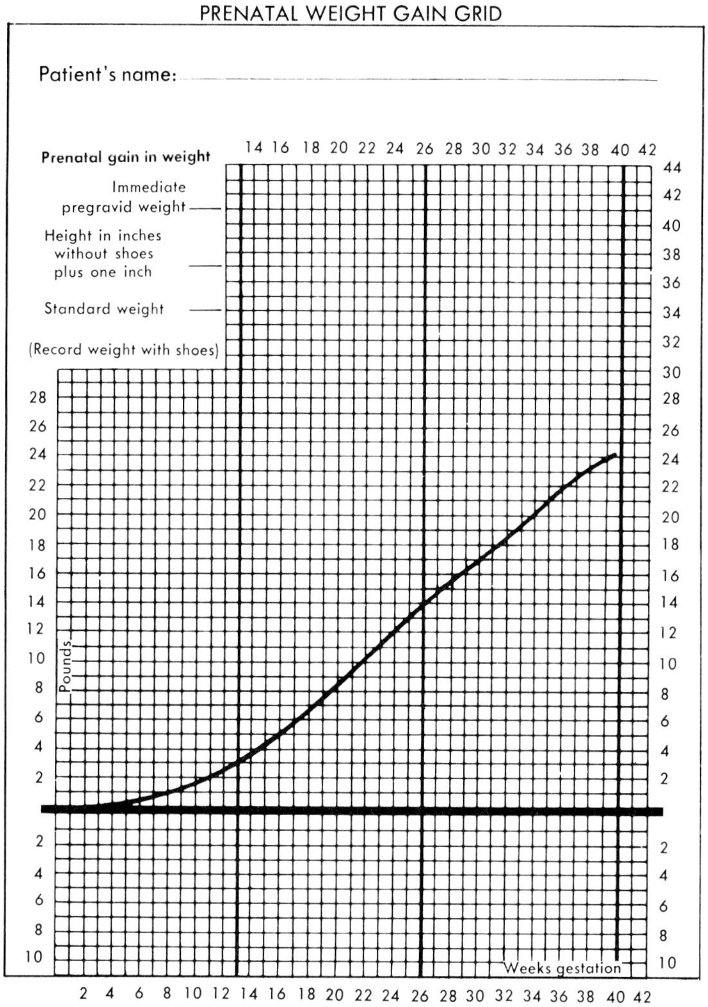

Fig. 4-4. Prenatal weight gain grid. (Courtesy of J.B. Lippincott Co.)

Increased uterine size	2.0 pounds (0.9 kilograms)
Increased blood volume	4.0 pounds (1.8 kilograms)
Increased breast size	0.9 pounds (0.4 kilograms)
Increased extracellular fluid	2.7 pounds (1.2 kilograms)
Other	3.5 pounds (1.6 kilograms)
Total	24.0 pounds (10.9 kilograms)

SIGNS AND SYMPTOMS

SIGNS OF PREGNANCY

The *presumptive* (presumed but not proved) signs and symptoms of pregnancy are mostly those that occur very early in pregnancy. The *probable* (likely but not definite) signs are those that occur generally after 6 to 8 weeks of pregnancy. The *positive* (no doubt about it) signs and symptoms appear after approximately the twentieth week of pregnancy.

Presumptive signs	Other causes
1. Amenorrhea (cessation of menses)	Could also result from hormone imbalance, emotional disturbance, disease, environmental changes, or excessive exercise
2. Frequency of urination	Could also be caused by a bladder infection, diabetes, a pelvic tumor, or congestive heart failure

3. Nausea and vomiting in the morning ("morning sickness")	Could have emotional causes, or be caused by a "flu" or a variety of intestinal disturbances
4. Quickening (first fetal life felt by mother)	Could be intestinal activity ("gas")
5. Enlargement of breasts	Could be caused by hormonal changes other than pregnancy
6. Pigmentation of the skin	May be present in all women
7. Chadwick's sign	Could be present when any pelvic congestion occurs

Probable signs	**Other causes**
1. Enlarged uterus and abdomen	Could also be fibroid tumor, ascites, or ovarian cysts
2. Braxton-Hicks' contractions	Probable indication
3. Hegar's sign	Probable indication
4. Ballottement	Could also occur with some tumors
5. Positive pregnancy test	Probable indication
6. Uterine souffle (a soft, blowing rhythm the same rate as the mother's pulse, caused by blood passing through large uterine vessels)	Audible after 16th week

Positive signs

1. Fetal heart beat—audible from 18th to 20th week on with stethescope; by 9 to 11 weeks with Doppler ultrasound
2. Fetal movement—palpable after 20 weeks
3. X-ray (taken only for specific reason)—will show fetal skeleton after 16 weeks gestation
4. Sonography—will show fetal outlines as well as movements by 5 to 6 weeks (occasionally at 4 weeks)

PRENATAL CARE

Because of the tremendous effect of pregnancy on the life of the woman and her family, it is important to know as soon as possible if she is indeed pregnant. The first visit to seek medical supervision is usually for confirmation of pregnancy.

Although pregnancy can usually be easily diagnosed once a women is well along in her pregnancy (simply by observing and palpating her distended abdomen), there are now simple examinations of the blood and urine that make it possible to diagnose pregnancy as early as 8 days after ovulation.

Pregnancy tests differ in their sensitivity, the time they take to complete, and whether urine or blood is used. Obviously, the more sensitive and sophisticated the test, the more it costs to do. All currently available tests detect levels of human chorionic gonadotropin (hCG), a hormone produced by the fertilized egg (see Unit II) that can be found in the pregnant woman's blood and urine. The urinary excretion of hCG doubles every 1½ to 2 days, and thus the more sensitive the test, the earlier pregnancy can be detected.

The five main types of pregnancy tests are latex agglutination inhibition (LAI), hemagglutination inhibition (HAI), radioreceptor assay (RRA), radioimmunoassay (RIA), and direct agglutination (DA). LAI tests are usually done by mixing a drop of urine onto a slide and agitating for 2 minutes. A clumped solution indicates a negative result (no pregnancy) and a milky-smooth solution indicates a positive result (pregnancy). LAI is cheap but is accurate only 21 to 24 days after conception. HAI tests are similar to LAI but usually require test tubes and take 1 to 2 hours. Most home pregnancy tests are of this type. A mat of debris at the bottom of the tube signals a negative result, and a ring at the tube base indicates a positive result. HAI is accurate from 14 to 18 days after ovulation. RRA tests, done in sophisticated laboratories, take about 1 hour to perform and can detect pregnancy approximately 14 days after ovulation. RIA tests, done on blood or urine, are the most sensitive of the currently available pregnancy tests and can detect pregnancy as early as 8 days after ovulation (actually *before* the missed menstrual period). Thus these are the tests of choice for assessment of ectopic pregnancies, hydatidiform mole, or threatened spontaneous abortions. DA tests, relatively recently introduced, are also very sensitive and accurate early in pregnancy.

Importance of prenatal care

EXPLAIN THE IMPORTANCE OF PRENATAL CARE

There is no doubt at all that improved prenatal care in this country has dramatically reduced maternal and infant morbidity and mortality. Detecting possible problems early leads to prompt treatment and greatly improved pregnancy outcome. Because so much of the wellness of pregnancy is dependent on the woman assuming responsibility for her own health maintenance with proper exercise, nutrition, and preventive measures, early diagnosis, assessment of the pregnancy, and a planned regimen of care are essential.

Nursing responsibilities

DESCRIBE NURSING RESPONSIBILITIES DURING PRENATAL EXAMINATIONS

When you first meet the pregnant woman and her family, remember that rapid physical and emotional changes are occurring, causing anxiety for the parents-to-be. A positive pregnancy test may not cause waves of joy for the woman. As mentioned in Unit I both men and women may have ambivalent feelings when pregnancy is confirmed. Frequently, your first introduction to the family will be to the woman only, since pregnancy has been considered "woman's business" in our society. If there is a mate, encourage his presence during prenatal visits. Through understanding the physiological and psychological changes the pregnant woman is experiencing, he is better able to offer help and support. Also, the expectant father has needs as he adjusts to his new role. It is not unusual for men to experience morning sickness, weight gain, and fatigue in early pregnancy. Such physiological changes may be cries for help on his part. Last but not least, consider the siblings and other family members. Including siblings in prenatal care may help to reduce sibling rivalry by a gradual introduction to the new family member through listening to the fetal heart beat, watching the uterus grow, and just not being excluded from this family event. Grandparents often feel left out because they have difficulty understanding today's trends toward natural childbirth and early discharge from the hospital. Remember that pregnancy is wellness. This is the family's pregnancy. Birth is the beginning or further growth of a family and you can contribute immeasureably to the experience.

Women alone may have considerably more need for emotional support and child care during visits than women with family support. Your role as nurse includes assessing the psychosocial needs of the childbearing people who seek your help and then determining how to meet these needs. Consultation from other members of the immediate health team may be necessary. Community resources should be sought out as well.

Medical history

A thorough medical and obstetric history is taken during the first examination to determine the present state of the mother's health. Although a complete medical, surgical, and psychosocial history should be taken, special emphasis is usually given to obstetrical and gynecological matters. The obstetrical history usually includes descriptions of each prior pregnancy, including dates of birth, sex, weight; lengths of labor and pregnancy; and complications. A commonly used form of obstetrical history abbreviation in clinics is as follows: number of pregnancies = gravida number, number of deliveries (alive or dead) = para number, number of abortions = "Ab" number. For example, a woman who was pregnant three times, delivered twice, had one abortion, and is now pregnant again would be: $gravida_4$ $para_2$ ab_1, or $G_4P_2Ab_1$. The history helps the medical and nursing team plan for the pregnancy and delivery and, if at all possible, prevent complications that may have occurred in previous pregnancies.

A careful recording of the woman's menstrual history will be essential in calculation of the data of delivery.

Calculation of estimated date of delivery

CALCULATING EDD USING NAEGELE'S RULE

An approximation of the estimated date of delivery (EDD) can be calculated by using *Naegele's rule:* (1) take date of last menstrual period (LMP), (2) subtract three months, (3) add 7 days and 1 year.

Example:	LMP = August 7, 1986	8/7/86
		− 3
		5/7/86
		+ 7/1
	EDD = May 14, 1987	5/14/87

The typical pregnancy lasts 40 weeks from the first day of the LMP.

Physical examination

After the psychosocial assessment and the woman's medical and obstetrical history are completed, she is ready for a physical examination. The nurse prepares the woman for a physical examination by first collecting a voided urine specimen to check it for sugar and albumin. The woman's temperature, pulse, respiration, blood pressure, and weight are also recorded. Vital signs should *not* be measured with the pregnant woman lying on her back, because compression of the inferior vena cava by the pregnant uterus may cause misleading values to be recorded. Next the nurse provides privacy for the woman in an examination room, instructs her to remove all clothing, provides a robe or drape for covering, and prepares all necessary equipment. If this is the first thorough physical and obstetrical examination for the woman, she may be very apprehensive. In this case the nurse will stay with the examiner to assist if necessary and to provide emotional support for the woman. If the expectant father is with the woman, encourage him to stay at the head of the examining table so that he can reassure her also. This is a very good time for the couple to learn together about the need for and meaning of the physical examination. It also gives him an opportunity for early involvement in the pregnancy.

The physical examination includes examination of all body systems and abdominal palpation (Fig. 4-5). The obstetrical examination includes examination of the external genitalia, the hymenal remnant (if present), the urethral orifice, the vagina, the cervix, the corpus of the uterus, the adnexal structures, and the rectum. It also includes a Papanicolaou smear for a cancer cytology test, measurements of the pelvis, and tests to detect sexually transmissible diseases (STDs) or infections if deemed necessary. Before the obstetrical examination, always be sure that the woman has emptied her bladder.

One *pelvic measurement* that is taken is the *diagonal conjugate* (Fig. 4-6) (from the inferior margin of the symphysis pubis to the sacral promontory). This is done on vaginal examination when the tips of the first two fingers of the examiner touch the sacral promontory. The point where the lower margin of the symphysis pubis rests on the finger is measured. An adequate size for vaginal delivery is considered to be 11.5 centimeters (Fig. 4-7). The *true conjugate* is obtained by subtracting 1.5 to 2.0 centimeters from the diagonal conjugate measurement. The normal measurement is 10 centimeters. The true conjugate measures the upper margin of the symphysis pubis to the sacral promontory and can be measured *directly* only by x-ray study (which is not recommended in pregnancy). *The prominence of the ischial spines*, the sloping of the pelvic walls, the curve or prominence of the sacrum, the mobility of the coccyx, and the angle of the pubic arch can be felt and estimated during vaginal examination. The *outlet* is measured by the distance between the ischial tuberosities *(intertuberous diameter)*, which averages 11 centimeters (see Fig. 2-13). This measurement is approximated with a pelvimeter or with four knuckles of the examiner's hand. The *posterior sagittal* measurement is made indirectly with a pelvimeter. Normal measurement is 8 to 9.5 centimeters. It is the distance between the midpoint of intertuberous diameter and tip of the sacrum.

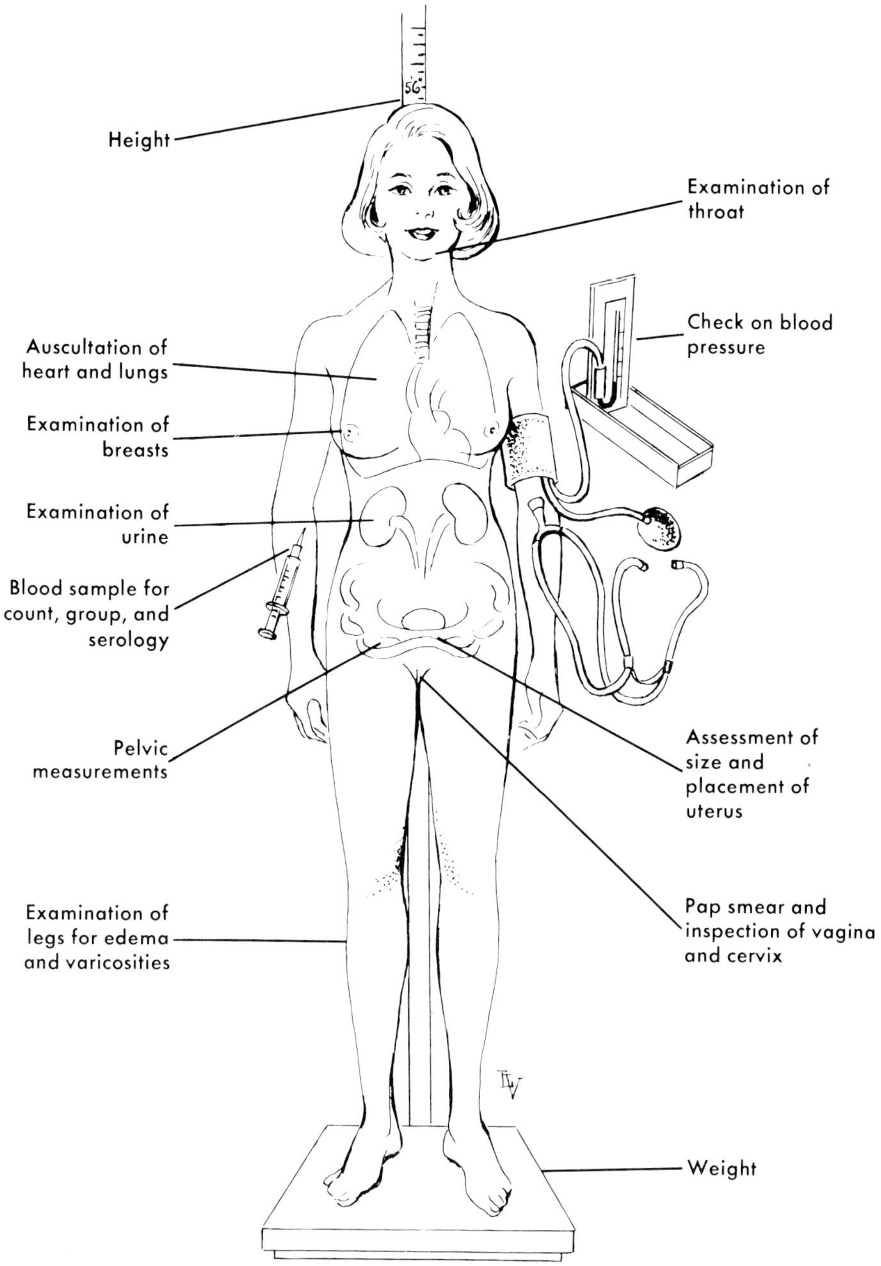

Fig. 4-5. Thorough physical examination. (From Lerch, C., and Bliss, V.J.: Maternity nursing, ed. 3, St. Louis, 1978, The C.V. Mosby Co.)

Laboratory tests. The following laboratory tests are routinely done:

NORMAL VALUES FOR LABORATORY TESTS COMMONLY DONE DURING THE ANTEPARTUM PERIOD

1. *Serology (VDRL)* is done to detect syphilis. If syphilis is present, the VDRL will usually be positive. It is often recommended that the serology test be repeated before labor begins.
2. *Rh factor* and *blood type* determinations are done to detect possible maternal-fetal blood incompatibilities. In the U.S. 85% of the population is Rh positive, which means that they have the Rh antigen in their blood; and 15% is Rh negative, which means that they lack the Rh antigen. A problem can exist if the mother is Rh negative and the father is Rh positive. A potential problem also exists if the mother is type O and the fetus is type A, B, or AB.

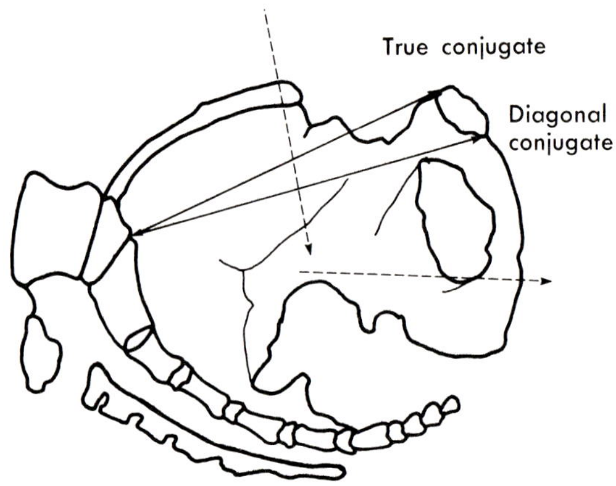

Fig. 4-6. Diagonal conjugate and true conjugate.

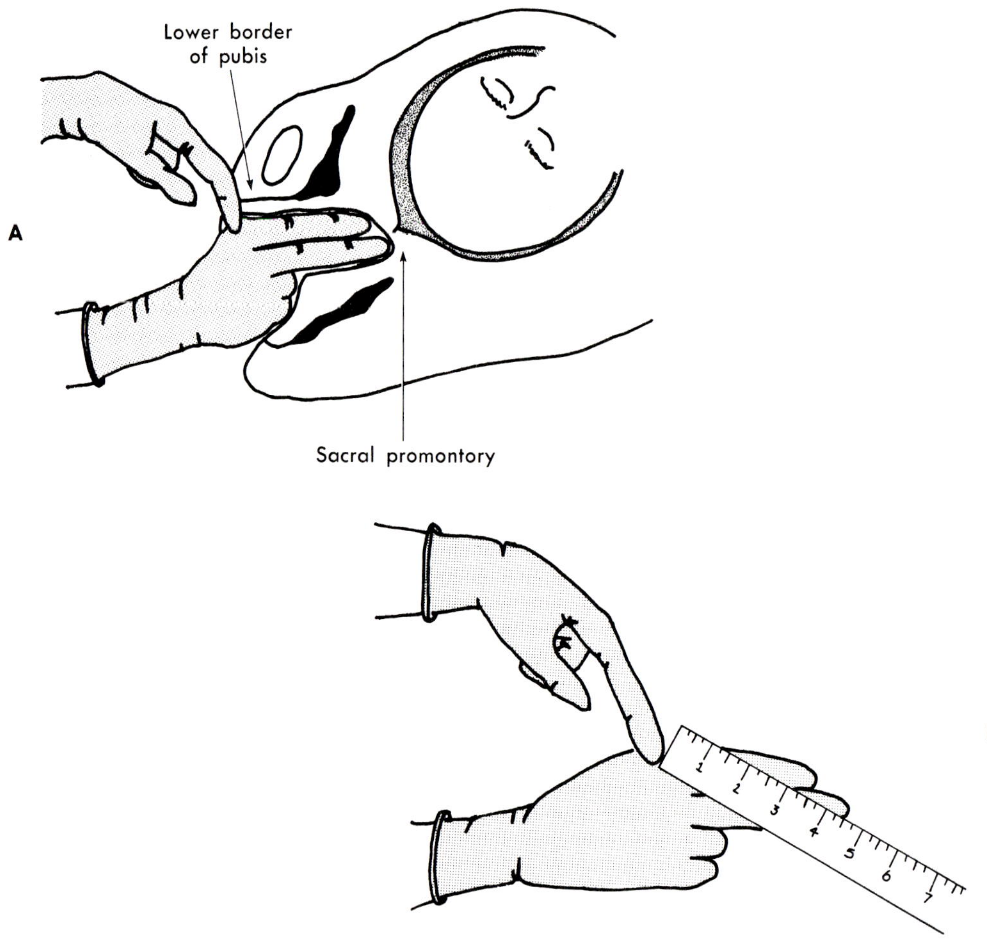

Fig. 4-7. Measuring diagonal conjugate.

3. *Normal hemoglobin and hematocrit levels* are as follows:

	Nonpregnant	**Pregnant**
Hemoglobin (Hgb)	>13 grams/100 milliliters	−12 grams/100 milliliters
Hematocrit (Hct)	>40%	−36%

Note: These values may vary slightly from laboratory to laboratory.

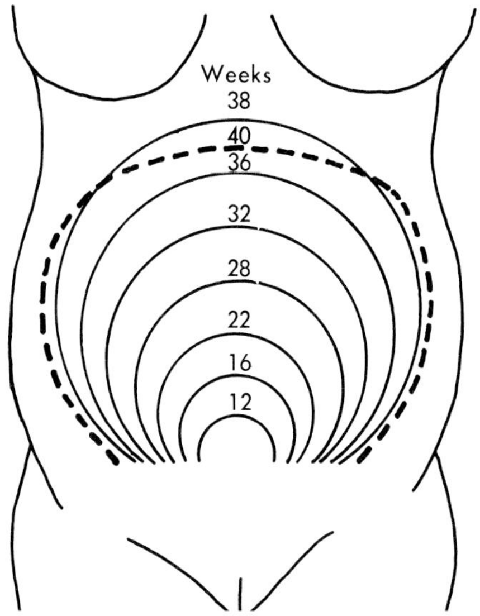

Fig. 4-8. Growth of uterus during pregnancy.

4. *Rubella screening* is usually routine to determine whether the woman is resistant to the rubella virus (German measles). A rubella antibody titer of between 1:8 and 1:20 (the exact cutoff point varies from laboratory to laboratory) *or greater* suggests immunity.
5. *Urine tests for sugar* are done to detect maternal diabetes. Urine should be free of sugar although in the latter part of pregnancy, sugar in the urine may occur as a result of increased amounts of lactose in the blood. Tests for *protein* are done to detect proteinuria, which is indicative of abnormal kidney functioning and toxemia. Urine should be free of protein.
6. *Sickle cell anemia* and *thalassemia* tests are done on women of African or Mediterranean heritage.
7. *Skin testing* for detection of tuberculosis should be done.
8. *Vaginal smears* to detect gonorrhea and laboratory testing for herpesvirus hominis and monilial and trichomonal infections are done if indicated.
9. *Papanicolaou test* (Pap smear) is a screening test to detect cervical cancer. This is usually done on the prenatal visit.

Further laboratory tests and repetitions of the above tests are done as indicated during the pregnancy.

Families are encouraged to return every 3 to 4 weeks during the first 7 months of pregnancy and every 2 weeks during the last 2 months or every week in the last month. At each visit, blood pressure, urine specimens, TPR, weight gain, height of uterine fundus (Fig. 4-8), fetal heart tones, and general physical and emotional status are assessed.

PERSONAL CARE

EXPLAIN RECOMMENDED PERSONAL CARE DURING PREGNANCY

When discussing the general hygiene of pregnancy with the woman and her family, the nurse should find out how much they already know, what they believe to be true, and what their cultural background has taught them. Next, the nurse should explain, discuss, clarify, reinforce, and share information, where appropriate, about what they do not know. Recommendations for care follow.

Bathing

Because the woman's sebaceous and sweat glands have become more active, she needs a daily bath. Either a tub bath or shower is all right. There is no danger if bath water enters the vagina. When bathing, she should not use soap and water on the nipples of her breasts because soap has a tendency to cause dryness and cracking. The expectant father or other family member could be encouraged to install safety strips or a nonslip bath mat in the tub or shower to make the area less slippery.

Clothing

Clothing should be nonconstricting. As the breasts enlarge, the bra size may need to increase, and the woman may choose a nursing bra before delivery. It is important to keep the breasts well supported during pregnancy to prevent overstretching of connective tissue, which could lead to sagging of the breasts. Pregnant women should never wear round or rolled garters because they constrict the leg vessels, slow down venous return, and thus cause edema and encourage the formation of varicose veins. Support stockings are helpful for women with varicosities. A girdle is usually not necessary, but does offer helpful support to the back and pelvis for some women. Shoes should have flat or medium heels because high heels tilt the body forward, upsetting the balance and causing increased curvature of the back to compensate for the forward tilt.

Oral hygiene

Daily oral hygiene is essential during pregnancy. A visit to the dentist early in pregnancy will detect any cavities that could make the mother more susceptible to infections. There is no truth in the old adage, "For every child, a tooth is lost."

Sexuality and feminine hygiene

As discussed at the beginning of this unit, unless contraindicated by a medical condition or complication of pregnancy, continuing usual sexual activity is encouraged during pregnancy. You might begin the discussion of sexuality by asking the couple what they have heard about sex during pregnancy.

Douching in pregnancy (or at any time) is not necessary unless done specifically under a physician's order to treat a vaginal irritation. It is not unusual to have increased vaginal secretions during pregnancy, and the woman needs to understand this. However, if the secretion is so copious as to require the wearing of a pad, the woman should seek medical attention. This could be indicative of a vaginal infection such as *Trichomonas vaginalis* infection (a profuse, yellowish green, irritating discharge with an unpleasant odor) or *Monilia* infection (a yeast infection causing a thick, white cheesy discharge with itching). Both of these infections tend to occur during pregnancy and are treatable.

Bowels

There is a tendency toward constipation as a result of decreased peristalsis. Decreased peristalsis causes the feces to remain longer in the bowel, thus increasing the water absorption from the feces. Encourage the addition to the diet of six to eight glasses of liquid per day, roughage, bran, and fruits and fruit juices. Explain to the woman that if constipation becomes a problem and if changes in her diet do not improve the condition, she may ask the doctor for a mild laxative. However, she should not medicate herself because harsh laxatives can stimulate the uterus to contract.

Exercise, travel, and employment

The pregnant woman should remain active during pregnancy, participating in her normal activities but avoiding activity that causes unnecessary fatigue. There are specific exercises that are helpful in maintaining the tone of the abdominal, back, and perineal muscles. Some of these exercises are illustrated in Fig. 4-9.

In today's world, many women continue to be employed outside the home during their entire pregnancy. If the family is dependent on the woman's income, or if she is supporting herself, it is totally unrealistic to encourage this woman to leave her job,

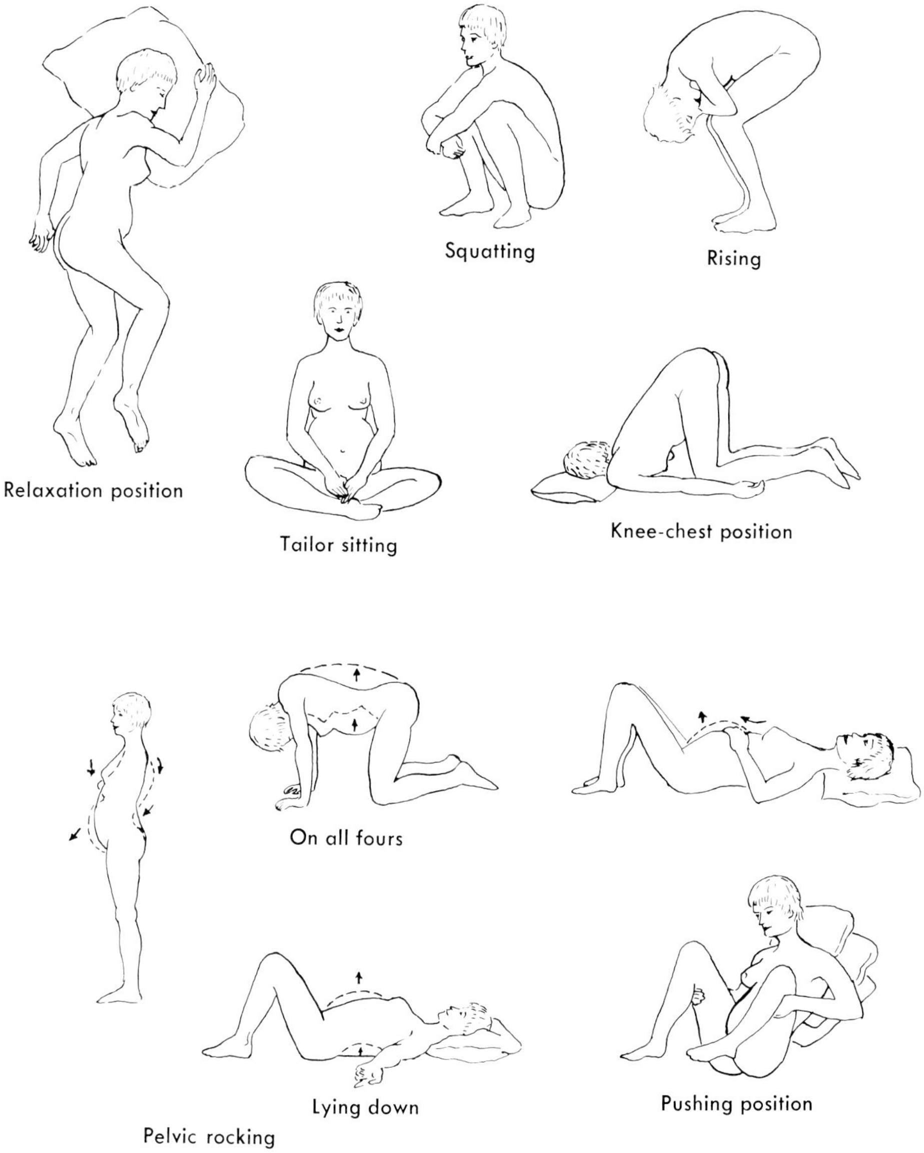

Fig. 4-9. Exercises for prenatal period. In the relaxation position all dependent parts are supported. Pelvic rock (which can be done standing, lying down, or on all fours) is very helpful in relieving backache. Squatting and tailor-sitting help to stretch perineal muscles. (From Hamilton, P.M.: Basic maternity nursing, ed. 4, St. Louis, 1979, The C.V. Mosby Co.)

unless absolutely essential for her health. The nurse can help the family or the single woman decide how to continue working but avoid becoming overtired.

NUTRITION

BASIC NUTRITIONAL NEEDS DURING PREGNANCY

An increase in the incidence of low birth weight babies and prematurity is directly related to an inadequate diet in pregnancy. Maternity texts prior to 1970 often discussed restricting weight gain in pregnancy and even described low calorie diets for the overweight pregnant woman. In 1970, the National Academy of Sciences issued a report stating that the nutrition of the mother directly affects the status of the infant; since this report, the emphasis on little or no weight gain in pregnancy has changed to concern for adequate nutrition in pregnancy, which often leads to a weight gain of 24 to 28 pounds, even in already overweight women.

The primary goal of nutritional management for any prenatal woman should be the optimal growth and development of the fetus! Families should be instructed in how to follow the new revised daily food guide (Table 4-1).

We speak in terms of RDAs (Recommended Dietary Allowances), which are defined as "levels of intake of essential nutrients considered, in the judgment of the Food and Nutrition Board on the basis of available scientific knowledge, to be adequate to meet the known nutritional needs of practically all healthy persons" (Tables 4-2 and 4-3).

Table 4-1. Revised daily food guide based on seven "index nutrients"

Food group	Number of servings		
	Nonpregnant woman	Pregnant woman	Lactating woman
Protein foods			
Animal*	2	2	2
Vegetable†	2	2	2
Milk and milk products	2	4	5
Breads and cereals	4	4	4
Vitamin C–rich fruits and vegetables	1	1	1
Dark green vegetables	1	1	1
Other fruits and vegetables	1	1	1

*One serving is two ounces (60 grams).
†Should include at least one legume.

Table 4-2. Recommended daily dietary allowances for pregnancy*

	Age			
	11-14	15-18	19-22	23-50
Body size				
Weight				
kg	46	55	55	55
lb	101	120	120	120
Height				
cm	157	163	163	163
in	62	64	64	64
Nutrients				
Energy, kcal	2700	2400	2400	2300
Protein, gm	76	76	74	74
Vitamin A, RE[1]	1000	1000	1000	1000
Vitamin D, μg[2]	15	15	12.5	10
Vitamin E, α TE[3]	10	10	10	10
Ascorbic Acid, mg	70	80	80	80
Folacin, μg	800	800	800	800
Niacin, mg[4]	17	16	16	15
Riboflavin, mg	1.6	1.6	1.6	1.5
Thiamin, mg	1.5	1.5	1.5	1.4
Vitamin B_6, mg	2.4	2.6	2.6	2.6
Vitamin B_{12}, μg	4.0	4.0	4.0	4.0
Calcium, mg	1600	1600	1200	1200
Phosphorus, mg	1600	1600	1200	1200
Iodine, μg	175	175	175	175
Iron, mg[5]	18+	18+	18+	18+
Magnesium, mg	450	450	450	450
Zinc, mg	20	20	20	20

*Adopted from Food and Nutrition Board, National Research Council, National Academy of Sciences, *Recommended Dietary Allowances,* Washington, D.C., 1979.
[1]RE = Retinol equivalent; IU = International Unit. The recommended unit of measure is RE. 1 RE = 10 IU. 1 RE = 1 μg retinol or 6 μg β-carotene.
[2]As cholecalciferol. 10 μg cholecalciferol = 400 IU vitamin D.
[3]α TE = α-tocopherol equivalent. 1 α TE = 1 mg d-α-tocopherol.
[4]Although allowances are expressed as niacin, it is recognized that on the average 1 mg of niacin is derived from each 60 mg of dietary tryptophan.
[5]This increased requirement for pregnancy cannot be met by ordinary diets; therefore, the use of supplemental iron is recommended.

The old outdated basic four food guide (based on 1953 RDA findings) is as follows:

1. Milk
2. Meat
3. Vegetables and fruits
4. Breads and cereals

It has several disadvantages:

1. It is meant as a foundation diet but is often taken to mean basic and *complete* nutrition.
2. It does not supply 100% of current RDA even when quality foods are added. Since 1953 the RDAs for calcium, vitamin A, vitamin C, and some B vitamins have changed. Recommendations have been added for magnesium, zinc, iodine, phosphorus, folacin, vitamin E, vitamin B_6, and vitamin B_{12}.
3. Nutrients may be present in different quantities or proportions in different foods within the same group. (For example, in the vegetables and fruit group, green beans and corn contain less vitamin A and vitamin C and folacin than do broccoli and collards.)
4. Many manufactured foods do not fit into any of the four groups.

Table 4-3. Recommended daily dietary allowances for lactation*

	Age			
	11-14	**15-18**	**19-22**	**23-50**
Body size				
Weight				
kg	46	55	55	55
lb	101	120	120	120
Height				
cm	157	163	163	163
in	62	64	64	64
Nutrients				
Energy, kcal	2900	2600	2600	2500
Protein, gm	66	66	64	64
Vitamin A, RE[1]	1200	1200	1200	1200
Vitamin D, μg[2]	15	15	12.5	10
Vitamin E, α TE[3]	11	11	11	11
Ascorbic acid, mg	90	100	100	100
Folacin, μg	500	500	500	500
Niacin, mg[4]	20	19	19	18
Riboflavin, mg	1.8	1.8	1.8	1.7
Thiamin, mg	1.6	1.6	1.6	1.5
Vitamin B_6, mg	2.3	2.5	2.5	2.5
Vitamin B_{12}, μg	4.0	4.0	4.0	4.0
Calcium, mg	1600	1600	1200	1200
Phosphorus, mg	1600	1200	1200	1200
Iodine, μg	200	200	200	200
Iron, mg[5]	18	18	18	18
Magnesium, mg	450	450	450	450
Zinc, mg	25	25	25	25

*Adopted from Food and Nutrition Board, National Research Council, National Academy of Sciences, *Recommended Dietary Allowances,* Washington, D.C., 1979.

[1]RE = Retinol equivalent; IU = International Unit. The recommended unit of measure is RE. 1 RE = 10 IU. 1 RE = 1 μg retinol or 6 μg β-carotene.

[2]As cholecalciferol. 10 μg cholecalciferol = 400 IU vitamin D.

[3]α TE = α-tocopherol equivalent. 1 α TE = 1 mg d-α-tocopherol.

[4]Although allowances are expressed as niacin, it is recognized that on the average 1 mg of niacin is derived from each 60 mg of dietary tryptophan.

[5]Continued use of supplemental iron for 2 to 3 months after parturition is advisable to replenish stores depleted by pregnancy.

The seven "index nutrients" identified in the revised daily food guide (Table 4-1) are described as follows. (Numbers in parentheses define the size of one serving.)

Protein foods include meat, poultry, fish (2 ounces), eggs (2); beans (1 cup cooked); nut butters (¼ cup), or nuts and seeds (½ cup); tofu (1 cup); or cottage cheese (½ cup). These foods build tissues in the baby and mother. They contain iron, protein, zinc, and many other nutrients.

Milk and milk products include nonfat, lowfat, or whole milk (1 cup); plain yogurt (1 cup); soymilk or tofu (1 cup); cheese (1½ to 2 ounces); nonfat milk powder (⅓ cup). Calcium builds healthy bones and teeth. The vitamins A and D and protein also make the baby healthy.

Breads and cereals include bread, rolls (1 slice); macaroni, rice, noodles (½ cup); hot cereal (½ cup); cold cereal (1 ounce); wheat germ (1 tablespoon). B vitamins for strong blood and nerves, iron and trace minerals, and natural fiber are present in breads and cereals.

Vitamin C–rich foods include orange or grapefruit juice (½ cup); 1 orange or ½ grapefruit; bell peppers, greens, tomato, cantaloupe, broccoli, cabbage, cauliflower (1 cup). Do not substitute artificially flavored canned fruit drinks. Vitamin C (ascorbic acid) develops and maintains connective tissue and improves normal connective tissue resistance to infection and disease.

Dark green vegetables include broccoli, Brussels sprouts, asparagus, cabbage, greens, red leaf or romaine lettuce, bok choy, watercress (1 cup raw or ¾ cup cooked). They provide folacin and iron for blood, vitamin A for soft skin and good eyesight, and vitamins E, C, K and natural fiber.

Other fruits and vegetables include all the others and their juices, such as apples, carrots, bananas, sweet potatoes, green beans (about ½ cup). Fruits and vegetables contain many different, healthy nutrients in various amounts. In addition, fats and oils should be used in moderation.

Daily guidelines call for 74-76 grams of protein, 2300 calories for those pregnant women between the ages of 23 and 50, 2700 calories for those pregnant females under age 15.

Families should be advised that a 24-pound weight gain during pregnancy is minimum. Such weight gains are associated with the lowest incidence of pre-eclampsia, low birth weight, and perinatal mortality. Pregnant women should *never* use weight reduction regimens! Restricting weight gain can cause maternal fat stores to be catabolized for energy, which results in ketonemia. Ketone bodies can be transported across the placental barrier. Ketosis is poorly tolerated by the fetus, and fetal acidosis can cause congenital anomalies and brain damage in the infant.

From 400 to 800 milligrams of folic acid is recommended as a daily supplement to help prevent the onset of megaloblastic anemia; from 30 to 60 milligrams of elemental iron is recommended as a daily supplement to prevent iron deficiency anemia.

Instead of sodium restriction in pregnancy, the use of iodized salt in moderation is recommended today. It has been recognized that women actually need more sodium in pregnancy than during the nonpregnant state. To maintain fluid balance and osmotic integrity when sodium is retained, water must be retained in pregnancy as well. This retained water contributes to the pregnant woman's weight gain. No longer are diuretics prescribed during pregnancy.

In addition to counseling pregnant families on the changes in approach to nutrition in pregnancy, the nurse needs to determine first what their diet is now. A nutrition questionnaire in addition to a diet interview and counseling session is very helpful here. The family can take the questionnaire home, discuss it, and complete it together. This exercise in itself is self-instructional. Also, the costs of foods should be discussed and appropriate alternatives to high-priced foods found.

The pregnant adolescent presents special problems in nutrition counseling because she frequently eats "junk food," and, in fact, may exist on colas, hamburgers, and french fries.

Early pregnancy classes (see Unit V) are an excellent way to discuss nutrition in pregnancy as well as common discomforts, sexuality, and ways to cope. When counseling any pregnant family, the nurse must keep in mind their attitudes, past experiences with foods, cultural influences on diet, and social, religious, and ethnic influences.

Many people do not consume adequate supplies of milk, which leads to an inadequate calcium and vitamin D (and possibly riboflavin) intake. One quart of milk supplies 100% of the daily requirements of calcium and vitamin D and almost 50% of the protein needed in one day. However, in the U.S., over two thirds of blacks, Latinos, Native Americans, Ashkenazic Jews, and Asians are lactose intolerant. Lactose is a constituent of milk, and lactose intolerance is the inability to digest and absorb lactose (a sugar) because of low level activity of the enzyme lactase. Symptoms of lactose intolerance are abdominal distention, discomfort, cramps and pain, loose stools, flatulence, and watery, fermentive acid diarrhea.

Persons who are lactose intolerant should (1) avoid milk and other dairy products except for hard or more aged cheese, such as Swiss and cheddar. These have less lactose than other types and can sometimes be tolerated in small amounts. Very cold milk may be tolerated; also cultured forms of milk, such as acidophilus milk and yogurt, are often tolerated by persons who are lactose intolerant. (2) Calcium and vitamin D supplements can be used. Phosphorus must always be present in the diet to balance calcium intake. (3) Protein foods should also be increased.

It is beyond the scope of this book to present detailed diets for all ethnic and religious groups; however, the California State Department of Public Health has published an excellent pamphlet on this subject (see Bibliography at the end of this unit).

COMMON DISCOMFORTS

COMMON DISCOMFORTS OF PREGNANCY AND WAYS TO ALLEVIATE THEM

Many of the symptoms that cause discomfort and concern can be alleviated and most will disappear as the months pass. For most women and their families a simple explanation of the cause of the discomfort and ways to possibly prevent it or to cope with it help tremendously in their acceptance and subsequent solution of the problem. Just knowing that the symptoms are not all psychological and that they will go away is very reassuring. The chart that follows summarizes these common discomforts, and suggests prevention and coping methods.

Discomfort	Prevention and coping
Nausea and vomiting	1. Eat six small meals a day. Avoid any food that might normally make you ill. Stay away from greasy, spicy food or foods that are hard to digest. 2. Drink a glass of milk before going to bed in order to have a source of some protein in the body before arising. 3. Leave crackers or juice at bedside to nibble on before getting out of bed. Have someone fix tea with honey or prepare food to be brought to you in bed. 4. Carry snacks in purse to anticipate times of nausea. 5. Try substituting crushed ice or sherbet for liquids. 6. Try separating intake of solids and liquids. 7. Try these measures and if still unable to cope with the situation consult your physician. *Do not* take home remedies or drugs without your physician's advice.
Heartburn	1. Frequent small feedings. 2. Avoid fatty foods and foods that produce gas. 3. Eat slowly. 4. Avoid eating just before bedtime.

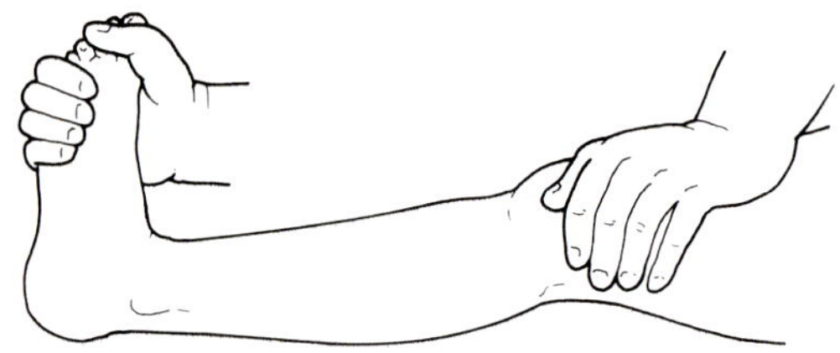

Fig. 4-10. To relieve leg cramps.

Constipation	1. Increase fluid intake. 2. Increase roughage intake (coarse cereal, whole wheat bread, leafy vegetables, salads, bran). 3. Regular unhurried bowel movements. 4. Increase physical activity. 5. Laxative may be prescribed if absolutely necessary.
Flatulence	1. Avoid gas-forming foods. 2. Regular bowel movements. 3. Increase physical activity.
Fatigue	1. Treat the symptom and rest when possible. 2. An afternoon nap is nice if convenient. 3. Laying your head down on your desk at work or elevating your feet when possible also helps. 4. An early bedtime will probably be a necessity.
Backache	1. Correct posture and exercise help most of all. 2. Bedboards under mattress may also help. 3. Massage and hot or cold packs.
Leg cramps	1. Increasing consumption of foods high in calcium may be helpful. 2. Straighten leg and force toes upward; push knee down (Fig. 4-10).
Pain in lower pelvis	1. Elevating feet and hips may help. 2. Pelvic rock. 3. Pelvic floor tightening.
Varicose veins	1. Stay off feet as much as possible. 2. Put legs up higher than hips. 3. Avoid tight garments such as girdles or supporters. 4. Avoid crossing legs, knees, or ankles. 5. If any redness, local soreness, or warmth develops in the veins, notify physician immediately.
Vaginal discharge	1. Liberally cleanse external genitalia with mild soap and water. 2. Seek medical help if irritation and itching are severe.
Itching and dry skin	1. Bathe with mild soap. 2. Use lotions.
Swelling of feet	1. Elevate legs and feet for short periods during day.
Excessive salivation	1. Treatment is limited. 2. Suck hard candy. 3. Chew gum. 4. Avoid starches.
Dyspnea (shortness of breath)	1. Sleep with head of bed elevated. 2. Stand and sit tall, head erect, shoulders slightly back.
Increased perspiration	1. Bathe frequently.

BREAST FEEDING

Unfortunately, many women who enter the hospital to give birth are still ambivalent about whether or not to breast feed. Research has shown that nurses and physicians can greatly influence a woman's decision. The prenatal period is the time to discuss the pros and cons of breast feeding and to assist the family in making a decision. Once again, the early pregnancy classes (Unit V) are an excellent place to start. However, during the antepartum period you can begin encouraging the woman and her family to think about how they will feed the baby. Try to find out what breast feeding means to the woman and her mate. Breasts are considered a sex symbol in our culture and frequently modesty says, "Keep them covered." For women and men who have a high degree of sexual anxiety, it may be more socially acceptable to bottle feed. Although breast feeding is recommended for healthy mothers and full-term infants, the mother should want to breast feed and should have support from her mate and family or a primary group such as the La Leche League. In helping the family, the following information may be useful:

LIST ADVANTAGES OF BREAST AND FORMULA FEEDING

Breast	Formula
Nutritional aspects	
1. Easily digested. 2. Uniquely suited to baby. 3. Colostrum = laxative. 4. Lower solute load. 5. More unsaturated fatty acids.	1. Cow's milk provides adequate amounts of vitamin A, thiamine, and riboflavin. 2. Formulas today simulate human milk.
Allergies	
May reduce allergic responses in infants.	
Immunological aspects	
Immunoglobulins supply antiviral and antibacterial antibodies to protect baby from certain diseases.	
Psychological aspects	
1. Prolactin (nature's own transquilizer) is active in breast feeding. 2. Creates closeness (skin-to-skin) between mother and baby.	1. Will not have to expose breasts. 2. Can hold baby close. 3. May be a tendency to overfeed, thus causing obesity problems in later life.
Economy	
1. Requires no buying of formula.	1. Will cost money. 2. Need bottles and supplies as well as formulas.
Safety	
1. Clean. 2. Not easily contaminated.	1. Can be contaminated.
Convenience	
1. No bottles to prepare.	1. Premixed formulas and disposable bottles are available.
Family	
1. Instant and natural sex education for older children. 2. Woman should not take oral contraceptives while breast feeding.	1. Other family members can feed baby. 2. Mother can take oral contraceptives.

If the family decides on breast feeding, it may be helpful to begin preparation of the breasts in the last few months of the antepartum period (see Figs. 4-11 to 4-13).

DESCRIBE THE CARE OF BREASTS IN PREPARATION FOR BREAST FEEDING

DANGER SIGNS IN PREGNANCY

DANGER SIGNS THAT MAY INDICATE COMPLICATIONS OF PREGNANCY THAT SHOULD BE REPORTED TO A PHYSICIAN

Alert the mother to report immediately any sign of the following:

1. Bleeding from the vagina
2. Swelling of face and fingers
3. Severe continuous headache
4. Blurring of vision
5. Pain in the abdomen
6. Persistent vomiting
7. Chills and fever
8. Sudden escape of a large amount of fluid from vagina
9. Scant urine

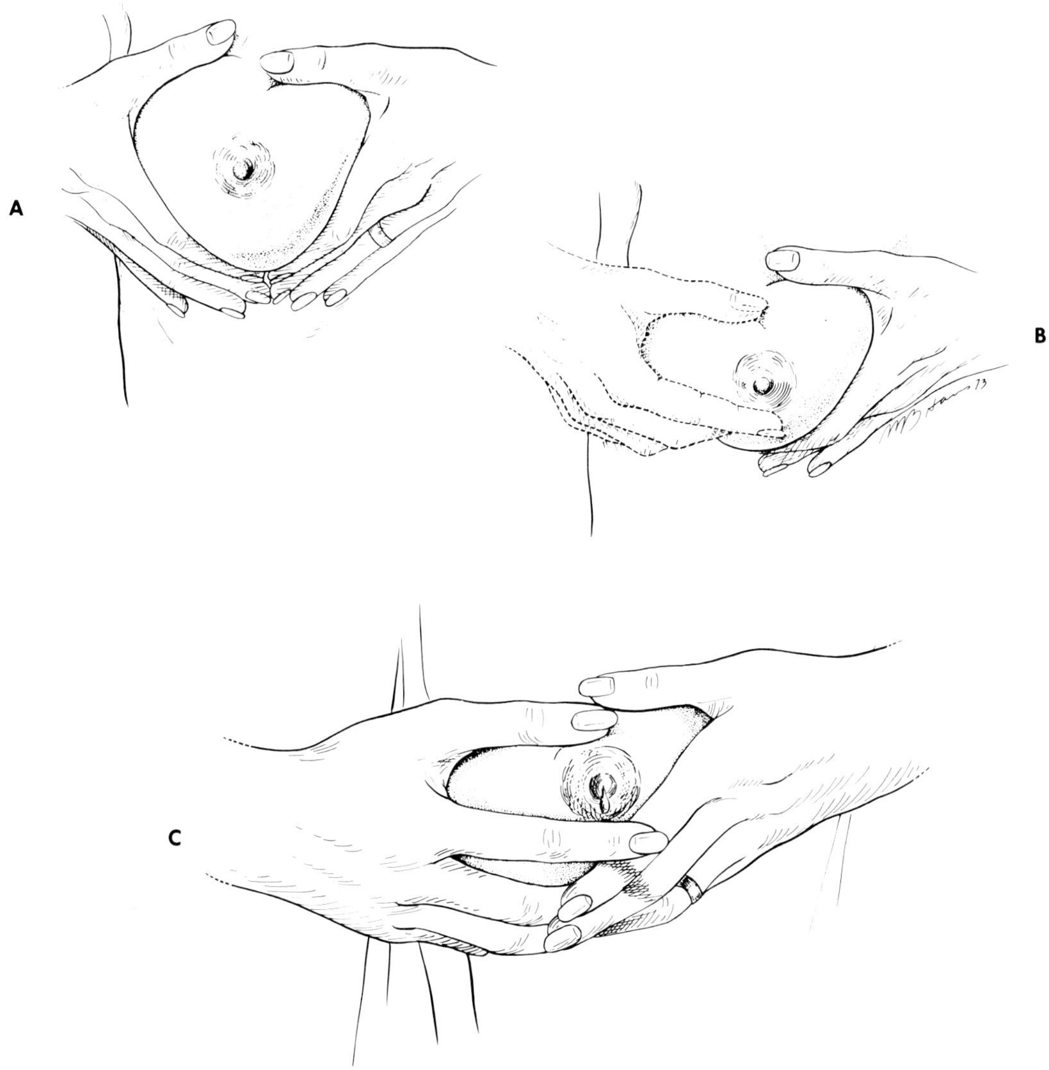

Fig. 4-11. Massaging and manual expression. (From Lerch, C., and Bliss, V.J.: Maternity nursing, ed. 3, St. Louis, 1978, The C.V. Mosby Co.)

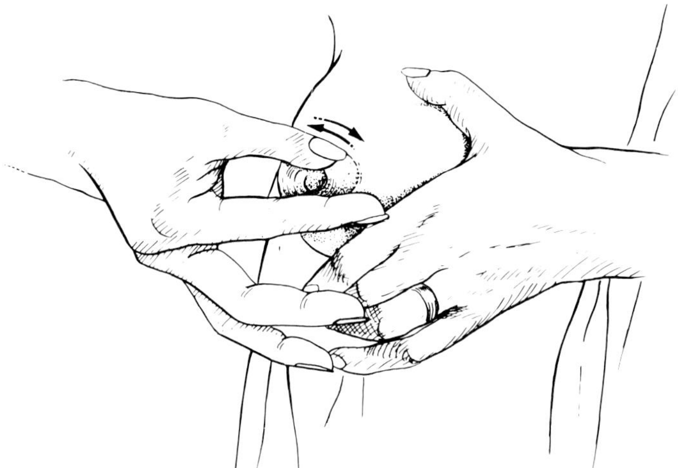

Fig. 4-12. Nipple rolling. (From Lerch, C., and Bliss, V.J.: Maternity nursing, ed. 3, St. Louis, 1978, The C.V. Mosby Co.)

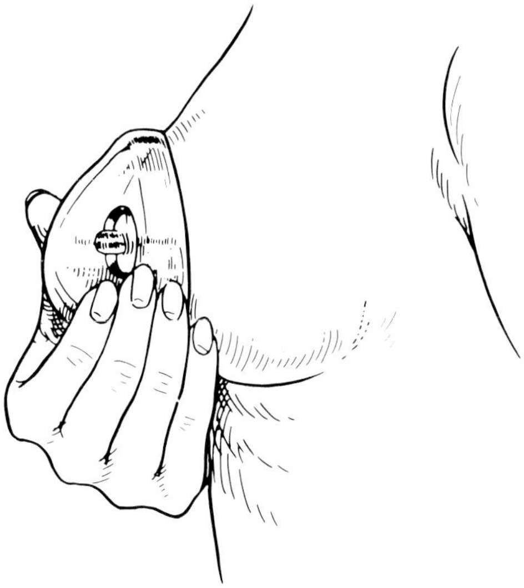

Fig. 4-13. Netsy milk cup. (From Lerch, C., and Bliss, V.J.: Maternity nursing, ed. 3, St. Louis, 1978, The C.V. Mosby Co.)

SUMMARY

Unit IV has concentrated on providing safe care for the pregnant family. Such care identifies psychologic and physical problems early so that they may be managed by the health care team and the family. An environment in which the family feels free to discuss any and all problems is essential. To this point, only the low-risk antepartum family has been considered. The high-risk antepartum family is discussed in Unit V.

BIBLIOGRAPHY

Berger, K.J., and Fields, W.L.: Pocket guide to health assessment, Reston, Virginia, 1980, Reston Publishing Co., Inc.

Bing, E., and Coleman, L.: Making love during pregnancy, New York, 1980, Bantam Books, Inc.

California State Department of Health, Maternal and Child Health Unit: Nutrition during pregnancy and lactation. Supplement to Standards and recommendations for public prenatal care, California State Department of Public Health, revised 1975.

Cohn, S.D.: Sexuality in pregnancy: a review of the literature, Nurs. Clin. North Am. **17**:91-98, March 1982.

Corruccini, C.G.: Food guidelines: their development, use, and specific changes suggested for "Nutrition During Pregnancy and Lactation," Maternal and Child Health Branch, California State Department of Health, June 1977.

Countryman, B.A.: Hospital care of the breast-fed newborn, Am. J. Nurs. **71**:2365-2367, December 1971.

Haynes, S., Jensen, D., and Rieger, C.: New family . . . new dimensions: a prenatal education manual for nurses, San Jose, Calif., 1976.

Knaff, K.: Conflicting perspectives on breast feeding, Am. J. Nurs. **74**:1848-1851, October 1974.

Kyndely, K.: The sexuality of women in pregnancy and postpartum: a review, J.O.G.N. Nurs. **7**:28-32, Jan./Feb. 1978.

Luke, B.: Lactose intolerance during pregnancy: significance and solutions, MCN **2**:93-96, March/April 1977.

Masters, W.H., and Johnson, V.E.: Human sexual response, Boston, 1966, Little, Brown & Co.

Moore, M.L.: Realities in childbearing, ed. 2, Philadelphia, 1983, W.B. Saunders Co.

Mueller, L.S.: Pregnancy and sexuality, J.O.G.N. Nurs. **14**:289-294, July/August 1985.

Otte, M.J.: Correcting inverted nipples—an aid to breast feeding, Am. J. Nurs. **75**:454-456, March 1975.

Pitkin, R.M., et al.: Maternal nutrition, a selective review of clinical topics, Obstet. Gynecol. **40**:777, Dec. 1972.

Reamy, K., and White, S.E.: Sexuality in pregnancy and the puerperium: a review, Obstet. Gynecol. Surv. **40**:1-13, Jan. 1985.

Rosenberg, F.J.: Lactose intolerance, Am. J. Nurs. **77**:823-824, May 1977.

Williams, S.R.: Nutrition and diet therapy, ed. 4, St. Louis, 1981, The C.V. Mosby Co.
Woods, N.F., and Woods, J.S.: Human sexuality in health and illness, ed. 2, St. Louis, 1979, The C.V. Mosby Co.
Worthington, B.S., and Williams, S.R.: Nutrition in pregnancy and lactation, ed. 2, St. Louis, 1981, The C.V. Mosby Co.

DEFINITIONS

Define the following terms:

antepartum	linca nigra
ballottement	*Monilia*
Braxton-Hicks' contractions	Naegele's rule
Chadwick's sign	Papanicolaou test
chloasma	para
colostrum	plasma
diagonal conjugate	prolactin
dyspnea	psychosocial
Goodell's sign	reflux
gravida	striae gravidarium
Hegar's sign	*Trichomonas vaginalis*
intertuberous diameter	trimester
lactose	true conjugate

LEARNING ACTIVITIES AND EXPERIENCES

1. Work in a pair with another student and practice taking a history with your fellow student assuming the role of a pregnant woman.
2. Plan a diet for a normal pregnant woman. Use a food value chart to analyze the diet for nutritive value. Such a chart is available from the Superintendent of Documents, U.S. Government Printing Office, Washington, D.C. 20402.
3. Determine what agencies or persons are available for pregnancy testing in your community. What are the costs?
4. Make a written 1-day food intake record on yourself, then calculate what changes would be needed if you were a lactating mother.
5. Interview an expectant father in a prenatal clinic. What are his plans for his new role?
6. View audiovisual aids and discuss.

SELF-ASSESSMENT

For questions 1 through 4, determine if the statements are true or false. Fill in the space to the left of the statement by indicating T for true and F for false.

______1. During the first trimester, there is frequently an increase in sexual desire and frequency of sexual intercourse.

______2. Sexual relations (intercourse) during pregnancy are all right unless the woman is uncomfortable.

______3. It is easy for couples to forego sexual activity for 6 weeks before birth and 6 weeks after birth.

______4. During the second trimester there is frequently an increase in sexual desire.

For questions 5 through 18, circle the best answer.

5. Constipation is best relieved by:
   a. regular use of laxatives
   b. maintenance of good posture
   c. increased roughage and fluid in the diet
6. Frequency of urination during early and late pregnancy is often caused by:
   a. decreased activity
   b. increased weight gain
   c. pressure exerted on bladder by uterus
7. Varicosities on the lower extremities in pregnancy are the result of:
   a. increased cardiac load
   b. pressure of the uterus impeding venous return
   c. increased blood volume
8. Weight gain during pregnancy should normally be:
   a. 24 to 28 pounds
   b. 8 to 10 pounds
   c. 12 to 20 pounds
   d. 10 to 15 pounds
9. A positive sign of pregnancy is:
   a. Chadwick's sign
   b. nausea and vomiting
   c. fetal heart sounds
   d. linea negra
10. Which one of these common signs and symptoms associated with pregnancy is a probable sign of pregnancy?
    a. cessation of menses
    b. frequent urination
    c. enlarged and tender breasts
    d. Hegar's sign
11. A positive sign of pregnancy is:
    a. a positive pregnancy test
    b. increase in abdominal size
    c. ballottement
    d. hearing fetal heartbeat

12. A presumptive sign of pregnancy is:
    a. enlargement of the uterus
    b. Braxton-Hicks contractions
    c. fetal heartbeat
    d. cessation of menses
13. Positive motivations for pregnancy include to:
    a. save a relationship
    b. share lives together
    c. please others
14. The pregnancy test is most accurate at the time of the highest level of hCG (human chorionic gonadotropin) in the urine, which is:
    a. 8 to 15 days after a missed period
    b. 2 days after a missed period
    c. 41 days after a missed period
15. Which of the following lunches would be the best for a pregnant woman?
    a. bologna sandwich, potato chips, cola
    b. cottage cheese, tossed salad and cracker, orange, glass of milk
    c. cold chicken, French fries, French roll, milk
    d. bowl of bean soup, crackers, glass of ice tea
16. Using Naegele's rule, if a pregnant woman's last menstrual period began on August 4, 1986, her estimated due date would be nearest:
    a. May 6, 1987
    b. May 11, 1987
    c. June 11, 1987
    d. May 17, 1987
17. A pregnant woman may develop constipation because of:
    a. diminished motility of the gastrointestinal tract
    b. pressure on the intestines from the enlarging uterus
    c. lack of adequate exercise
    d. lack of adequate fluid intake

    Answer (circle one): 1. a, b, and d
    2. c, b, and d
    3. a, b, and c
    4. all of these
18. Improved prenatal care in the U.S. is responsible for:
    a. the population explosion
    b. the increase in pregnancies
    c. dramatically reduced maternal mortality

Supply the correct answer(s) for items 19 through 31.

19. Four aims of prenatal care are:
    a.
    b.
    c.
    d.
20. Advantages of breast feeding include:
    a.
    b.
    c.
21. Define gravida. ______________________________
22. Define para. ______________________________
23. Identify the normal findings for the following three laboratory tests in pregnancy:
    a. Hct (hematocrit) and Hgb (hemoglobin) ______________________________

b. urinalysis
(1) sugar ______________________________
(2) protein ______________________________

24. What are four myths you have heard associated with childbearing and birth?
a.
b.
c.
d.

25. Explain how a nurse can help to reduce a woman's anxiety on her first visit to the physician to confirm pregnancy.

26. What would you suggest for relief of varicose veins?

27. How many servings of each group of food listed below should be included in the pregnant woman's diet daily?
a. milk and milk products ______________________________
b. breads and cereals ______________________________
c. dark green vegetables ______________________________
d. vitamin C–rich fruits and vegetables ______________________________
e. other fruits and vegetables ______________________________
f. protein foods ______________________________

28. What can be done to cope with leg cramps in pregnancy?

29. Preparation of the nipples for breast feeding includes:
a.
b.

30. Advantages of formula feeding include:
a.
b.
c.

31. List nine danger signs of pregnancy:
a.
b.
c.
d.
e.
f.
g.
h.
i.

32. On the line to the left of each item in Column A match the physiologic change occurring in pregnancy with the body system in which that change occurs.

Column A	Column B
______1. respiratory system	a. linea nigra
______2. integumentary system	b. relaxation of pelvic joints
______3. circulatory system	c. depends on prepregnant state
______4. GI system	d. blood volume increase
______5. skeletal system	e. constipation
______6. urinary system	f. enlarging uterus
______7. endocrine system	g. urinary frequency
______8. reproductive system	h. difficulty breathing
	i. increase in basal metabolic rate

For questions 33 through 38, fill in the blanks:

33. Wearing high-heeled shoes in pregnancy may cause ______________________________.

34. When a pregnant woman's feet swell at the end of the day, the edema is probably the result of ______________________________.

35. If a pregnant woman's hands and face are swollen in addition to her feet, you would ____.

36. When washing her breasts, a pregnant woman should not use ______________ on her nipples, since it has a tendency to dry them.

37. The blood volume ________ but the hemoglobin ________ during pregnancy.

38. A woman is $G_5P_4Ab_1$; this means she has been pregnant ________ times, has delivered ________ children, and has had ________ abortions.

UNIT V
The antepartum family with complications

GOALS

This unit is designed to provide the reader with information that will:

□ promote awareness of deviations from normal in the antepartum period.
□ explore the nursing role in common complications in the antepartum period.

STUDENT OBJECTIVES

After studying this unit, you should be able to:

1. Indicate at least two factors in each of the following categories that classify a woman as high risk in pregnancy: (1) general physical, social, and demographic factors, (2) past complications associated with pregnancy, (3) complications of current pregnancy, and (4) coexistent medical-surgical-psychiatric disorders.
2. Design a plan to illustrate how the nurse can help the high-risk family adapt to the tasks necessary during illness in pregnancy.
3. Briefly describe signs and symptoms of hypertensive states in pregnancy and describe nursing responsibilities.
4. Explain the causes of Rh incompatibility, types of treatment available (before and after birth), and nursing responsibilities with families who have Rh incompatibilities.
5. Distinguish between the meaning of the term *abortion* to the layperson and to professional health personnel.
6. Plan supportive nursing care for women experiencing the three common causes of bleeding problems in early pregnancy.
7. Discuss the significance of diabetes to pregnancy.
8. Describe five common diagnostic tests used in high-risk maternity care and the nursing responsibilities in preparing the family for these tests:
   a. ultrasonography
   b. amniocentesis
   c. estriol test
   d. contraction stress test (CST)
   e. nonstress test (NST)

Unit I discussed a two-tiered maternity model, designating two levels of care: (1) normal (a simple, humanistic model for healthy women and their families) and (2) high risk (a more complex but still humanistic model for women with medical complications and/or complications of pregnancy, and their families). Also mentioned was the concept of regionalization of nursing care, which provides levels of care appropriate for each level of the childbearing population.

This unit will introduce you to the high-risk population for whom, ideally, the regional center would provide care.

IDENTIFICATION OF THE HIGH-RISK MOTHER

A high-risk pregnancy is one in which the prospects for optimal outcome for either the mother or the fetus are reduced. High-risk mothers and infants have a greater incidence of morbidity and mortality than the general population of mothers and infants. A pregnancy is classified as high risk if certain conditions are present that have been identified as dangerous to the health and life of the mother and infant. These conditions include:

FACTORS THAT CLASSIFY A WOMAN AS HIGH RISK IN PREGNANCY

1. General physical, social, and demographic factors
2. Coexistent medical-surgical-psychiatric disorders
3. Past complications associated with pregnancy
4. Complications of current pregnancy

The following factors contribute to reproductive risk. The presence of any one or more of these factors merits further assessment and evaluation.

1. General physical, social, and demographic factors:
   a. Maternal age of 15 years or younger
   b. Maternal age of 35 years or older
   c. Markedly underweight or overweight
   d. High parity
   e. Small maternal size (under 5 feet)
   f. Poor socioeconomic status
   g. Lack of prenatal care
   h. Inadequate human support resources
   i. Continual presence of stressful situations
   j. Teratogen exposure (radiation, drugs, chemicals, viral infections)
   k. Emotional and/or psychological disorders
   l. Maternal social habits (drug ingestion, alcohol consumption, cigarette smoking)
   m. Family history of hereditary disease or congenital anomaly
   n. Some cultural and ethnic practices
2. *Coexistent medical-surgical-psychiatric disorders:*
   a. Infertility of more than 2 years duration
   b. Genital tract abnormalities
   c. Chronic medical disease that adversely affects general health of mother:
      i. cardiac
      ii. vascular
      iii. respiratory
      iv. neurologic
      v. chronic hypertension
      vi. chronic renal problems
      vii. diabetes
      viii. thyroid disease
      ix. hematologic disorders
      x. malignancy
   d. Psychiatric disturbances
   e. Drug addiction or alcoholism
   f. Infection (maternal and neonatal)
   g. Parental rejection of pregnancy, particularly maternal
   h. Major family upheaval or stress
3. *Past complications associated with pregnancy: Maternal*
   a. Previous premature labor
   b. Previous cesarean or midforceps delivery
   c. Borderline or contracted pelvis
   d. Premature delivery with incompetent cervix

e. Previous pre-eclampsia or eclampsia
f. Prior fetal malpresentation
g. Medical indication for termination of prior pregnancy

Infant

a. Previous stillborn or neonatal loss
b. Two or more spontaneous abortions
c. Previous infants who were excessively large (over 4000 grams) or excessively small (under 2500 grams)
d. Known congenital or familial problems
e. Previous infant requiring special neonatal intensive care

4. *Complications of current pregnancy:*
   a. Suspected ectopic pregnancy
   b. Suspected abortion
   c. Suspected trophoblastic disease
   d. Anemia
   e. Hyperemesis gravidarum
   f. Infections (maternal or fetal)
   g. Diabetes of pregnancy
   h. Pregnancy-induced hypertension (PIH)
   i. Inappropriate fetal growth
   j. Hemorrhage (maternal or fetal)
   k. Hydramnios
   l. Abruptio placentae
   m. Placenta previa
   n. Rh isoimmunization
   o. Multiple pregnancy
   p. Malpresentation of fetus
   q. Premature rupture of membranes
   r. Premature labor
   s. Postdate pregnancy (gestation of longer than 42 weeks)
   t. Dysfunctional labor
   u. Intrauterine fetal demise

Risk scoring

Risk scoring in pregnancy helps to identify those pregnancies that have a significantly greater statistical risk of perinatal morbidity and mortality. As a result, those women identified may receive appropriate management. Numerous attempts have been made to quantify obstetrical risk. The usual approach uses scoring systems that range from 100 factors to 5 or 10 factors that identify pregnancies of low, high, or extreme risk. An example of a risk scoring system is integrated into Hollister's maternal/newborn Record System.

Reasons for avoidance of prenatal care

STATE SEVERAL REASONS WHY WOMEN DO NOT SEEK PRENATAL CARE

A study was undertaken at the University of Nebraska Hospital in the latter half of the 1960s to determine why mothers did not seek prenatal care. In a sample of 64 mothers, approximately 30% felt that prenatal care was not important; however, 70% of the women had very real reasons for not availing themselves of prenatal care on an "ability to pay" schedule. Problems cited were:

1. Babysitter problems
2. Financial problems
3. Newness to community
4. Transportation problems

5. Working during clinic hours
6. Fear
7. Other

Frequently, clinics serving the poor offer fragmented, depersonalized care with long waiting periods (often all day) in crowded, unattractive, depressed surroundings. Prenatal clinics are usually open during the same hours women and their families must work; to complicate the issue even more, these clinics are often geographically distant from the women's homes. It is also important to remember that acceptance of preventive prenatal health care may be incompatible with people's cultural beliefs and practices.

These social factors offer a challenge to health care providers. When the University of Nebraska Hospital improved the services to indigent women as a result of the survey cited, there was a significant reduction in the numbers of women who did not seek prenatal care.

According to recent studies, preventive health programs that provide prenatal care have been found to be cost-effective. Because these programs reduce the incidence of infant mortality and low-birth-weight babies, the additional costs of providing comprehensive care are more than recovered. It is possible to change the grim statistics. Comprehensive prenatal care that includes prenatal education and supplemental nutrition programs for low-income pregnant women can significantly improve pregnancy outcome.

Preparatory tasks

HOW THE NURSE CAN HELP THE HIGH-RISK FAMILY ADAPT TO THE TASKS NECESSARY DURING ILLNESS IN PREGNANCY

As stated in Unit I, the following preparatory tasks should be completed by the parents-to-be in preparing for the birth: (1) acceptance of the pregnancy, (2) establishment of a bond with the fetus, and (3) adjustment to the role of change of woman (daughter) and man (son) to mother and father.

The high-risk mother and family must work through all of these normal preparatory tasks of pregnancy and also those tasks necessary during conditions deviating from normal. Because pregnancy represents a major life change, it is a period of crisis even for the normal family. When the high-risk condition is added, there is a serious crisis for this family because they must also cope with an uncertain outcome.

Nursing care

The nurse can be extremely helpful to the high-risk family by actively listening to their concerns; by being sure they understand the reasons for all the tests, treatments, and medicines used; and by being open and honest, giving no false assurances or promises. During hospitalization, the nurse can help by giving the woman and her family a chance to control their environment and by helping them prepare for the baby with feeding plans and care instructions for the high-risk infant. It is often difficult for high-risk families to establish a bond with the fetus because the outcome of the pregnancy is so uncertain. It is not unusual for them to come to the hospital without baby clothes or articles to care for the baby. They may not even choose a name for the baby until they are certain the baby will live.

The danger signals during pregnancy are listed in Unit IV. Take a few minutes to review that list.

MAJOR COMPLICATIONS OF PREGNANCY

Hypertensive states of pregnancy can be classified as follows:

1. Pre-eclampsia/eclampsia (pregnancy-induced hypertension—PIH). Accounts for 70% to 75% of hypertensive disorders of pregnancy.
2. Chronic hypertension. Accounts for 15% to 20% of hypertension disorders of pregnancy.
3. Chronic hypertension with superimposed PIH. Accounts for 6% of hypertensive disorders of pregnancy.

Pre-eclampsia

SIGNS AND SYMPTOMS OF HYPERTENSIVE STATES IN PREGNANCY

Pre-eclampsia is a condition occurring after the twentieth week of pregnancy in 6% to 7% of all pregnancies. Pre-eclampsia is characterized by edema, hypertension, and proteinuria. The term *toxemia* has been used to describe pre-eclampsia and eclampsia but is now considered obsolete because no toxin has yet been found to be the cause of this syndrome.

Pathophysiology. Although the most current tenable theory involves a disorder of prostaglandin synthesis, the etiology of pre-eclampsia remains obscure. Pre-eclampsia occurs primarily during first pregnancies in women under 20 or over 35 years of age. Factors associated with risk include multiple pregnancy, vascular disease, polyhydramnios, hydatidiform mole, malnutrition, inadequate prenatal care, poor health care, and family history of pre-eclampsia, eclampsia, or hypertension. In pregnancy-induced hypertension, a generalized spasm of the arteries causes a gradual rise in blood pressure and results in decreased blood flow to the kidneys, uterus, liver, and eventually the brain. There is also decreased plasma volume with most of the fluid in the extracellular spaces, resulting in an increased hematocrit. A further complicating factor is central nervous system (CNS) irritability evident first as jitteriness, hyperactive reflexes, and visual disturbances. CNS irritability can eventually lead to seizures.

Mild pre-eclampsia. In mild pre-eclampsia there is an elevation in blood pressure of 30 mmHg systolic and/or 15mmHg diastolic over the woman's usual blood pressure observed on two or more occasions 6 hours apart with the woman at rest. (A blood pressure of 140/90 usually arouses concern and indicates the need for further evaluation.) In addition, there is abnormal fluid retention, generalized edema, and weight gain of more than 2 pounds per week. Proteinuria of 1+ or greater may be found on a clean catch urine specimen.

The primary objectives of treatment are (1) prevention of convulsions, (2) control of blood pressure, and (3) safe delivery of a viable infant. Treatment usually includes bed rest in the left lateral position and close observation and recording of baseline reflexes, urine protein, intake and output, blood pressure, daily weight, and fetal status. Close medical supervision, perhaps requiring sedation, and instruction of the woman and her family concerning diet and treatment regimens are essential. The nurse can be a great help in counseling the woman on the importance of strict adherence to the prescribed treatment by making sure she understands the treatment.

Severe pre-eclampsia. If mild pre-eclampsia is not checked, the woman's blood pressure may be recorded at 160/110 or above on two or more observations 6 hours apart. Proteinuria will be equal to or greater than 3+ or 4+ on routine urinalysis and the edema will worsen. At this point there may be cerebral or visual disturbances and oliguria of 400 ml or less per 24 hours. Treatment for severe pre-eclampsia includes hospitalization with strict bed rest, sedation, a high-protein diet without added salt, and close monitoring of fetal well-being.

Nursing care. Nursing care becomes extremely important for cases of severe pre-eclampsia and includes the following (1) placing the woman in a quiet room, padding the bedrails, and keeping the environment quiet; (2) weighing the woman daily; (3) monitoring fluid intake and output hourly; (4) administering medications according to the physician's orders; (5) having eclamptic precautions ready (for example, padded tongue blade, seizure medicines, O_2); (6) checking urine for protein; (7) collecting any other necessary laboratory specimens: (8) checking patellar reflexes and clonus at least four times daily and inquiring about other symptoms such as epigastric pain, headache, and visual disturbance; (9) checking blood pressure every 4 hours; (10) monitoring fetal well-being; and (11) accurately recording and immediately reporting any sudden deviations from the baseline in any of the areas outlined to observe.

This family will be anxious and probably very worried about the pregnancy outcome. There may be problems such as financial and child care needs that must be addressed as the nurse helps to alleviate the woman's anxiety. The contributions of the social service member of the health care team may be vital in helping this woman and her family to cope with the crisis of hospitalization, which may be for days or even weeks.

Eclampsia

If the symptoms of pre-eclampsia continue until the woman experiences convulsions, coma, or both, the woman is said to be *eclamptic*. Symptoms and signs suggesting impending eclampsia include epigastric pain; severe headache; confusion and disorientation; visual symptoms such as bright spots, flashes, blurring; increasing acitvity of reflexes, and accelerating hypertension and tremulousness.

Nursing care. The care of an eclamptic woman requires (1) intensive nursing care in a quiet room, (2) hourly recording of vital signs, (3) hourly notation of urine volume (an indwelling catheter), (4) protective care during convulsions, (5) constant fetal monitoring, (6) frequent checking of reflexes, (7) administration of medications as ordered, (8) supportive care of the family, and (9) explanations of treatment and management to the family and to the woman if she is responsive.

An acute psychosis may develop in the eclamptic woman 2 to 3 days following delivery. Eclamptic precautions should be continued after delivery for at least 48 hours, since there is still a danger of convulsions as long as central nervous system irritability exists.

Medical treatment. Medications prescribed to treat pre-eclampsia or eclampsia include:

1. Magnesium sulfate, intravenously or intramuscularly, to prevent or control seizures by decreasing central nervous system irritability
2. Calcium gluconate to reverse magnesium toxicity should it occur
3. Hydralazine (Apresoline) to lower diastolic pressures greater than 110 mmHg
4. The use of diuretics in treating pregnancy-induced hypertension is contraindicated

The specific therapy of eclampsia is delivery, which is often accomplished by induction or cesarean birth when the physician has determined that the infant is better off out of the uterus than in. In eclampsia the rate of maternal mortality may be 5% to 10%. The fetus is usually small for gestational age (SGA) and may die in utero.

In most women signs and symptoms of pregnancy-induced hypertension disappear within the first week following delivery. In counseling on future pregnancies, the family should be informed that if a woman has been eclamptic, she may develop eclampsia in subsequent pregnancies. Of course, the real solution to the problem of eclampsia is prevention. The nurse can be very helpful here in counseling on the importance of prenatal care and a high protein (> 80 gm/day) diet in the pregnancy to help prevent pre-eclampsia.

Chronic hypertensive vascular disease

DIFFERENTIATE BETWEEN THE HYPERTENSIVE STATES IN PREGNANCY

Chronic hypertensive vascular disease includes (1) hypertension known to exist before pregnancy, (2) hypertension discovered before the twentieth week of pregnancy, and (3) hypertension secondary to maternal medical disease (hypertension discovered after the twentieth week of pregnancy). This form of hypertension will also persist for more than 6 weeks postpartum.

Nursing care. The woman with chronic hypertension may have been advised against pregnancy and may have many guilt feelings to work through in addition to carefully following a treatment regimen. In fact, how well the woman and her family accept the antihypertensive treatment regimen may be directly connected to their feelings about the pregnancy. The nurse's support, attentive listening, and teaching can be very helpful in this situation. In hypertensive pregnancies, management of the fetus is of prime importance because it frequently suffers from distress in utero and/or intrauterine growth retardation.

Hypertension with superimposed pre-eclampsia is development of symptoms and findings of pre-eclampsia or eclampsia in a woman with chronic hypertension.

Rh factor

CAUSES OF Rh INCOMPATIBILITY, TYPES OF TREATMENT AVAILABLE, AND NURSING RESPONSIBILITIES WITH FAMILIES WHO HAVE Rh INCOMPATIBILITIES

An Rh-negative woman lacks the D antigen on her red blood cells. When an Rh-negative woman is carrying an Rh-positive baby (the baby's father is Rh positive) as occurs in 10% of all pregnancies, a few fetal red blood cells may enter the mother's circulation during labor or delivery, causing the mother's immune system to produce antibodies against the fetal D antigens. Because fetal and maternal blood normally do not mix during pregnancy, the first Rh-positive infant of an Rh-negative mother usually does not have problems. However, if a few fetal cells of an Rh-positive baby enter the bloodstream of an Rh-negative mother during the birth of the first baby, the mother will be sensitized (formation of serum antibodies). Between 1% and 2% of all Rh-negative women develop anti-D antibodies during their first pregnancy. If this sensitized Rh-negative mother subsequently becomes pregnant with an Rh-positive fetus, the antibodies she has formed cross the placenta, coat the red blood cells of the fetus, and cause their destruction *(erythroblastosis fetalis)*. As the red blood cells are destroyed, the fetus becomes anemic and may go into heart failure. In the most severe form of Rh sensitization, the fetus becomes severely edematous, develops pleural effusion and ascites *(hydrops fetalis)*, and may die in utero or, if born alive, may die in a few days.

Treatment. If the fetus is too immature to survive outside the uterus, it may be given intrauterine transfusions of group O, Rh-negative erythrocytes. The blood type is compatible with that of the mother. The transfusion, which can be repeated often, is given into the peritoneal cavity of the fetus.

Sometimes transfusions are not necessary in erythroblastic infants until 24 hours after birth. When this happens, exchange transfusion of the infant may be done using Rh-negative blood. If Rh-positive blood were used, the anti-Rh positive antibodies already circulating in the infant's blood would destroy the new red cells. Exchanging one set of positive cells for another set of positive cells is not the answer.

Tests. It is possible to determine whether a pregnant woman has anti-Rh positive antibodies (anti-D antibodies) in her blood by tests on her serum during pregnancy. Antibody-titer or anti-Rh titers can be used, as well as the enzyme-linked antiglobulin assay and the acid elution test.

Antenatal prophylaxis. Researchers have shown that prenatal administration of anti-Rh positive globulin (RhoGAM) to Rh-negative pregnant women can reduce the incidence of women sensitized during pregnancy from between 1% and 2% to 0.1%. Established protocols for prenatal prophylaxis recommend administering Rho (D) immune globulin at 28 to 32 weeks of gestation and again within 72 hours after delivery to an Rh-negative mother with no evidence of anti-D antibodies in her bloodstream.

Postpartum treatment. An injection of RhoGAM into Rh-negative mothers within 72 hours after delivery of an Rh-positive infant suppresses the formation of Rh antibodies. To receive RhoGAM, the mother must be Rh negative and have no Rh antibodies in her serum, and the baby must be Rh positive and have a negative direct Coombs test. Once the mother has been sensitized to factor D, RhoGAM is of no value (Fig. 5-1).

Nursing care. The nurse has a very important role in making sure that each woman who should get RhoGAM is treated. Nursing care for the Rh-negative woman and her family also includes recognition of their fears about the uncertain outcome of pregnancy and realistic support and teaching. The woman or man may suffer guilt feelings for having the "wrong" blood type or for even mating at all. The couple needs a chance to work through these feelings if they exist, and the nurse is in an excellent position to afford the childbearing couple the help they need.

ABO incompatibility

A much more common kind of blood incompatibility is *ABO incompatibility*, in which the father is blood type A, B, or AB and the mother is type O. If the fetus inherits the

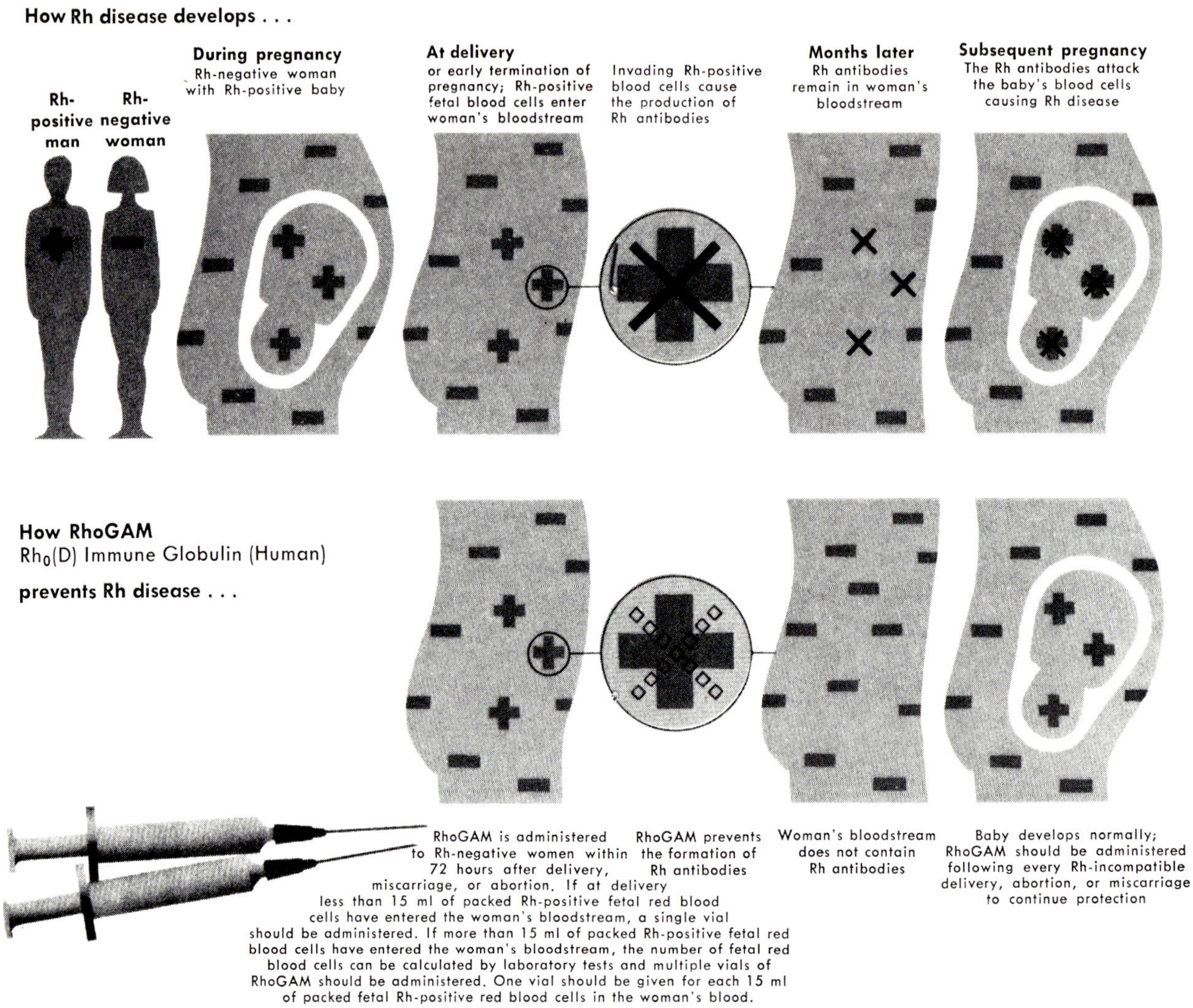

Fig. 5-1. How Rh disease develops and how RhoGAM prevents Rh disease. (Reprinted by permission of Ortho Diagnostics, Inc., Raritan, N.J.)

blood type from the father, fetal blood may cross the placenta and cause the mother to be sensitized to antigens of the foreign blood type. The complications of this type of incompatibility are usually not severe. However, because there is no adequate method of antenatal diagnosis, careful observation is crucial in the neonatal period.

Bleeding in early pregnancy

Any bleeding during pregnancy is abnormal. When bleeding occurs early in pregnancy, the most common causes are abortion, ectopic pregnancy, and hydatidiform mole.

MEANING OF THE TERM *ABORTION* TO THE LAYPERSON AND TO PROFESSIONAL HEALTH PERSONNEL

Abortion. To the layperson, the term *abortion* frequently means inducing the end of pregnancy, and the term *miscarriage* means spontaneous termination of pregnancy. The obstetrical definition of abortion is the termination of pregnancy before the fetus has become viable, which generally occurs at 20 weeks of gestation and 500 grams of weight. The great majority of these abortions occur in the first trimester. Abortion may be *spontaneous* (through natural causes) or *induced* (by mechanical or medical agents).

The types of spontaneous abortion are:

1. *Complete*—spontaneous expulsion of all products of conception.
2. *Incomplete*—partial expulsion of products of conception.
3. *Threatened*—signs and symptoms of abortion present but no passage of tissue from the vagina; this abortion could be reversed.

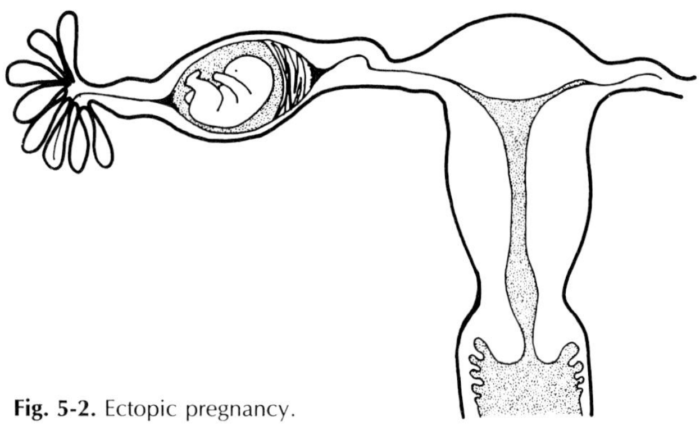

Fig. 5-2. Ectopic pregnancy.

4. *Inevitable*—vaginal bleeding, usually with cramps and dilation of the internal os; cannot be reversed.
5. *Habitual*—abortion of three successive pregnancies.
6. *Missed*—fetal death occurred, but products of conception still in uterus for over 8 weeks.

An induced abortion is the voluntary ending of a pregnancy. An induced abortion may be therapeutic (for medical reasons) or elective (for social reasons).

A *septic abortion* is any abortion complicated by intrauterine infection and fever. Although secondary infections of a spontaneous abortion or induced abortion are possible, criminal induction can be assumed to have taken place in essentially all septic abortions.

IDENTIFY THE SIGNS AND SYMPTOMS OF ECTOPIC PREGNANCY

Ectopic pregnancy. An *ectopic pregnancy* is any pregnancy occurring outside the uterine cavity. The most common cause is previous pelvic inflammatory disease (PID). Of all pregnancies that occur outside the uterus, 95% occur in a fallopian tube (Fig. 5-2). The fallopian tube stretches to accommodate the growing embryo, but because it is not elastic enough, the tube cannot stretch much. If the tubal pregnancy is not diagnosed and removed surgically, the distended tube will rupture. Early in the ectopic pregnancy the woman will complain of abdominal pain on one side and usually will have vaginal bleeding, although it is possible to show no outward signs of bleeding. With a ruptured ectopic pregnancy, the woman will exhibit signs and symptoms of shock (cold, moist skin; fall in blood pressure; a rapid, weak pulse; thirst; apprehension; pallor; weakness; and "air hunger"). These signs of shock will not be proportional to blood loss because of the enormous pain.

Hydatidiform mole. *Hydatidiform mole* is a developmental anomaly of the placenta causing vaginal bleeding in the first trimester. In 1 in every 2000 pregnancies in the United States, abnormal trophoblastic growth causes higher than normal human chorionic gonadotropin (hCG) levels. The uterus enlarges rapidly, although there is no fetal heart tone, fetal movement, or palpable fetus (Fig. 5-3). Signs and symptoms of preeclampsia may be present as well as vaginal bleeding, often brownish in color. When a hydatidiform mole is suspected, no fetal skeleton is seen.

Treatment consists of immediate evacuation of the uterus and follow-up for possible malignancy (approximately 20% of cases progress to invasive *choriocarcinoma*). If there is a metastasis, treatment with chemotherapy is effective. Another pregnancy is contraindicated for 1 year, over which time the chest radiograph and radioimmune assay for the beta-subunit of hCG should have returned to normal.

NURSING CARE FOR WOMEN EXPERIENCING THE THREE COMMON CAUSES OF BLEEDING IN EARLY PREGNANCY

Nursing care. Abortion, ectopic pregnancy, and hydatidiform mole, the common causes of bleeding problems in early pregnancy, require supportive nursing care from nurses knowledgeable about these conditions and their potential complications. The woman and her family expected a healthy baby and instead are experiencing loss of that baby and loss of a healthy body image at the same time. The resolution of grief can begin

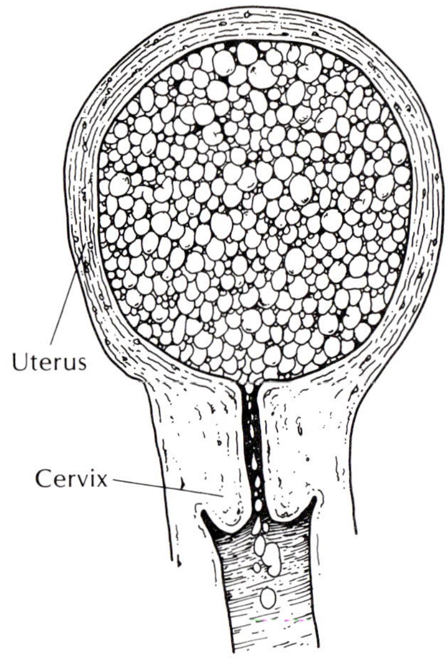

Fig. 5-3. Hydatidiform mole.

in the hospital as the nurse helps the mother and family to work through the grief process of denial, anger, bargaining, depression, and acceptance.

Bleeding in late pregnancy

TYPES OF PLACENTA PREVIA AND NURSING CARE

Placenta previa. *Placenta previa* is the most common cause of bleeding during the second half of pregnancy. The bleeding is painless, fresh vaginal bleeding. Instead of being implanted in the upper portion of the uterus, the placenta develops in the lower uterine segment either partially or completely covering the cervix in approximately 8 out of 1000 pregnancies.

There are three types of placenta previa, according to the degree to which the placenta covers the cervix: (1) partial, (2) marginal, and (3) complete (Fig. 5-4). With placenta previa there is painless vaginal bleeding after the twenty-eighth week of pregnancy. The dangers to the mother from placenta previa include hemorrhage, infection (because the area of placental implantation is close to the cervix and susceptible to infection from the outside), and lowered resistance secondary to hemorrhage. The dangers to the baby include premature birth and hypoxia and/or asphyxiation from the oxygen supply being reduced or cut off.

Nursing care. It is important for the nurse to alert the woman and her family to the significance of *painless bleeding*, which is an early sign of placenta previa, and to stress the importance of reporting this to the physician. The mother will probably be hospitalized immediately. The nurse should not administer an enema or do a rectal or vaginal examination because it is possible to put an examining finger right through a placenta previa or dislodge it, thus causing life-threatening hemorrhage.

If the bleeding of placenta previa is not severe, the woman may be kept on bed rest in the hospital for observation. As with the care of the hospitalized pre-eclamptic woman, the nurse must assess the family situation and offer supportive care.

DESCRIBE ABRUPTIO PLACENTAE AND NURSING CARE

Abruptio placentae. *Abruptio placentae* is premature separation of the normally implanted placenta late in pregnancy or during labor. Premature placental separation occurs in approximately 1% of deliveries. With abruptio placentae there may be (1) partial separation with concealed bleeding, (2) complete separation with concealed bleeding, or (3) partial separation with apparent hemorrhage (Fig. 5-5). The severity of separation may range from being so mild that there are no clinical symptoms to severe separation with

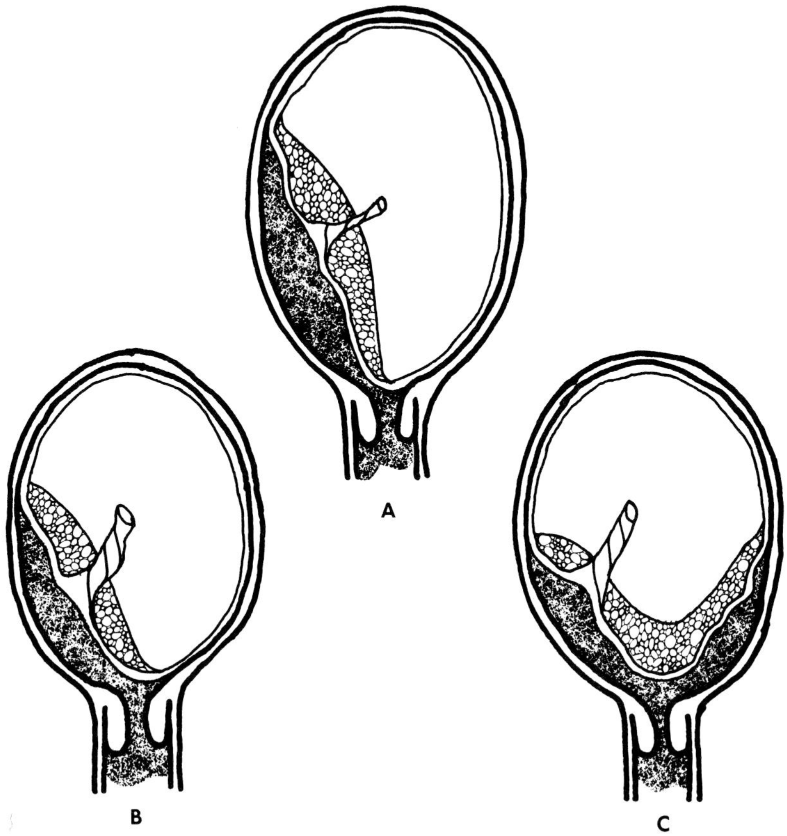

Fig. 5-4. Placenta previa. **A,** Marginal implantation. **B,** Partial placenta previa. **C,** Complete placenta previa.

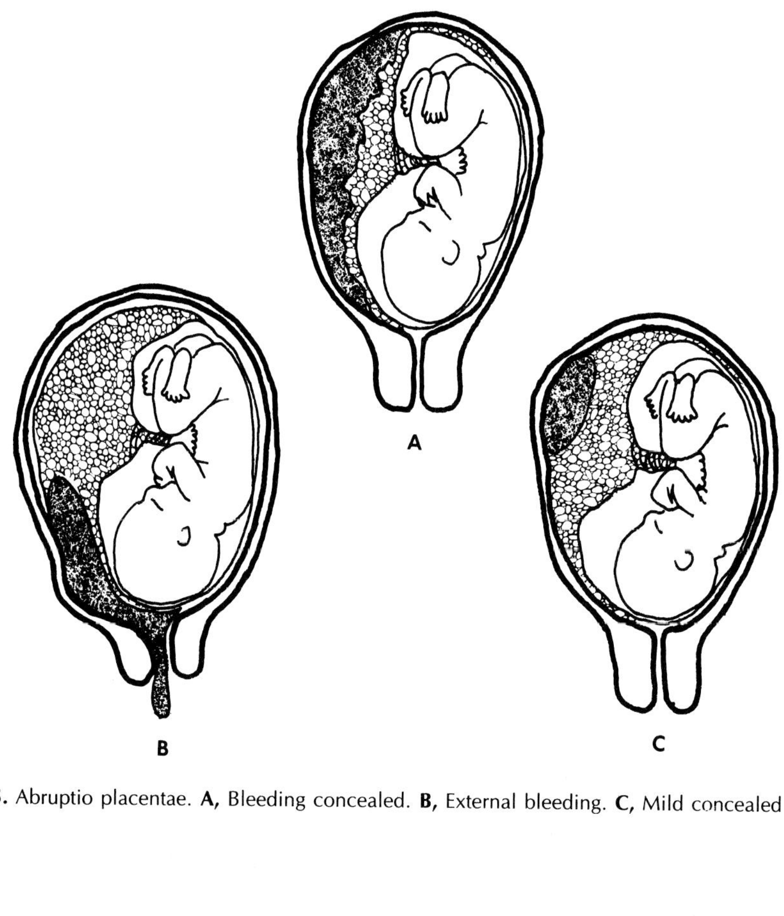

Fig. 5-5. Abruptio placentae. **A,** Bleeding concealed. **B,** External bleeding. **C,** Mild concealed bleeding.

maternal shock. In the case of a mild abruption of the placenta the only evidence may be a scar on the maternal side of the placenta found after delivery. In the more severe instances of abruptio placentae the woman complains of uterine tenderness and pain and the uterus becomes rigid. The woman may experience nausea and vomiting. The fetal heart rate may indicate distress or may be absent. For severe abruptio placentae there is no delayed treatment as in placenta previa because delay can result in severe hemorrhage with anemia, fetal death, and the serious coagulation disorder of disseminated intravascular coagulation (DIC). Cesarean birth is usually the method of delivery in severe abruptio placentae.

Nursing care. A family experiencing severe abruptio placentae is usually very aware of the acute emergency situation they are facing. As the nurse prepares the woman for emergency surgery (blood for type and cross-match, Foley catheter in place, recording vital signs, shaving abdomen in preparation for surgery, fetal heart monitoring, signature of surgery consent forms), it is important to be aware of the fear and shock the woman and her family are experiencing. The woman should not be left alone and should have all procedures explained before or as they are being done.

DIFFERENTIATE BETWEEN HYPEREMESIS AND "MORNING SICKNESS"

Hyperemesis gravidarum

Hyperemesis gravidarum is frequent, uncontrollable vomiting in early pregnancy. In Unit IV, it was stated that the nausea and vomiting ("morning sickness") in pregnancy are usually caused by the high levels of circulating hormones. However, when the nausea and vomiting become severe or continue beyond the first few months of pregnancy, a psychological component is often suspected. This woman may become severly dehydrated and have electrolyte imbalances. Also, she may be malnourished, with weight loss.

If the condition is severe, the treatment consists of hospitalization with intravenous feeding and antiemetic tranquilizing medications. Psychiatric consultation may also be requested.

Nursing care. Realizing that the cause of hyperemesis may be psychological, the nurse should provide an understanding environment, giving the woman a chance to verbalize her problems and feelings. Communication with the entire family is essential, because family problems or attitudes about the pregnancy itself may be the causative factor.

Diabetes in pregnancy

Diabetes is a complex systemic disorder of carbodydrate, fat, and protein metabolism due to a relative or complete lack of insulin secretion by beta cells of the pancreas. Diabetes is the most common endocrine disorder complicating pregnancy, with the incidence reported to be as high as 2%.

DESCRIBE THE CARE OF DIABETIC PREGNANT WOMEN

Pregnancy is characterized by an exaggerated rate and amount of insulin release but with insulin resistance at the cellular level so that the actions of insulin are restricted. As pregnancy progresses, more and more anti-insulin factors are produced by the placenta, and there is more and more stress on the maternal pancreas. Normally, the mother meets this stress with increased insulin. If a woman's pancreatic reserve is low, her insulin production may be inadequate for the first time in her life. This woman is classified as a gestational diabetic. Gestational diabetes accounts for 90% of diabetes in pregnancy.

Two other classifications of diabetes are type I, insulin-dependent diabetes, and type II, non-insulin dependent diabetes. However, type II diabetes invariably requires insulin during pregnancy.

The adverse effects of diabetes on the mother during pregnancy include increased incidence of pre-eclampsia, eclampsia, infection, oversized infants, difficult delivery, premature labor, hydramnios, and postpartum hemorrhage. Adverse effects on the fetus include increased mortality, respiratory disease, hypoglycemia, major congenital defects, and ketoacidosis.

Complicated diabetic pregnancies are frequently terminated prior to term because of the large size of the fetus and because of maternal complications. Tests of placental function and fetal maturity are done to choose the appropriate date for delivery.

The baby of a diabetic mother is placed in neonatal intensive care and treated according to current practice until stable. The infant is at risk for developing rebound hypoglycemia and, if untreated, brain damage and even death.

Nursing care. Comprehensive antepartum education plays a major role in the management of a pregnancy complicated by diabetes. The most successful programs start preconceptually and involve the family as active members of the health care team to promote optimum outcomes for mother and baby. Overall objectives include (1) keeping maternal blood glucose levels as close to normal as possible, (2) providing adequate nutrition for normal development of the fetus, (3) preventing progression of maternal vascular disease, and (4) preventing premature delivery and fetal or neonatal complications.

Multiple pregnancy

LIST NURSING ACTIONS WHEN MULTIPLE PREGNANCY OCCURS

Identical twins *(monozygotic)* result from the union of one sperm and one ovum; fraternal twins *(dizygotic)* result when two ova are fertilized by two sperm (Fig. 5-6). With fraternal twins, there are two amniotic sacs and two placentas. With identical twins, there are two amniotic sacs and one placenta. Approximately 1 in 90 births in the United States is a twin birth. Because of overdistention of the uterus, twins usually deliver prior to term and have extended hospital stays. Twins may be double joy but also double responsibility and more expense than for one baby. The parents need a great deal of support both before and after the twins arrive. It is possible to breast-feed twins. However, the woman who plans to do this needs help with her other responsibilities because breast-feeding will consume a lot of her time.

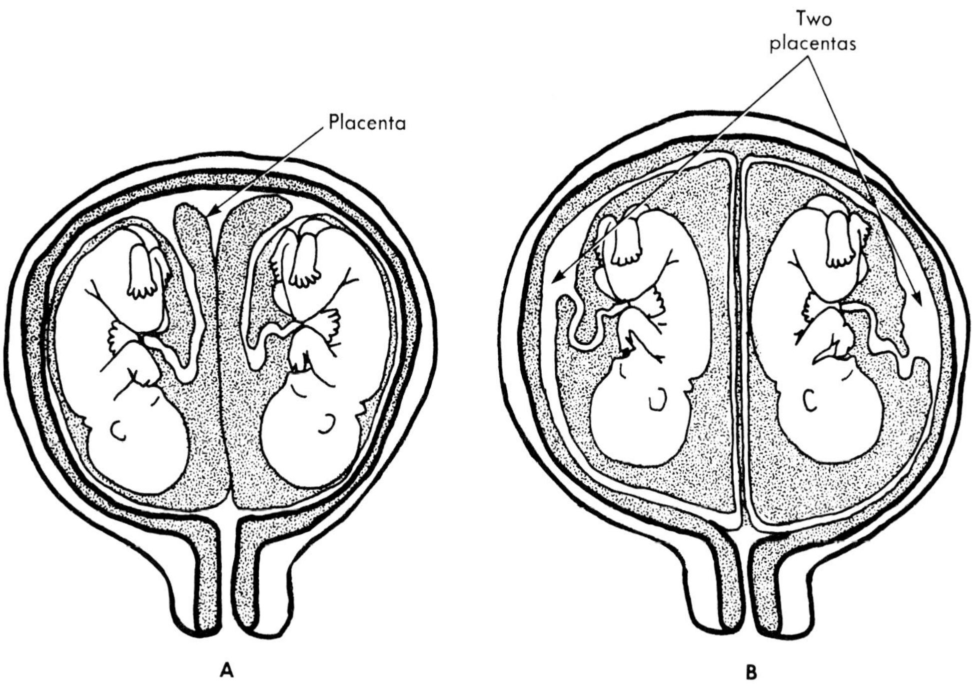

Fig. 5-6. Multiple pregnancy. **A,** Identical (monozygotic) twins: two sacs, one placenta. **B,** Fraternal (dizygotic) twins: two sacs, two placentas.

DESCRIBE THE CARE OF A PREGNANT WOMAN WITH HEART DISEASE

Heart disease

Heart disease complicates pregnancy because the diseased or damaged heart may not be able to meet the demands of the increased cardiac workload of pregnancy. Approximately 1% of all pregnant women have some form of heart disease. The majority of these women have heart disease either as a congenital lesion or caused by rheumatic fever. Just as the woman with diabetes should be under close medical supervision during pregnancy, so should the woman with heart disease. Early antepartum care and frequent and regular visits to an obstetrician and a cardiologist should be stressed for this woman. Adequate rest and avoidance of activities that cause shortness of breath and fatigue are essential for the pregnant woman with heart disease. Also, excessive weight gain, which could put more strain on the heart, must be avoided.

The woman with heart disease may experience heart failure at any time during pregnancy. The symptoms of heart failure are difficult breathing *(dyspnea)*, paroxysmal nocturnal dyspnea (awakening at night short of breath), orthopnea (sleeping on 2 to 4 pillows because of shortness of breath), nocturia (awakening at night to void), and peripheral edema. She is also at risk for contracting respiratory infections and should seek prompt treatment for a cold or sore throat.

Nursing care. The nurse can be very helpful by encouraging the woman with heart disease to follow the physician's orders. The nurse can also work with the woman and her family in restructuring family chores and activities to reduce the woman's workload and also help the family plan their food intake to reduce salt in the woman's diet. Also, continuous psychological support is essential.

Anemia

Anemia is a condition in which there is a reduction in the oxygen-carrying capacity of the blood because of a reduction in red cells and/or hemoglobin.

If the pregnant woman's hemoglobin level falls below 11.0 grams and the hematocrit falls below 31% in the second trimester, *iron-deficiency anemia* is suspected. In iron-deficiency anemia inadequate hemoglobin production is the result of decreased heme synthesis. Iron supplementation of 300 milligrams three times per day should be recommended when iron deficiency is the cause of anemia.

Folic acid–deficiency anemia may result from malabsorption of folate from the intestine, poor intake of folate, liver damage, or frequent pregnancies in which the woman cannot replenish body folate stores. Iron-deficiency anemia can be associated with folate deficiency. Folate supplementation of 400 micrograms of folic acid daily in pregnancy should prevent folate deficiency.

Thalassemia primarily affects people of Mediterranean and Southeast Asian origin. In this form of anemia there is inadequate hemoglobin production plus an excessive breakdown of the defective red cells that are produced. The stress of pregnancy frequently worsens the anemia in thalassemia. Iron therapy is *not* recommended.

Sickle cell trait is a sickling of red blood cells found in approximately 8% of black childbearing women. These women are susceptible to urinary tract infections, and the fetus may be at risk for hypoxic stress. Of the pregnant women who have sickle cell trait, less than 1% have *sickle cell anemia.* In pregnancy complicated by sickle cell anemia, the maternal mortality rate can be as high as 70% and the perinatal mortality rate as high as 50%. Iron and folic acid supplementation should be prescribed, and the sources of both should be increased in the diet.

Drug addiction

Addiction to drugs can cause severe problems for both the mother and baby. A large percentage of addicted pregnant women experience chronic anxiety and depression and lack confidence and hope for the future. If a woman is addicted to an illegal drug, she may avoid prenatal care in an effort to prevent detection. Some of the drugs abused are LSD, cocaine, marijuana, alcohol, amphetamines, nicotine, barbiturates, codeine, diazepam, and narcotics. Heroin addiction is a problem in maternity populations of large metropolitan hospitals. Of the infants born to heroin-addicted women, 60% to 90% show signs of withdrawal. Infants born to women on methadone at the time of delivery will also have withdrawal symptoms. The severity of symptoms and the time of onset are related to the duration and type of maternal addiction as well as the mother's drug level prior to giving birth. Because the drug-dependent baby is only physically dependent, the chance for complete recovery is good. However, the drug-dependent mother will need long-term supportive therapy if she is to live drug free.

Hydramnios

Hydramnios is the accumulation of excessive amounts (2000 milliters or more) of amniotic fluid. Hydramnios is associated with a high incidence of fetal abnormalities (40%). The condition is often suspected by the seventh month of pregnancy and can be confirmed by ultrasound screening. When the diagnosis is made, further testing is done to see if the fetus has a major abnormality, that is, anencephaly, spina bifida, or myelomeningocele.

An amount of 100 to 200 milliliters of amniotic fluid is called *oligohydramnios* and is associated with renal anomalies.

DIAGNOSTIC TECHNIQUES

Numerous diagnostic and monitoring procedures are in use today for determining fetal well-being and fetal growth and maturity. New technologies are frequently integrated into systems of care before a long-term major analysis is completed. Professional reluctance to criticize a "revolutionary tool," especially when it represents a major technological advance, may make it difficult to collect objective scientific data once the intervention has been generally accepted.

Ultrasonography

COMMON DIAGNOSTIC TESTS USED IN HIGH-RISK MATERNITY CARE AND NURSING RESPONSIBILITIES IN PREPARING THE FAMILY FOR THESE TESTS

Approximately half the pregnant women in the United States routinely receive ultrasound scans to determine the age of the fetus and location of the placenta. In recent years the benefit-to-risk ratio for use of routine ultrasound in pregnancy has been questioned. This concern has led to a panel report by the National Institutes of Health (NIH) and the publication of a position paper by the International Childbirth Education Association (ICEA). The ICEA Position Paper is reproduced in Appendix H.

Ultrasonography (sonography, sonogram, scan) is a painless technique in which ultra high frequency soundwaves (too high to be heard) are beamed into the body (Fig. 5-7). These soundwaves bounce off soft tissue in different ways, sending out echos, which can be recorded on an oscilloscope and photographed for permanent records in Polaroid photographs. One scanning technique can measure the size of the fetal head to determine whether the fetus is growing normally. Another technique can monitor continuous fetal activity, watch the fetal heart beating, measure fetal breathing and even observe the fetus sucking its thumb. Other uses for ultrasound are to localize the placenta in suspected placenta previa or before doing amniocentesis, so that the operator will not place the needle into the placenta. Sonography can also pick up some fetal anomalies, a hydatidiform mole, twins, or tumors in the uterus.

Nursing care. Ultrasonography is one test in which the success of the technique is heavily dependent on the woman having a full bladder. For 1½ hours before the test, the nurse encourages the woman to drink a full glass of water every 15 minutes. The full

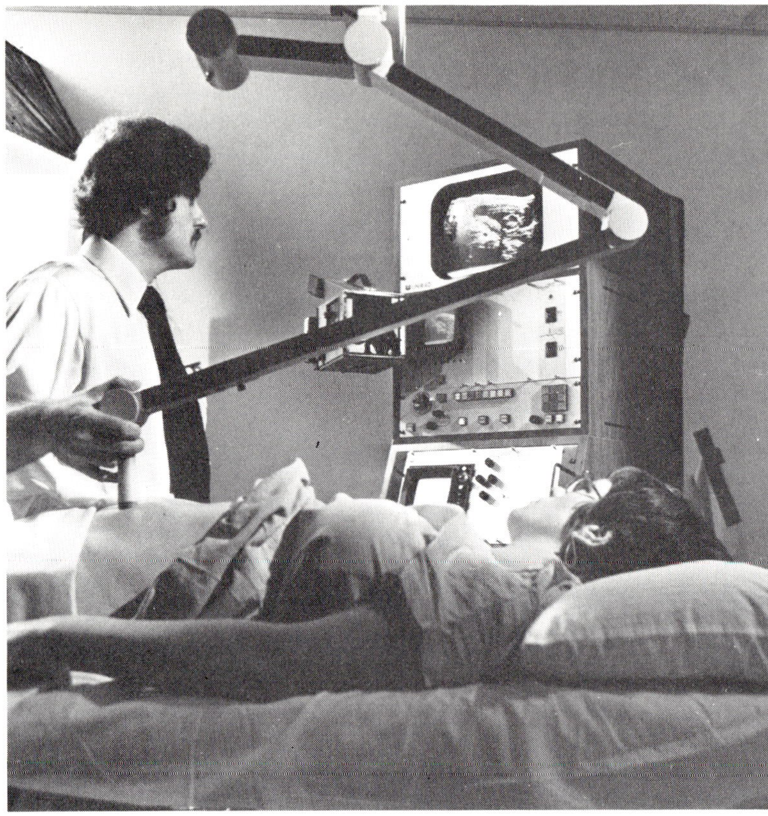

Fig. 5-7. Ultrasonography. (Permission to reproduce this publication has been granted by The National Foundation—March of Dimes as the copyright holder of the original publication.)

bladder both helps to push the uterus upward and serves as an amplifier for sound. Because a full bladder can make the pregnant woman very uncomfortable, she needs a thorough explanation of the reasons involved.

Amniocentesis

Amniocentesis is the removal of amniotic fluid from the amniotic cavity by needle puncture (Fig. 5-8). The risks involved with amniocentesis are abortion of approximately 1% of the pregnancies and trauma to the fetus or placenta resulting in bleeding, infection, and Rh sensitization from fetal bleeding into the maternal circulation. Even though these risks are slight, the fact that they are possible rules out amniocentesis as a routine screening procedure. It is the physician's responsibility to inform the woman and her family of the risks of amniocentesis and to obtain a signed consent form if a decision is made that the benefits from the procedure outweigh the risks. (The need to obtain amniotic fluid to accurately determine fetal maturity or to determine the presence of Down's syndrome or other suspected genetic defects in the population at risk are accepted reasons for amniocentesis.)

Nursing care. For amniocentesis, the placenta is localized by ultrasound and fetal position determined. The nurse records the fetal heart rate and prepares the woman's abdomen as for a minor surgical procedure. From 20 to 30 milliliters of amniotic fluid are withdrawn by the physician and placed in taped or amber test tubes to protect the specimen from light. On conclusion of the procedure, the nurse places an adhesive bandage over the puncture site and again listens to the fetal heart tones and watches for any outward symptoms. Prior to the procedure, the nurse explains what will happen to the woman and her family, clarifying anything they do not understand. During the proce-

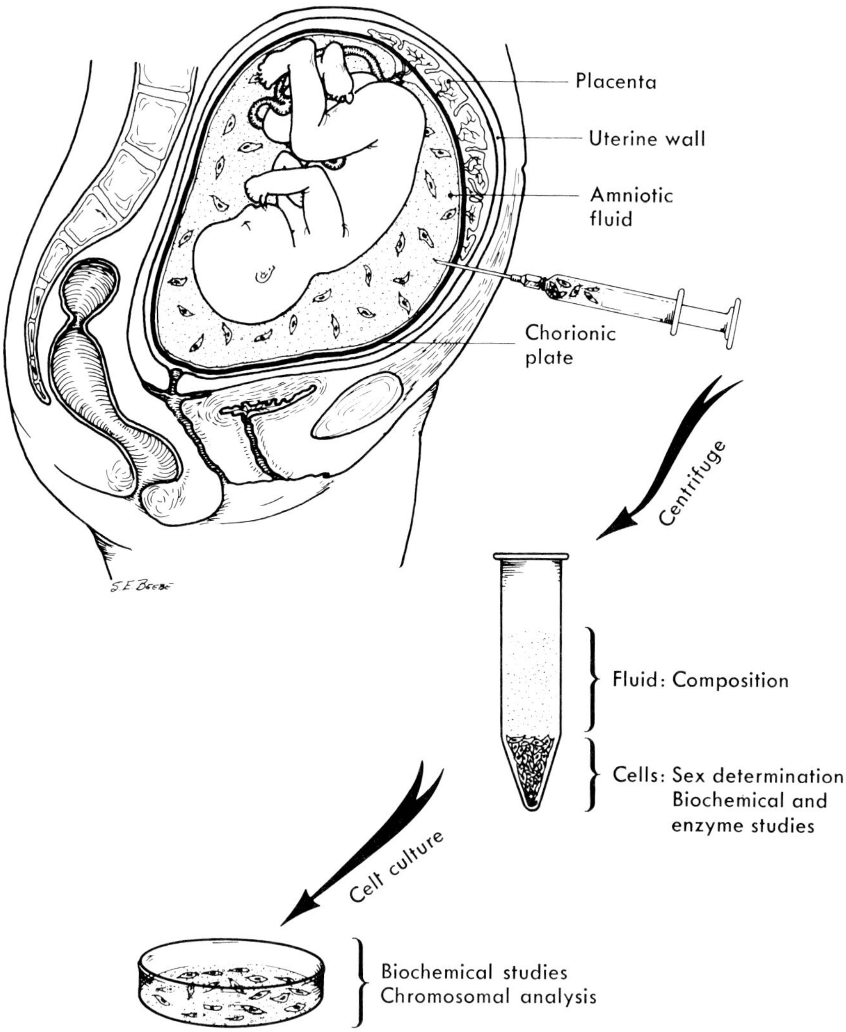

Fig. 5-8. Amniocentesis. (From Tucker, S.M.: Fetal monitoring and fetal assessment in high-risk pregnancy, St. Louis, 1978, The C.V. Mosby Co.)

dure, the nurse has the key role in supporting the woman. The Rh^- woman with an Rh^+ partner receives 300 micrograms of anit-Rh immunoglobulin (RhoGAM) after the test.

Amniotic fluid studies

Chromosomal abnormalities such as Down's syndrome, the sex of the fetus, and certain genetic defects can be detected by culturing the cells from amniotic fluid and studying them.

Alpha-fetoprotein (AFP) studies can detect neural tube malformations such as hydrocephalus, spina bifida, and microcephaly.

Lecithin-sphingomyelin ratios (L/S ratios) can be done on amniotic fluid to determine maturity of the fetal lungs. Lecithin and sphingomyelin are the predominant phospholipids making up *surfactant*, which is the complex detergent-like substance lining the alveoli of the lungs. This surfactant lowers the surface tension in the alveoli and keeps the alveolar walls from collapsing on themselves. L/S are present as a ratio, changing predictably as the pregnancy progresses (Fig. 5-9). When the ratio of lecithin to sphingomyelin is 2.0 or greater, the fetal lung is considered mature. Phosphatidylglycerol is another phospholipid in surfactant. Absence indicates pulmonary immaturity.

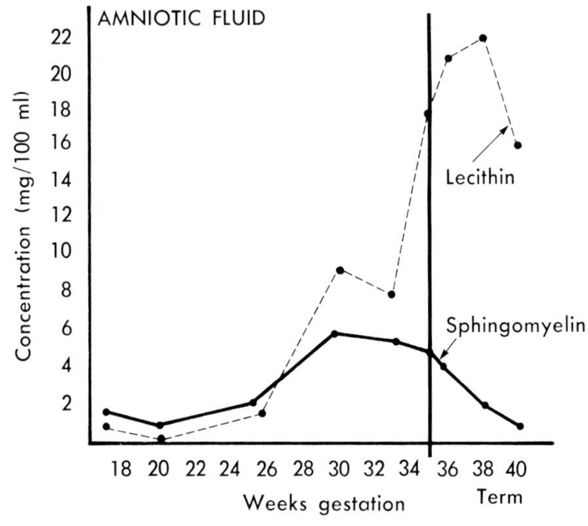

Fig. 5-9. Lecithin/sphingomyelin (L/S) ratio.

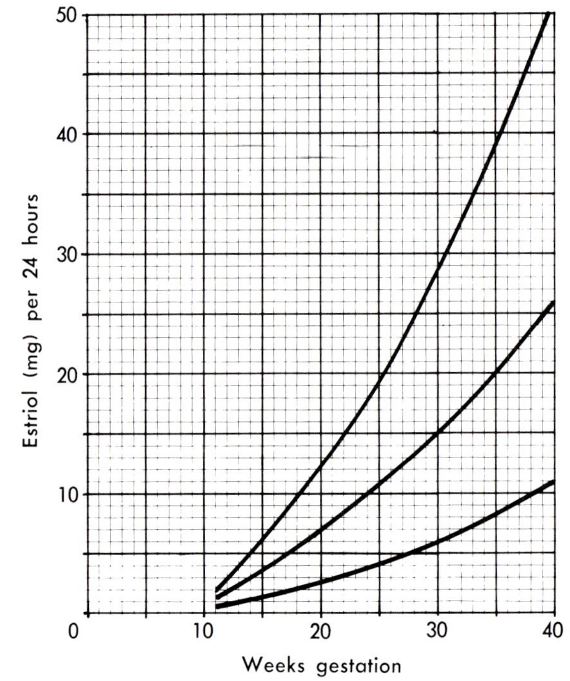

Fig. 5-10. Average excretion of urine estriol throughout pregnancy is depicted by the middle line.

Creatinine levels, bilirubin levels, and *the percentage of fat cells* present in the amniotic fluid can also indicate fetal maturity.

Estriol test

Estriol is a major metabolite of estrogen and is found in relatively large quantities in maternal urine in the last half of pregnancy. The fetus contributes to the maternal urinary estriol, through its adrenals, to the placenta and then into the maternal blood. The synthesis of estriol requires a normal placenta and fetal adrenal cortex. Estriol levels excreted in maternal urine should rise predictably throughout pregnancy (Fig. 5-10). A fall in estriol levels usually signals trouble in the fetal-placental unit and possible impending fetal death. A single estriol level alone is of limited value, but a falling estriol along with other tests indicating a compromised fetal-placental unit is a diagnostic tool. Estriol tests done on the mother's plasma are much faster than the 24-hour urine collection. Because serial estriol determinations alone are not always an accurate indicator of fetal well-being, they should be used in conjunction with other tests.

Nursing care. In addition to collecting the specimens (whether 24-hour urine or maternal blood), once again the nurse plays the role of explaining to the woman and her family the need for the estriol test and the significance of the test results.

Contraction stress test

In a *contraction stress test* (CST), continuous fetal monitoring is used to test placental respiratory function and reserve. Oxytocin is given intravenously using an infusion pump until the woman experiences three uterine contractions within a 10-minute period. The fetal heart rate is observed in relation to the contractions. If the heart rate remains stable during contractions, the test is negative; however, if late decelerations in the fetal heart rate appear, the test is positive. A negative test means that the present status of the fetus is satisfactory and the pregnancy can continue for another week when the test should be repeated. If other tests of fetal status are positive, a positive CST may indicate the need for prompt termination of the pregnancy.

Breast or nipple stimulation tests

Many perinatal centers are now using breast stimulation instead of oxytocin for inducing uterine activity. Manual or breast pump stimulation of the nipple and breast releases oxytocin from the pituitary, thus stimulating contractions of the uterine musculature. Because breast stimulation is a potent stimulator of uterine contractions, it should be performed only unilaterally and for short periods of time.

Nonstress test

During the last part of pregnancy women may also be monitored using a *nonstress test* (NST). It is a sign of fetal well-being if the fetal heart accelerates in response to fetal movement. The fetus may move spontaneously or with a Braxton-Hicks' contraction or by external manipulation, such as rubbing the woman's abdomen.

A reactive NST pattern is fetal movement associated with two accelerations of fetal heart that last 15 seconds or more and achieve a zenith of 15 beats per minute in one of two 20-minute periods.

The reactive NST and negative CST are highly predictive of fetal well-being. However, controversy exists as to which test should be used as the primary screening test.

Nursing care. The CST, the NST, and breast stimulation require thorough explanations for the woman and her family both before and during the procedures. Following the tests, the nurse makes sure that the woman and her family understand the results of the tests and implications for further care.

Fetal movements

Monitoring fetal motion is worthwhile in predicting fetal distress in high-risk pregnancies. Since the beginning of time, pregnant women have been known to experience decreased fetal activity prior to fetal death. Because there is a wide variation in the number of daily movements, each mother needs to determine what is normal for her baby. After 24 weeks of gestation, pregnant women could be instructed to concentrate on fetal movements for specified periods of time daily (according to their risk potential). Noticing fewer than three movements in 8 hours or movements changing from strong to weak should be communicated to the health care team immediately. Cessation of fetal movement places the fetus in a high-risk category and should alert the care providers to the need for an NST.

Table 5-1. How to interpret fetal well-being from BPS scores

Biophysical variable	Normal (BPS = 2)	Abnormal (BPS = 0)
Fetal breathing movements	At least one episode of FBM of at least 30 seconds duration in 30 minutes observation	Absent FBM or no episode of ≥30 seconds in 30 minutes
Gross body movement	At least three discrete body-limb movements in 30 minutes (episodes of active, continuous movement considered a single movement)	Two or fewer episodes of body–limb movements in 30 minutes
Fetal tone	At least one episode of active extension with return to flexion of fetal limb(s) or trunk (opening and closing of hand considered normal tone)	Either slow extension with return to partial flexion or movement of limb in full extension or absent fetal movement
Reactive FHR	At least two episodes of FHR acceleration of ≥15 bpm and of at least 15 seconds duration associated with fetal movement in 30 minutes	Fewer than two episodes of acceleration of FHR or acceleration of <15 bpm in 30 minutes
Qualitative AFV	At least one pocket of AF that measures at least 1 centimeter in two perpendicular planes	Either no AF pockets or one pocket <1 centimeter in two perpendicular planes

Reproduced with permission from Contemporary OB/GYN 25 [1] xxxx.
FBM - fetal breathing movement
FHR - fetal heart rate
bpm - beats per minute
AFV - amniotic fluid volume
AF - amniotic fluid

Biophysical profile (BPS)

Fetal biophysical scoring begins with detailed dynamic ultrasound scanning of a pregnant woman (over 26 weeks of gestation) who has had high-risk factors identified. Five fetal biophysical variables—fetal breathing movements, fetal movements, fetal tone, qualitative amniotic fluid volume, and the NST—are measured and scored according to fixed criteria. Each variable is assigned an arbitrary score of 2 (if normal) or 0 (if abnormal). When all variables are normal (BPS = 10) or the amniotic fluid volume and at least three other variables are normal (BPS = 8), the fetus is considered nonasphyxiated. See Table 5-1 for criteria used to interpret fetal well-being from BPS scores.

SUMMARY

Because this is a basic text, this unit has presented only an introduction to the care of the high-risk woman and her family. Although the major complications of pregnancy were introduced, some of the less common high-risk conditions were not included. As pregnancy screening for identification of high-risk pregnancies becomes more refined and diagnostic techniques more sophisticated, the need for nurses with special education in the care of high-risk families will increase. In regionalized high-risk centers, continuous in-service education will be needed to update the nursing care provided. As we continue to expand both knowledge and skills, we must not lose sight of the goal of the high-risk level of the new maternity model—that is, to provide a more complex but still humanistic model for women with medical complications or complications of pregnancy.

BIBLIOGRAPHY

Alonso, B.K.: Hypertensive disorders of pregnancy, NAACOG Update Series, vol. 3, lesson 3, Princeton, 1985, CPEC.

Baca, J.E.: Some health beliefs of the Spanish speaking, Am J. Nurs. **69**:2172-2176, 1969.

Beeson, D., Douglas, R.: Prenatal diagnosis of

fetal disorders, part 1: technological capabilities, Birth **10**(4):227-232, 1983.
Beeson, D., Douglas, R., and Lunsford, T.F.: Prenatal diagnosis of fetal disorders, part II: issues and implications, Birth **10**(4):233-240, 1983.
Capeless, E.L., and Mann, L.I.: Use of breast stimulation for antepartum stress testing, Obstet. Gynecol. **64**(5):641-645, 1984.
English, J.T.: The dimensions of poverty, Am. J. Nurs. **69**:2424-2428, 1969.
Finnegan, L.P., and MacNew, B.: Care of the addicted newborn, Am. J. Nurs. **74**:685–693, 1974.
Geiger, H.J.: The endlessly revolving door, Am. J. Nurs. **69**:2436-2445, 1969.
Goldstein, A., and Dumars, K.W.: Minimizing the risk of amniocentesis for prenatal diagnosis, J.A.M.A. **237**:1336-1338, 1977.
Hammer, R.M., Bower, E.J., and Messina, L.J.: The prenatal use of Rho(D) immunoglobulin, MCN **9**:29-31, Jan./Feb. 1984.
Hoffmaster, J.E.: Detecting and treating pregnancy-induced hypertension: a review, MCN **8**:398-405, Nov./Dec. 1983.
ICEA Position Paper: Diagnostic ultrasound in obstetrics, ICEA News **22**:2, March 1983.
Leppert, P.C., and Namerow, P.B.: Costs averted by providing comprehensive prenatal care to teenagers, Journal of Nurse-Midwifery **30**:285-289, Sept./Oct. 1985.
Manning, F.A.: Fetal biophysical profile scoring predicts trouble—when it counts, Contemporary Ob/Gyn, **20**:126-137, Jan. 1985.
McNerney, W.J.: Changing the health care system, Am. J. Nurs. **69**:2428-2435, 1969.
Moore, M.L., and Davis, O.S.: Realities in childbearing, Philadelphia, 1978, W.B. Saunders Co.
Moore, M.L.: Realities in childbearing, ed. 2, Philadelphia, 1983, W.B. Saunders Co.
National Institutes of Health: The use of diagnostic ultrasound imaging in pregnancy, Consensus Development Conference, Consensus Statement, Bethesda, Md., Feb. 6-8, 1984.
Oakes, G.K., Chez, R.A., and Morelli, I.C.: Diet in pregnancy, Am. J. Nurs. **75**:1134-1136, 1975.
Pardue, S.F.: Hydatidiform mole: a pathological pregnancy, Am. J. Nurs. **77**:836-838, 1977.
Portale, A.M.: Diabetes in pregnancy, NAACOG Update Series, vol. 3, lesson 5, Princeton, N.J., 1985, CPEC.
Rayburn, W.F.: Clinical implications from monitoring fetal activity, Am. J. Obstet. Gynecol. **144**:967-980, 1982.
The risk of diagnostic ultrasound—a literature survey and a response, Birth Fam. J. 4(3):127-130, 1977.
Schuler, K.: When a pregnant woman is diabetic: antepartal care, Am. J. Nurs. **79**:456-459, 1979.
Slatin, M.: Why mothers bypass prenatal care, Am. J. Nurs. **71**:1388-1389, 1971.
Sonstegard, L.: Toxemia update. Pregnancy-induced hypertension: prenatal nursing concerns, MCN **4**:90-95, March/April 1979.
State of California, Department of Health: Family Health Bulletin, Spring 1977.
Tichy, A.M., and Chong, D.: Toxemia update. Placental function and its role in toxemia, MCN **4**:84-89, March/April 1979.
Wetzel, S.K.: Are we ignoring the needs of the woman with a spontaneous abortion? MCN **7**:258-259, July/Aug. 1982.

DEFINITIONS

Define the following terms:

abortion
abruptio placentae
alpha-feto-protein
antibodies
bilirubin
clonus
demographic
diabetogenic state
diastolic
diuretics
dizygotic
eclampsia
ectopic pregnancy
electrolyte
estriol
gestational diabetes
hyperemesis gravidarum
immunoglobulin
incompatibility
incompetent cervix
induction
isoimmunization
ketoacidosis
monozygotic
oscilloscope
oxytocin
placenta previa
pregnancy-induced hypertension
proteinuria
regimen
RhoGAM
sensitization
systolic
titer
ultrasonography

LEARNING ACTIVITIES AND EXPERIENCES

1. Group discussions.
2. Guest speakers: a nurse from a high-risk maternity clinic.
3. View audiovisual aids, listen to tapes, and discuss.

ENRICHMENT/IN-DEPTH STUDY

1. Discuss the pros and cons of a two-tiered maternity model.
2. Discover community resources for high-risk prenatal care in your community.
3. Investigate resources in your community that provide financial aid to pregnant families in need of such aid.

4. Determine the average cost of prenatal care in your community.
5. Determine the average cost of the hospital stay for delivery and post-delivery care in your community.
6. Investigate community resources for continued schooling, prenatal education, and preparation for birth available in your community for teenage mothers and fathers.
7. Discuss the emotional reactions a family may experience when receiving results of amniocentesis indicating that the fetus has Down's syndrome or neural tube malformations.

SELF-ASSESSMENT

For questions 1 through 4, circle the best answer.

1. In which of the following situations is Rh isoimmunization possible?
   a. mother is Rh negative; father is Rh(D) positive
   b. mother is Rh(D) positive; father is Rh negative
   c. both parents are Rh(D) positive
   d. both parents are Rh negative
2. Careful follow-up of the woman who has had a hydatidiform mole is important because she:
   a. will probably have twins next pregnancy
   b. will become infertile
   c. may develop choriocarcinoma
3. After delivery from the diabetic mother, the baby is usually placed in the neonatal intensive care unit for close observation because the baby often develops:
   a. hyperglycemia
   b. hypoglycemia
   c. Rh problems
   d. anemia
4. The ratio of lecithin to sphingomyelin indicates the maturity of the:
   a. fetal lungs
   b. fetal kidneys
   c. placenta

For questions 5 through 21, fill in the blanks:

5. The nonstress test uses fetal heart acceleration in response to ______________ as a point of reference.
6. A pregnant woman about to undergo ultrasonography needs a(n) ____________ bladder.
7. For amniocentesis, the placenta is localized by ______________.
8. A fall in estriol levels during pregnancy could mean ____________________________.
9. The procedure by which a specimen of amniotic fluid is collected for laboratory tests is called ____.
10. When fetal blood cell damage is occurring in utero, the fetus may be given __________ __________.
11. One test that can indicate the severity of fetal blood cell damage during the pregnancy of a sensitized woman is known as the ____________________________.
12. If the Rh-positive infant shows signs of erythroblastosis after birth, the treatment of choice will probably be ___________________ __________________.
13. The anti-Rh positive globulin that suppresses the formation of Rh antibodies is ____________________ ______________________________________.
14. To a layperson the term *abortion* may mean ____________________________.
15. The obstetrical definition of *abortion* is ____________________________.
16. For a woman whose pregnancy is complicated by heart disease, ____________ is essential.
17. Twins usually deliver prior to term because ____________________________.

18. Under the category of age and parity, the major high-risk groups are women under the age of ________ or over the age of ________, as well as women who have given birth to more than ________ babies.
19. Indicate two previous pregnancy problems that would classify a woman as high risk.
    a.
    b.
20. Medical conditions that would classify a pregnant woman as high risk include ____________________ and ____________________.
21. In the eclampsias an elevated blood pressure is detected ____________ the twentieth week of pregnancy. In the chronic hypertensive states of pregnancy an elevated blood pressure is detected ____________ the twentieth week of pregnancy.

Supply the correct answer(s) for items 22 through 33.

22. Women experiencing abortion, ectopic pregnancy, or hydatidiform mole are also experiencing loss of their expected baby. Explain supportive nursing care for these women.
23. Why is close medical supervision necessary for the pregnant diabetic woman?
24. Which is the most common variety of diabetes in pregnancy?
25. Nursing responsibilities with families who have Rh incompatibilities include:
    a.
    b.
    c.
26. List three common causes of bleeding in early pregnancy:
    a.
    b.
    c.
27. List two common causes of bleeding in late pregnancy:
    a.
    b.
28. What are some reasons why women may *not* seek prenatal care?
    a.
    b.
    c.
29. The high-risk pregnant woman has to accomplish specific tasks to achieve stability in a complicated pregnancy. How can the nurse help this woman and her family adapt? Propose a plan of care for a woman and her family when the woman has been hospitalized in the eighth month of pregnancy for treatment of severe pre-eclampsia.
30. What would the nurse advise a woman who wants to breast-feed twins?
31. What are three signs of early pre-eclampsia?
    a.
    b.
    c.
32. When a woman with severe pre-eclampsia has been admitted to the hospital, the nursing care should include:
    a.
    b.
    c.
    d.

e.

f.

g.

h.

i.

33. The classifications of placenta previa are:

a.

b.

c.

34. Match Column A with Column B. Each item in Column B may be used more than once, or not at all.

Column A	Column B
______1. eclampsia	a. blood pressure 160/110
______2. severe pre-eclampsia	b. 3+ to 4+ proteinuria
______3. mild pre-eclampsia	c. elevation of blood pressure
	d. generalized edema
	e. convulsions

35. Match Column A with Column B. Each item in Column B may be used once or more than once.

Column A	Column B
______1. "morning sickness"	a. uterine tenderness and rigidity
______2. hyperemesis gravidarum	b. nausea and vomiting
______3. ectopic pregnancy	c. abdominal pain on one side and vaginal bleeding
______4. placenta previa	d. dehydration and electrolyte imbalance
______5. abruptio placentae	e. painless bleeding

UNIT VI
Preparation For Childbirth

GOALS

This unit is designed to provide the reader with information that will:

- □ promote awareness of common factors inherent in all prepared childbirth techniques.
- □ increase appreciation of the need for physical and psychological support for the laboring family.
- □ develop an understanding of the role of the support team with both prepared and unprepared childbearing families.

STUDENT OBJECTIVES

After studying this unit, you should be able to:

1. List the six major techniques that most instructors include in their preparation for childbirth classes.
2. Describe at least five helpful actions the support person may use when offering verbal or "hands on" support to a couple who have prepared for labor.
3. Demonstrate the following specific exercises widely used in preparation for childbirth classes:
   a. controlled relaxation
   b. concentration-relaxation
   c. slow chest breathing
   d. rapid superficial breathing
   e. pant and blow breathing
   f. expulsion breathing
4. Describe types of classes offered to childbearing families.

HISTORICAL OVERVIEW

Since colonial times in America, women have shared their information on childbirth with other women. In the nineteenth century, male physicians gradually came to be recognized as experts to whom women went for information about birth. By 1900 physicians finally usurped women's age-old skills concerning childbirth and became, for many, the sole authorities.

However, as early as 1908 the American Red Cross recognized the need to teach mothers about hygiene and good health practices. In the United States the first formal classes in childbirth education were offered nationally in 1913 by the American Red Cross. Maternity Center Association in New York City followed with classes for expectant parents as early as 1919. Literature on these early attempts at childbirth education revealed that the first classes for childbirth were developed out of a public health need to teach mothers basic hygiene.

An English physician, Dr. Grantly Dick-Read, published two books in which he theorized that pain in childbirth is caused by a fear-tension-pain syndrome. His first book, *Natural Childbirth,* was published in 1933. Dick-Read's second book, *Childbirth Without Fear,* was published in the United States in 1944. Dick-Read's work became the foundation for the first organized programs of preparation for childbirth and teacher training. The first of such groups to organize was the International Childbirth Education Association (ICEA) founded in 1960.

At about the same time, the Lamaze method, also known as psychoprophylaxis (PPM), was gaining popularity in the United States. PPM opened new perspectives into preparation for childbirth by emphasizing mind control. Marjorie Karmel introduced PPM to the United States in her book, *Thank You, Dr. Lamaze,* which was published in the United States in 1959. Others have written extensively on PPM. This system grew out of Pavlov's work on the higher nervous activity of humans and animals in which he proposed that every vital activity of an organism is a complex reflex process capable of conditioning.

In 1960 the American Society for Psychoprophylaxis in Obstetrics (ASPO) was formed in New York as a national organization to promote use of the Lamaze method and prepare teachers of the method. Childbirth Without Pain Education League, Inc. (CWPEL) was formed in 1970 to teach the Lamaze method and prepare teachers. The Council of Childbirth Education Specialists, Inc. (CCES) was founded in New York City in 1971 and offered teacher training seminars through the United States.

A Denver obstetrician, Dr. Robert Bradley, published *Husband-Coached Childbirth* in 1965. In this book he advocates what he proposes is the true natural childbirth, without any form of anesthesia or analgesic, and with a "husband-coach" and breathing techniques for labor. The American Academy of Husband-Coached Childbirth (AAHCC) was founded to make the Bradley method available and to prepare teachers.

Of the other techniques developed, the most widely known include the work of Kitzinger and Wright, developed in England. Wright's work is based on PPM, described as "levels of breathing." Kitzinger's work is designed around a psychosexual approach, which proposes that birth is a sexual experience. As such, birth is perceived as a normal physiological process in which the woman works in harmony with her body.

Inevitably, components of one method have been combined with those of others until there are now numerous methods of childbirth preparation. Hypnosis, autogenic training, yogic childbirth, the Gamper method, the Swiss method, and Russian hydrotherapy are examples of the proliferation in techniques to prepare for birth. Although the techniques are more alike than different, explanations of their effectiveness can vary dramatically.

EFFECTIVENESS OF METHODS

Chertok summarized and evaluated the effectiveness of preparation for birth and suggested that all preparation techniques had three components: (1) psychophysical techniques, (2) psychological components, and (3) intellectual components.

Psychophysical. Various studies have been undertaken to determine the physiological effectiveness of prepared childbirth methods in terms of the amount of pain experienced during labor and birth, maternal and fetal complications, and the length of labor. Chertok and Velvovsky reviewed many studies in which investigators demonstrated the effectiveness of preparation-for-birth approaches to pain relief during childbirth. Huttel reports observations of less "complaint" and "tension" behaviors among women who were prepared for birth compared with women who did not attend preparation classes. Huttel suggested that preparation for birth enables the mother to experience a shorter labor.

Psychological. Although the physiological benefits of prepared childbirth are important, additional benefits have been claimed. A review of the literature by Buxton in 1962 concluded by emphasizing the critical importance of the psychological benefits of preparation for birth. Unlike some of the contradictory material found on physiological effects, research on psychological effects continues to be overwhelmingly in agreement. Tanzer found that prepared women had a more positive subjective experience during delivery. It is particularly notable in this research how many of the women stressed the importance of having either their husband or another support person present during labor. Tanzer's results indicate that the women experience a positive and highly desirable effect when their mates are present during birth. Other studies report that support and participation in labor and birth by the infant's father contribute to positive perceptions of the birth experience.

Intellectual. The intellectual components of preparation for childbirth are closely tied to the psychological components, since research has indicated that the more knowledge a woman gains concerning pregnancy, labor, and birth as a result of childbirth preparation classes, the more favorable will be her resultant attitude toward the pregnancy and labor and delivery experience. A woman's perception of maintaining control is closely associated with satisfaction, according to a study of 145 women. Although the mechanisms by which preparation for childbirth classes affect the birth experience are not yet fully understood, it is clear that these classes affect the subjective experience in a positive manner.

METHODS OF CHILDBIRTH PREPARATION

Dick-Read method: childbirth without fear

Psychophysical techniques. Relaxation and controlled breathing are taught as a way to cope with contractions. Dr. Dick-Read basically recommended three techniques: deep breathing in both abdominal respirations and thoracic respiration, shallow breathing, and breath-holding for the second stage of labor.

Psychological component. According to Dick-Read: "Fear, tension, and pain are three veils opposed to the natural design which have been concerned with preparation for and attendance at childbirth. If fear, tension, and pain go hand in hand, then it must be necessary to relieve tension and to overcome fear in order to eliminate pain. The implementation of my theory demonstrates the methods by which fear can be overcome, tension may be eliminated and replaced by physical and mental relaxation" (Dick-Read, 1959, p. 39).

Intellectual component. Dick-Read's program educates women to exchange understanding and confidence for fear of the unknown. Adequate prenatal education includes information on nutrition, basic hygiene, and labor and birth.

Lamaze (PPM) method

Psychophysical techniques. Controlled muscular relaxation and breathing techniques combine in the Lamaze method. PPM emphasizes conditioning and repetition.

Psychological component. According to this method, pain in labor is a conditioned response and women can be conditioned not to experience this pain. The essential elements of Lamaze include an external focus of attention and a series of relaxation and breathing exercises with a coach.

Intellectual component. The Lamaze method emphasizes understanding the body and how it works.

Bradley method

Psychophysical techniques. Breath control, diaphragmatic breathing, and general body relaxation are used in the Bradley method. Working in harmony with the body is emphasized.

Psychological techniques. The importance of the husband's support is foremost in this method. Women are helped to find their own ways to relax and give birth in their own fashion.

Intellectual component. Preparation for birth teaching concentrates on minimizing the need for analgesics or anesthetics.

NURSING ACTIONS

Most methods include one or all of the following:

1. Relaxation
2. Breathing techniques
3. Pushing techniques
4. Second-stage coping
5. Good posture and body mechanics
6. Genital and pelvic floor awareness

DESCRIBE THE OVERALL PHILOSOPHY OF EDUCATION IN PREPARATION FOR CHILDBIRTH

Finally, as an umbrella covering all methods of preparation for birth is the philosophy that knowledge can liberate people from the chains of fear of the unknown. Therefore, all childbearing people need knowledge of pregnancy, birth, and parenting. When people are informed of all the options open to them, they should be able to make informed choices, thus becoming intelligent consumers of maternity care.

Even if the laboring woman and her partner (or family or support persons) are well prepared, the nurse is still an important member of the childbirth team. Labor is a crisis time, and all people, no matter how well prepared, enter labor with some level of anxiety. Women respond differently to labor depending on the pain associated with their labor, fears, coping styles, and goals and expectations. Remember that labor is stress even if the couple is prepared. They need you. Do not leave them totally alone. Provide support when they need it—and privacy when they need it.

The following are some helpful actions the nurse as a support person may use to offer both verbal and "hands on" support during labor:

ACTIONS SUPPORT PERSON MAY USE WHEN OFFERING SUPPORT TO COUPLE PREPARED FOR LABOR

1. Encourage moving around during labor. If labor is progressing slowly, walking may accelerate it. Changing position frequently from sitting to standing to hands and knees to lying down to walking will help relieve pain.
2. Talk of contractions, not pains. Remember, the woman is having "contractions"!
3. Relax and get as near to the woman's level as possible. If she is lying down, sit by the bedside. Do not tower over her. Touch!
4. The labor bed should provide for comfortable positions. She should never be flat on her back because the weight of the uterine contents puts too much pressure on major blood vessels, thus reducing the blood flow back to the brain. Use pillows to support all dependent body parts.
5. Use comfort measures such as cold cloths, backrubs, and massages. Give ice chips and fruit juices for hydration. Keep the room warm, with bright lights dimmed but still enough light in the room for her to see the "focal point" if she is using one.
6. Carry on a conversation only between contractions if necessary.
7. Talk with the father or other support person. Give reassurance and remember that the father has needs for nourishment, rest, and elimination as well as the mother. Let him know where the bathroom is and where he may purchase food. Also, reassure him that you will stay with the laboring woman if he needs to leave for a while to tend to his own needs.
8. Do not ask irrelevant questions. Keep talk to a minimum. It uses energy needed to cope. Be aware of attitudinal changes as labor progresses.
9. Keep your voice well modulated at all times.
10. Remind the mother to urinate frequently. A full bladder can slow the descent of the baby.
11. Encourage rest between contractions.
12. Keep the couple and family members informed of what is happening: how many centimeters dilated, station, effacement, and fetal position.
13. Assure the mother she is doing well, offer encouragement, agree with her if she says it hurts but offer positive comments too.

14. Do not distract her during contractions. Wait until a contraction is over to do a nursing procedure.
15. Remember that the time period just before complete dilatation may be the most intense time in labor. Because the woman may fall asleep between contractions, they may overpower her. She may become very irritable.
16. During the actual birth stage, trust her and work with her body. This is not an athletic contest; the goal is pelvic floor release and relaxation. Encourage a series of quick breaths, holding one for 5 seconds while pushing and then again. Give verbal support such as: "Beautiful! Go with it! Let it flow! Open up below! Soft and loose! Open the door!" You might even give the woman a mirror so that she can watch her own progress as she pushes the baby out.
17. If the birth will occur in a delivery room, give the father or other support person the clothes to wear in the delivery room well in advance so that there is no last minute rush.

DISCUSS SUPPORT FOR FATHER DURING LABOR

18. As you encourage relaxation, encourage release toward your touching hand on her body. This will help the woman to increase her body awareness.
19. Always encourage the breathing that feels right for each woman. She may have practiced one type of breathing before labor only to find that it is not helpful during a certain part of labor. If this happens, be flexible. Encourage her to find what is working for her and stick with it.
20. There is no failure! Some people who have prepared faithfully for a "natural" childbirth will not be able to achieve that goal because of circumstances beyond their control. They may need analgesia, anesthesia, or a cesarean birth. If they are disappointed, encourage them to talk about their disappointment and then help them to work through it by emphasizing that there is no failure. When they have achieved a meaningful and safe birth experience, they have achieved their goal.
21. And last, but maybe most important, throughout the entire labor process be constantly and consistently aware of the needs of the fetus. When the couple have prepared diligently for labor and are extremely intent on what they are doing, it is often easy for the support person to get caught up in that intensity and feel reluctant to do any procedure that might "spoil" their experience. Continually think of yourself as a fetal advocate and use your knowledge and skills to make sound judgments that will lead to a meaningful and safe birth experience for all family members.

CHILDBIRTH EXERCISES

The nurse who has a basic understanding of the exercises widely used in preparation for childbirth classes will be able to work effectively with laboring people. Therefore, you should practice each of the prepared childbirth exercises that follow. You may find it easier and more fun to practice the exercises by working in a team with a fellow student while one of you pretends to be the woman in labor and the other assumes the role of support person. Find a quiet, comfortable place where you will not be disturbed for about an hour. Because the best way to practice is on the floor, you will probably be most comfortable on a carpeted floor or on a mat.

Exercises for the pelvic floor (Kegel exercise)

DESCRIBE THE KEGEL EXERCISES FOR PELVIC FLOOR

Many women are not aware of the muscles of the pelvic floor until it is pointed out that these are the muscles used during urination and sexual intercourse and are therefore consciously controlled. Because pelvic floor muscles ring the outlet through which the baby must pass, it is important that they be exercised, because an exercised muscle can stretch and contract readily at the time of birth. To locate these muscles, a woman can practice stopping the flow and starting it again while urinating.

Once the muscles are located, this exercise needs to be practiced many times a day to be effective. A good time to practice is during trips to the bathroom, but additional practice at other times is even more beneficial. Because it is not obvious when a woman is practicing, she might practice anytime and anywhere.

The procedure is to tighten the pelvic floor muscles as in holding back urine, hold for 10 seconds, and then release. Or think of the vagina as an elevator and practice ascending and descending slowly. This exercise can be done 10 times in a row, 5 to 10 times or more a day. Although some people recommend doing this exercise as many as 100 times in a row, this only fatigues the pelvic floor muscles. After delivery, this exercise helps the pelvic floor muscles return to normal and should be begun immediately after delivery.

Controlled relaxation

Relaxation is the foundation for all other techniques in labor. The first step in learning how to relax is knowing the difference between relaxation and tension.

EXERCISES WIDELY USED IN PREPARATION FOR CHILDBIRTH CLASSES

1. Find a position that can support your body completely. Do not have a part of you resting on any other part, and do not have any of your joints straight. Support all your dependent parts by placing a pillow under head, knees, and arms if necessary (Fig. 6-1).
2. Breathe slowly and naturally. When you first begin to learn relaxation, it is important that you relax systematically by tightening muscles in a structured order and then letting them go slowly so that you can feel the contrast.
   a. Start with your left foot; tighten it and then relax it; tighten your left leg next, keeping your left foot relaxed; now relax your left foot and leg.
   b. Next tighten your left hand and then relax it; tighten your left arm, keeping your left hand relaxed; now relax your left arm and hand.
   c. At this point, your left foot and left leg, left hand and left arm should be relaxed.
   d. Now work on the right side of your body in the same order: right foot to right leg; right hand to right arm.
   e. When both feet and legs and hands and arms are relaxed, gently and firmly pull in on the abdomen, draw the buttocks tightly together, and then release gradually.
   f. Continue to breathe slowly and easily, trying to make your mind a blank slate.

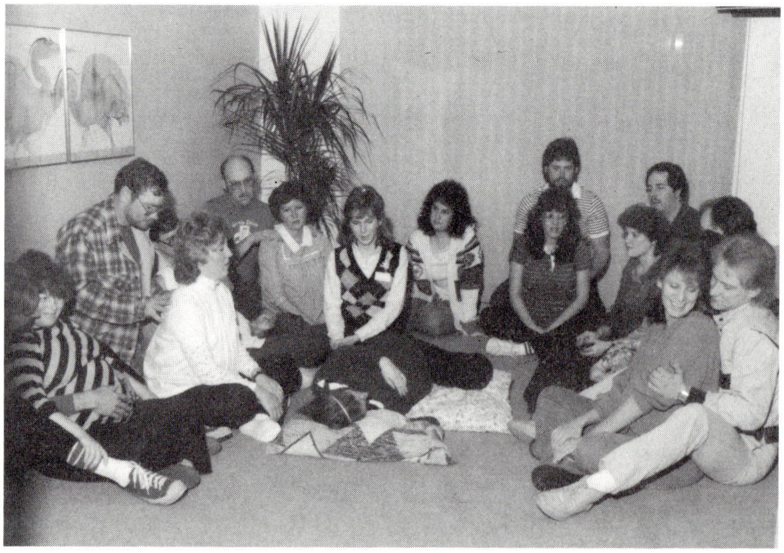

Fig. 6-1. Practicing relaxation. (Courtesy Valley Hospital and Medical Center, Spokane, Wash.)

Don't permit thoughts to enter in. If you find this difficult, concentrate completely on one simple, pleasant thought, excluding all others. Count sheep, if that helps.

g. Now draw your shoulders and back firmly upward and release slowly.

h. Last, make a face by tightening your face and neck muscles, pinching your mouth and eyes closed. Release your mouth, neck, and eyelids, letting the lower jaw fall loosely. Now work on the upper half of your body. Draw your shoulders and back firmly upward, clench fists and tighten arms. Release slowly. Finally, tighten your face and neck muscles by frowning, clenching your eyes closed, wrinkling your nose upward, clenching your jaws, drawing your lips back over your teeth, and pressing neck muscles together. Release your jaws, lips, neck, cheeks, and nose, letting your lower jaw fall slack and tongue hang loose. Let your eyelids and brow fall smooth, so that your eyes remain gently closed.

i. When entirely relaxed, your bones, muscles, and joints feel heavy at first; later, there is little or no feeling. It is as though you had "melted away" or sunk into the floor. When a woman uses this controlled relaxation when having contractions, much energy is conserved, and the working uterus is enabled to do a more efficient job (Fig. 6-2).

Different positions will be necessary for comfort as the baby moves through the birth canal. Relaxation should be practiced in many positions, including standing, sitting, semisitting, getting on hands and knees, squatting, and lying on your side.

Concentration-relaxation exercise

Lie on the floor; put a pillow under your head and another under your knees so you are completely supported. Relax your body using the relaxation techniques just prac-

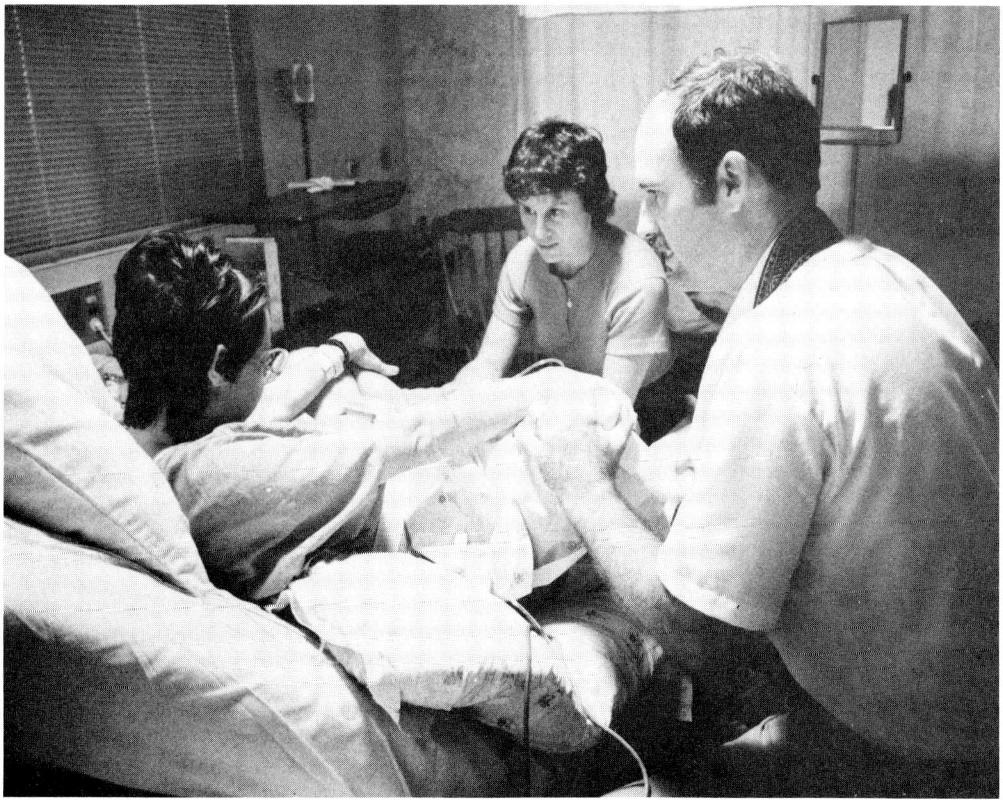

Fig. 6-2. Team work. (Photo by Paul O'Mara, courtesy Sharon and Vance Baker.)

ticed. Now, with the rest of your body as completely relaxed as possible, contract your right arm: tighten your shoulder, elbow, fist, and raise your arm. Release it; let your entire arm go limp and let it fall to the floor. Contract your left arm in the same way—release. Contract your right leg, tighten your entire leg, release. Contract your left leg—release. Contract your right arm and left leg—release. Do not tighten the other limbs. *Continue to keep the rest of your body relaxed.*

If you are practicing in a team, the support person should check to see if the opposite limbs are relaxed when they should be; for example, if the right arm and left leg are contracted, the left arm and right leg should be totally relaxed. (Practice by alternately contracting and relaxing opposite limbs.)

Slow chest breathing

Slow chest breathing is the easiest and most relaxing of the techniques and is used in early labor.

Sit comfortably on the floor with legs relaxed and pillows supporting all dependent parts. Assume a contraction is beginning. Take a deep *cleansing breath* (inhale through your nose and exhale through your mouth). Following the cleansing breath, breathe deliberately and slowly with your chest, inhaling through your nose and exhaling through your mouth. Take six to nine breaths in 1 minute. Relax completely and focus on an object in the room or your support person as you breathe. This will be your focal point. When the contraction is over, take another cleansing breath and rest. (To begin a "practice" contraction, simply look at the second hand on a clock or watch and choose a starting time. Allow the contraction to last 60 seconds.)

After you can breathe comfortably with slow chest breathing, use a light circular stroke *(effleurage)* to massage the abdomen to the rhythm of your breathing. Hold your hands just above your pubic bone and stroke with your fingertips upward over your abdomen while breathing in and down again to the starting point while blowing out (Fig. 6-3).

(The support person could give definite directions at beginning and end of contraction by signaling "contraction begins" and "contraction ends" and should check for relaxation of all muscles during the contraction, while offering encouragement and a concerned touch.)

Rapid, superficial breathing

For active labor a more active, superficial breathing is often helpful. Begin with a deep breath in and blow it out (cleansing breath). Then keep both nose and mouth open and move only your chest, as little as possible. Breathe lightly, rapidly, and evenly, accenting the out breath for 1 full minute and ending with a deep cleansing breath. Exchange the air as superficially as possible. Keep your body relaxed, and open your mouth slightly. Repeating "he, he, he" as you exhale will help you establish a rhythm. You may find that counting will help, "1-2-3-4, 1-2-3-4," putting emphasis on the "one" as you exhale.

After you have mastered this breathing, adjust your timing to the "wavelike" flow of contractions. Start breathing slowly as the contraction begins, then speed up your breathing as the contraction increases in strength, and slow down again as it goes away (Fig. 6-4). As the contractions get longer, stronger, and closer together, breathing becomes shallower and faster. Remember to keep your eyes open and focus on an object in the room while you practice and to keep your body relaxed. If you should feel lightheaded, you may be hyperventilating. Simply rebreathe your own air by breathing into a paper bag.

The support person could continue to signal "contraction begins" and "contraction ends," timing the contraction to last 60 seconds.

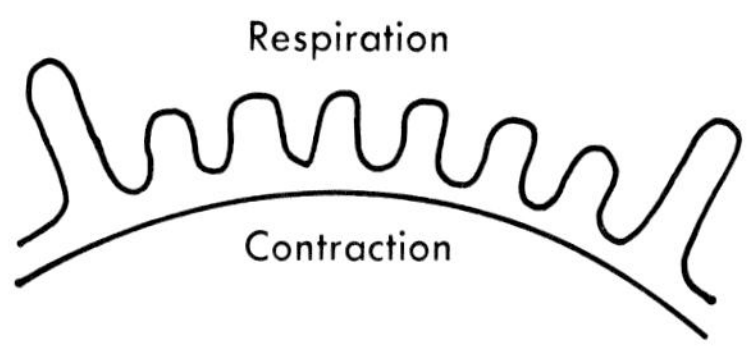

Fig. 6-3. Slow chest breathing.

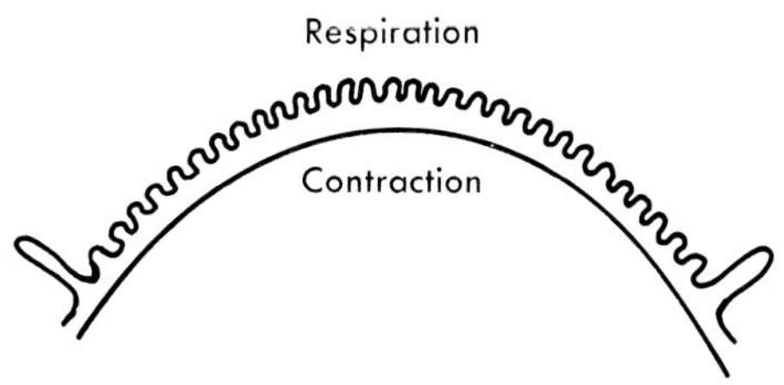

Fig. 6-4. Rapid, superficial breathing.

In addition to being the timer, the support person should continue to check for complete relaxation and offer verbal and "hands on" support.

Concentrate on keeping your breathing slow, controlled, relaxed, and rhythmical—between 25 and 60 breaths per minute. Your breathing is like a steam engine pulling out of the train station. As your contraction gradually peaks, your breathing accelerates. As your contraction subsides, your breathing gradually slows like the steam locomotive slows down arriving at the next station.

Pant and blow breathing

Pant and blow breathing is for the transition stage of labor, which is often the most stressful time. It is like rapid, superficial breathing but with forced blowing out at intervals.

Begin by taking a cleansing breath. Then take four light, shallow breaths, counting as you exhale—"1-2-3-4." Now breathe in another shallow breath and as you exhale, blow out forcefully through your mouth. Return to light, shallow breaths and blow out forcefully according to the 1-2-3-4 pattern established.

Transition contractions may last 60 to 90 seconds, with only short intervals between them. The support person may find it necessary to encourage two or three forceful BLOWS to block an early urge to push.

Expulsion breathing

To push the baby down through the vagina, when the contraction begins, assume a comfortable position. Because of the detrimental effects of the supine position, more and more women are choosing positions of comfort for the delivery of the baby. Semisitting, kneeling, squatting, lying on one's side, standing, and semistanding are all positions women choose. Remember that to push effectively along the axis of the curved birth canal, you must be in a position complementing this curve. The baby moves down, forward, and out as though descending on a sliding board. Breathe in and out very slowly (so not to waste your energy by pushing too soon). Again, breathe in slowly and hold onto your breath, fixing your diaphragm downward, and push downward using your abdominal muscles. Again, remember to keep the muscles of your pelvic floor relaxed. Continue to push for the count of 4 or 5, then take another breath. Repeat this effort until the contraction is gone. When the contraction has ended, breathe in and out several times, assume a comfortable position, and rest (Fig. 6-5).

Sometimes you will hear people helping women push by saying, "Push as though you were going to have a bowel movement." Remember this woman is pushing a baby out through the vagina and needs to relax the vagina and pelvic floor to do this. Talking to her about having a bowel movement may only serve to confuse her pushing efforts.

Also, sometimes you will hear helping people ask a woman to "hold her breath" and push as long as she can before coming up for air. When a woman holds her breath for more than 6 or 7 seconds as she pushes, there is greatly reduced exchange of gases across the placenta to the fetus. This reduction in perfusion could be dangerous to the fetus by

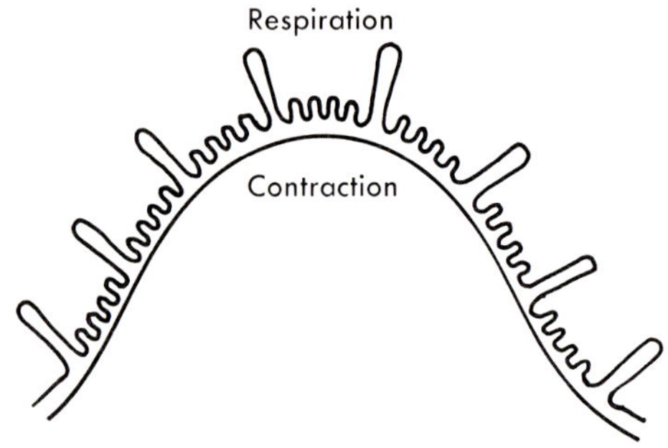

Fig. 6-5. Expulsion breathing.

causing a reduced oxygen supply. So when you push or help women to push, encourage them to push as *they* feel like pushing, without holding their breath more than 5 seconds at a time, if at all possible.

After you have practiced each of these six specific exercises, exchange roles so that the support person becomes the laboring woman and vice versa.

Because these exercises may not be exactly like those being taught in your community, attend a series of preparation for birth classes so that you can become acquainted with what expectant parents are being taught.

Now that you have experienced breathing patterns for birth, you are probably thinking that preparation for childbirth is a lot of work—and you are right. It is! Breathing exercises are only a part of the birth preparation and should be practiced daily in the last weeks of pregnancy. In addition to the breathing exercises, childbirth preparation classes usually include information on the anatomy and physiology of labor, the mechanisms of labor, pain relief methods available, ways of coping with the stress of labor, characteristics and care of the newborn, and of course, emotional preparation for parenting.

PREPARATION FOR PARENTING PROGRAMS

Classes in preparation for the birth itself are only a small part of an extensive preparation for parenthood program that should be available to all childbearing people, whether single or in couples. Such a program recognizes that pregnancy is not a disease state but is a state of wellness, during which people move from the role of expectant parents to the role and responsibilities of parents of a new baby, as a new family. Pregnancy can be a meaningful growth experience and can increase the family's self-confidence with the help of education for parenting.

TYPES OF CLASSES

A typical preparation for parenthood program recognizes that childbearing people have different interests and information needs as the pregnancy progresses; consequently, the program is designed to meet the concerns of the people at the three major stages of pregnancy, plus after birth.

Early pregnancy ("early bird") classes. Early pregnancy classes provide fundamental information about early development, physiological and emotional changes of pregnancy, human sexuality, and the nutritional needs of the mother and fetus.

Midpregnancy classes. Midpregnancy classes provide information on preparation for breast- and bottle-feeding, basic hygiene, health maintenance (rest, exercise, nutrition), and infant health.

Late pregnancy classes. Late pregnancy classes include the preparation for childbirth classes already discussed.

Throughout the series of classes there is discussion of support systems people can use during pregnancy and after delivery, so that they can function independently and effectively by developing their own health awareness and health maintenance behavior. During all the classes the open expression of feelings and concerns about any aspect of pregnancy, birth, and parenting is welcomed.

After birth classes ("What do we do now?"). After birth classes include coping mechanisms for the reality of parenting, support systems, infant care and growth and development, birth control methods, human sexuality, and adapting to new roles (wife/lover⇆mother and husband/lover⇆father).

Preparation for parenthood programs are multiplying throughout the country as more and more satisfied new parents tell friends, neighbors, and families about their prepared births. It is really very exciting to watch well-informed, interested people become active, intelligent consumers of health care. Table 6-1 presents an excellent prenatal teaching guide.

Prenatal classes for repeat parents. Prenatal classes for repeat parents are especially for expectant parents who already have children. The focus is on preparing the older child for the arrival of the new baby as well as reviewing previously used childbirth preparation techniques. In addition, the classes deal with the physical, social, and emotional changes unique to the growing family.

Sibling preparation classes. Sibling preparation classes are designed to ease the anxiety children face when mother goes to the hospital or birth center to give birth. Children are prepared for the role of big brother or big sister, thereby enhancing the experience for the entire family (Fig. 6-6).

Grandparenting classes. The content of grandparenting classes includes looking at the changing role of being a grandparent. The role of grandparent is compared with and contrasted to the role of parent. The content includes an update on childbirth, the role of the father as active participant, and "new" infant care trends.

Other classes. Other classes in a comprehensive program might be on cesarean preparation, adolescent family classes, prenatal exercise, pregnancy after 30, preparation for vaginal birth after cesarean, blended family, breast-feeding, and parenting and adult living. There are also orientation classes to specific hospital programs. Involving families in mother and baby care programs can be an effective educational approach.

Although the emphasis in this unit has been on labor support for the prepared couple, not all couples come to labor prepared and not all laboring women have partners for support. The helpful actions for labor support given in this unit are still very useful for all laboring people. However, if there is no family or friend to support the laboring woman, then the nurse's role becomes even more crucial. A woman should never have to labor alone! If the realities of staffing shortages prevent your constant attendance to women laboring alone, you could seek labor support persons from community volunteer groups. A few days spent in teaching and preparation of these volunteers could provide countless hours of labor support for women alone at this crisis time in their lives. Until labor support groups can be formed, you can communicate openly and honestly with women laboring alone. Inform them of the constraints on your time and let them know where you will be when you leave their side, how they can communicate with you, and when you will be coming back.

Women alone or couples who have not attended preparation for birth classes can learn relaxation and slow chest breathing techniques with your help during labor. Inform them that there are ways to cope with labor and that you can help them to learn these techniques right then and there. A motivated learner is the best learner, and most laboring women are highly motivated for relief of discomfort.

There are times when no matter how much support you offer and no matter what you do, the woman or couple will choose not to cope with labor and request analgesia and/or anesthesia (total or partial). Each person has a right to labor and give birth in whatever way she chooses, provided the way is safe for both mother and baby. Unit VII discusses

Table 6-1. Prenatal teaching guide

1st-12th Weeks Woman more concerned with herself, physical changes with pregnancy, and her feelings about the pregnancy	**12th-24th Weeks** Woman has usually resolved the issue of the pregnancy and becomes more aware of the fetus as a person	**24th-32nd Weeks** Woman becomes more interested in baby's needs as a corollary to her own needs now and after birth
Changes that are normal for pregnancy	Growth of fetus	Fetal growth and status
Breast fullness	Movement	Presentation and position
Urinary frequency	FHT	Well-being—FHT
Nausea and vomiting	Personal hygiene	Personal hygiene
Fatigue	Comfortable clothing	Comfortable clothing
EDC—calculate and explain	Breast care and supportive bra	Body mechanics and posture
Compare with uterine size	Recreation, travel	Positions of comfort
Expectation for care	Vaginal discharge	Physical and emotional changes
Initial visit	Employment or school plans	Sexual needs and changes. Intercourse
Subsequent visits	Method of feeding baby	
Clinic appointments	Breast or bottle	Alleviation of backache
Need for iron and vitamins	Give literature re methods	Braxton Hicks contractions
Resources available	Avoidance or alleviation of	Dyspnea
Education	Backache	Round ligament pain
Dental evaluation	Constipation	Leg ache or edema
Medical service	Hemorrhoids	Confirm infant's feeding plans
Social service	Leg ache, varicosities, edema, cramping	Prepare for breast or bottle feeding
Emergency room		Nipple preparation
Danger signs	Round ligament pain	Massage and expression of breast
Drugs, self-medication	Nutritional guidance	
Spotting, bleeding	Weight gain	Preparation for baby
Cramping, pain	Balanced diet	Supplies
	Special nutritional needs	Household assistance
		Danger signs
		Pre-eclampsia
		Headache, excessive swelling, blurred vision
		Tubal ligation (papers prepared ahead)

From Roberts, J.: Prenatal teaching guide, J. Obstet. Gynecol. Neon. Nurs. **5:**17-20, May/June 1976.

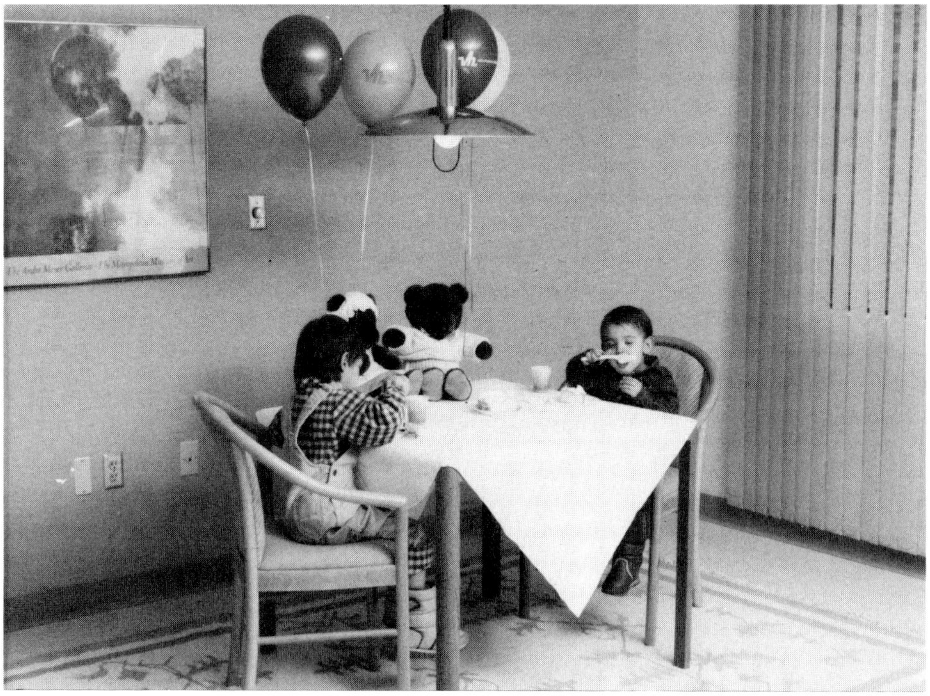

Fig. 6-6. Sibling party. (Courtesy Valley Hospital and Medical Center, Spokane, Wash.)

32nd-36th weeks Woman anticipates approaching labor and caring for baby after birth.	36th week to term Woman should feel "ready" for labor and for the assumption of care-taking responsibilities for baby, even though she may feel anxious about both of these as well.

Fetal growth and status
Personal hygiene
  Positions of comfort
  Rest and activity
  Vaginal discharge
Alleviation of discomfort
  Backache
  Round ligament pain
  Constipation or hemorrhoids
  Leg ache or edema
  Dyspnea
Recognition of "false labor"—Braxton Hicks contractions
  How to cope and "practice" with these
Nature of "true labor" signs. Difference between "bloody show" and bleeding
What happens during labor
  Labor contractions and progress
  What she will experience
Relaxation techniques
Breathing techniques
  Abdominal
  Accelerated pattern
  Panting and pushing
Involvement of husband or significant other
Provision for needs of other children
  Anticipation of baby
  Care for children at home while mother is in hospital
	Review signs of labor (or teach)
	Review or continue instruction regarding relaxation and breathing techniques
	Finalize home preparations
	Anticipation of hospitalization
	  Admission (ER and labor admitting room)
	  Examination, IV, shave, possible enema
	  Care in labor
	  Medication and anesthesia available
	  Postpartum care
	  Supplies needed: bra, personal items, money
	  May have two visitors
	  Tour of maternity unit
	Confirm plans to get to hospital; care of other children.
	  When to go and where
	Consider family planning needs
	Emergency arrangements
	  Precipitate delivery
	  Premature rupture of membranes with or without contractions
	  Care away from home
	  Vaginal bleeding

analgesia and anesthesia used for labor and delivery and responsibilities of the helping person.

SUMMARY

This unit has given you an opportunity to become familiar with some of the exercises widely used in preparation for childbirth classes and support techniques for labor so that you will be able to work effectively with childbearing couples. This unit on preparation for childbirth has been presented before the discussion of intrapartum care, which contains the mechanisms of birth, so that you can begin to get the feeling of the birth experience before you learn the mechanics of it. To become a skilled maternity nurse, you will need to develop feelings and sensitivity for this profound experience in addition to many skills.

BIBLIOGRAPHY

American Society of Psychoprophylaxis in Obstetrics: You want to be a certified childbirth educator? 1979.

Andersen, J.: A clarification of the Lamaze method, J. Obstet. Gynecol. Neon. Nurs. 7(2):53-54, 1977.

Barker-Benfield, G.L.: The horrors of the half-known life, New York, 1977, Doubleday.

Beals, P., editor: ICEA teacher's guide, ed. 2, Milwaukee, 1975, International Childbirth Education Association.

Bernardini, J.Y., Maloni, J.A., and Stegman, C.E.: Neuromuscular control of childbirth-

prepared women during the first stage of labor, J. Obstet. Gynecol. Neon. Nurs. **12**:105-111, March/April 1983.
Bing, E.: Six practical lessons for an easier childbirth, New York, 1969, Bantam Books.
Bradley, R.: Husband-coached childbirth, New York, 1965, Harper & Row, Publishers, Inc.
Buxton, C.L.: A study of psychological methods for relief of pain in childbirth, Philadelphia, 1962, W.B. Saunders Co.
Bylaws of the Childbirth Without Pain League, Riverside, Calif., May 15, 1979.
Chabon, I.: Awake and aware, New York, 1966, Dell Publishing Co., Inc.
Chertok, L.: Psychosomatic methods of preparation for birth, Am. J. Obstet. Gynecol. **98**(5):698-707, 1967.
Copstick, S., and others: A test of a common assumption regarding the use of antenatal training during labor, J. Psychosom. Res. **29**(2):215-218, 1985.
Cronenwett, L., and Newmark, L.: Father's responses to childbirth, Nurs. Res. **23**(3): 210-217, 1974.
Deutsch, R.M.: The key to feminine response in marriage, New York, 1968, Random House, Inc.
Dick-Read, G.: Childbirth without fear, ed. 2, New York, 1959, Harper & Row, Publishers, Inc.
Ehrenreich, B., and English, D.: For her own good: 150 years of the experts' advice to women, New York, 1978, Harper & Row, Publishers, Inc.
Ewy, D., and Ewy, R.: Preparation for childbirth, New York, 1972, New American Library.
Hassid, P.: Textbook for childbirth educators, ed. 2, Philadelphia, 1984, J.B. Lippincott Co.
Hathaway, T., and Hathaway, M., editors: The Bradley method, Sherman Oaks, Calif., American Association of Husband Coached Childbirth, 1985.
Henderson, J.S.: Effects of a prenatal teaching program on postpartum regeneration of the pubococcygeal muscle, J. Obstet. Gynecol. Neon. Nurs. **12**(6):403-408, 1983.
Hommel, F.: Painless childbirth. In Childbirth education, J. Am. Soc. Psychoproph. Obstet. **2**:4, 1969.
Huprich, P.A.: Assisting the couple through a Lamaze labor and delivery. MCN **2**(4):245-253, July/Aug. 1977.
Huttel, F.A., and others: A quantitative evaluation of psychoprophylaxis in childbirth, J. Psychosom. Res. **16**:81, 1972.
Jimenez, S.M., Jones, L.C., and Jungman, R.G.: Prenatal classes for repeat parents: a distinct need, MCN **4**:305-308, 1979.
Kitzinger, S.: The experience of childbirth, Middlesex, England, 1970, Pelican Publishing Co., Inc.
Klopher, F., Cogan, R., and Henneborn, W.: Second stage medical intervention and pain during childbirth, J. Psychosom. Res. **19**:289, 293, 1975.
Lamaze, F.: Painless childbirth: the Lamaze method, Chicago, 1970, Henry Regnery Co.
McKay, S., and Roberts, J.: Second stage labor: what is normal? J. Obstet. Gynecol. Neon. Nurs. **14**(2):101-106, 1985.
McKay, S.: Second stage labor—has tradition replaced safety?, Am. J. Nurs. **81**:1016, 1019, 1981.
McKay, S.: Squatting: an alternative position for the second stage of labor, MCN **9**:181-183, 1984.
Melzack, R.: The myth of painless childbirth (the John J. Bonica Lecture), Obstet. Gynecol. Surv. **40**(5):297-298, 1985.
Noble, E.: Childbirth with insight, Boston, 1983, Houghton Mifflin Co.
Otto, S., editor: ICEA 1978 biennial report, Milwaukee, 1978, International Childbirth Education Association.
Phillips, C.R.: Preparation for birth class outlines, 1984.
Preparation for parenthood, NAACOG technical bulletin, no. 3, 1978.
Sasmor, J.L.: Childbirth education: a nursing perspective, New York, 1979, John Wiley & Sons, Inc.
Smith, B.A., Priore, R.M., and Sterm, M.K.: The transition phase of labor, Am. J. Nurs. **74**:448-450, 1973.
Tanzer, D.: Why natural childbirth? New York, 1972, Doubleday & Co., Inc.
Tanzer, S.: The psychology of pregnancy and childbirth: An investigation of natural childbirth, doctoral dissertation, 1967, Brandeis University.
Vadurro, J.F., and Butts, P.A.: Reducing the anxiety and pain of childbirth through hypnosis, Am. J. Nurs. **82**(4):620-623, 1982.
Velvovsky, I., and others: Painless childbirth through psychoprophylaxis, Moscow, 1960, Foreign Languages Publishing House.
Wertz, R.W., and Wertz, D.C.: Lying in: a history of childbirth in America, New York, 1977, The Free Press.
Willmuth, L.R.: Prepared childbirth and the concept of control, J. Obstet. Gynecol. Neon. Nurs. **4**(5):38-41, 1975.
Wright, E.: The new childbirth, New York, 1966, Hart Publishing Co., Inc.

DEFINITIONS

Define the following terms:

analgesia

anesthesia

Bradley method	Kegel exercise
cleansing breath	Lamaze method
disassociation	natural childbirth
effleurage	perfusion
fetal advocate	psychoprophylaxis
fetus	Dick-Read method
focal point	transition

LEARNING ACTIVITIES AND EXPERIENCES

1. Group practice sessions.
2. Guest speakers: Bradley instructor, Dick-Read instructor, Lamaze instructor, a couple who experienced a prepared childbirth.
3. Visit a preparation for birth class in your community and report your impressions.
4. View audiovisual aids and discuss.
5. Determine the types of classes offered to childbearing families in your community.

ENRICHMENT/IN-DEPTH STUDY

1. Read: Chabon, L.: Awake and aware, New York, 1966, Dell Publishing Co.
   Dick-Read, G.: Childbirth without fear, ed. 2 (rev.), New York, 1959, Harper & Row, Publishers, Inc.
   Karmel, M.: Thank you, Dr. Lamaze, Philadelphia, 1959, J. B. Lippincott Co.
   Lamaze, F.: Painless childbirth: the Lamaze method, New York, 1972, Pocket Books.
2. Write a short, thoughtful paper on: "Should everyone try natural childbirth?"
3. Work through *The Lamaze Experience,* three 33⅓ rpm records, workbook, and chart.
4. Listen to: *Practice for Childbirth,* a 33⅓ rpm record, 15 minutes.

SELF-ASSESSMENT

1. List the six broad categories that most preparation for childbirth methods include in their teaching:
   a.
   b.
   c.
   d.
   e.
   f.

Situation: A laboring couple, Catherine and Duncan, have attended preparation for childbirth classes at the local YWCA and are now in the early stages of labor. Catherine is relaxing well and using the slow breathing pattern. Questions 2 through 7 relate to this situation. Circle the best answer.

2. As a member of this team, you would be sure Catherine is in the best position for early labor, by:
   a. rolling her bed down flat so that she is flat on her back
   b. encouraging Catherine to assume a position of comfort
   c. placing pillows to support Catherine's head
3. Between uterine contractions, you would:
   a. carry on a polite conversation
   b. encourage rest
   c. explain to Catherine and Duncan the activities going on in the maternity department
4. During a long, intense contraction, Catherine says, "Oh, that one really hurt!" Your best response would be:
   a. "No, it doesn't hurt. You must be losing control."
   b. "Would you like an anesthetic now?"
   c. "Would you like medicine to relieve your pain?"
   d. "That was really a good contraction that probably helped your progress very much, even though it did hurt a bit."
5. You would encourage Catherine to urinate every hour during labor because a full bladder can:
   a. cause urine to leak on the bed during a contraction
   b. cause painful uterine contractions
   c. slow down the descent of the baby
6. As labor progresses, it is necessary for you to have Catherine sign a consent form for use of the delivery room. You would do this:
   a. quickly at the peak of a contraction
   b. between contractions
   c. just as the contraction is ending
7. During the labor process, Duncan needs your support, too. Recognizing this, you would:
   a. ask him to sit down, rest, and conserve his strength because he is not needed now
   b. encourage him to go to the visitors' waiting room to rest
   c. offer him nourishment, inform him of the rest and bathroom areas, and offer him encouragement

For questions 8 and 9, circle the best answer.

8. The overall philosophy of preparation for childbirth education includes
   a. developing muscle strength by calisthenics to prepare for labor as an athlete would prepare for a race
   b. preparing for labor so one never has to take drugs for pain relief
   c. sharing information with people about pregnancy, birth, and parenting, so that they can make informed choices
9. The procedure to use when doing the Kegel exercise is:
   a. to breathe in slowly through the nose and out the mouth six to nine times a minute
   b. to breathe out, abdominally, holding the abdominal wall up off the uterus for 30 seconds
   c. to tighten the pelvic floor muscles as in holding back urine, hold for 10 seconds, and then release
10. Before completing this unit of study, demonstrate the following to your instructor during a group meeting held for return demonstration purposes:
    a. controlled relaxation
    b. concentration-relaxation
    c. slow chest breathing
    d. rapid superficial breathing
    e. pant and blow breathing
    f. expulsion breathing

UNIT VII
The intrapartum family

GOALS

This unit is designed to provide the reader with information that will:

□ promote an understanding of the birth process.

□ develop an awareness of individualized nursing care during labor and birth.

STUDENT OBJECTIVES

After studying this unit you should be able to:

1. Recognize circles representing dilation from 1 to 10 centimeters.
2. Distinguish among the four stages of labor and briefly describe what occurs in each stage. (Include usual duration for a primigravida and a multipara.)
3. Name the two main phases of cervical dilatation during stage one of labor and indicate their average duration for a primigravida and a multipara.
4. Describe a uterine contraction in terms of (1) increment, (2) acme, (3) decrement, (4) duration, and (5) time interval between contractions.
5. Recognize the average blood loss during the third stage of labor.
6. Demonstrate a basic understanding of fetopelvic relationships by:
   a. defining lie and presentation
   b. identifying the following bones composing the fetal head:
      (1) occipital
      (2) parietal
      (3) temporal
      (4) frontal
   c. identifying the anterior and posterior fontanels
   d. recognizing fetal position according to the four quadrants of the mother's pelvis
7. Distinguish among six types of fetal position and identify the letters of the alphabet used to designate each.
8. Demonstrate an understanding of the stress of labor by:
   a. identifying the psychologic stressors in labor
   b. discussing coping behaviors of women in labor

The physiological and psychological care a family receives during labor and birth is termed intrapartum care (*intra*, during; *partum*, birth).

ONSET OF LABOR

GIVE SEVERAL FACTORS ASSOCIATED WITH ONSET OF LABOR

Just exactly what causes labor to begin is not known. It is probably caused by one or more of the following factors: (1) Near term the placental production of progesterone drops. It is thought that progesterone is essential for the maintenance of the pregnancy. (2) Any hollow organ distended to an extreme extent will atempt to empty itself. At term (or before in the case of twins or polyhydramnios) the uterus is certainly distended; frequently, at this point, the uterine muscles contract. (3) Laboring women have increased levels of oxytocin, which causes the uterus to contract. (4) Prostaglandins, found in amniotic fluid during labor and in the plasma of pregnant women in labor, may play a role in causing labor to begin. (5) The pressure of the fetal presenting part on the cervix and the nerves around the cervix may stimulate labor. (6) The fetus itself may decide the time to be born. It has been proposed that at the proper time, the fetal adrenal glands release a pair of substances that trigger the release of other chemicals in the mother's uterus to begin labor. The human fetus may indeed be in control of its own destiny with respect to the onset of labor.

Although labor technically begins when the cervix starts to dilate, it is difficult to identify the exact moment when that happens. Because labor is unique, careful questioning of the woman about when and how she felt that labor had begun usually gives a fairly accurate estimation of the onset time.

Prelabor

DIFFERENTIATE BETWEEN TRUE LABOR AND PRELABOR

Throughout pregnancy the uterus contracts at slightly irregular intervals, about every 15 to 20 minutes, and lasting for about 25 seconds. These contractions may be felt as tightening of the abdomen, but they are not painful. They were described by Braxton Hicks many years ago and have become known as Braxton Hicks contractions. Sometimes women will be aware of Braxton Hicks contractions occurring on and off for hours, days, or even weeks before true labor begins. Most of the time they are felt only in the front of the abdomen and do not increase in intensity. These contractions usually are not regular or rhythmical and can often be relieved or even stopped by walking or by taking a warm shower or bath.

True labor

As labor begins, the woman will usually feel uterine contractions different from the Braxton Hicks contractions she has experienced during much of the pregnancy. The contractions of labor are more uncomfortable and rhythmical and recur at regular intervals (every 5 to 15 minutes, lasting 30 seconds or more). As these regular contractions continue, the interval between them gradually grows shorter. Also, true labor contractions usually become stronger when a woman walks around.

There are other signs that may be present when labor begins. (1) "Show," a small amount of blood-tinged, thick, stringy mucus escaping from the vagina. This mucous plug filled the cervix during pregnancy. (2) Rupture of the "bag of waters" with a trickle or gush of clear fluid from the vagina. This bag of waters is the transparent sac (amnion and chorion) in which the fetus floated during the pregnancy. Although the bag may rupture 10% to 15% of the time before labor, it frequently remains intact until labor has progressed almost to the birth. (3) Diarrhea with no apparent cause. (4) Low backache that often starts in the lower back and encircles the abdomen like a tight band. However, for labor to have begun, the preceding signs must be associated with contractions of the uterus and dilation of the cervix.

Proof that labor has begun may have to be a vaginal or rectal examination to check for dilation of the cervix. If the cervix has begun to dilate, true labor has begun. However, even though dilation has started, true labor may stop for a few hours or even days.

PROCESS OF LABOR

Pregnant and nonpregnant uterus and cervix

Both the uterus and cervix undergo remarkable changes during pregnancy. Briefly review the divisions of the cervix (refer to Fig. 2-2, p. 27). Note that the cervix is composed of a canal, with an internal os at the upper position, separating the cervix from the uterine cavity, and an external os below, which closes the cervix from the vagina. The cervix is about 2.5 centimeters long. The area between the internal and external ossa is the cervical canal.

The cervix is composed mostly of connective tissue interspersed with muscle fibers. In the nonpregnant state, it feels firm, somewhat like the tip of one's nose. During pregnancy, the cervix softens and feels somewhat like the lower lip. (Feel your lips and your nose. Note the difference?) This softening is caused by increased vascularity, edema, and hyperplasia of the cervical glands. Ripening is the softening of the cervix that takes place in late pregnancy.

Cervical dilation

Dilation (or dilatation) of the cervix means the enlargement of the external os from an orifice of 0.5 centimeters to an opening large enough to permit passage of the fetus—that is, to a diameter of about 10 centimeters.

Fig. 7-1 is an exact reproduction of a ruler showing centimeters on one side and inches on the other. Put the tip of your index finger on a centimeter. Does the tip of your finger cover the centimeter? Note that:

6 inches = approximately 15 cm
1 inch = approximately 2½ cm
½ inch = approximately 1¼ cm

DILATION

At the beginning of dilation, the cervix usually admits one finger easily (the tip of the index finger is approximately 1 centimeter wide). The cervix at the beginning of true labor is 1 centimeter dilated. At the end of the first stage of labor, the cervix is dilated to 10 centimeters.

Cervical effacement

EXPLAIN CERVICAL DILATION AND EFFACEMENT

Effacement is the shortening of the cervical canal from a structure of 2.5 centimeters in length to one in which no canal at all exists, but merely a circular orifice with almost paper-thin edges.

Fig. 7-2 shows the length of the area between the internal os and external os before labor. This is the area that shortens (or effaces). Note the edges of the internal os drawn several centimeters upward, drawn up even more, and, finally, the completely effaced cervix.

Effacement is determined during a pelvic examination and is measured in percentages from 0% to 100%. "Zero percent effacement" means the cervix has not begun to thin; "80% effacement" means that the cervix is almost completely thinned. For a primigravida, most of the effacement has usually occurred before dilatation begins. Multigravidas usually experience dilation and effacement at the same time.

Effacement can be compared with a funneling process in which the whole length of a moldable tube (the cervical canal) is converted into a very large, flaring funnel, with only a small circular orifice for an outlet.

Fig. 7-3 is a schematic drawing illustrating the change in the uterus during effacement. It is as if a gallon bottle has been converted into a gallon jar.

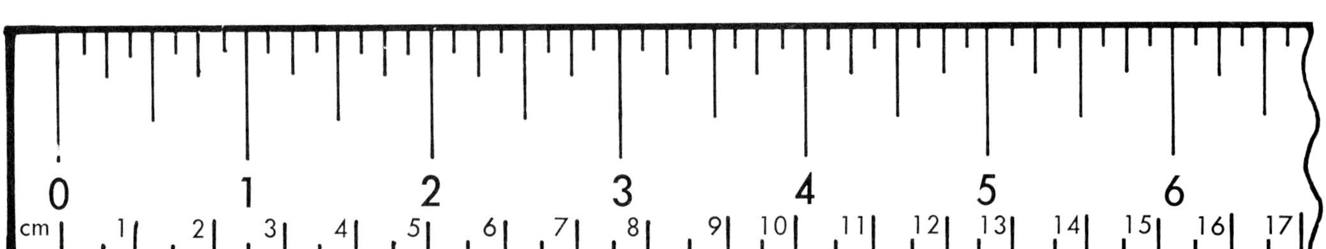

Fig. 7-1. Exact reproduction of a ruler.

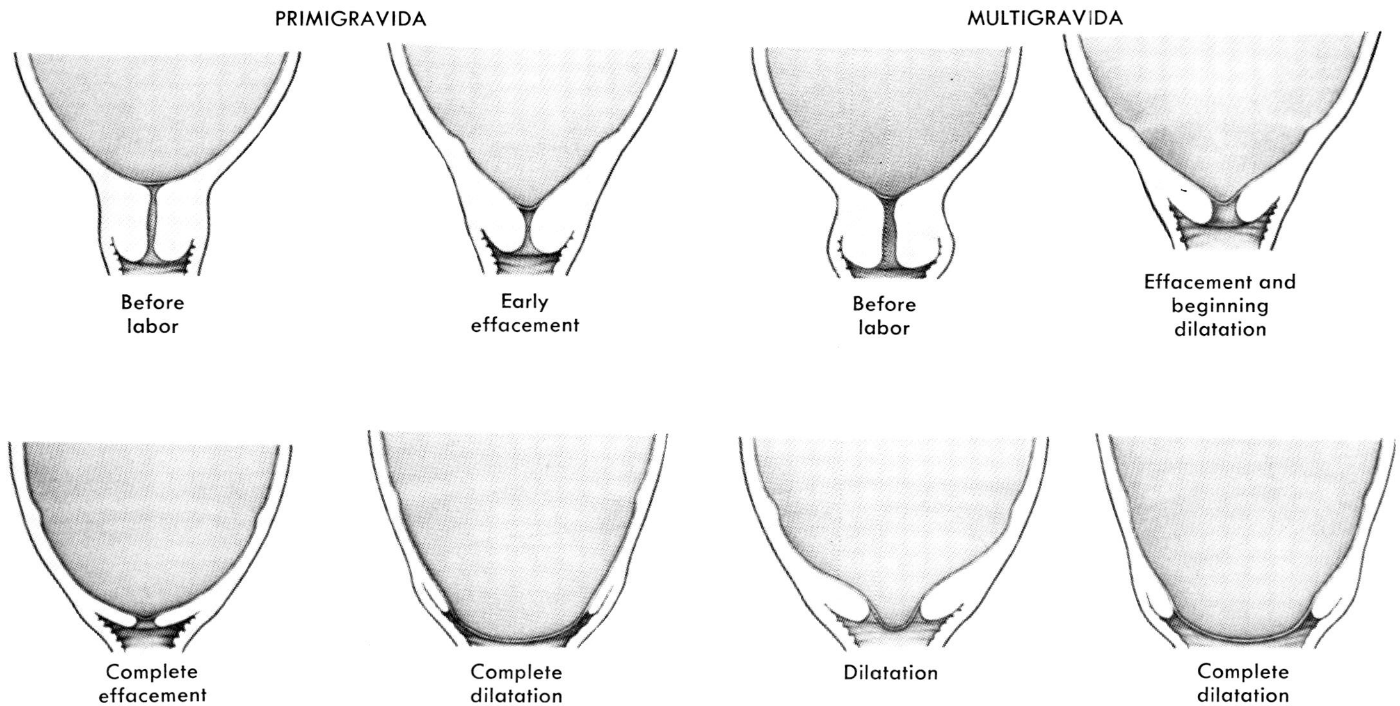

Fig. 7-2. Cervical effacement and dilation. (From Mechanisms of normal labor, Ross Laboratories Clinical Education Aid No. 13, Ross Laboratories, Columbus, Ohio.)

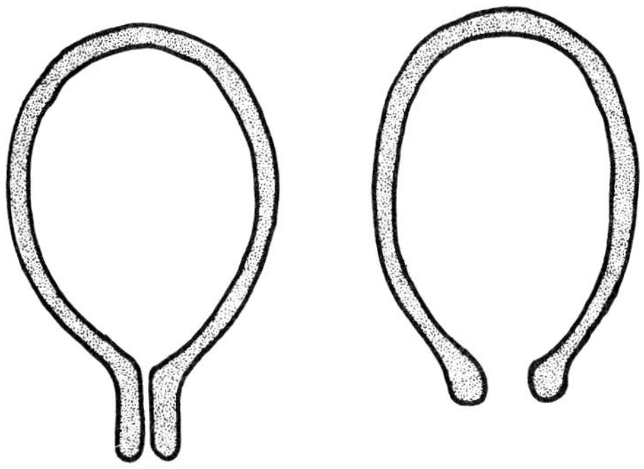

Fig. 7-3. Schematic illustration of effacement. **A,** Uneffaced cervix. **B,** Effaced cervix.

THE FOUR STAGES OF LABOR

Stage one

IDENTIFY SIGNS OF EACH STAGE OF LABOR

The first stage of labor is the stage of dilation and effacement of the cervix. It begins with true labor contractions and ends with complete dilation of the cervix (average 10 centimeters) (Fig. 7-4). This is the longest and most tedious stage for everyone concerned (8 to 12 hours in a primigravida and 6 to 8 hours in a multipara). The entire first stage of labor is not under voluntary control, and the only thing the woman can do is relax and work with labor at the same time. Although as labor begins contractions may be 15 to 20 minutes apart (lasting 30 seconds), toward the end of the first stage they are usually coming every 2 to 3 minutes and lasting 60 to 90 seconds.

PHASES OF STAGE ONE OF LABOR

The first stage of labor can be divided into two main phases of cervical dilation: the latent phase and the active phase. The *latent phase* is the long, slow climb during which the cervix dilates to 3 to 4 centimeters. The *active phase* has been subdivided further into an acceleration phase, a phase of maximum slope, and a deceleration phase (Fig. 7-5).

The deceleration phase can also be known as *transition.* This transition phase represents the last 1 or 2 centimeters of cervical dilation and is often the peak of intensity, pain, and difficulty. The woman's body is still in the first stage but is showing signs of moving into the second stage.

The cervix dilates as the uterus contracts from top to bottom (Fig. 7-6). A contraction is stimulated by pacemakers in cells of the myometrium near the right or left insertions of the fallopian tubes and moves down the uterus in a triple descending gradient (strongest at the top, intermediate strength in the middle, and weakest at the bottom). As labor progresses the uterus is divided into two distinct portions: (1) an active upper portion or segment (fundus and body of the uterus) and (2) a passive lower portion or segment (isthmus and cervix). As the muscles of the upper uterine segment contract and become thicker, reducing the size of the upper uterine cavity, the muscle fibers of the lower uterine segment become thinner and longer, increasing the area of the lower uterine cavity. When the uterus contracts, it rises up by a pull of the ligaments that support it; consequently, during a contraction the long axis of the uterus is in line with the axis of the birth canal. This change in the shape and angle of the uterus causes the fetus to be forced farther down into the mother's pelvis. At the same time, the cervix dilates and effaces as the muscle fibers of the uterus are pulled tight and up.

UTERINE CONTRACTIONS

Uterine contractions come and go like ocean waves, and have great force just like waves in the ocean. Each uterine contraction has three phases: (1) the *increment* phase, during which the intensity of the contraction builds, (2) the *acme*, or peak, of the contraction, and (3) the *decrement* phase, during which the intensity decreases (Fig. 7-7).

Fig. 7-4. Dilation of 1 to 10 centimeters.

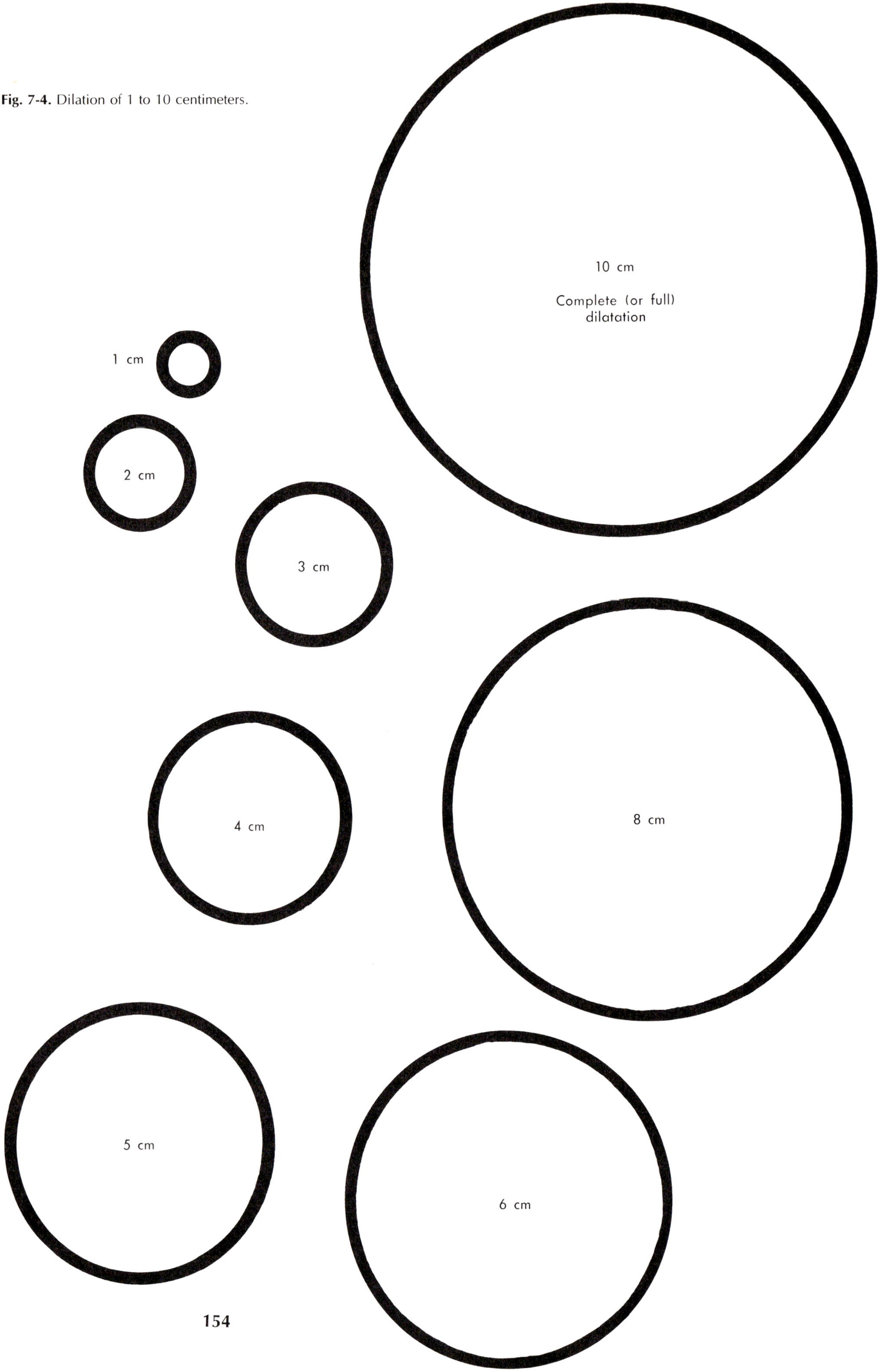

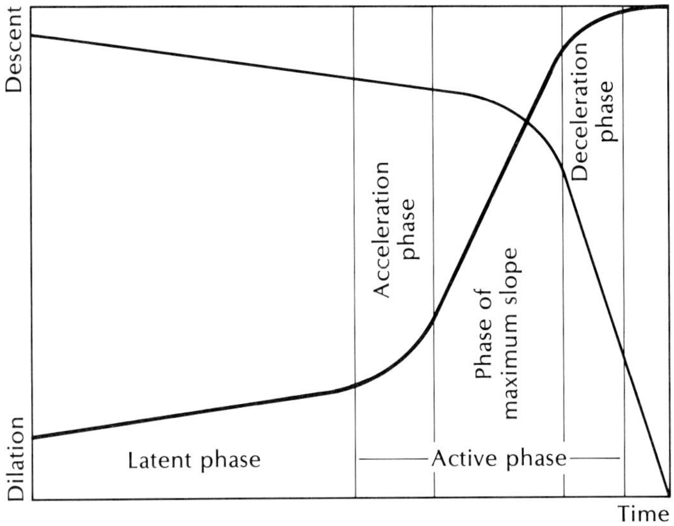

Fig. 7-5. Normal labor curve, with functional divisions.

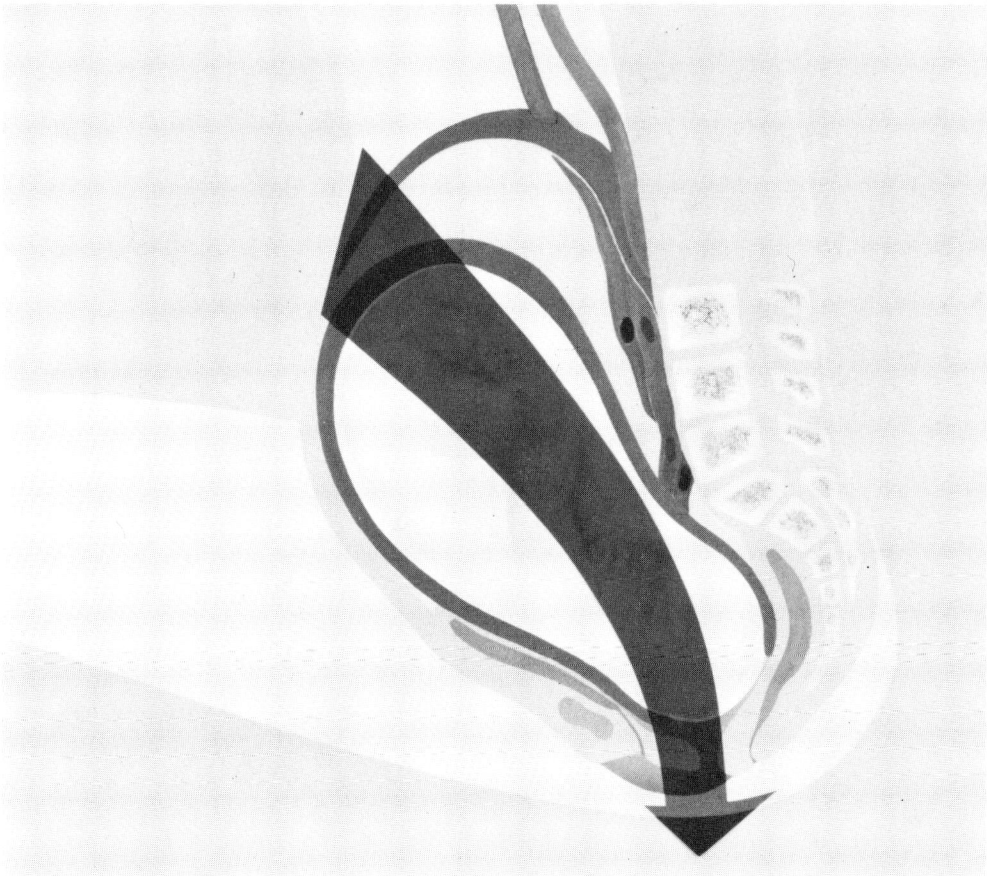

Fig. 7-6. The uterus contracts from top to bottom. (Courtesy of the Borning Corporation, Spokane, Wash.)

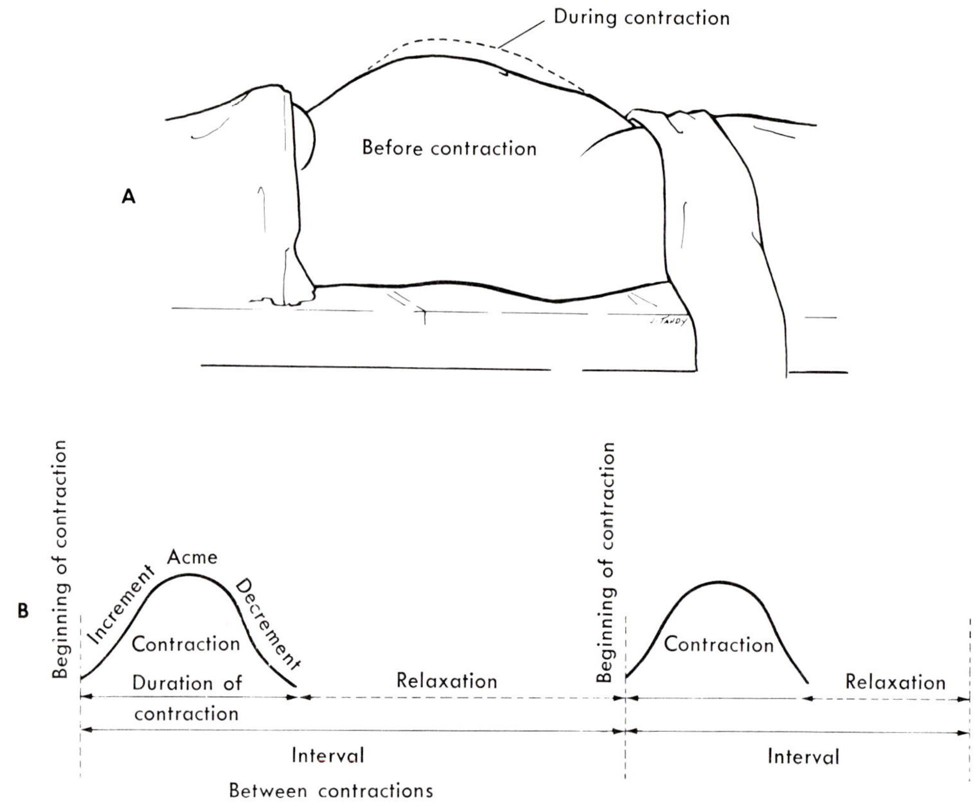

Fig. 7-7. Uterine contraction. (From Jensen, M., and Bobak, I.M.: Maternity and gynecologic care, the nurse and the family, ed. 3, St. Louis, 1985, The C.V. Mosby Co.)

The duration of a contraction is from the beginning of the increment to the end of the decrement. The frequency, or interval between contractions, is defined as being from the beginning of one contraction to the beginning of the next contraction.

Stage two

The second stage of labor is the stage of *expulsion*. It begins with complete dilation of the cervix and ends with the birth of the baby. It usually takes 30 minutes to 2 hours in a primigravida and 5 to 30 minutes in a multipara. The uterine contractions change in character and become very strong but slightly farther apart. The woman can actively participate in this stage by pushing the baby out, using her abdominal muscles. As the second stage begins, the fetus leaves the uterus and begins its descent into the birth canal, pushed forward by the contractions of the thickened upper uterine segment and the voluntary pushing of the woman. The vaginal tissue bulges (*bulging*), the rectum dilates, the pelvic floor muscles stretch, and a small part of the head of the fetus will appear at the vaginal opening. When the widest diameter of the fetus's head is visible at the vaginal opening, it is said to be *crowning*. Then with additional effort, a baby is born.

PRESENT THREE REASONS WHY EPISIOTOMY MAY BE DONE

Episiotomy. When the head crowns, an episiotomy may be done if it is decided that the fetal head needs more room so as not to tear the perineum as the head extends. An *episiotomy* is an incision into the perineum and may be made (1) midline (ML), (2) right mediolateral (RML), or (3) left mediolateral (LML) (Fig. 7-8). Episiotomies are also done to facilitate delivery when fetal distress occurs and to relieve prolonged pressure of the fetal head against the perineum in a long, difficult second stage.

There is much debate on the necessity for episiotomy. Many times massaging the perineum with warm oils, applying warm compresses, and stretching the perineum by the attendant's fingers prior to delivery will prevent tearing. Also, stretching, perineal

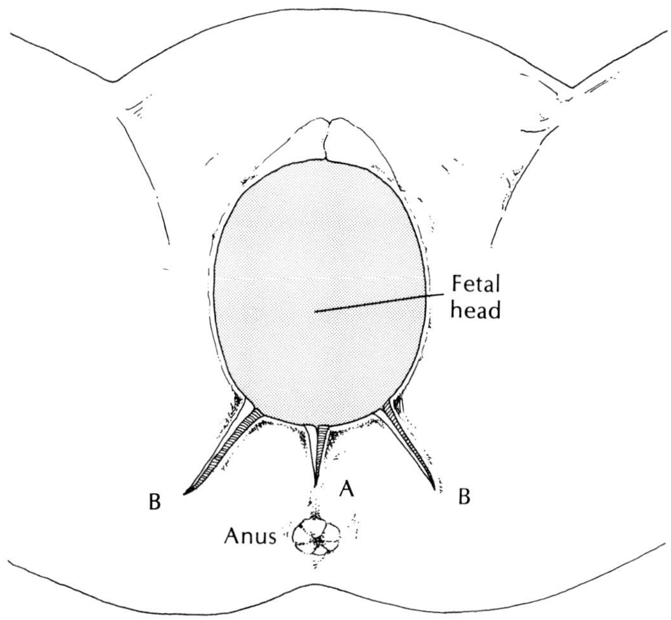

Fig. 7-8. Episiotomy. **A,** Median or midline. **B,** Right or left mediolateral. Fetal head is crowning.

massage, and Kegel exercises performed during pregnancy often permit the mother to relax her perineal muscles at birth, thus allowing the fetal head to emerge over an intact perineum.

Stage three

The third stage of labor is the *placental stage,* consisting of two phases: (1) placental separation and (2) placental expulsion. It begins with the birth of the baby and terminates with the delivery of the placenta. During this stage the membranes are separated and expelled from the body. This may require from 5 to 30 minutes. With the fetus gone, the uterus is now smaller and the fundus lies at or just below the umbilicus. Because the uterus is smaller, the placenta will no longer fit in it without buckling on itself. The spongy layer of the lining of the uterus gives way, and the placenta separates from the uterine wall. The signs that indicate the placenta is separating are bleeding from the vagina, a lengthening of the umbilical cord protruding from the vagina, and a globular shape to the uterus, which may rise up in the abdomen (Fig. 7-9).

INDICATE THE TWO PHASES OF STAGE THREE OF LABOR

Uterine contractions plus voluntary pushing by the mother will expel the placenta from the lower uterine segment and then the vagina. When the uterus is empty, it becomes firm and hard and the fundus can be felt at the umbilicus.

The average blood loss accompanying the third stage is 200 to 500 milliliters. If the placenta is not expelled in an hour after delivery and uterine massage and downward pressure on the fundus do not cause the placenta to be expelled, manual removal is necessary.

AVERAGE BLOOD LOSS DURING THIRD STAGE OF LABOR

Stage four

The fourth stage of labor is the period following delivery of the placenta until the mother's condition is stabilized. This usually requires 1 to 2 hours for both primiparas and multiparas. If anesthesia was used or if labor was complicated, this fourth stage may last longer. This is a very important stage for close observation because if the uterine muscles do not contract, the blood vessels running through them will not constrict, causing hemorrhage.

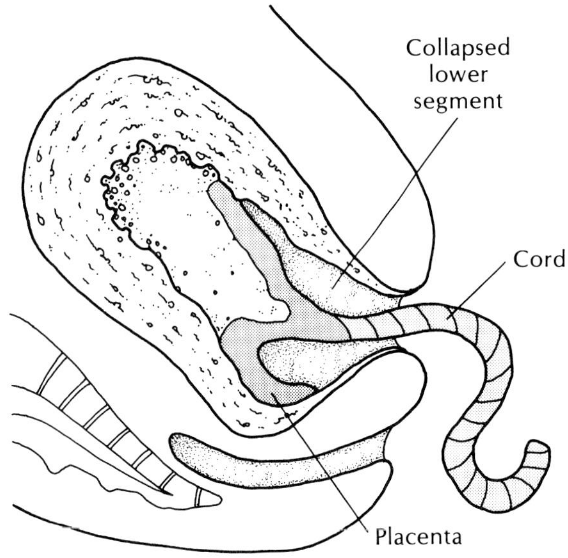

Fig. 7-9. Placental separation.

FETOPELVIC RELATIONSHIPS

Lie

FETOPELVIC RELATIONSHIPS

The lie refers to the relationship of the fetus to the long axis of the mother. In most cases, the long axis of the fetus is parallel to the long axis of the mother and is called *longitudinal.* Rarely, the long axis of the fetus lies across the mother's pelvis and is termed *transverse* (Fig. 7-10).

Presentation

In approximately 95% of all births the fetal head is the part that enters the birth canal first. Thus the head is most often the *presenting part.* When the head presents, the presentation is termed *cephalic presentation.* When the buttocks present, the presentation is termed *breech presentation.* A third type of presentation is *shoulder* (Fig. 7-11).

FETAL PRESENTATION

Fetal skull

The fetal head is composed of the bony skull and the face. The bones making up the fetal skull are two *frontal* bones, two *parietal* bones, two *temporal* bones, and one *occipital* bone (Fig. 7-12). Joining these bones are membranous attachments known as *sutures:* the *sagittal* suture joins the two parietal bones; the *lambdoidal* suture joins the parietal and occipital bones; and the *coronal* suture joins the parietal and frontal bones. The *fontanels* are the areas where several sutures meet: the anterior fontanel ("soft spot") is diamond shaped, and the posterior fontanel is triangular. Because the relatively thin bones of the skull are joined together by these membranous attachments, they can override and mold to fit through the birth canal.

The three distinct sections of the fetal skull are (1) the *vertex,* the area between the anterior and posterior fontanels; (2) the *occiput,* the occipital bone; and (3) the *brow,* the area between the anterior fontanel and the eyes. The widest transverse diameter of the fetal skull is the biparietal diameter. The smallest diameter of the head is the suboccipitobregmatic. When the fetus flexes its head onto its chest, it presents the smallest diameter of its head to the birth canal.

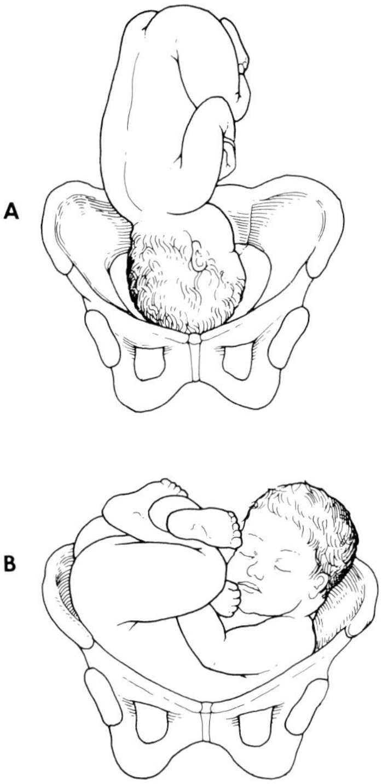

Fig. 7-10. A, Longitudinal lie. **B,** Transverse lie.

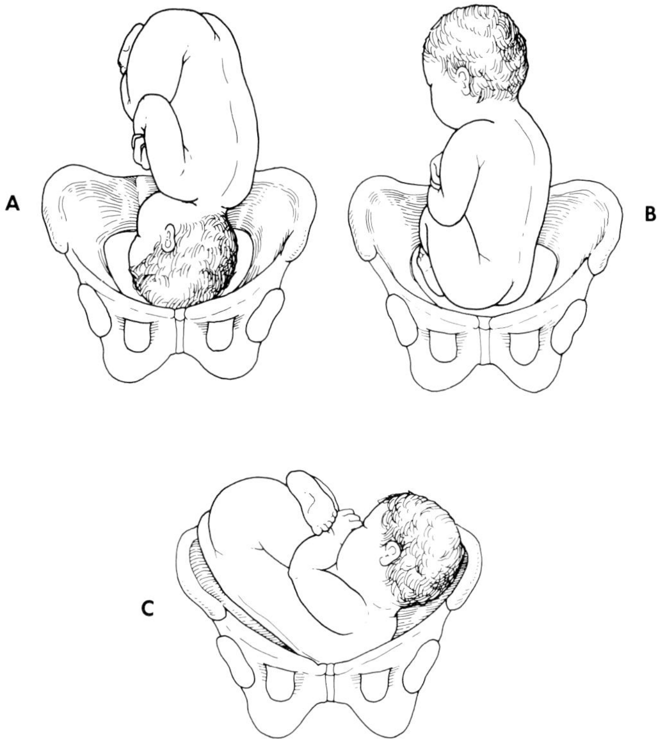

Fig. 7-11. A, Cephalic. **B,** Breech. **C,** Shoulder presentation.

Position

Position refers to the relation of the presenting part to the four quadrants of the mother, right or left, front (anterior) or rear (posterior). There are six positions for each presentation (Fig. 7-13). When the head (occiput) is presenting, it is designated by the letter O for occiput. Its position in relation to the mother's quadrants may be left occiput anterior (LOA), left occiput posterior (LOP), or left occiput transverse (LOT). On the right, it may be right occiput anterior (ROA), right occiput posterior (ROP), or right occiput transverse (ROT). The LOA position is the most common. A buttocks presentation is designed by the letter S for sacrum; a face presentation is designated by the letter M for mentum; and a shoulder by the letters SC for scapula.

Lightening and engagement

When the largest diameter of the presenting part of the fetus descends into the true pelvis, passing the pelvic inlet, *engagement* has occurred. In primigravidas, the fetus usually drops into the pelvis (engages) 2 weeks before labor begins. When this happens it is called *lightening.* The mother truly feels lighter since there is more room in the abdominal cavity and she can breathe deeply again. However, in multiparas, engagement may not happen until after labor begins. Fetal descent is presented diagrammatically in Fig. 7-14.

EXPLAIN LIGHTENING, ENGAGEMENT, AND STATION

Station

Station is the relationship of the presenting part to an imaginary line drawn between the ischial spines and is used to indicate the degree of advancement of the presenting part through the pelvis.

Stations are expressed in centimeters above (minus) and below (plus) the level of the ischial spines (zero).

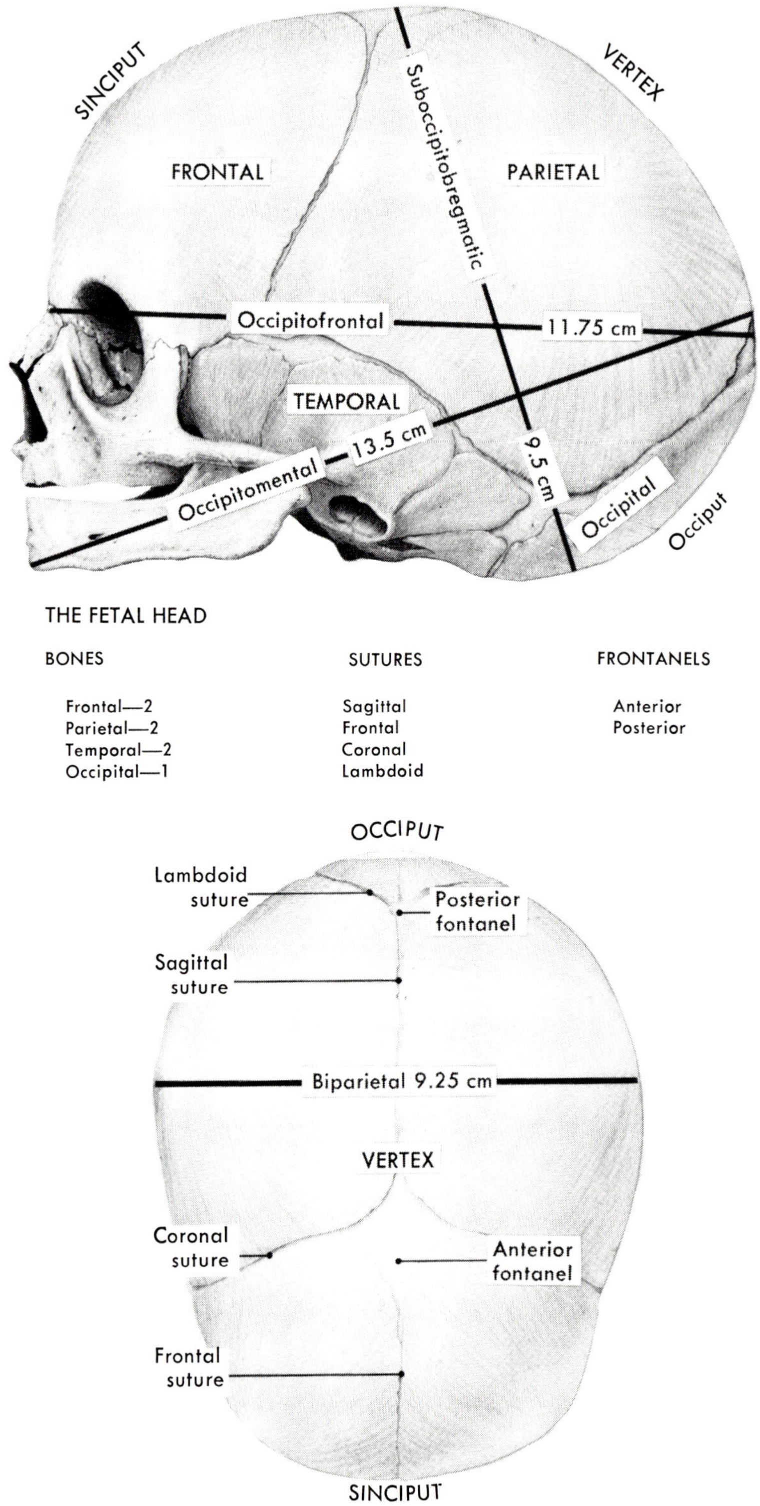

Fig. 7-12. The fetal head (From Mechanisms of normal labor, Ross Laboratories Clinical Education Aid No. 13, Ross Laboratories, Columbus, Ohio.)

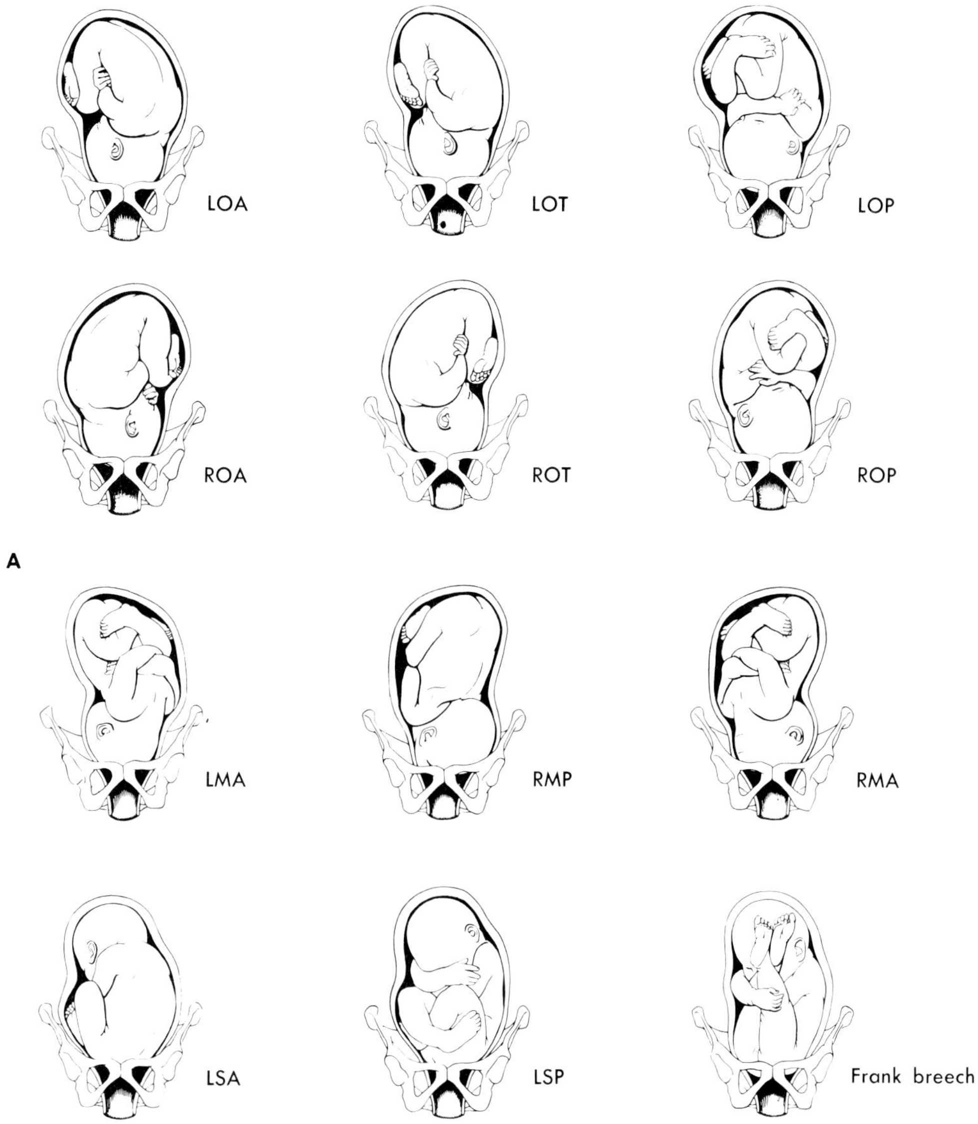

Fig. 7-13. A, categories of presentations. (From Obstetrical presentation and position, Ross Laboratories Nursing Education Service, Ross Laboratories, Columbus, Ohio.)

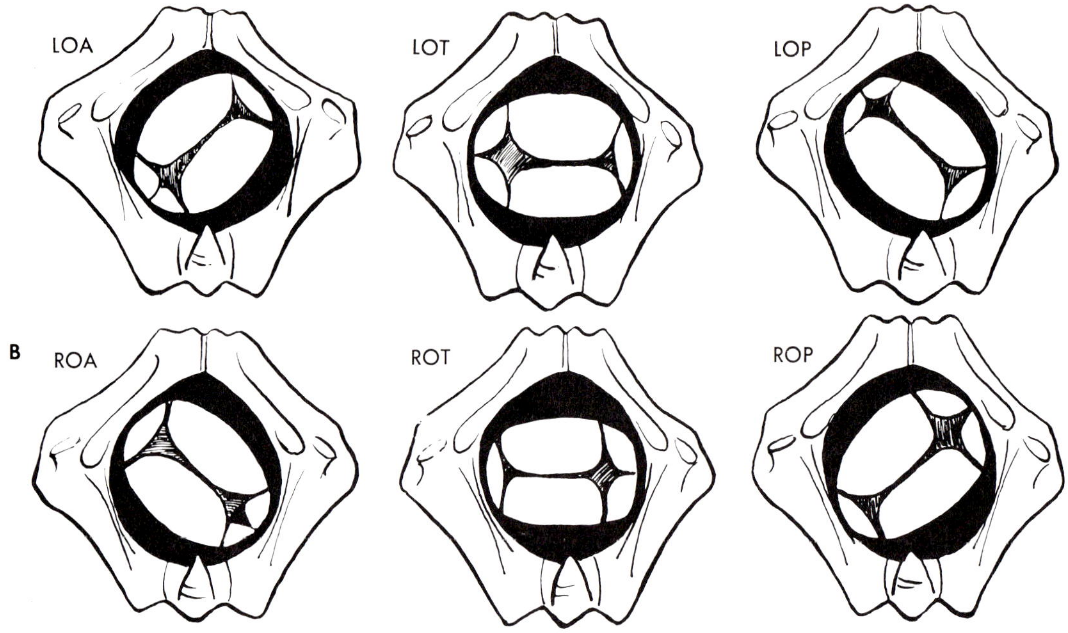

Fig. 7-13. B, Positions of occipital presentation as seen looking upward from the outlet. (From Lerch, C.: Maternity nursing, St. Louis, 1978, The C.V. Mosby Co.)

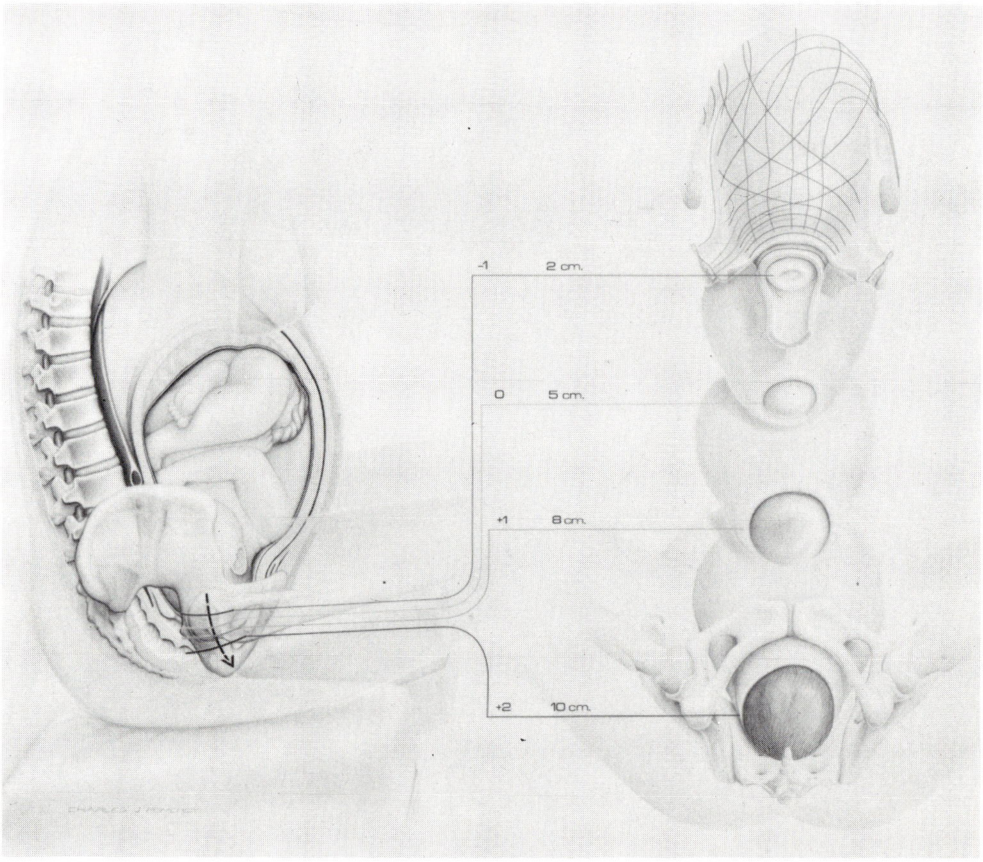

Fig. 7-14. Fetal descent. (Drawing by Charles Pomeroy is courtesy of the Borning Corporation, Spokane, Wash.)

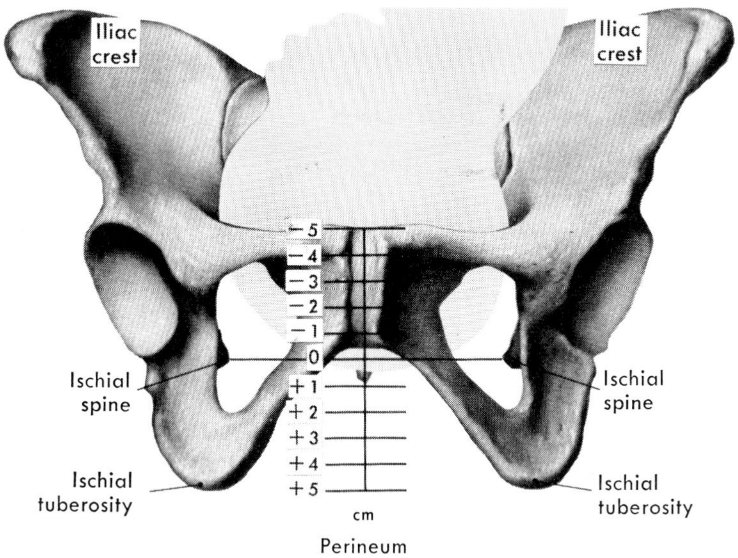

Fig. 7-15. Station zero. (From Mechanisms of normal labor, Ross Laboratories Clinical Education Aid No. 13, Ross Laboratories, Columbus, Ohio.)

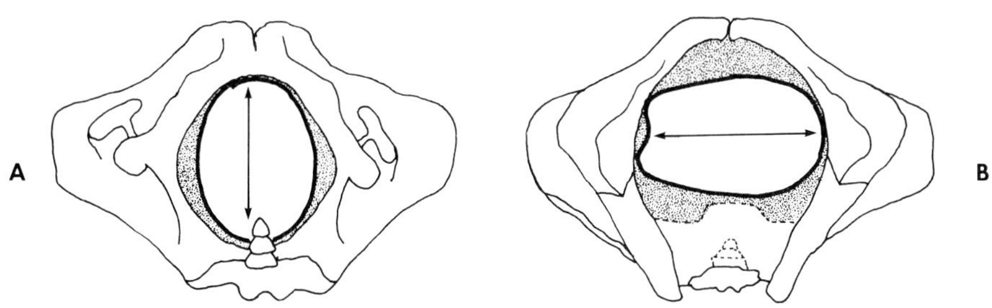

Fig. 7-16. A, Anterior-posterior (front to back) diameter of outlet. **B,** Transverse (side to side) diameter of inlet.

In Fig. 7-15 note that the fetal head is at zero station. Observe the minus and plus stations in relation to the ischial spines. Women who start labor with the fetal head high usually have lesser degrees of cervical dilation. A low station may be associated with a cervix that is more effaced and dilated, both at the onset of labor and in the beginning of the active phase.

MECHANISMS OF LABOR

The largest diameter of the inlet to the pelvis is transverse (side to side), while the largest diameter of the outlet is anterior-posterior (front to back) (Fig. 7-16). The fetal head enters the pelvis in a transverse position and during labor turns its head to emerge from the outlet in an anterior-posterior position, with the occiput up and the face looking at the floor. The series of passive, adaptive movements that the fetal head and shoulders make through the birth canal are called the *mechanisms of labor* (Fig. 7-17). In these mechanisms, the fetus adjusts itself so that its smallest diameter is presented to the irregular shape of the mother's pelvis, thus encountering as little resistance as possible.

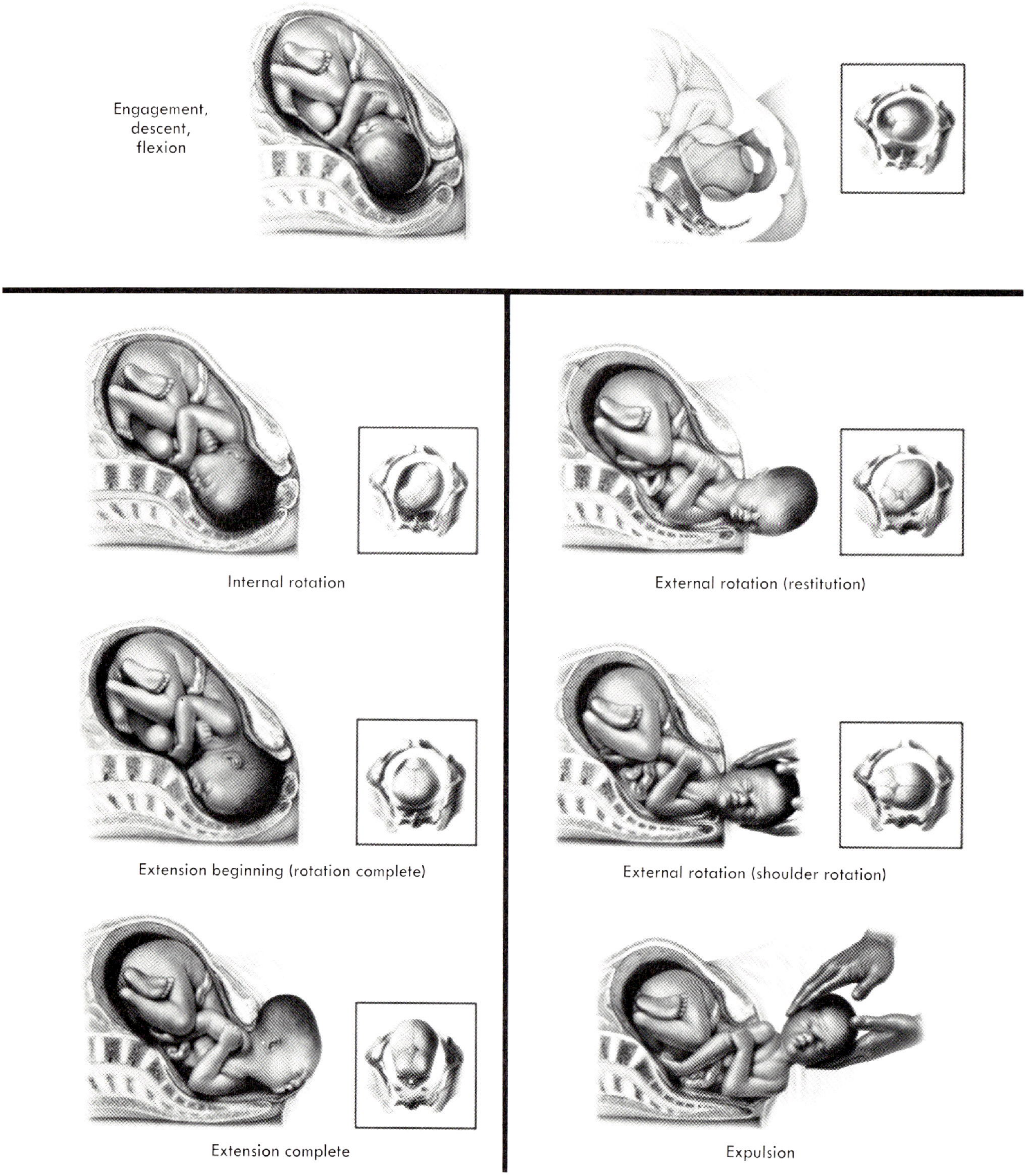

Fig. 7-17. Mechanism of labor. (Courtesy Ross Laboratories, Columbus, Ohio.)

Although these seven cardinal movements do not occur in separate steps, but rather overlap or occur in combination, they can be listed in their most frequent order of happening:

LIST SEVEN CARDINAL MOVEMENTS OF FETUS THROUGH BIRTH PROCESS

1. *Engagement:* With a vertex presenting, the head is engaged when the biparietal diameter (largest diameter) has cleared the pelvic inlet.
2. *Descent*: Occurring intermittently with contractions.
3. *Flexion:* A forward tipping of the fetal head on the chest to present the smallest diameter.
4. *Internal rotation:* The occiput usually rotates anteriorly to the midline under the symphysis, being brought about by twisting of the neck, *not* by any movement of the shoulders.
5. *Extension:* The head sweeps upward and forward under the symphysis.
6. *Restitution:* The head untwists, returning to its original right or left position.
7. *Expulsion:* Usually the anterior shoulder presents and delivers first with the posterior next, and then the rest of the body is born.

PSYCHE

To this point in this unit, the discussion has centered on the physical, physiological, and mechanical aspects of labor; or we could say on the *passage*, the *passenger*, and the *powers*. However, our discussion is not complete until we also consider the factors that contribute to the psychological stress of labor and the ways in which women react to labor.

STRESSES OF LABOR

When a woman and her mate and/or family enter a hospital to give birth, they are confronted with many strange faces, sounds, and smells in an unfamiliar environment. Glaring lights, hospital routines, and equipment can be extremely disconcerting. The woman may be asked to give up her own clothing and to put on a small, unattractive hospital gown that exposes most of her body. She may have to relate to numerous nurses and hospital personnel. There is a definite lack of privacy as these hospital personnel go in and out of the labor room. If the woman has been in early labor during her normal sleeping hours, she may be very tired and feel irritable. All of these factors are environmental stressors over which the woman usually has very little control. The father or other people with the woman experience similar environmental stressors. The sights, sounds, and smells are new to them as well, and they may feel anxious and fearful as efficient hospital personnel come and go, often without speaking to them.

Hospital labor rooms are often narrow, dark, windowless, cell-like rooms designed for the "twilight sleep" era of 20 to 30 years ago. A woman may have to labor in such a cell without a bathroom. The other extreme is laboring in a large ward with other laboring women and only curtains between the labor beds. Such an environment for labor does not offer privacy or adequate space to walk around or have family members present.

To add to this dehumanizing environment, most women are still moved from labor bed to stretcher and transported down a hall to a delivery room for birth. Then once again they must lift their heavy bodies from stretcher to delivery table to give birth. This is a painful and often frightening and humiliating experience for women. Is it any wonder that women in labor often find it difficult to use the techniques they have learned in prenatal classes?

If the couple have prepared for the birth, as discussed in Unit VI, they will begin to cope with the stress of the environment and the discomfort by using the techniques they have practiced. However, if the laboring woman is unprepared or not yet ready for labor and delivery, the stimulus of pain can bring all of her unresolved feelings, fears, and attitudes about labor to the surface. Remembering previous experiences with hospitals can stir up old fears. A woman's unresolved feelings about femininity and motherhood may threaten her feelings about herself as the reality of labor and fast-approaching motherhood crowd in on her. If the relationship of the couple is unstable, many unresolved feelings may come between them, and their communication system may literally break down.

Adapting

COPING BEHAVIORS

In spite of all these stressors on the psyche, women do cope with labor and have done so since the beginning of time no matter what their environmental stressors are.

During the latent phase (0 to 3 centimeters of dilation), the uterine contractions are usually mild. The woman usually seems happy that labor has finally begun and smiles, talks, and answers questions freely. She may be anxious but can verbalize her anxiety.

As labor progresses and the cervix is about 4 centimeters dilated (beginning part of active phase), the contractions get closer together (every 5 minutes) and last longer (35 to 40 seconds). The woman's face may flush, her respiration deepen, and her anxiety increase. She may start to feel that there is a force outside of her body that is controlling her, and thus may start to feel helpless. She may use aggressive and hostile behavior to maintain control at this point.

At 6 centimeters of dilation, the woman usually becomes serious, talks less, and focuses on herself. Her breathing may become labored, and she may become restless, exhibiting moderate to severe anxiety. She may verbalize a fear of abandonment. At this point, the contractions are coming every 3 to 5 minutes and are lasting 40 to 50 seconds.

LIST FOUR SIGNS THAT TRANSITION HAS BEGUN

Between 8 and 10 centimeters (*transition*) the mother may feel that labor is never going to end and she simply wants to stop the whole process and go home. She may perspire heavily, shake, have chills, hiccups, and nausea and vomiting. She will become more withdrawn, focusing on herself, and become very restless. At the same time, she may be amnesic and actually sleep between contractions. The contractions may be coming every 1 to 3 minutes and last 60 to 90 seconds.

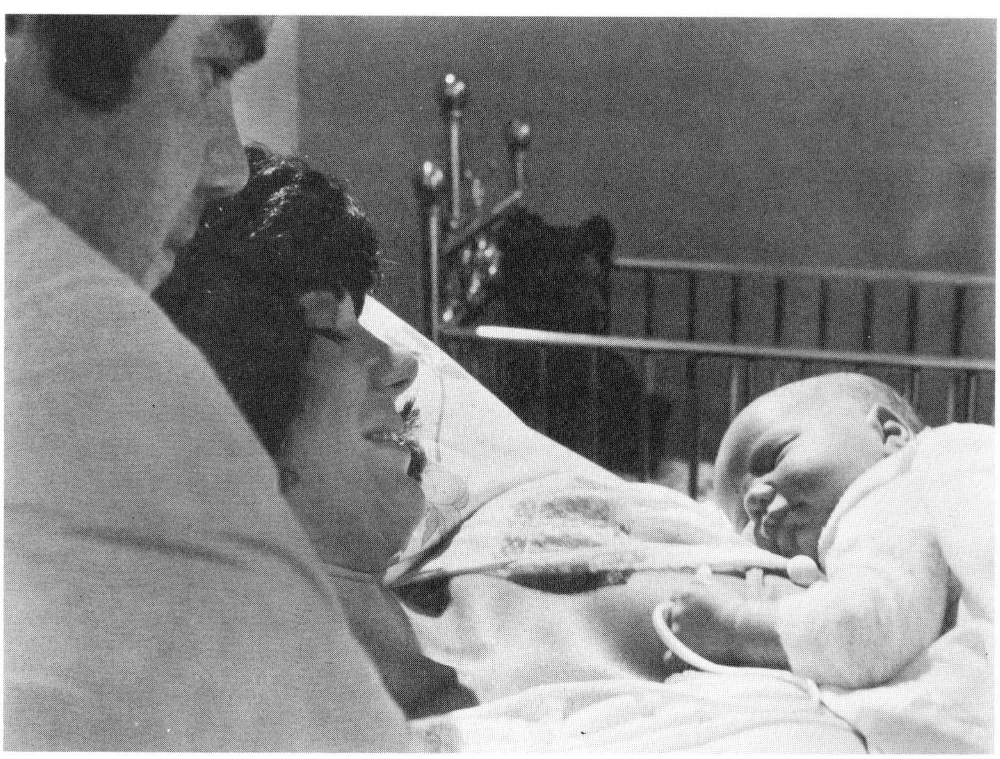

Fig. 7-18. Joy. (Courtesy the Borning Corporation, Spokane, Wash.)

As the second stage begins, the woman may feel she has to move her bowels. She may verbalize the urgent need to bear down and become very anxious if she is restrained from pushing. As she bears down, her face becomes flushed, the veins in her neck protrude, and she may grunt and groan, making gutteral noises with each expulsive effort. This is hard work, and everyone around her knows it. Some women have told of experiencing a prolonged and intense sexual orgasm as the baby's head crowns. Other women tell of how they felt like they were splitting apart as the head was born. The father or other support person may become very worried by the noises the woman makes as she pushes, especially if he is not prepared for them.

IDENTIFY A LABORING WOMAN'S SEXUAL FEELINGS DURING LABOR

Immediately after the baby is born, most women and their partners experience a moment of pure joy—unlike anything they have ever experienced before (Fig. 7-18.).

SUMMARY

In this unit you have been introduced to the dynamic events of the intrapartum experience—perhaps the most exciting and rewarding experience of a lifetime, although certainly not without dangers. Unit VIII will help you to learn the meaning of individualized care for the intrapartum family.

BIBLIOGRAPHY

Anderson, B.G., and Shapiro, P.J.: Obstetrics for the nurse, Albany, N.Y., 1979, Delmar Publishers.

Ingalls, J.A., and Salerno, N.C.: Maternal and child health nursing, ed. 4, St. Louis, 1979, The C.V. Mosby Co.

Moore, M.L.: Realities in childbearing, ed. 2, Philadelphia, 1983, W.B. Saunders Co.

Oxorn, H., and Foote, W.R.: Human labor and birth, ed. 3, New York, 1975, Appleton-Century-Crofts.

Pritchard, J.A., MacDonald, P.C., and Gant, N.F.: Williams obstetrics, ed. 16, Norwalk, Conn., 1985, Appleton-Century-Crofts.

Wiedenbach, E.: Family-centered maternity nursing, ed. 2, New York, 1967, J. Putnam's Sons.

Wiggins, J.D.: Childbearing physiology, experiences, needs, St. Louis, 1979, The C.V. Mosby Co.

DEFINITIONS

Define the following terms:

acme
active phase
axis
biparietal diameter
Braxton Hicks contractions
bulging
cephalic
crowning
decrement
effacement
engagement
episiotomy
flexion
fontanels
hyperplasia
increment
latent phase
lie
lightening
occiput
presentation
prostaglandins
restitution
ripening
"show"
station
sutures
transition
vertex

LEARNING ACTIVITIES AND EXPERIENCES

1. Group discussions.
2. Guest speakers: a midwife or obstetrician to discuss their experiences with normal labor; a new mother to relate her experience.
3. View audiovisual aids and discuss.

ENRICHMENT/IN-DEPTH STUDY

1. Demonstrate the mechanisms of the passage of the fetus down the birth canal by twisting, turning, and thus manipulating a pliable rubber doll through an imaginary delivery. You might sketch the uterus and birth canal in chalk on the board or on the floor and move the doll through it.
2. Study Ross Laboratories' charts on the mechanisms of labor.

SELF-ASSESSMENT

1. The percentage of births that occur with a cephalic presentation is
   a. 20 percent
   b. 8 percent
   c. 95 percent
   d. 5 percent
2. Painless, intermittent uterine contractions are known as
   a. Braxton Hicks contractions
   b. colostrum
   c. true labor
   d. "show"
3. The only sure sign of true labor is
   a. pain
   b. bleeding
   c. cervical dilation
   d. Braxton Hicks contractions
4. The first stage of labor covers the time period from the first true labor contraction until ____________ of the cervix.
5. What is the average length of time of the first stage of labor in a primigravida? ____________ ; in a multipara? ____________
6. The second stage of labor covers the time from complete dilation of the cervix until ________________________.
7. What is the average length of the second stage of labor in a primigravida? ____________ ; in a multipara? ____________
8. The third stage of labor is the ____________ stage.
9. What is the average length of time of the third stage of labor in a primigravida? ____________ ; in a multipara? ____________
10. The fourth stage of labor is the period following ________________.
11. What is the average length of time of the fourth stage of labor? ____________
12. The distance of the presenting part above or below the level of the ischial spines is known as ____________.
13. A woman's ways of coping with stresses of labor include all of the following behaviors: ____________, ____________, ____________, ____________, ____________, and ____________.
14. Give a brief description of true prelabor contractions.
15. Identify the cervix that is completely effaced. A or B?

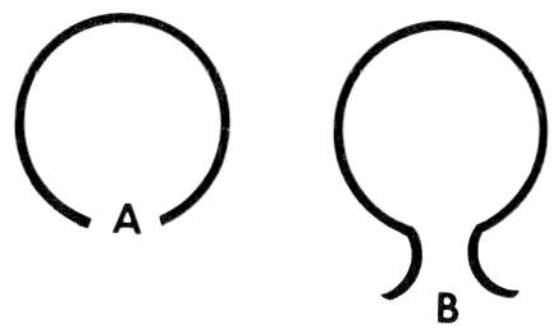

16. A completely dilated cervix is open to the diameter of how many centimeters?

17. Approximately how many centimeters does the circle A below measure?

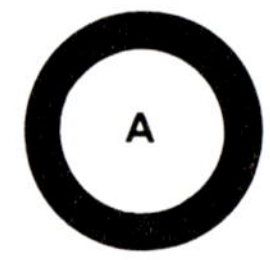

18. Approximately how many centimeters does the circle B below measure?

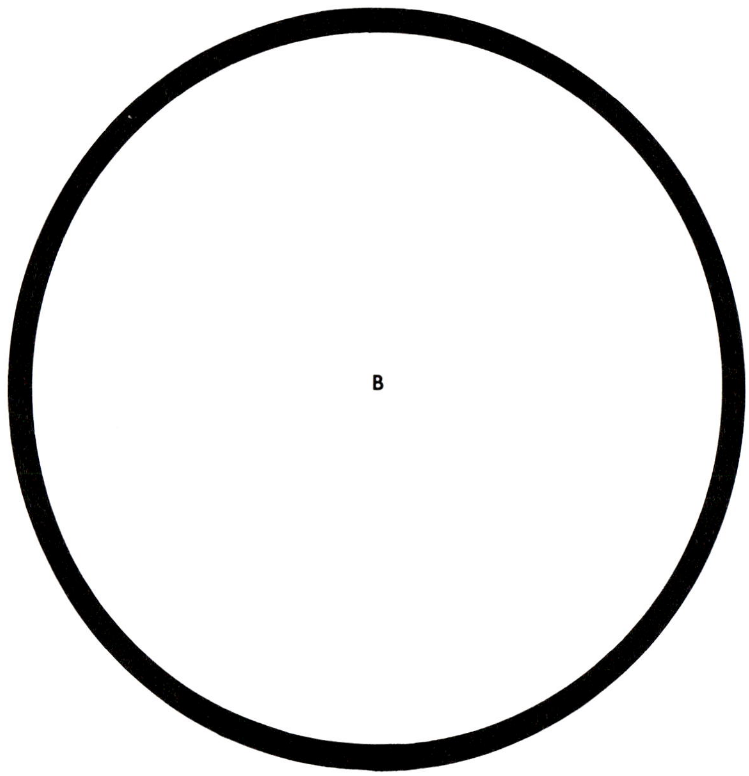

19. The nurse can identify the transition period of labor by signs the woman presents. Four of these signs are:
    a.
    b.
    c.
    d.
20. A woman has confided in you that she experienced sexual orgasm during the birth of her child and is concerned that she is "weird." How would you respond?

21. Explain why the head of the fetus must rotate in the birth canal to be born.

22. List the seven cardinal movements of the fetus through the birth process to delivery.
    a.
    b.
    c.
    d.
    e.
    f.
    g.

23. The fetus can present to the birth canal in four different ways. What are they?
   a.
   b.
   c.
   d.
24. What is the average blood loss during the third stage of labor?
25. What are three reasons why an episiotomy may be done as the fetal head crowns?
   a.
   b.
   c.
26. During what stage of labor may the woman be an active participant?

27. After the placenta is expelled, in what condition should the uterus be?

28. The widest transverse diameter of the fetal skull is:
   a. biparietal
   b. bitemporal
29. When the long axis of the fetus is parallel to the long axis of the mother, the lie is called ____________________.
30. The presenting part is usually the ____________________.

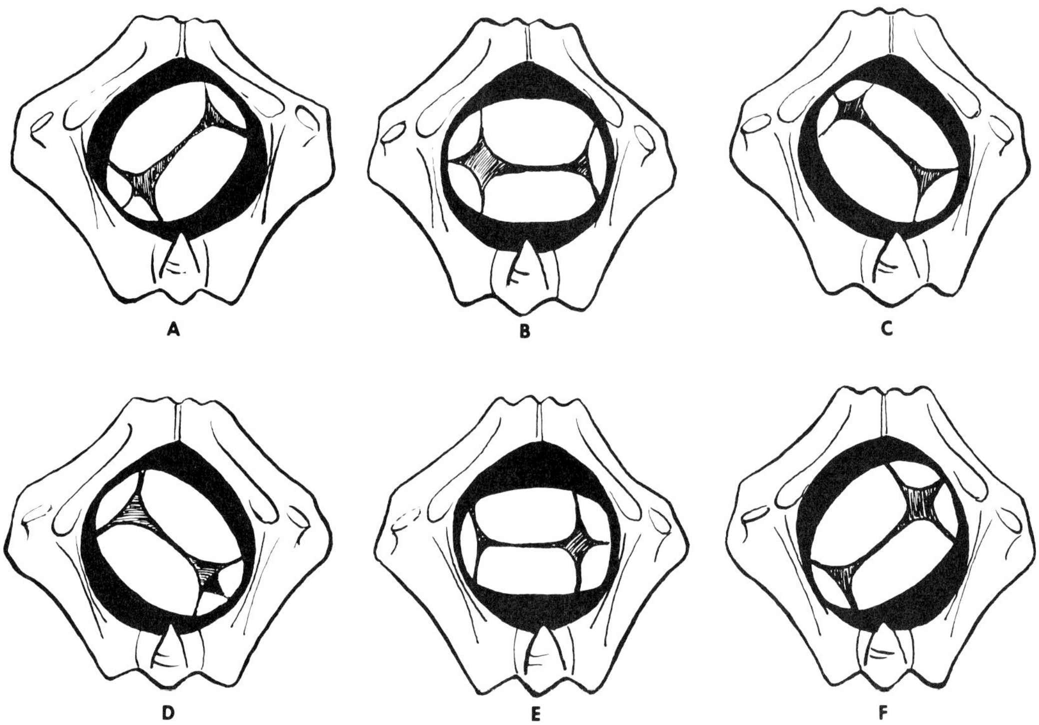

31. On the line to the left of each item in Column A match the appropriate positions of the fetal occiput (see fig.) from Column B.

Column A	Column B
_____A	ROA
_____B	ROP
_____C	LOA
_____D	LOP
_____E	ROT
_____F	LOT

32. On the line to the left of each item in Column A match the appropriate designation from Column B.

Column A	Column B
Designation of the presenting part:	
______1. head	a. shoulder (Sc)
______2. breech	b. sacrum (S)
______3. face	c. mentum (M)
	d. occiput (O)

UNIT VIII
The intrapartum family and the nurse

GOALS

This unit is designed to provide the reader with information that will:

□ promote awareness of nursing care responsibilities for intrapartum families.
□ develop an understanding of the meaning of individualized care for the intrapartum family.

STUDENT OBJECTIVES

After studying this unit, you should be able to:

1. Identify information about the progress of labor that can be assessed by a nursing history.
2. Demonstrate Leopold's maneuvers for determining fetal position.
3. Identify (a) the normal fetal heart rate range during labor, and (b) nursing responsibilities for regular and periodic checking.
4. Differentiate among three common types of periodic changes (early, late, and variable) in the fetal heart rate during labor and give nursing care for each.
5. Give one advantage and one disadvantage for both external and internal fetal heart rate monitoring.
6. Describe the normal appearance of amniotic fluid and two common variations from normal appearance, explaining the significance of these variations.
7. Differentiate among the characteristics of the four degrees of perineal lacerations.
8. List three common drugs used to cause uterine contractions in the third and fourth stages of labor. Include dosages and methods of administration.
9. Discuss the most frequent causes of excessive bleeding in the fourth stage of labor. Include signs and symptoms, treatment, and nursing care.

ADMISSION PROCEDURES

Although admission procedures vary from hospital to hospital, the laboring woman and her family undergo common examinations and receive the basic care discussed in this unit.

Admission consent

RECOGNIZE THE USUAL CONTENT OF PREADMISSION FORMS

All hospitals have permission or consent forms for the woman to sign upon admission to the hospital. These forms authorize the performance of routine procedures that may be necessary during labor and delivery. Whether these consent forms are signed in a centrally located admissions office or in the labor area, the woman and her family need a thorough explanation of what they are signing (see Pregnant Patient's Bill of Rights in Unit I).

Prenatal records

Ideally, a copy of the woman's prenatal records, containing a health history, pregnancy profile, and prenatal flow record, will be sent to the birth site several weeks before the woman's due date. These prenatal records should be checked immediately upon admission since they are very important.

Preadmission records

It is advisable for people to preregister with the hospital or birth center of their choice 1 month before the due date to complete all the other necessary forms for identification and financial matters when not under the stress of labor. An additional preadmission form that is very helpful is a "preference profile," in which the woman and her family designate what they expect from their childbirth experience. For example, they may request the delivery area light to be dimmed or no episiotomy to be done or no student nurses to be present in the delivery area. Whenever these predesignated preferences do not interfere with the safety of the birth experience, they *must* be respected by nurses and physicians. By having these preferences spelled out clearly in advance of labor, the staff can communicate with the family about any preference listed that might compromise the safety of either mother or baby. In this way, problems in matching the desires of the woman and family with the goals and expectations of the nursing and medical staffs can be averted. (See Appendix C for a preference profile.) If notified in advance of the woman's arrival the nurse can thoroughly review the prenatal and preadmission records before greeting the woman, thus personalizing and individualizing the greeting and welcome. However, whether or not there has been time to review the preadmission records, the nurse should greet the woman and her mate and family (if present) in a warm and friendly manner, remembering that labor is a crisis time for them. A warm, relaxed, welcoming introduction will do much to reduce anxiety for both the nurse and the laboring woman and family.

Nursing history

LIST THE BASIC INFORMATION TO BE GATHERED FIRST WHEN ADMITTING A WOMAN IN LABOR

While assisting the woman to undress and either put on her own gown or a hospital gown, some basic information can be obtained. If not known by prenatal record, it is important to determine first how many babies she has had and the duration of previous labors. Time may be important in working with a multipara who has a history of rapid labors. Next, the following information is determined:

1. Mother's general condition (frightened? fatigued? relaxed?)
2. When contractions began; their frequency and duration
3. Presence of blood-tinged mucus from the vagina (show) or vaginal bleeding
4. Whether or not membranes have ruptured; time of rupture and color of fluid
5. Due date (EDD); last menstrual period (LMP)
6. Time of last meal; food eaten
7. Mother's age and nutritional status
8. Knowledge base: prenatal classes
9. Any complications during the pregnancy

After making these first pertinent observations, the nurse would report any significant deviations from normal immediately.

If the woman is using any preparation for birth techniques to cope with labor, she needs her mate or other family member or friend to remain with her at all times. It can be extremely stressful for her to be without her support person for even a brief examination. Even if the woman has not prepared herself for birth, it may be very important that she not be separated from her family or friend. The nurse can determine this from the preadmission preference profile or simply by asking the woman. When policies, procedures, rules, and regulations seem to get in the way of meeting needs expressed by laboring women, it is often helpful to remember: Whose baby is this?

After making the initial observation, the nurse can complete a maternity nursing care history, determining information not previously gathered about the woman and her family. This information will be helpful in deciding on a plan of care during the entire hospital stay.

At some time during the admission procedures, it is necessary to care for the woman's personal items by labeling all her clothing carefully and listing all her valuables. Many hospitals have a special envelope for valuables, which can be locked in a safe place. If such a service is not available, it is advisable to have a family member take the valuables home.

FIRST STAGE OF LABOR: NURSING CARE

An evaluation of general physical status includes checking the mother's weight, general physical condition, vital signs, and taking blood and urine specimens for laboratory examination.

Vital signs

EXPLAIN NURSING CARE IN EARLY LABOR

Vital signs are recorded hourly during routine labor or more frequently during abnormal labor. An elevated temperature may mean infection. An elevated pulse rate may mean infection or dehydration. Blood pressure is usually checked and recorded on admission and every 2 hours during labor unless otherwise indicated. If the blood pressure is elevated abnormally (over 140/90), it may be checked and recorded as often as every 15 minutes. An elevated blood pressure may indicate pre-eclampsia. Report any abnormalities immediately.

Urine specimen

A clean voided urine specimen is checked on admission for the presence of blood, sugar, and albumin. If the woman's membranes are ruptured, it may be impossible to obtain a urine specimen free of amniotic fluid. Albumin, blood, or sugar in the urine should be reported immediately.

Timing uterine contractions

DESCRIBE THE PROCESS OF MONITORING INTENSITY OF UTERINE CONTRACTIONS BY TOUCHING

The nurse records and reports the frequency, duration, and intensity of uterine contractions on admission and through labor. As explained in Unit VII, a uterine contraction has three phases: (1) a period of increasing intrauterine pressure, known as *increment*; (2) a period of peak intensity, called *acme*; and (3) a period of decreasing pressure, known as *decrement* (see Fig. 7-7, p. 156). The length of contraction *(duration* is measured from the increment through the acme and to the end of the decrement. The *frequency* is measured from the beginning of one contraction to the beginning of the next.

The nurse can actually feel the muscular contractions of the uterus by gently touching the fundus. Because the contractions begin at the fundus, there will be a tightening in this area first, which will gradually move down the uterus, from top to bottom. At the time of the acme, the uterus will be firm all over but tightest at the fundus. Also, the abdominal wall will rise with a contraction and relax again between contractions. Between contractions the uterus will feel soft. With strong uterine contractions, the uterine wall cannot be indented by the examiner's fingers. With moderate contractions, the uterus will feel moderately firm. When the uterine contractions are mild, practically no difference in uterine tone can be detected by gentle palpation.

INDICATE THE AVERAGE DURATION OF A UTERINE CONTRACTION IN FIRST STAGE OF LABOR

During the first stage of labor the average contraction lasts 40 to 60 seconds. It would be abnormal for a contraction to last longer than 80 seconds or for the uterus not to relax between contractions. Any deviations from normal contractions should be reported immediately.

Abdominal palpation (Leopold's maneuvers)

LEOPOLD'S MANEUVERS

By first determining the position of the fetus, the nurse can locate the fetal heart tones quickly, since they are best heard through the baby's back. Palpating the woman's abdomen to check the position and presentation of the baby is called *Leopold's maneuvers.*

Before palpating the abdomen, the nurse first inspects it without touching. In most pregnancies, the uterus at term is egg shaped with lengthwise enlargement, and the bulk or mass of the fetus is obvious on either the mother's right or left side. The nurse looks for fetal movement, particularly feet and hand movement. The obvious mass is probably the fetal back and the gentle movements are probably the extremities.

With the mother lying on her back with her knees slightly bent and a pillow or a lift to raise her trunk to a 35 to 45 degree angle, the nurse stands facing her and with warm hands palpates the uterine fundus (*first maneuver*) to determine what part of the fetus lies in the upper part of the uterus. The fetal head is hard and round and can be moved from side to side on the neck. The buttocks (breech) are larger, softer, and cannot be moved like the head. The fetal head in the fundus indicates a breech presentation. The fetal buttocks in the fundus indicate a cephalic or vertex (head first) presentation.

To determine on which side of the uterus the long axis (back) of the fetus is located, the nurse's hands move down each side of the uterus at the same time (*second maneuver*). A long, smooth, curved surface is the fetal back. Small irregular bumps and lumps, which often move and kick, are the legs and arms.

Still facing the woman the nurse presses with one hand over the symphysis pubis (*third maneuver*), feeling for the presenting part. If the fetal head is not engaged, it can be felt like a small hard round object above the symphysis. Also, gentle pressure can move it.

For the last maneuver, the nurse turns and faces the woman's feet. To confirm that the fetal head is presenting, the nurse presses downward on both sides of the woman's uterus, about 2 inches above the symphysis pubis (*fourth maneuver*). In this maneuver, the nurse is feeling for the brow of the baby, which should be on the side opposite from where the back was located (Fig. 8-1).

If the fetus is in the LOA position, the fetal heart should be heard best in the left lower quadrant. (The head is presenting with the occiput at the left front and the brow facing the right back. The fetal back is on the left.) However, if the fetus is in the LOP position, the fetal heart is heard best slightly below the upper outer border of the left hip bone. (The head is presenting with the the occiput at the left back and the brow facing the right front. The fetal back is on the right.)

With breech presentations, the fetal heart will be heard at or above the level of the mother's umbilicus (Fig. 8-2).

Fetal heart tones

NORMAL FETAL HEART RATE RANGE DURING LABOR

Fetal heart tones are heard with the use of special stethoscopes: a fetoscope (Fig. 8-3) worn on the examiner's head, or a Leff's stethoscope (Fig. 8-4). An ultrasound fetoscope, or Doppler instrument (Fig. 8-5), is a special electronic device for amplifying the sounds of the fetal heart beat. The normal fetal heart rate (FHR) is from 120 to 160 beats per minute. The fetal heart rate is checked and recorded on admission, every half-hour during early labor (latent phase), every 15 minutes during active labor, and every 5 minutes or more often in the second stage of labor. In addition to this regular checking,

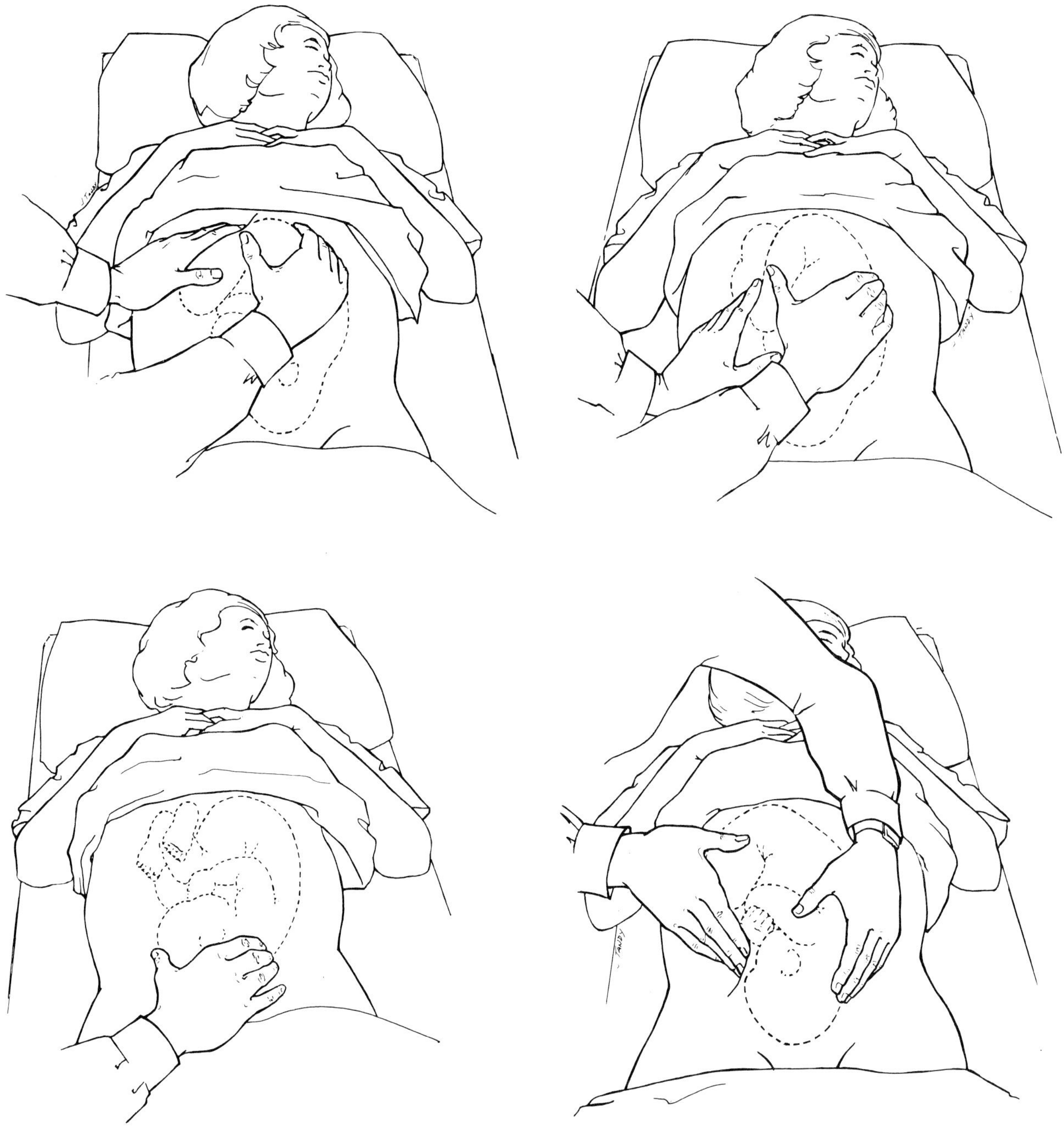

Fig. 8-1. Leopold's maneuvers. (From Jensen, M., and Bobak, I.M.: Maternity and gynecologic care: the nurse and the family, ed. 3, St. Louis, 1985, The C.V. Mosby Co.)

the FHR is checked and recorded after any examination or treatment, immediately following rupture of the membranes, and immediately after administration of analgesia or anesthesia. When listening to the fetal heart with a stethoscope, the nurse should listen for at least a full minute from the acme of the contraction, through the decrement, and into the interval between contractions. Because of the tightened uterine muscle, it is often uncomfortable for the mother when the nurse listens to the fetal heart during the most intense part (acme) of the contraction. The FHR normally either slows down or speeds up by about 10 beats at the height of the contraction but returns to normal within 10 seconds of the end of a contraction. To be sure that the mother's pulse is not being heard through the stethoscope, the mother's radial pulse can be palpated at the same

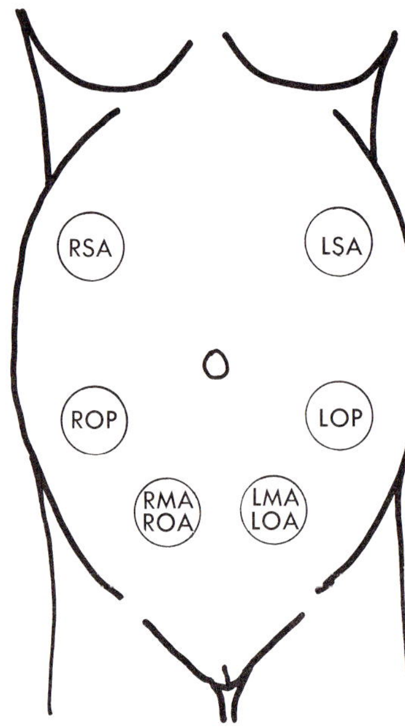

Fig. 8-2. Location of fetal heart.

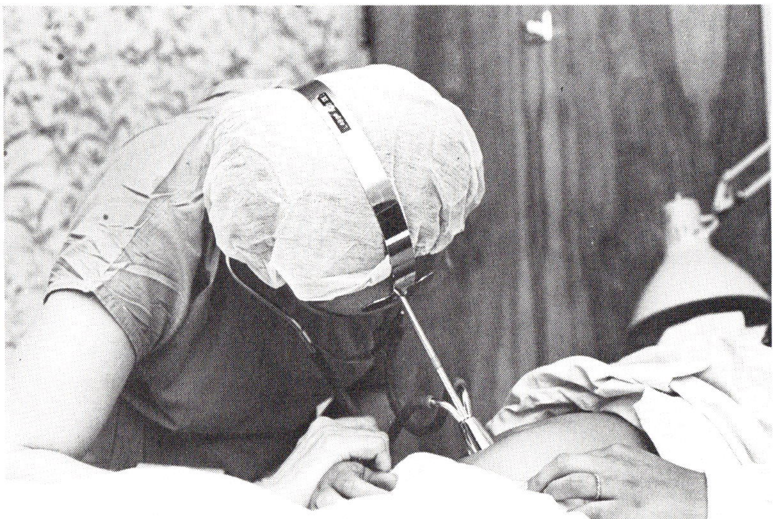

Fig. 8-3. Fetoscope worn on examiner's head.

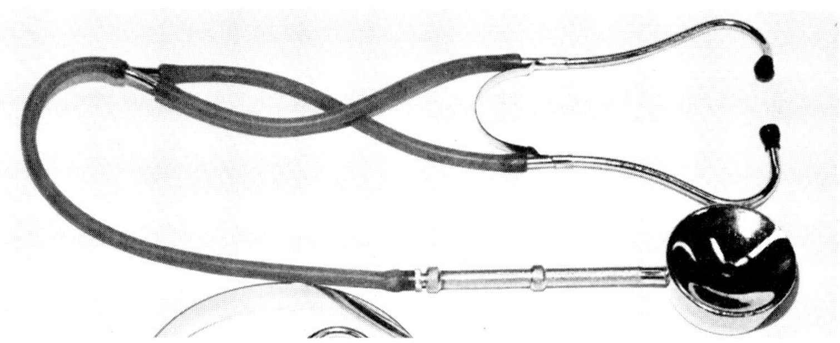

Fig. 8-4. Leff's stethoscope. (From Ingalls, A.J., and Salerno, M.C.: Maternal and child health nursing, ed. 6, St. Louis, 1987, The C.V. Mosby Co.)

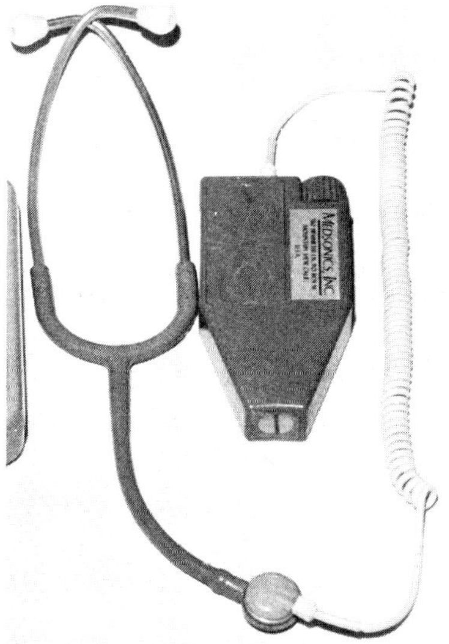

Fig. 8-5. Ultrasonic fetoscope operates on Doppler effect, reflecting echoes or sounds from moving interfaces. (From Ingalls, A.J., and Salerno, M.C.: Maternal and child health nursing, ed. 6, St. Louis, 1987, The C.V. Mosby Co.)

time the fetal heart rate is checked. A comparison of what is being felt at the mother's wrist with what is being heard with the stethoscope will indicate whose heart is being monitored with the stethoscope.

Any abnormalities in FHR (irregular rhythm, rate over 160 or below 120) should be reported immediately.

Continuous electronic fetal heart monitoring

EXPLAIN THE PURPOSE OF CONTINUOUS FETAL MONITORING

Modern technology has made available electronic monitors that record uterine contractions and fetal heart activity simultaneously and continuously throughout labor (Fig. 8-6). The purpose of continuous fetal monitoring is to pick up early warning signs of fetal distress so that appropriate measures can be taken if necessary.

PERIODIC CHANGES IN FETAL HEART RATE DURING LABOR

Because contractions represent sources of repetitive stress to the fetus, signs of fetal distress may first appear as changes in the FHR in relation to the pressure of uterine contractions. There are three basic periodic changes in FHR in relationship to uterine contractions; early decelerations, late decelerations, and variable decelerations (see Fig. 8-7 for descriptive illustrations, causes, and nursing actions for each periodic change in rate).

Fetal bradycardia and/or a pattern of late decelerations or variable decelerations may indicate fetal distress. When any of these patterns is detected, the following actions should be taken to treat the cause of the distress. (1) If oxytocin is being administered, it should be discontinued. The oxytocin may be causing the uterus to contract too strongly or not to relax enough between contractions, thus interfering with placental circulation. (2) The woman's position should be changed to relieve pressure on the umbilical cord. (3) Oxygen should be administered to the mother by mask. (4) The woman's blood pressure should be taken to rule out hypotension. (5) The umbilical cord should be checked for prolapse.

In addition to detecting periodic changes in FHR in relationship to uterine contractions, the fetal monitor can provide other data that could indicate fetal well-being. The monitor will also detect fetal *tachycardia* (baseline fetal heart rate more than 160 beats per minute lasting longer than a 10-minute period) or fetal *bradycardia* (baseline FHR less than 120 beats per minute lasting longer than a 10-minute period) very early in its onset. Both fetal tachycardia and fetal bradycardia may be indicative of fetal distress.

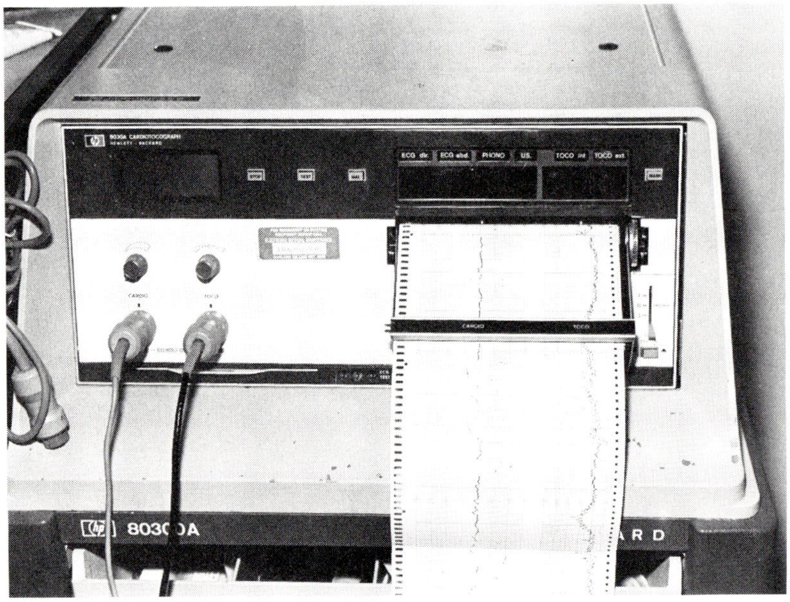

Fig. 8-6. Electronic fetal monitor. (Courtesy Kaiser-Permanente Medical Center, Santa Clara, Calif.)

EXPLAIN BASELINE FETAL HEART RATE

Baseline FHR is the heart rate between contractions. The FHR baseline is usually 120 to 160 beats per minute in the normal full-term fetus. Variability is the beat-to-beat difference between successive fetal heart beats. Normal variability is 6 to 10 beats per minute. With increased variability, the baseline FHR varies more than 10 beats per minute. With decreased variability the baseline FHR varies less than 6 beats per minute.

EXPLAIN THE RELATIONSHIP OF GOOD FETAL HEART VARIABILITY TO WELLNESS OF FETAL NERVOUS SYSTEM

Variability in the FHR reflects the interplay of the parasympathetic (cardiodeceleration) and sympathetic (cardioacceleration) divisions of the fetal nervous system as it responds to stress. The fetal heart speeds up under sympathetic stimulation and slows under parasympathetic stimulation, so that an average variation of beat-to-beat variability is a sign of a healthy, adaptable fetal nervous system. Increase of variability or no variability or decrease in variability as labor progresses following a previously average reading could be a sign of fetal distress.

Fetal monitoring can be done by internal or external methods or a combination of both. *External* monitoring consists of two parts: (1) an ultrasound system or microphone amplification technique to pick up the fetal heart and record it on graph paper and (2) a

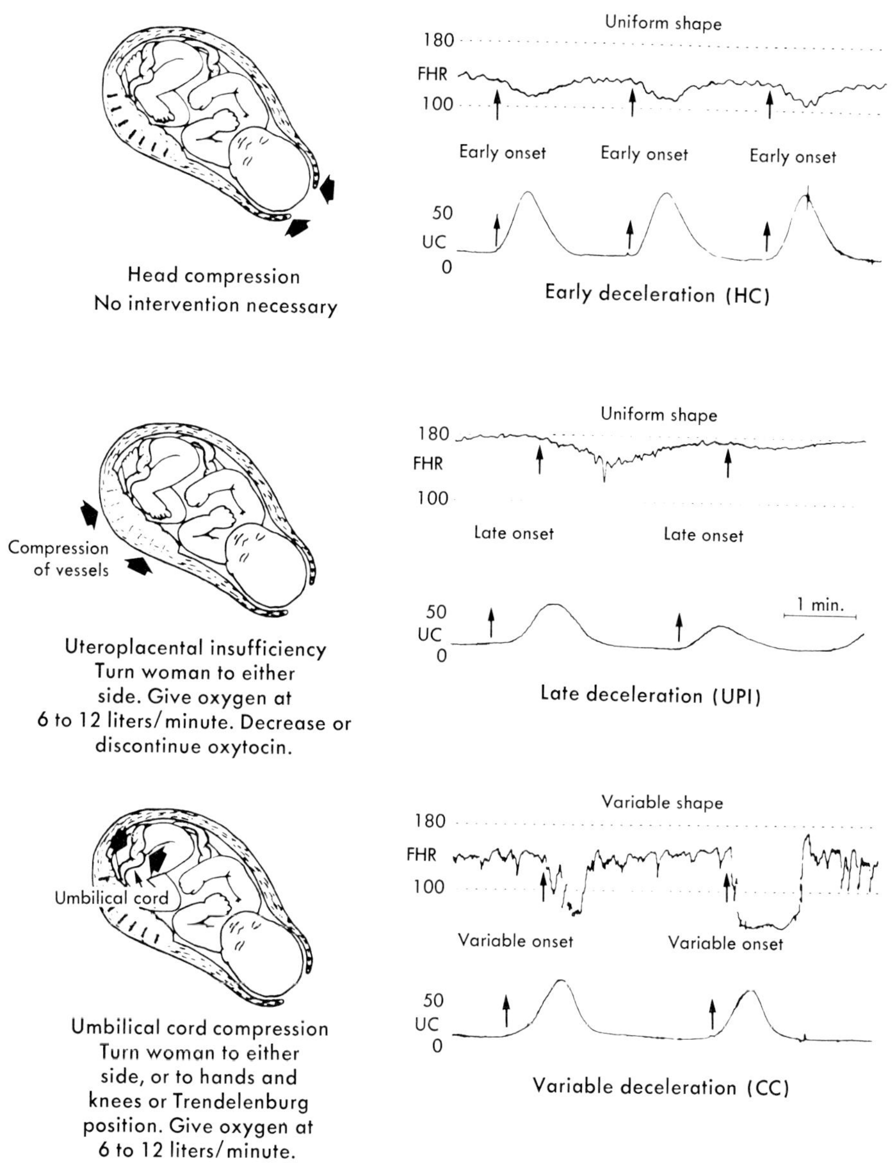

Fig. 8-7. Periodic changes in fetal heart rate. (From Hon, E.H.: An introduction to fetal heart rate monitoring, Wallingford, Conn., Corometrics Medical Systems, Inc.)

EXTERNAL AND INTERNAL FETAL HEART RATE MONITORING

pressure-sensitive transducer that measures the tension on the abdominal wall when the uterus contracts (Fig. 8-8). The advantages of external monitoring are that it does not require rupture of the membranes and that it can be used in early labor or for tests of fetal status such as the oxytocin challenge test (OCT), nipple stimulation test, and the nonstress test discussed earlier. However, external monitoring is much less accurate than internal monitoring and is more difficult to keep in adjustment. The mother's movement is often restricted when adjustment is a problem.

Internal monitors also consist of two parts: (1) a tiny wire (ECG electrode), which is attached to the scalp of the fetus to record fetal heart beat, and (2) a soft polyethylene catheter filled with distilled water that is placed inside the uterus to record intensity, duration, and frequency of uterine contractions, and resting tone of the uterus (intrauterine pressure between contractions) (Fig. 8-9). Internal monitoring has the advantage of being accurate and easy to adjust. The major disadvantage is that the cervix must be dilated 3 to 4 centimeters and the membranes must be ruptured, thus making it an invasive technique. Invasive techniques increase the risk of maternal and fetal infections.

It is important for the nurse to recognize that the fetal monitor is only a tool and not a replacement for the nurse. The uses and working of the monitor should also be explained to the laboring woman and her family.

The Food and Drug Administration of the U.S. Department of Health and Human Services has recommended that diagnostic ultrasound not be advertised as unequivocably safe until adequate human studies of possible adverse effects can be conducted.

Because it is beyond the scope of this book to discuss fetal monitoring in detail, the bibliographic sources at the end of this unit are recommended for further study where appropriate.

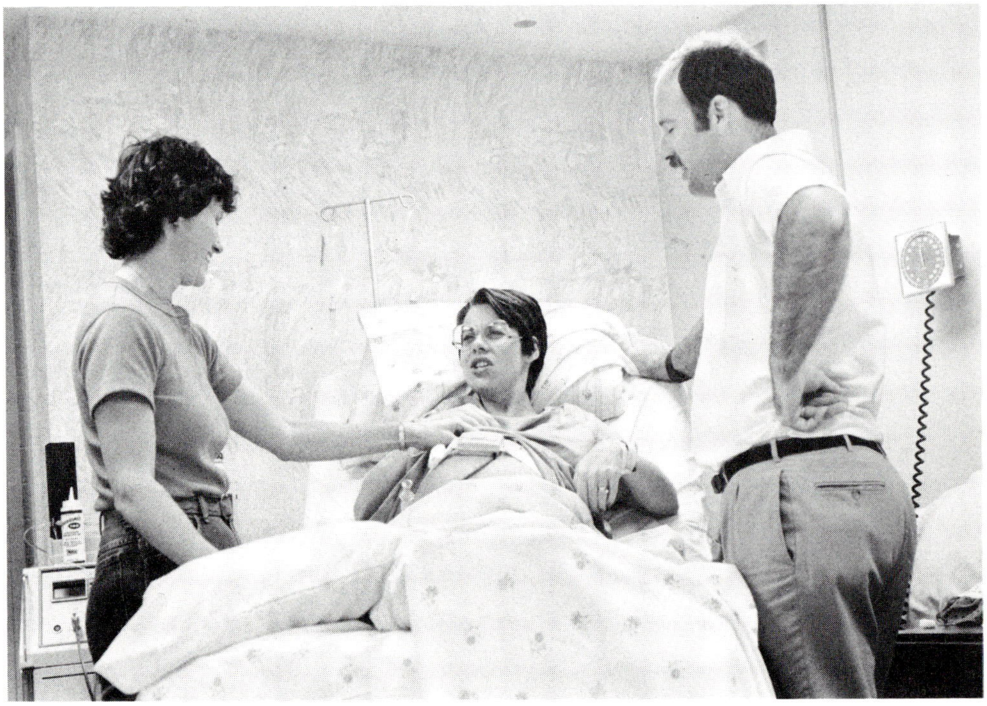

Fig. 8-8. External monitoring. (Photo by Paul J. O'Mara, Rome, Georgia. Courtesy Vance Simpson and Sharon Baker.)

Fetal blood sampling

If the signs of fetal distress do not respond to treatment as outlined, fetal status can be assessed by obtaining a sample of capillary blood from the presenting part, either scalp or buttocks. With membranes ruptured, an endoscope is inserted into the vagina. A knife blade with a long handle is used to puncture the fetal scalp or buttocks. Capillary blood is collected in long heparinized glass capillary tubes. A fetal scalp pH of 7.20 to 7.25 is considered borderline and should be repeated within 20 minutes. Two successive fetal scalp pHs less than 7.20 may indicate acidosis and the need for immediate delivery. (A normal fetal scalp pH would be more than 7.25.) Some high-risk maternity centers are using sensors that can be attached to the fetal scalp for continuous pH monitoring.

Vaginal and rectal examination

INDICATE THE PURPOSE FOR VAGINAL OR RECTAL EXAMINATIONS IN LABOR

Upon admission and when necessary during labor, a vaginal examination is done to determine the state and progress of labor. Using a sterile glove, antiseptic solution, and aseptic techniques, the examiner gently inserts one or two fingers into the woman's vagina to ascertain the dilation, station, effacement, presenting part, and position of the presenting part. A rectal examination can also be done to determine the state and progress of labor, but a rectal yields less accurate information because of the intervening recto-vaginal wall; it also increases the chances of infection.

In some hospitals vaginal examinations are the responsibility of the physician only, while in others vaginal examinations are nursing responsibilities.

Rupture of membranes

Sometimes during a vaginal examination, the bag of waters may be found bulging down into the cervix with great pressure. The physician or midwife may decide to rupture the membranes with an Allis's clamp or membrane hook, thus performing an *amniotomy*. There is disagreement over the necessity of this procedure, however, because it is believed that the bulging bag of waters fits into the cervical opening and serves as a hydrostatic wedge to dilate the cervix. Also, with the bag of waters gone, the cushioning effect of the waters for the head of the fetus is lost. Those who favor amniotomy believe that labor is accelerated by this procedure, thus reducing the length of time the fetus is stressed. The woman and her family should be told the pros and cons of artificial rupture of membranes (ARM) in birth preparation classes so that they can give informed consent for the procedure.

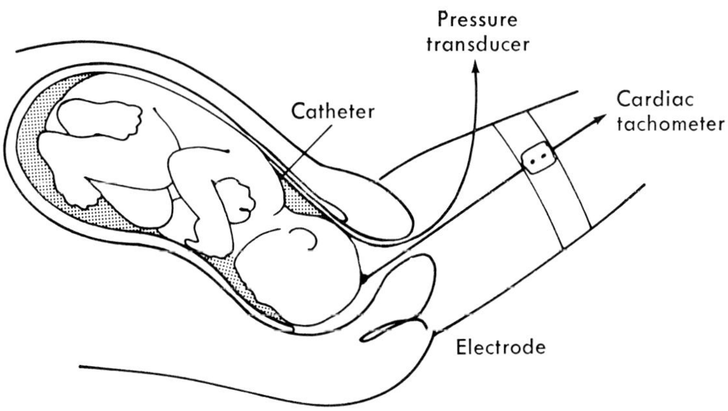

Fig. 8-9. Internal monitoring. (From Wiggins, J.: Childbearing; physiology, experiences, needs, St. Louis, 1979, The C.V. Mosby Co.)

APPEARANCE OF AMNIOTIC FLUID

Whether the membranes are ruptured artificially or spontaneously in labor, the fluid should be clear and colorless. If it is not clear and colorless, the physician should be notified immediately. A yellowish, foul-smelling fluid may be indicative of infection of the amniotic sac (*amnionitis*). If the presentation is vertex, thick greenish or brownish fluid may mean that the fetus has passed meconium (fetal stool) into the fluid and may be in distress. If the fetus suffers from a lack of oxygen in utero, the anal sphincters may relax and dilate, releasing meconium into the amniotic fluid. With a breech presentation, meconium-stained fluid may be normal.

If a woman suspects possible ruptured membranes, fluid from her vagina can be tested for pH with nitrazine paper. A positive result for amniotic fluid turns the paper dark blue since amniotic fluid has a pH of 7.0 to 7.5. With a negative result, the nitrazine paper would be yellow or brown since vaginal secretions have a pH of 3.8 to 5.5. Blood and some antimicrobial solutions and lubricants could yield false-positive results. Another test for ruptured membranes is the ferning (or arborization) test. In this test a few drops of fluid dry on a clean glass slide, and then the slide is examined microscopically. A positive result would occur when the sodium chloride in amniotic fluid crystallizes on the slide into a fern-like pattern.

EXPLAIN NURSING ACTION FOLLOWING ARTIFICIAL RUPTURE OF MEMBRANES

The risk of amnionitis may increase as the time the membranes have been ruptured increases. Sometimes, if the membranes have been ruptured for 24 hours and good labor has not begun, an induction is started. The fetal heart must always be checked immediately after rupture of membranes. The sheet under the woman's buttocks should be kept clean and dry.

Perineal preparation

Perineal preparation was done in the past because of the belief that it provided a clean field for delivery. Many physicians no longer believe that shaving the perineum is necessary; some order a half, or "mini," preparation (perineal area only) if episiotomy repair is necessary and perineal hair is troublesome. An examination of the origin and procedure of perineal shaving has provided evidence that shaving pubic hair to prevent infection is not necessary. In fact, shaving compromises the integrity of the skin by inflicting multiple small abrasions. The procedure of perineal shaving is also humiliating and frightening for many women.

Enema

IDENTIFY TWO REASONS NOT TO GIVE ENEMA TO WOMAN IN ACTIVE LABOR

Either a rectal suppository or a small disposable enema may be given in early labor for the following purposes: (1) to prevent contamination of the perineum by feces that may be expelled with delivery of the baby, (2) to provide more room in the pelvis for the passage of the fetus, and (3) to help stimulate uterine contractions. An enema is not given if the woman has an unusual amount of vaginal bleeding or is rapidly approaching the second stage of labor. As with the perineal preparation, an enema is not necessary for all women in labor and each case should be evaluated on an individual basis.

Bladder

DISCUSS THE IMPORTANCE OF EMPTY BLADDER IN LABOR

It is important to keep the laboring woman's bladder as empty as possible because a full bladder mechanically impedes the descent of the fetal head. If the woman is up and about, she should be helped to the toilet often. If she is on bed rest, she should be offered the bedpan at frequent intervals. A full bladder can be observed and palpated as a soft balloon full of water above the symphysis pubis (Fig. 8-10). If all attempts at voiding fail and the bladder is definitely distended, catheterization is necessary.

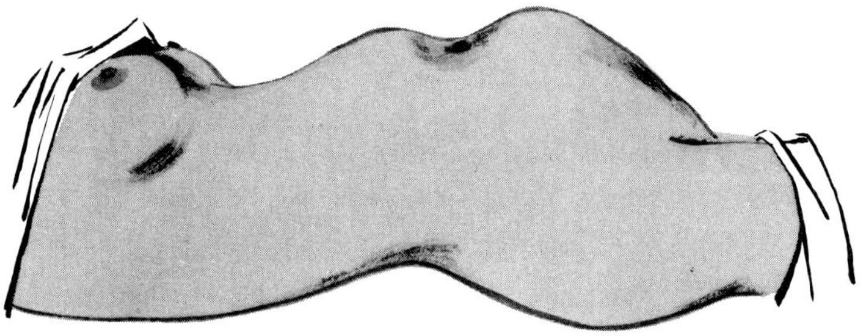

Fig. 8-10. Full bladder. (From Lerch, C., and Bliss, V.J.: Maternity nursing, ed. 3, St. Louis, 1978, The C.V. Mosby Co.)

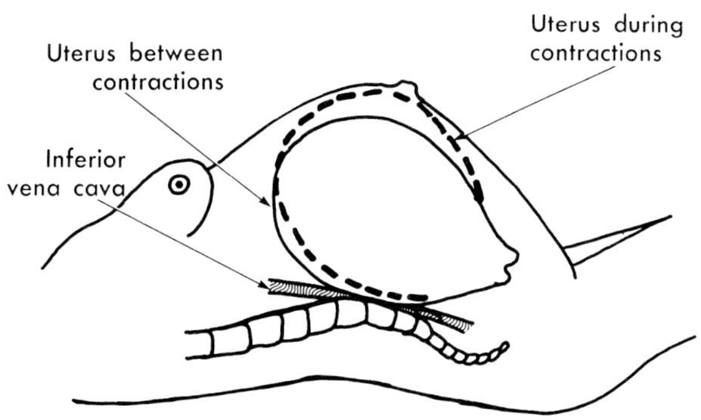

Fig. 8-11. Supine hypotensive syndrome.

Activity

DESCRIBE THE CAUSE AND PREVENTION OF SUPINE HYPOTENSIVE SYNDROME

If the woman's membranes have ruptured early in labor and the presenting part is not yet engaged, she should remain in bed because of the possibility of an umbilical cord prolapse. However, if the membranes are intact or if the presenting part is tight against the cervix after membranes are ruptured, she may be more comfortable walking around, taking a warm shower, sitting, or rocking. She should be able to assume a position of comfort even if that means getting on all fours and rocking her pelvis up and down. Never should the woman labor flat on her back because the pressure of the full uterus on the vena cava and other major vessels can slow down the venous return blood flow to her brain, causing *supine hypotensive syndrome* (Fig. 8-11). Ambulation during labor is not only more comfortable for the woman but also can facilitate labor. It is important to evaluate each woman's labor individually to determine the most comfortable, safe, and efficient positions for her. Labor is not a static process, and neither should the woman's position be static (see Fig. 8-12).

Food

Because gastric mobility decreases during labor and digestion slows, solid food is usually not given during labor. Food eaten up to 12 hours before the onset of labor may remain in the stomach. However, water or ice chips are usually recommended, and sucking on hard candy helps to keep the woman's mouth moist. Fruit juices, broths, or teas with added sugar or honey can help maintain the woman's level of hydration as well as her blood sugar level. A record of fluid intake and output must be kept during labor.

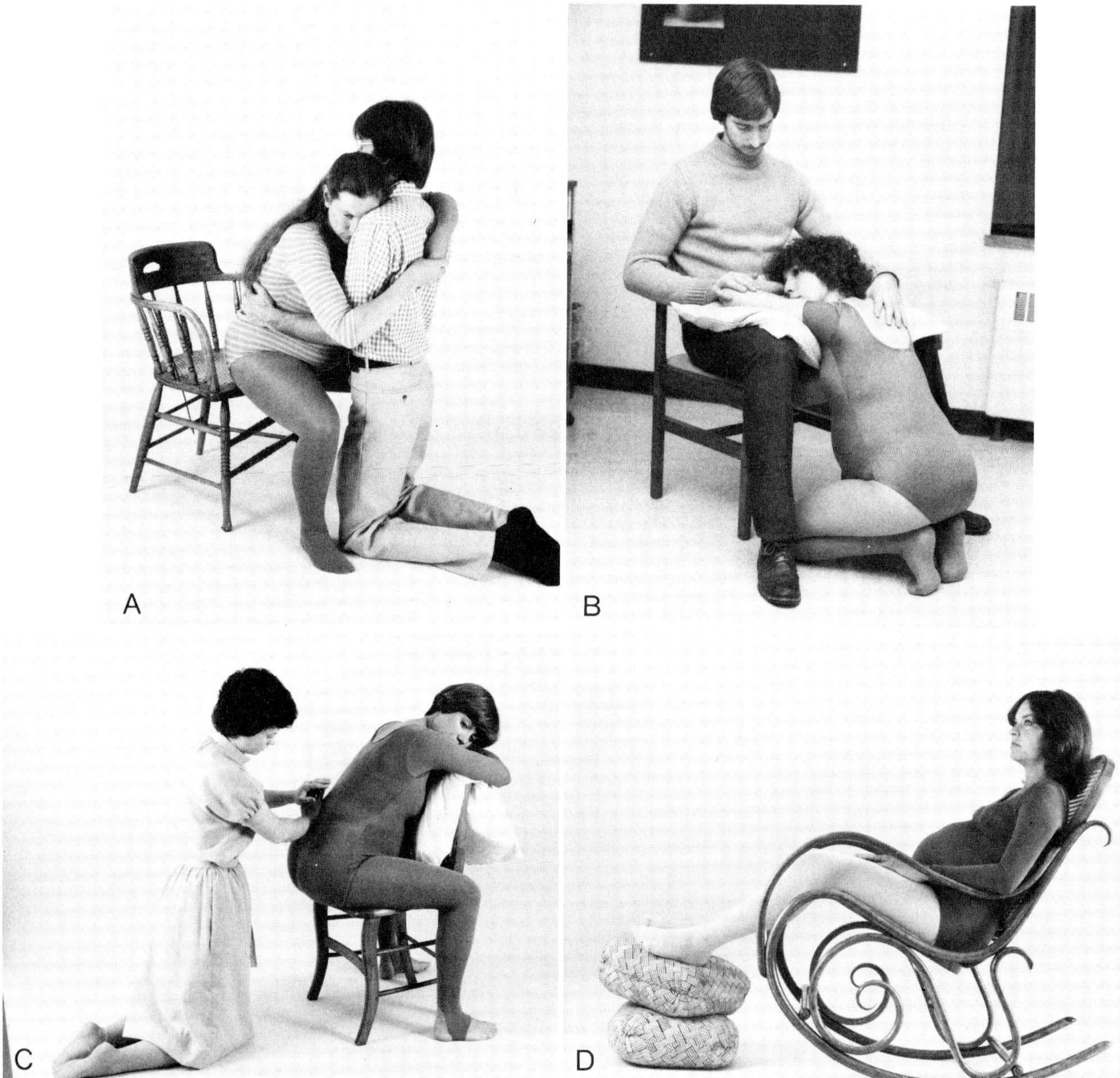

Fig. 8-12. Positions for labor. **A,** Sitting forward with her partner supporting her may offer flexibility for a woman during labor. **B,** While squatting during labor, a woman can support her balance by leaning against her partner. **C,** Firm pressure on the sacral area of the mother's lower back often relieves back pain that accompanies some labors. **D,** Many women find rocking during labor to be both relaxing and comfortable. **E,** Effleurage (light rhythmic stroking) may be soothing during labor and can be perfomed by the woman or her support person. **F,** Many women find that relaxing in a tub of warm water relieves discomfort in early labor. **G,** Laboring in a shower during early labor may be comforting for a woman. Warm water streaming against her back may relieve back pain. **H,** Assuming a hands-and-knees position and rocking her pelvis may help a woman to relieve back pain during labor. **I,** During labor, a position of comfort may be side lying, with pillows supporting the woman's shoulders and legs.

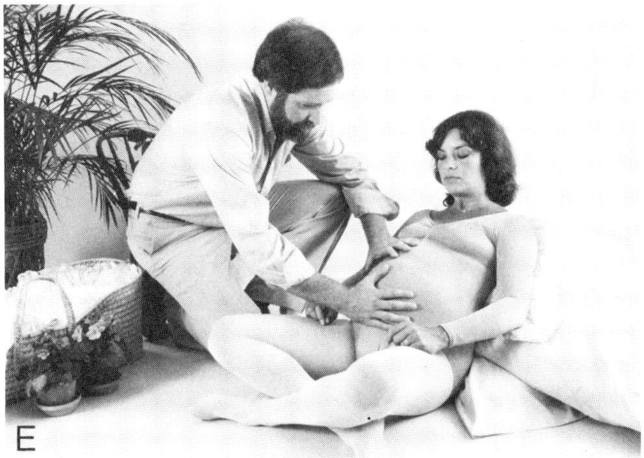

E

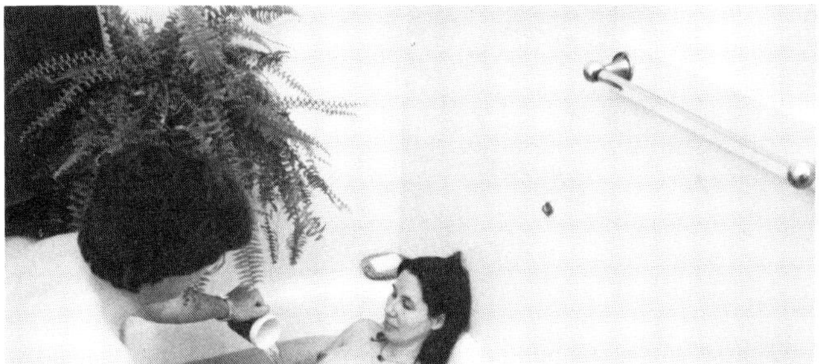

F

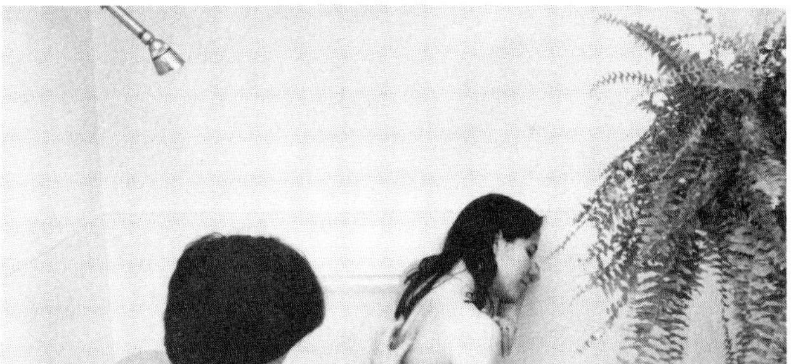

G

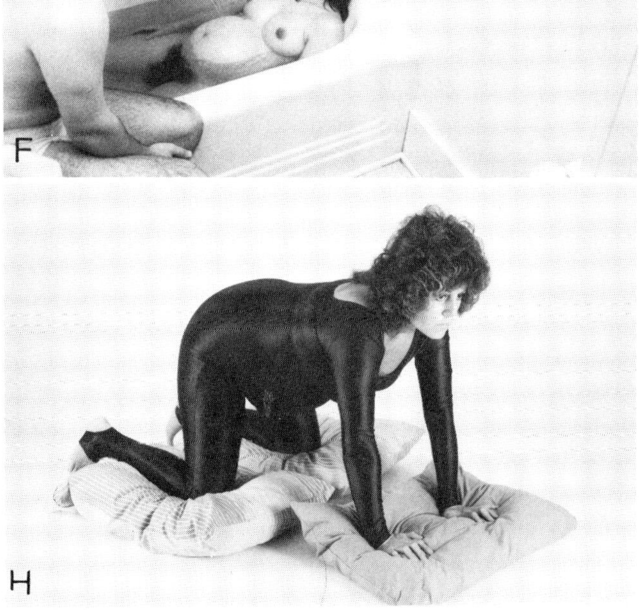

H

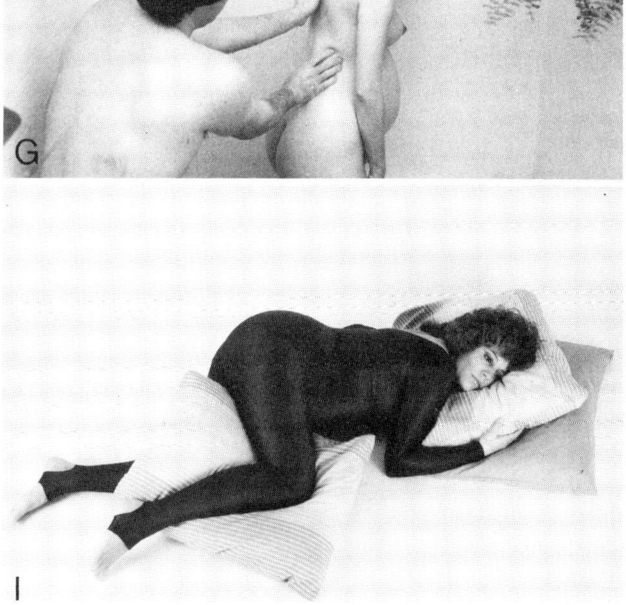

I

Intravenous therapy may be necessary for hydration and/or medication. If nausea and vomiting are present, the risk of aspiration is a concern. Sometimes it is helpful to give antacids to neutralize gastric juices and thus reduce the risk of possible aspiration pneumonitis.

Comfort measures

General comfort measures as simple as replacing soiled bed linen are very important. Many of these measures were discussed in Unit VI. This would be a good time to review that unit.

Whenever any procedures or examinations are done, the privacy and comfort of the woman should always be considered. Keeping her covered or draped, explaining all procedures to her, and obtaining her permission to perform them are essential nursing responsibilities. Table 8-1 summarizes nursing care during labor.

SECOND STAGE OF LABOR: NURSING CARE

RECOGNIZE THE SIGNS AND SYMPTOMS INDICATING APPROACH OF SECOND STAGE OF LABOR

The second stage of labor begins with complete dilation of the cervix and ends with delivery of the baby. Signs and symptoms indicating the approach of the second stage include: (1) an increase in bloody show, (2) nausea and vomiting, (3) a feeling of needing to defecate, (4) short grunting respirations with bearing down reflex efforts by the mother, and (5) a bulging perineum.

Delivery room preparation

The actual moment when a woman is moved from the labor room to the delivery room varies, but generally primigravidas are moved to the delivery room when the fetal head is visible. Multiparas are moved to the delivery room when fully dilated or when about 7 to 8 centimeters dilated if labor is rapid. More and more women and their families are requesting to deliver in their labor beds or in "birthing rooms"; in labor, delivery, recovery rooms (LDRs); or in labor, delivery, recovery, postpartum rooms (LDRPs) (Fig. 8-13) to avoid having to move at a very uncomfortable moment in the birth process. (Discussion of these contemporary settings for birth can be found in the final unit of this book.) If these options are not available, the delivery room can be set up within 12 hours ahead of time with the delivery table, sterile instrument table, sterile basins, an incubator, or an infant warmer unit of some kind, plus resuscitation equipment for the baby (Fig. 8-14). All of the sterile linen and equipment can be covered with sterile drapes, which are removed at the time of delivery. Adequate preliminary preparation eliminates last minute hustle and bustle and subsequent anxieties.

Delivery table

Unfortunately, many women and health care providers have been socialized to birth lying down. Also, many health care providers promote the lithotomy position for birth because of its convenience for monitoring FHR, doing and repairing episiotomies, and administering anesthetics and its utility for obstetric intervention. Re-education is necessary for all involved because the disadvantages of the lithotomy position far outweigh the advantages. Disadvantages include aortocaval compression; risk of venous thrombosis in legs from pressure of stirrups; back pain; decreased pushing ability; rigidity and tightening of the perineum; and fetal distress secondary to maternal hemodynamic changes. In addition, it is difficult for the mother to see and hold her baby, and she has less control of the birth itself.

LIST NURSING ACTIONS WHEN POSITIONING WOMAN ON DELIVERY TABLE

If obstetrical intervention is imperative and it is absolutely essential to have a woman in lithotomy position for second stage, when elevating the woman's legs into the stirrups on the delivery table it is important to put both legs up in stirrups at the same time to prevent straining of ligaments. Pillows or a lift under the head of the table or mattress

Table 8-1. Nursing care during labor

Nursing care	Stage one of labor		Stage two	Stage three	Stage four
	Latent phase	Active phase			
Emotional support	Continuous support, encouragement, reassurance, and information.		Same as stage one.	Same as stage one.	Same as stage one.
Enema	May be given in early labor if no unusual vaginal bleeding.				
Bladder	Encourage women to void frequently.	Void frequently.	May have to catheterize.		Keep bladder empty.
Intake	Encourage fluids and ice chips unless contraindicated; no solid foods.		Same as stage one.	Same as stage one.	Fluids high in CHO.
Activity	Walk, sit, assume position of comfort as long as safe to do so.				Probably bed rest.
Comfort	Wash face and hands with cool water; apply cream, lotion or Chapstick to lips; apply back pressure to small of woman's back; encourage relaxation.	Cool cloth to face and hands; instruct and assist with bearing down for expulsion; explain what is happening; relieve leg cramps if necessary by forcing the foot upward with pressure on the knee.			Check uterus.
Temperature, pulse, respiration	Check every hour unless abnormal (temperature $>100^\circ$ F; pulse >100 or <60; respirations >30 or <12).				Check pulse and respirations every 15 minutes (first hour), then every 30 minutes (second hour); check temperature once.
Blood pressure	Check every 2 hours unless abnormal: blood pressure over 140/90 is abnormal.			Before giving oxytocic drugs or any other medication.	Check every 15 minutes (first hour) then every 30 minutes (second hour).
Fetal heart tones	Check every 30 minutes (normal, 120–160 beats/minute).	Check every 15 minutes.	Check after every contraction or every 5 minutes.		
Measure contractions	Time uterine contractions every 30 minutes; check for intensity, frequency, and duration.	Check contractions every 15 minutes.	Time each contraction.		Check uterus frequently for excessive bleeding; make sure uterus remains firm.
Record data		Continuous recording of data.			

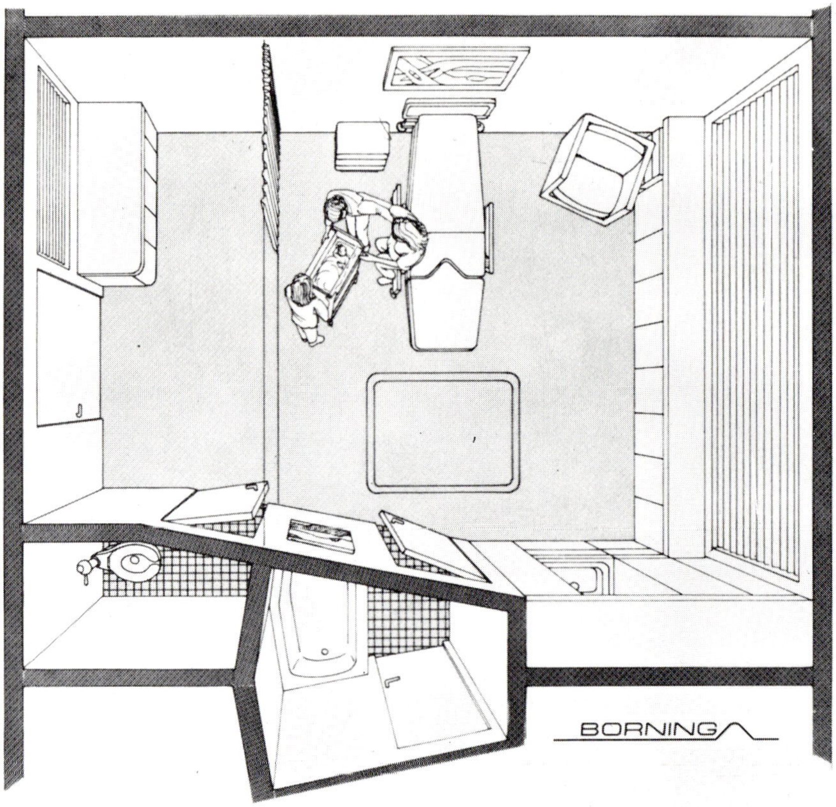

Fig. 8-13. Labor, delivery, recovery, postpartum room (LDRP) after the birth and mother and baby are stable. (Drawing by Charles Pomeroy. Photo courtesy of the Borning Corporation, Spokane, Washington.)

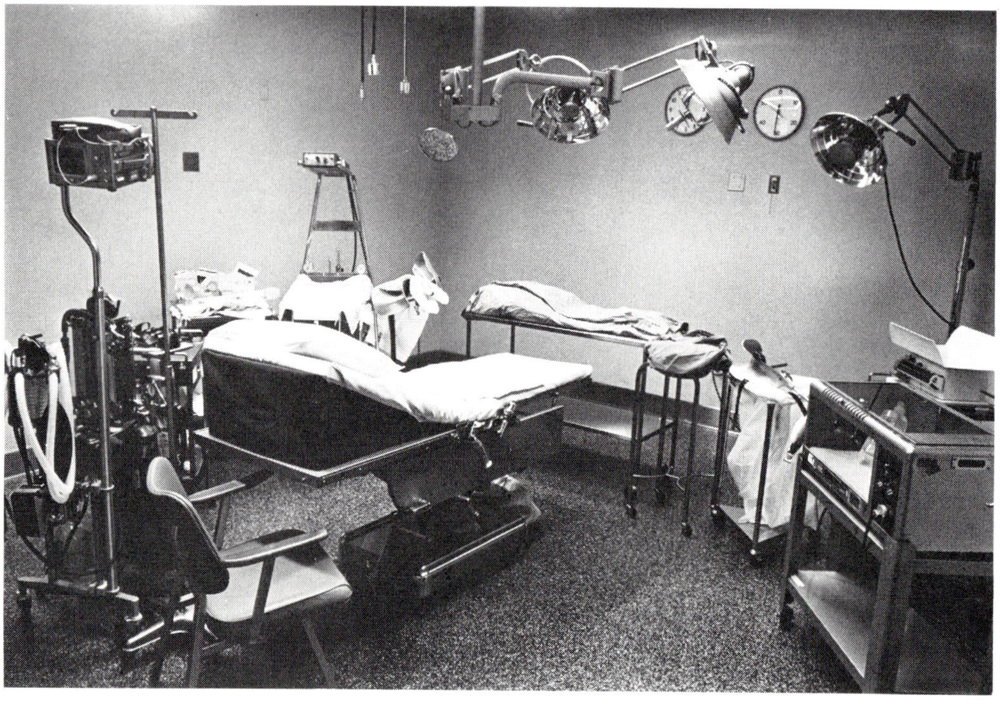

Fig. 8-14. Delivery room set-up. (Courtesy Kaiser-Permanente Medical Center, Santa Clara, Calif.)

enable the woman's trunk to be at a 35- or 45-degree angle. This position is vital to facilitate her pushing efforts and to keep the weight of the uterus and its content off the woman's major blood vessels, as discussed previously.

Perineal preparation

A perineal scrub with bactericidal solution is usually done before sterile drapes are arranged on the woman. For this perineal cleansing, the nurse wears a sterile glove.

Delivery

As the baby's head crowns, the woman must be encouraged to "pant" so that the expulsion of the baby can be controlled. At this point, the doctor or midwife may perform an episiotomy if deemed necessary to prevent tearing of the perineum. The nurse notes and records the exact time of the delivery of the baby.

The woman's partner, support person, or other family members can be very helpful at delivery (Fig. 8-15). However, these persons also need positive reinforcement, recognition, and support from the staff. It is their experience also and can have profound meaning for them. If the family has decided to include young siblings at the birth, a support person should be present for each sibling.

IDENTIFY THE IMMEDIATE NEEDS OF NEWBORN

Immediately after birth, the baby is dried, and a clear airway is assured using a bulb suction or DeLee's mucus trap if necessary. Then the baby is placed on the mother's abdomen. Some mothers want to reach down and help their baby out into the world. The mother can do this "gentle assist" even in a sterile delivery room with the nurse's careful assistance. The cord is usually tied or clamped in two places and cut in between when it stops pulsating. Some physicians give the scissors to the baby's father and en-

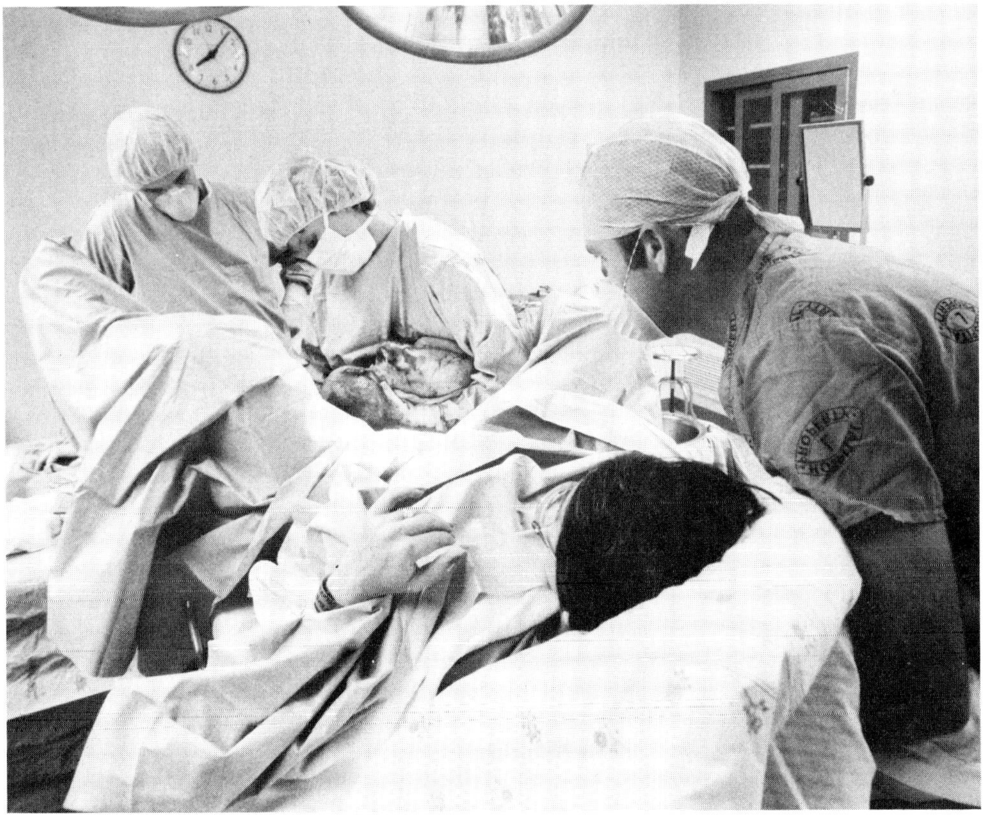

Fig. 8-15. Delivery. (Photo by Paul J. O'Mara, Rome, Georgia. Courtesy Vance Simpson and Sharon Baker.)

courage him to cut the cord. There is a lot of symbolism in this gesture as he seems to be freeing his child (Fig. 8-16) and thus accepting the responsibilities of parenthood.

Apgar scoring

NAME THE FIVE SIGNS SCORED IN APGAR SYSTEM

The Apgar scoring system is used to evaluate the general condition of the baby at 1 minute of life and again at 5 minutes. Apgar scores are based on five signs: heart rate, respiratory effort, muscle tone, reflex response, and color. Each sign is given the score of 0, 1, or 2 points. A perfect Apgar is 10 at 1 minute and again at 5 minutes (Fig. 8-17).

Immediate care of the newborn

If the infant is dried, covered with a warm blanket, and placed in skin-to-skin contact with the warm mother or father and is apparently responding and breathing normally, the first 15 or 30 minutes of life can be a family time without interruption by the staff. If there are any deviations from normal, the baby will have to be placed in an incubator or infant warmer for close observation and proper treatment. Fortunately, most infants are well and normal and have Apgar scores of 8 or better and thus can remain with the mother or father for the initial acquaintance or bonding process described in Unit I. Some mothers like to breast-feed their babies immediately after birth. If the baby is alert, well, sucking, and wanting to feed, this is an excellent time to begin.

EXPLAIN THE PURPOSE OF INSTILLING SILVER NITRATE IN NEWBORN'S EYES

After this initial bonding period, the nurse can weigh and measure the baby, take its temperature, remove superficial blood and mucus, and instill two drops of 1% silver nitrate (Credé treatment) in each conjunctival sac using two ampules, one for each eye. This Credé treatment is required by law to prevent blindness caused by gonococcal organisms that may be present in the vagina. It is recommended by the U.S. Centers for

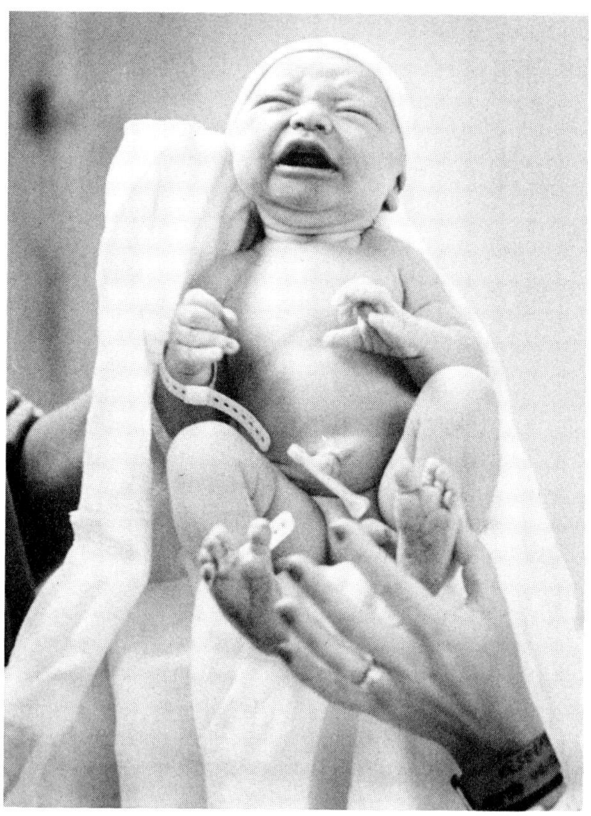

Fig. 8-16. Cord cutting is completed. (Photo by Paul J. O'Mara, Rome, Georgia. Courtesy Vance Simpson and Sharon Baker.)

Disease Control (CDC) that the baby's eyes not be irrigated after instilling the silver nitrate (Fig. 8-18).

Other acceptable prophylactic agents that prevent ophthalmia neonatorum include:

1. Erythromycin (0.5%) ophthalmic ointment in drops in single-use tubes or ampules
2. Tetracycline (1%) ophthalmic ointment in drops or single-use tubes or ampules

Erythromycin and tetracycline ointment and drops have also been found to prevent chlamydial ophthalmia neonatorum, which is a common problem now. In 1983, the American Academy of Pediatrics recommended instillation of erythromycin or tetracycline ointment or drops shortly after birth in all infants.

Identification

The mother and baby must be identified before leaving the delivery room. Plastic bands having the same number on them are attached to the mother's wrist and to the baby's wrist and ankle. All three bands contain the baby's sex, date and time of birth, mother's name, and physician's name. Some hospitals footprint the baby and also take the mother's fingerprints; however, these are not legally identifying data.

THIRD STAGE OF LABOR: NURSING CARE

The third stage of labor begins after the delivery of the baby and ends with the discharge of the placenta. The nurse is responsible for recording the time the placenta is delivered. After the placenta is expelled, the physician or midwife inspects it to be sure that it is intact. The physician may order an oxytocic drug after the placenta is expelled to aid in stimulating contractions of the uterine muscles. The average blood loss in the third stage of labor is 300 milliliters. The nurse must observe the mother for hemorrhage and shock and massage the uterus if it relaxes. If blood loss reaches 500 milliliters, it is considered a hemorrhage. If this occurs, grasp the uterus and massage it gently but firmly until it becomes hard again.

Lacerations

Even in the most carefully controlled delivery, lacerations or extensions of the episiotomy may occur. Usually the same anesthetic used for the episiotomy can be used to repair lacerations. Sometimes a local anesthetic is administered.

APGAR SCORING CHART

Sign	0	1	2
HEART RATE	Absent	Slow (below 100)	Over 100
RESPIRATORY EFFORT	Absent	Weak cry, hypoventilation	Good strong cry
MUSCLE TONE	Limp	Some flexion of extremities	Well flexed
REFLEX RESPONSE 1. Response to catheter in nostril (tested after oro-pharynx is clear)	No response	Grimace	Cough or sneeze
2. Tangential foot slap	No response	Grimace	Cry and withdrawal of foot
COLOR	Blue, pale	Body pink, extremities blue	Completely pink

Fig. 8-17. Apgar scoring chart. Category condition: 0–3, poor, critical, severely depressed; 4–6, moderately depressed; 7–10, good.

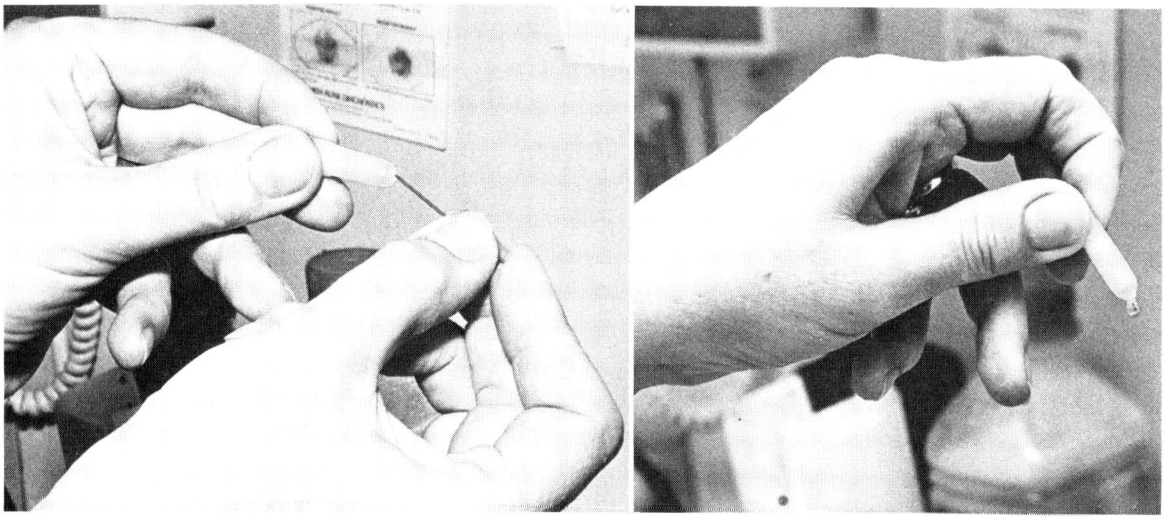

Fig. 8-18. Silver nitrate for Credé's treatment. A, Puncturing wax ampule containing 1% silver nitrate ophthalmic solution with pin. B, Squeezing out a drop to instill in each conjunctival sac of newborn.

CHARACTERISTICS OF FOUR DEGREES OF PERINEAL LACERATION

Lacerations are classified according to the extent of the tear as first, second, third, or fourth degree. First-degree lacerations are fairly common and involve tearing of the skin and mucous membrane only. Lacerations involving skin and muscles are called second degree. Third-degree lacerations involve skin, muscles, and tearing into the rectal sphincter (Fig. 8-19). Fourth-degree lacerations involve all of these structures and the anal wall.

Immediate postdelivery care

Cleansing the perineal area after the delivery, applying clean perineal pads, covering the mother with warm dry blankets, and, if she is in stirrups, bringing both legs down at the same time are nursing responsibilities.

The woman's blood pressure and pulse, firmness of the uterus, and amount of vaginal bleeding are checked and recorded before she is transferred to the recovery area. It is this time that the baby may be taken to the nursery in traditional hospital procedures.

FOURTH STAGE OF LABOR: NURSING CARE

EXPLAIN APPROPRIATE NURSING ACTIONS DURING FOURTH STAGE OF LABOR

CAUSES OF EXCESSIVE BLEEDING IN FOURTH STAGE OF LABOR

The first few hours after delivery until the mother's vital signs are stable can be called the fourth stage of labor. During this time the nurse checks the woman's blood pressure and pulse every 15 minutes for the first hour and every 30 minutes for the second hour after delivery. The firmness and location of the uterus and amount of vaginal bleeding are also checked frequently. The fundus immediately after delivery should be firm and slightly above the level of the umbilicus. If the uterus relaxes and bleeds excessively, the nurse should massage the uterus until it becomes firm. If the uterus does not contract, there may be clots forming at the site of placental separation, or there may be retained placental pieces. These clots can be expressed by gentle, firm, downward pressure on the uterus fundus. Overstimulation of the uterus by vigorous massage is not recommended because it may cause uterine relaxation instead of contraction. If massage does not cause the uterus to contract, it may be necessary to "hold" the fundus. This is accomplished by placing one hand over the woman's symphysis pressing inward and then up toward her head. The other hand grasps and holds the fundus (Fig. 8-20). Again,

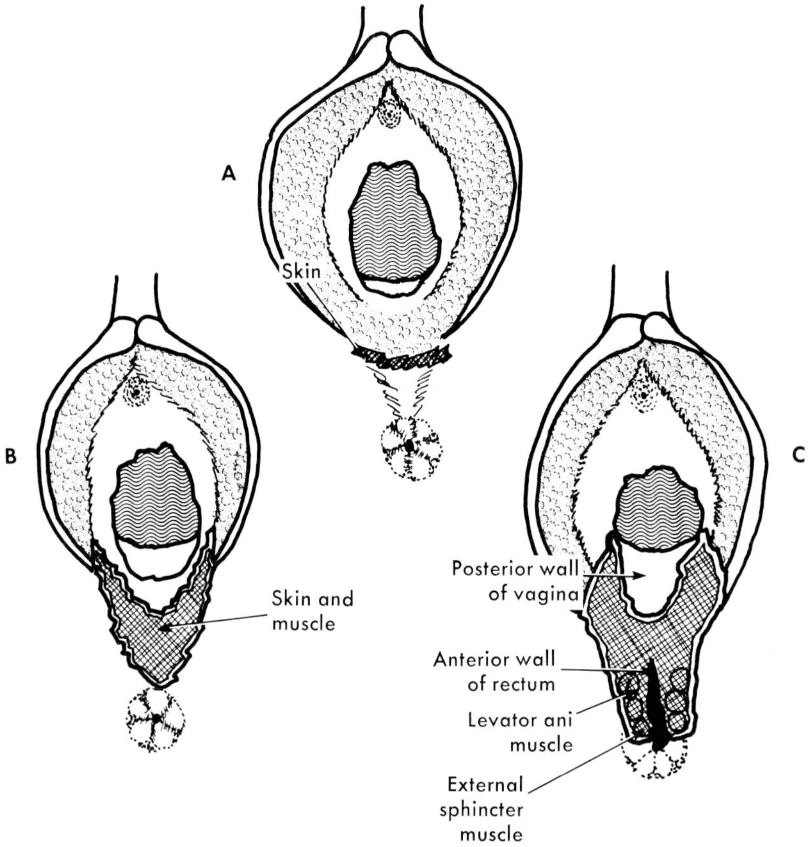

Fig. 8-19. Perineal lacerations. **A,** First-degree. **B,** Second-degree. **C,** Third-degree.

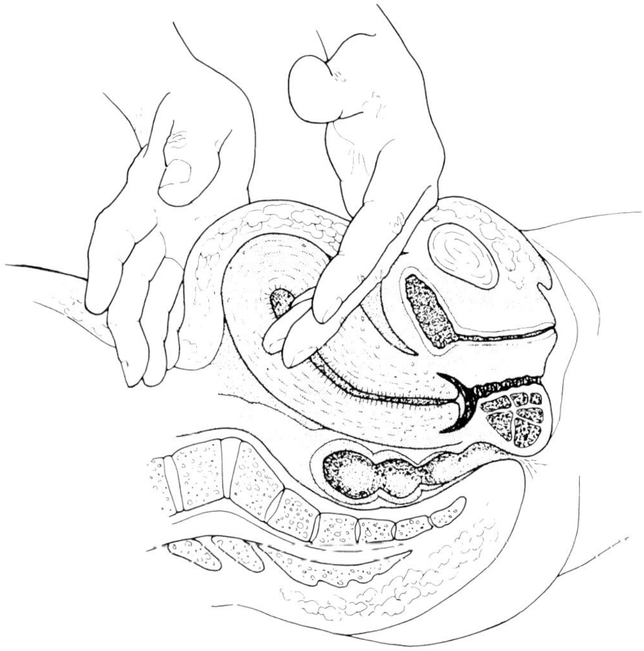

Fig. 8-20. Holding the fundus. (From Jensen, M., and Bobak, I.M.: Maternity and gynecologic care: the nurse and the family, ed. 3, St. Louis, 1985, The C.V. Mosby Co.)

COMMON DRUGS TO CAUSE UTERINE CONTRACTIONS IN THIRD AND FOURTH STAGES OF LABOR

oxytocic drugs may be needed to stimulate the uterus to contract. These are:

- Synthetic oxytocin
  - Pitocin:
    - 10 to 40 units intravenous infusion in 500 to 1000 milliliters of intravenous solution and using a controlled infusion device
  - Syntocinon:
    - 10 units intramuscularly
- Ergot derivatives
  - Ergonovine maleate (Ergotrate):
    - 0.2 milligrams intramuscularly or orally
  - Methylergonovine maleate (Methergine):
    - 0.2 milligrams intramuscularly or orally

Methergine and Ergotrate are given intravenously only for life-threatening, extremely severe uterine bleeding. If administered intravenously, Methergine and Ergotrate can cause acute hypertensive and cardiac crises, nausea and vomiting, dizziness, headache, tinnitus, dyspnea, diaphoresis, and palpitations. If given intravenously ergot derivatives should be diluted in 50 ml or more of fluid and given over a period of not less than 1 minute.

Because ergonovine has a vasoconstricting effect, it can cause elevated blood pressure. Always take the woman's blood pressure before giving ergonovine. It is never given to women with hypertension or pre-eclampsia, nor is it ever given before the placenta is expelled because it can cause the uterus to contract forcibly and thus trap the placenta inside.

Methylergonovine can also raise blood pressure, and consequently, is never given to a woman with hypertension. Injectable Ergotrate and Methergine must be refrigerated because they deteriorate when exposed to heat and light.

Oxytocic agents, such as pitocin, are potent drugs and can cause uterine contractions lasting more than 90 seconds *(tetanic contractions)*. The most common method of administering pitocin is in an intravenous infusion with an infusion pump. Close supervision is necessary.

When checking the perineal area for vaginal bleeding, any suture line should be checked for possible formation of a *hematoma* (a collection of blood in tissue) (Fig. 8-21). Each time the perineal pads are changed, the amount of bleeding and appearance of suture lines should be recorded. Ice compresses applied to sutured areas help to reduce swelling and pain.

Diaphoresis occurs after birth so that the woman may appreciate a sponge bath. Also, after birth the bladder fills up quickly with urine and must be checked for distention frequently. A distended bladder can interfere with uterine contraction and thus cause bleeding.

During the fourth stage of labor, the woman's mate and family can offer her warm support and assist with comfort measures (Fig. 8-22). Often this is the time the new father chooses to telephone anxious family and friends and share the news of the new family member.

SUMMARY

In this unit, common nursing care and procedures for use during the stages of labor were discussed. Step-by-step procedures were not presented since they differ from hospital to hospital. This unit is a general overview of how the nurse interacts with the intrapartum family when providing basic nursing care.

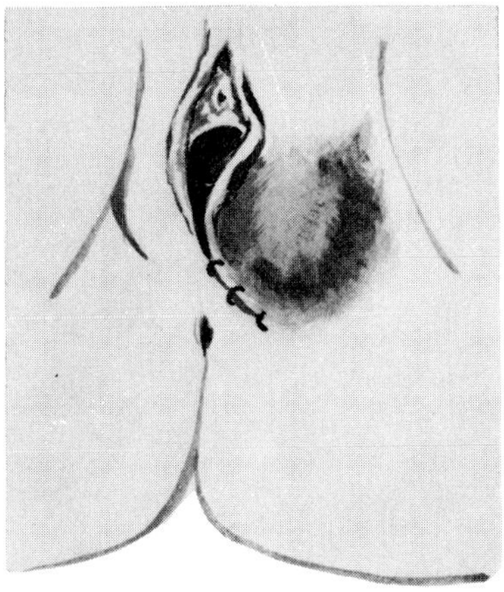

Fig. 8-21. Perineal hematoma. (From Lerch, C., and Bliss, V.J.: Maternity nursing, ed. 3, St. Louis, 1978, The C.V. Mosby Co.)

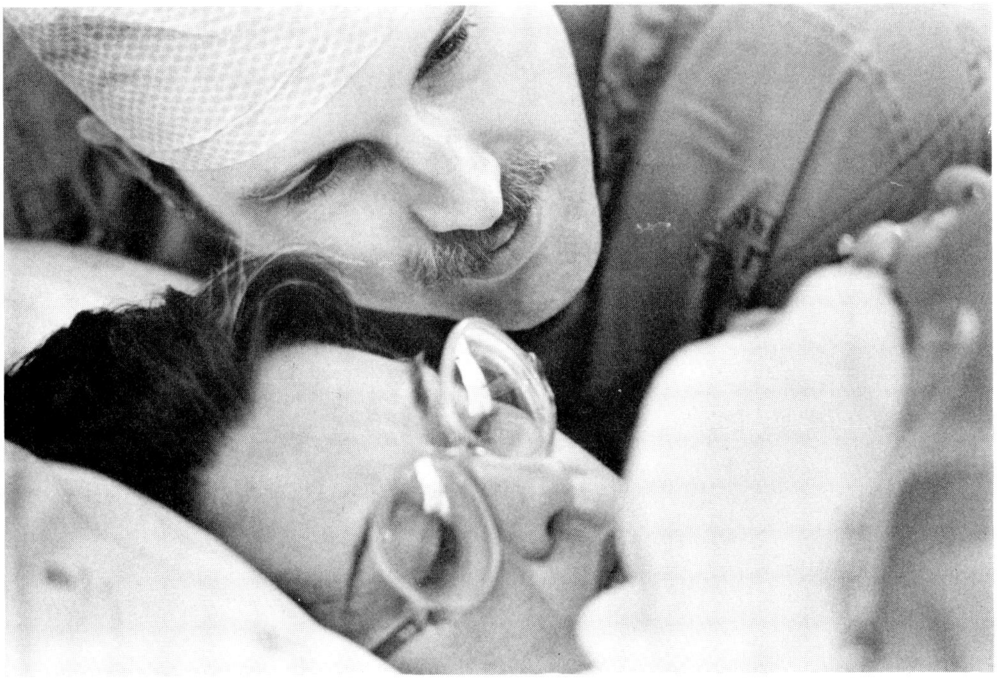

Fig. 8-22. Warm support. (Photo by Paul J. O'Mara, Rome, Georgia. Courtesy Vance Simpson and Sharon Baker.)

BIBLIOGRAPHY

American Academy of Pediatrics: Prophylaxis and treatment of neonatal gonococcal infections, Pediatrics **65**(5): 1047-1048, 1980.

American Academy of Pediatrics and American College of Obstetricians and Gynecologists: Guidelines for perinatal care, Evanston, Ill., AAP, and Washington, D.C., ACOG, 1983.

Anderson, B.G.: Obstetrics for the nurse, ed. 4, New York, 1983, Delmar Publishers.

Caldeyro-Barcia, R.: Some consequences of obstetrical interference, Birth Fam. J. **2**:2, 1975.

Caldeyro-Barcia, R., and others: Effect of position changes on the intensity and frequency of uterine contractions during labor,

Am. J. Obstet. Gynecol. **80**:284-290, August 1960.
Cohen, W.R.: Steering patients through the second stage of labor, Contemp. OB/GYN **24**:122, July 1984.
Drug Information, 84, American Society of Hospital Pharmacists, 1345-1347.
Fetal and maternal monitoring, a CEU offering, Am. J. Nurs. **78**:2097-2116, 1978.
Food and Drug Administration, Bureau of Radiological Health: Draft notice of intent to propose rules and develop recommendations related to diagnostic ultrasound equipment, U.S. Department of Health, Education, and Welfare, April 27, 1973.
Greenberg, M., and Morris, N.: Engrossment: the newborn's impact upon the father, Am. J. Orthopsychiatry **44**:520-531, 1974.
Intrapartrum evaluation of the fetus, JOGN Nurs. **5**(5):suppl., 1976.
Liu, Y.C.: Effects of an upright position during labor, Am. J. Nurs. **74**(12):2202-2205, 1974.
Mahan, C.S., and McKay, S.: Are we overmanaging second-stage labor? Contemp. OB/CYN, XX:37-63, Dec. 1984.
Mahan, C.S., and McKay, S.: Preps and enemas—keep or discard, Contemp. OB/GYN, XX:241-248, Nov. 1983.
McKay, S., and Mahan, C.S.: Laboring patients need freedom to move, Contemp. OB/GYN XX(24):90, July 1984.
Moore, M.L.: Realities in childbearing, ed. 2, Philadelphia, 1983, W.B. Saunders Co.
Tucker, S.M.: Fetal monitoring and fetal assessment in high-risk pregnancy, St. Louis, 1978, The C.V. Mosby Co.
U.S. Department of Health, Education, and Welfare, Centers for Disease Control: Morbidity and Mortality Weekly Report, vol. 27, March 31, 1978.

DEFINITIONS

Define the following terms:

amnionitis	Kreiselman's crib
amniotomy	laceration
Apgar score	late deceleration
aspiration pneumonitis	LDR
baseline fetal heart rate	LDRP
bradycardia (fetal)	Leff's stethoscope
Credé treatment	Leopold's maneuvers
deceleration	meconium
DeLee's mucus trap	nursing care history
diaphoresis	ophthalmia neonatorum
early deceleration	oxytocin
ergot derivatives	stethoscope
ferning	tachycardia (fetal)
fetal heart rate	umbilicus
fetoscope	uteroplacental insufficiency
hematoma	variability
incubator	variable deceleration

LEARNING ACTIVITIES AND EXPERIENCES

1. Group discussions
2. Guests: admissions office personnel or volunteer who helps with maternity admissions to explain procedures
3. Visit hospital admissions office and observe hospital preadmissions procedures for maternity patients.
4. View audiovisual aids and discuss.

ENRICHMENT/IN-DEPTH STUDY

1. Review basic nursing procedure for: enema, catheterization, medical and surgical asepsis.
2. Practice sterile gowning and gloving techniques.
3. Visit facilities that offer labor, delivery, recovery rooms (LDRs), or labor, delivery, recovery, postpartum rooms (LDRPs).

SELF-ASSESSMENT

1. If the woman preregisters for labor and delivery, she can complete what pre-admission forms before hospitalization?

2. When admitting a woman in labor, what information should the nurse gather first?
   a.
   b.
   c.
   d.
   e
   f.
3. In the first stage of labor, temperature, pulse, and respiration (TPR) are taken and recorded every ________ hours. Blood pressure is taken and ________ every ________ hours.
4. ________________ in the urine specimen may be a sign of ____________.
5. In the first stage of labor, it would be abnormal for a uterine contraction to last longer than ________ seconds.
6. Because uterine contractions begin at the fundus, the nurse can monitor the contraction by gently touching the fundus. Describe how to estimate whether the contraction is strong, moderate, or mild: ____
____
____
7. When performing Leopold's first three maneuvers on a woman in labor, the nurse would stand at the woman's side facing her ______________. The first maneuver includes palpating her ______________. The second maneuver determines on which side of the uterus the ______________ of the fetus is located. In the third maneuver, one hand is pressed over the ______________. Before beginning the fourth maneuver, the nurse must turn around to face the woman's ______________.
8. The normal fetal heart rate is ________ beats per minute.
9. In addition to the regular checking of the fetal heart rate, name three other instances when the heartbeat should be checked:
   a.
   b.
   c.
10. How would you explain the purpose of continuous fetal monitoring to an expectant couple? ____
____
____

11. Match Column A with Column B:

Column A	Column B
_____ _____1. early deceleration	a. late onset
_____ _____2. variable deceleration	b. early onset
_____ _____3. late deceleration	c. uteroplacental insufficiency
	d. head compression
	e. cord compression
	f. variable onset

12. The fetal heart rate (FHR) present between uterine contractions is identified as the ____________________ FHR.
13. Match Column A with Column B

Column A	Column B
_____ _____1. short-term variability	a. fluctuations occurring two to six times each minute
_____ _____2. long-term variability	b. averages 5 to 15 beats per minute
	c. averages 6 to 10 beats per minute
	d. beat-to-beat variability

Circle the correct answers for questions 14 through 20.

14. To accurately evaluate the resting tone of the uterus between contractions, the contractions must be monitored by:
    a. external methods
    b. internal methods
15. The major disadvantage of internal monitoring is:
    a. membranes must be ruptured
    b. it is difficult to keep in adjustment
16. Loss of variability or decrease in variability as labor progresses in a previously average reading could be:
    a. a good sign
    b. an ominous sign
17. Vaginal or rectal examinations are done in labor to:
    a. determine the state and progress of labor
    b. speed cervical dilation
18. Following artificial rupture of membranes (amniotomy), the nurse should immediately:
    a. listen to and record fetal heart rate
    b. perform Leopold's maneuvers
19. The normal appearance of amniotic fluid is:
    a. clear and colorless
    b. thick and greenish
20. A pregnant woman is being admitted to the hospital in early labor. When preparing to give an enema ordered routinely for all laboring women, the nurse notices bright-red vaginal bleeding. The nurse would:
    a. cleanse the vaginal area and give the enema as ordered
    b. not give the enema and notify the physician

Fill in the blanks for questions 21 through 32.

21. Describe the significance of the following findings in relation to a woman in labor:
    a. a full bladder ____________________
    b. the woman lying flat on her back ____________________
    c. meconium-stained amniotic fluid ____________________
    d. a woman's complaint of rectal pressure ____________________
22. What are the signs of the beginning of the second stage of labor? ____________________

    ____
23. When elevating the woman's legs into the stirrups on the delivery table, the nurse

should put ________________ in the stirrups at the same time to prevent ________________.

24. The Credé treatment involves the instillation of ________________ into the newborn's eyes.
25. How would you tell expectant parents about the Credé treatment? ________________
____
26. Perineal lacerations are sometimes unavoidable. What areas are involved in the following:
    a. First degree: ________________
    b. Second degree: ________________
    c. Third degree: ________________
    d. Fourth degree: ________________
27. Complete the following chart for oxytocic drugs used to cause uterine contractions in the third stage of labor:

	Drug used	Common dosage	Method of administration
a.			
b.			
c.			

28. The Apgar score assesses the following five signs:
    a.
    b.
    c.
    d.
    e.
29. Describe the care given to the baby as soon as it is born (immediate needs): ______
____
30. In fourth stage of labor, the mother's pulse, respiration, and blood pressure are checked every ________________ until stabilized.
31. If the mother begins to bleed excessively in the fourth stage of labor, the first thing to do is ________________.
32. When bleeding in the fourth stage of labor reaches ________________ milliliters, it is considered a hemorrhage.

UNIT IX
The intrapartum family with complications

GOALS

This unit is designed to provide the reader with information that will:

□ develop an awareness of deviations from normal in the intrapartum period.
□ explore the nursing role in common complications in the intrapartum period.

STUDENT OBJECTIVES

After studying this unit, you should be able to:

1. Differentiate between hypotonic and hypertonic uterine inertia and give the treatment for each.
2. Recognize several causes of uterine dysfunction in the latent phase of labor and identify the main cause.
3. Distinguish between the kinds of breech presentations possible, identifying the most common.
4. Identify signs of emergencies during labor and appropriate emergency nursing measures (prolapsed cord, abruptio placentae, placenta previa).
5. Discuss the causes, prevention, treatment, and nursing care for preterm labor.
6. Describe postmaturity syndrome and identify the risk to neonates.
7. Describe the three basic types of cesarean birth, and identify the incision most likely to rupture with a subsequent labor.
8. Differentiate between forceps delivery and vacuum extraction delivery.
9. Discuss the usual dose, effects, possible side effects for both mother and baby, and nursing care when giving the following analgesics, sedatives, and tranquilizers during labor:
   a. meperidine (Demerol)
   b. pentobarbital sodium (Nembutal)
   c. promethazine (Phenergan)
10. Discuss the mode of administration, the area anesthetized, possible side effects for both mother and baby, and nursing care for the following regional anesthetics:
    a. paracervical block
    b. caudal and lumbar epidural
    c. saddle block (low spinal)

As discussed in Unit I, 80% to 95% of women have normal childbirth, and the rest have complications. In Unit V we discussed the complications apparent in the antepartum period. Those complications that could be predicted would be best cared for in the high-risk centers described earlier. Statistics have shown that a fetus transported to such a center *in utero* has a better chance for survival than one transported by ambulance or helicopter following delivery. However, most of the complications explored here do not happen until labor is beginning or has begun.

COMPLICATIONS OF LABOR

Dystocia

DEFINE DYSTOCIA

If the labor pattern does not follow the normal time frame for latent and active phases as described in Unit VII, it is probably the result of abnormalities in the "powers," the "passenger," the "passage," or the psyche. The term given to difficult labor is *dystocia.*

HYPOTONIC AND HYPERTONIC UTERINE INERTIA

Uterine dysfunction. Abnormalities in the powers (uterine contractions) cause uterine dysfunction (also called *uterine inertia*). Labor is a dynamic process. Uterine dysfunction in any phase of cervical dilation is characterized by lack of progress. According to Friedman, prolongation of the latent phase of labor is defined as greater than 20 hours in nulliparas and 14 hours in multiparas. A protracted active phase of labor is defined by Friedman as cervical dilation of less than 1.2 centimeters per hour in nulliparas and 1.5 centimeters per hour in multiparas. Abnormal contractions may be *hypotonic* (*primary inertia* occurring in the latent phase) or *hypertonic* (*secondary inertia*, usually occurring in the active phase). In primary inertia the contractions are weak, irregular, and uncoordinated and the cervix fails to dilate. Treatment for hypotonic contractions during the latent phase is usually sedation. After the woman is rested, contractions may begin spontaneously. In secondary inertia, the contractions become irregular and infrequent and are of poor quality. Treatment is uterine stimulation by intravenous administration of oxytocin after the possibility of fetopelvic disproportion is ruled out. The main cause of uterine dysfunction is ill-timed and too much analgesic. Other causes are minor degrees of pelvic contracture, malposition of the fetus, overdistention of the uterus, a distended urinary bladder or rectum, decreased efficiency of the uterine muscle (many pregnancies), chronic disease, and extreme fear and tension.

CAUSES OF DYSFUNCTION

PROPOSE NURSING INTERVENTION WHEN LABOR IS COMPLICATED BY UTERINE INERTIA

Nursing care. The woman and her family may become very worried when their expectations of labor are not met. Consequently, they need a thorough explanation of what is happening. Early recognition of uterine dysfunction is essential so that treatment can begin before the fetus is in distress or the mother is exhausted. A deviation from the normal lengths of time for the average latent and active phases of labor indicates that uterine inertia may be present. Graphing the progress of labor on a labor curve can be very helpful in determining whether the labor is of normal duration. Because abnormal labor may cause the fetus to be distressed, the nurse must monitor the fetal heart tones often whenever labor deviates from the normal pattern. Preferably, continuous fetal monitoring is used. The nurse must be aware that too much medication too soon in labor is the major cause of uterine inertia in the latent phase. Under ordinary circumstances, it is wise for the woman to wait until her cervix is at least 3 centimeters dilated before receiving medications for pain.

Disproportion. Variations from normal in either the passenger (baby) or the passage (pelvis) or both can cause dystocia. A contracted pelvis is a narrowing in any of the three planes of the bony pelvis (see Fig. 2-12). A contracture in any of the planes may make the fetal passage difficult, particularly if the fetus is large. When there is a disproportion between the size of the fetus and the birth canal, *fetopelvic disproportion,* which is often called CPD for cephalopelvic disproportion, exists. A long, difficult labor may result, and forceps delivery or cesarean birth may be necessary.

Abnormal fetal positions. As discussed, the most favorable position for the fetus is right occiput anterior (ROA) or left occiput anterior (LOA). However, when the fetus is a breech, brow, face, or shoulder presentation or when its position is right or left occiput posterior (ROP or LOP) (Fig. 9-1), labor can be long and difficult. Face and brow presentations occur less than 0.5% of the time and usually cause prolonged labors. The

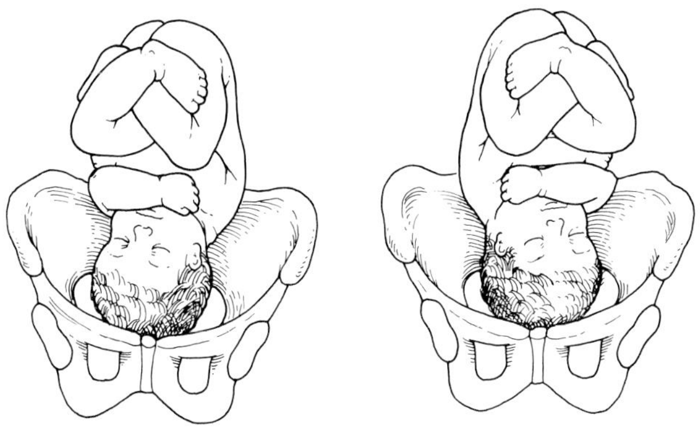

Fig. 9-1. Occipitoposterior positions. **A,** Left occipitoposterior. **B,** Right occipitoposterior.

shoulder presentation (transverse lie) occurs in about 1 time in 500 births. Virtually all shoulder or persistent brow presentations require cesarean delivery because of the high rate of perinatal morbidity with vaginal delivery. For a face presentation a vaginal delivery may occur if labor happens normally and the pelvis is adequate. A baby born with a face presentation will usually have a swollen and bruised face. The parents need reassurance that this is only a temporary condition. A posterior position causes more contractions because the fetus must rotate through a larger arc (two times the rotation needed for an occiput anterior). A posterior labor is termed *back labor* because the woman experiences severe backache as this long arc rotation occurs.

Approximately 25% of the time the fetal head enters the pelvis with the occiput directed posteriorly. However, during labor anterior rotation occurs spontaneously in 70% of the instances. This rotation can be encouraged by having the mother change position often (every 20 to 30 minutes). Have the mother lie on the side opposite the side to which the fetal occiput is directed, or place her in the knee-chest position for three to four contractions at a time. The weight of the baby plus gravity will encourage anterior rotation of the occiput posterior baby. Also, because squatting causes maximum enlargement of the pelvic outlet, this position may provide enough room for an occiput posterior baby to rotate. If rotation does not occur spontaneously, the physician may rotate the fetal head at the time of delivery, either manually or with forceps.

Counterpressure on the painful area will help relieve the back pain. Back massage, cold or hot packs on the low back, and hot showers are helpful. The woman experiencing an occiput posterior labor needs support and encouragement because she and her family will be fatigued and feel frustrated because the labor is longer and more painful.

BREECH PRESENTATIONS

Breech. About 3% of all births are breech presentations. There are three varieties: frank (the most common), complete, and footling (Fig. 9-2). With a breech birth there is a higher fetal risk because the cord can easily prolapse and be compressed. Also, because the head is larger than the buttocks, the buttocks can pass through a cervix that is not dilated enough for the head to pass; thus the head can actually become trapped. In recent times, a cesarean birth has frequently been the method of choice to deliver a breech baby—particularly if the woman is a primigravida with a large baby. However, there is a growing controversy over whether all breech presentations are best managed by cesarean delivery. Individualization and sound clinical judgment are indispensable in making decisions about the method of delivery for breech presentations. If a vaginal birth of a breech is chosen, Piper forceps are used exclusively for the delivery (see Fig. 9-6).

EXPLAIN THE DANGERS OF BREECH PRESENTATIONS

An attempt to turn the fetus externally *(external version)* is sometimes made in the third trimester. Ultrasonography is used to locate the placenta and fetus and to look for abnormalities. Intravenous tocolytic drugs are given to the mother to relax the uterus

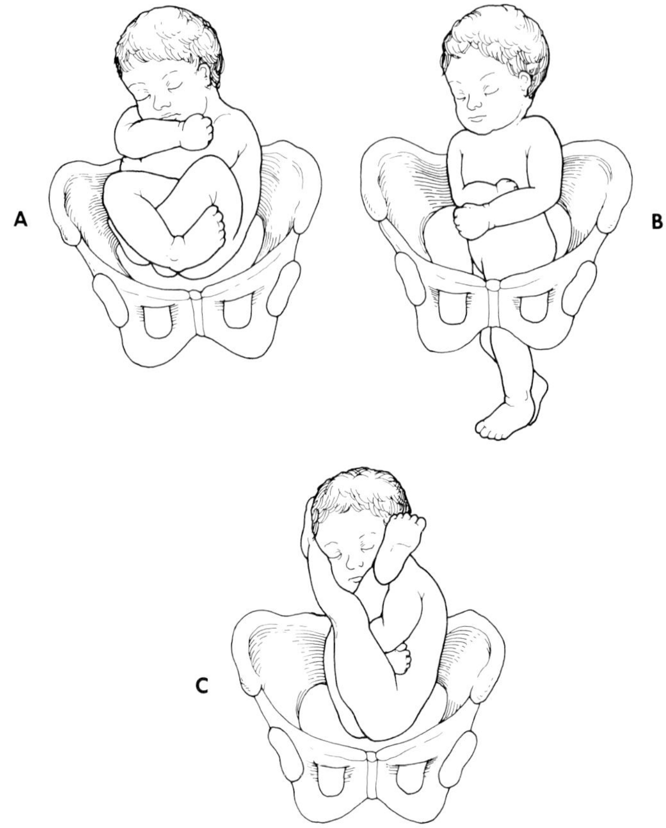

Fig. 9-2. Three variations of breech presentation. **A,** Complete breech. **B,** Footling breech. **C,** Frank breech.

prior to the external version. While the fetus is still floating in the amniotic fluid, it can be manipulated manually and sometimes turned from a breech to a cephalic presentation. Also, having the woman lie on her back with her buttocks elevated on two or three pillows for 20 to 30 minutes several times a day while the fetus is still floating has been reported to assist the fetus in turning itself from breech to cephalic presentation.

Labor accidents

Although some complications such as placenta previa can be detected before labor begins, some conditions occur during labor without warning.

SIGNS OF EMERGENCIES DURING LABOR

Prolapsed cord. A rare obstetric emergency that occurs about once in every 400 cases is prolapse of the umbilical cord. Factors that increase the risk of cord prolapse include polyhydramnios, abnormally long cord, low implantation of the placenta, breech presentation, transverse lie, unengaged fetal presenting part, and delivery of the second twin. Premature rupture of the membranes (especially if the presenting part is not engaged) can cause the umbilical cord to lie alongside or below the presenting part after the membranes have ruptured. As a result, the oxygen supply to the fetus can be impaired or totally cut off (Fig. 9-3). This is a serious emergency, and the pressure must be relieved from the cord quickly.

Nursing care. Nursing actions include changing the woman's position to take the pressure off the cord by placing her in a knee-chest position or in the Sims' position with her hips elevated on pillows so that they are higher than her chest. She may also be placed in deep Trendelenburg's position. Upward pressure on the presenting part by sterile gloved fingers in the vagina may keep the cord pulsating until delivery is possible. The woman may become frightened because of the danger to her baby and thus needs

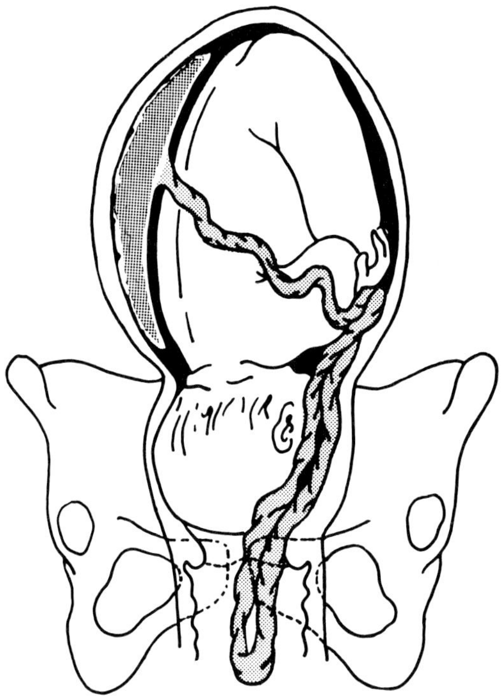

Fig. 9-3. Prolapsed cord. (From Hamilton, P.M.: Basic maternity nursing, ed. 4, St. Louis, 1979, The C.V. Mosby Co.)

constant attendance and reassurance. Oxygen by mask to the mother will probably increase the amount of O_2 the fetus receives. Delivery by vaginal or cesarean birth should occur as quickly as possible.

Abruptio placentae. Abruptio placentae and placenta previa were discussed in Unit V (see Figs. 5-4 and 5-5). These conditions occur in the antepartum period but may not be apparent until the intrapartum period.

When abruptio placentae occurs in labor, the uterus feels tense and hard all the time instead of relaxing between contractions. The woman complains of a great deal of pain. If the hemorrhage is concealed, there may be no vaginal bleeding but the uterus will increase in size. If the hemorrhage is apparent, there will be a lot of dark blood from the vagina. The woman may go into shock.

Nursing care. Intravenous fluids and blood replacement must be started quickly and vital signs, fetal heart tones, urinary output, and amount of vaginal bleeding must be monitored closely. Labor is often very rapid when the placenta abrupts; however, if the woman does not deliver quickly, a cesarean birth is in order. The woman and her family need to know what to expect and need emotional support.

Placenta previa. When a woman with a placenta previa is in labor, the nurse must be alert for any increased bright red vaginal bleeding, a drop in blood pressure, and change in fetal heart tones. It is a good idea to save all perineal and hip pads if the woman bleeds heavily. With this evidence, blood loss can be estimated accurately. When blood loss is estimated by weighing pads, 1 gram equals 1 cubic centimeter.

Precipitate labor

A very rapid labor lasting one hour or less is a precipitate labor. These labors usually occur in multiparous women who have very strong contractions. The danger in these labors is to the fetus because of the extreme force with which it is propelled through the birth canal. These babies may have bruises on their faces and cerebral injuries. There is also a risk of tearing the mother's perineum because of the force with which the baby's head is born. Women who have precipitate labors are at risk for postpartum hemorrhage as a result of a hypotonic uterus.

Preterm labor

DISCUSS THE CAUSES, PREVENTION, AND TREATMENT FOR PRETERM LABOR

Preterm labor is the onset of rhythmical uterine contractions that produce cervical change, effacement, and/or dilation after fetal viability is established but before fetal maturity is achieved. Preterm labor usually occurs between the twenty-sixth and thirty-seventh weeks of gestation. A *preterm birth* is any birth that occurs prior to 37 completed weeks of pregnancy. Preterm labor and delivery continue to be the major causes of perinatal morbidity and mortality in the United States.

The incidence of preterm births is a reflection of the general socioeconomic status of the population, the education level of the parents, the proportion of nonwhite populations, and whether the mother received prenatal care. Health care professionals cannot predict with certainty which women are likely to begin labor prematurely. The following factors are known to increase the risk, however:

1. A previous preterm labor or delivery
2. Twins or triplets
3. Repeated miscarriages or abortions (particularly in the second trimester)
4. Age under 18 or over 40 years
5. Obesity or very low weight
6. Heavy cigarette smoking
7. Heavy use of alcohol or drugs
8. Prenatal exposure to diethylstilbestrol (DES)
9. Premature thinning or dilation of the cervix
10. Maternal medical illness such as kidney infection, liver disease, or heart ailments
11. High blood pressure
12. Strenuous physical work, a long commute, fatiguing childcare responsibilities
13. Unusual emotional stress

Identifying women at risk for preterm labor and teaching them life-style modifications and self-examination procedures to help them recognize early danger signals of preterm labor can promote prompt treatment to stop labor or delay it. A Preterm Prevention Program at the University of California Medical Center, San Francisco, has reduced by 73% yearly premature births in 1150 women studied from 1978 to 1980. In fact, the program, developed in 1977 by obstetrician Robert K. Creasy, has proved so successul that the March of Dimes is funding similar studies at other medical centers.

If preventive measures fail, the treatment for true preterm labor is bed rest in lateral position, hydration, and labor-inhibiting drugs. The advantages and disadvantages of inhibiting labor in each case are weighed before drug therapy is begun.

Tocolytic therapy. Drugs that inhibit uterine contractions are called *tocolytic agents*. Several medications, such as ethyl alcohol, prostaglandin synthesis inhibitors, magnesium sulfate ($MgSO_4$), and beta-adrenergic receptor stimulants, have been used to inhibit premature labor, with varying degrees of success. The most widely used beta-adrenergic receptor stimulants in use in the United States are isoxsuprine (Vasodilan), terbutaline (Brethine), and ritodrine hydrochloride (Yutopar). However, the only one of these drugs approved as a tocolytic agent by the U.S. Food and Drug Administration (1980) is ritodrine hydrochloride (Yutopar). Basically, these drugs are smooth muscle relaxants that relax the contracting uterine muscles. Initial therapy is intravenous followed by oral maintenance. Corticosteroids are frequently given at the same time to hasten fetal lung maturity while tocolytic therapy delays delivery.

NURSING CARE OF WOMAN IN PRETERM LABOR

Nursing care. This family may be under exceptional stress, unprepared for early labor, and grieving a possible loss of their expected full-term baby. In addition to suffering emotional stress, the woman receiving alcohol intravenously presents all the special problems of intoxication: for example, nausea, vomiting, and mood swings. She must receive nothing by mouth because of the danger of aspiration. The woman receiving terbutaline or ritodrine may experience hypotension, tachycardia, nausea, nervousness, and sweating. Close observation and recording of vital signs, fetal heart tones, intake and output of fluids, and emotional status plus constant and consistent emotional support are vital nursing actions.

Postterm pregnancy

A postterm pregnancy is one that persists for 42 weeks (294 days) or more from last menstrual period (LMP), assuming a 28-day cycle. Currently, management of postterm pregnancy falls into three major categories: (1) routine induction, (2) fetal assessment with intervention if evidence of fetal compromise, and (3) no intervention or assessment of the postterm pregnancy.

DEFINE POSTTERM PREGNANCY

Although postterm pregnancies represent 7% to 11% of all pregnancies, they account for over 15% of all perinatal mortality. Postmaturity syndrome is the abnormal condition of a fetus or newborn resulting from postterm pregnancy. Approximately 20% of postterm babies have this syndrome which includes wrinkled, peeling skin, alert facies, creases over the entire surface of the sole of the foot, and absence of vernix or lanugo. The literature is clear regarding the compromised status of most postmature infants. They are at risk for developing serious problems resulting from chronic or acute placental insufficiency and asphyxia at birth.

DESCRIBE POSTMATURITY SYNDROME, AND IDENTIFY THE RISK TO NEONATES

Management of the postterm pregnancy requires accurate dating of the pregnancy. (Often postdate pregnancies have been found to be misdated and not truly prolonged pregnancies.) Second, fetal evaluation using fetal movement counting (FMC), nonstress tests (NSTs), contraction stress tests (CSTs), and a fetal biophysical profile will help to determine the fetus at risk for the problems associated with postmaturity.

Nursing care. Postterm pregnancy is accompanied by feelings of fatigue, frustration, anger, and disappointment. Many women experience guilt and loss of control. There is fear concerning the baby's well-being and future development. The fetal evaluation testing itself can become anxiety provoking because it emphasizes concern over fetal well-being. Family relationships can be severely strained. It is important not to ignore, minimize, or treat casually any feelings expressed by the pregnant woman and her family. They need an opportunity to express all feelings in an environment of acceptance and support.

If careful dating and fetal evaluation indicate that the pregnancy is in need of termination, labor can be stimulated or induced.

Induction of labor

Induction of labor is causing labor to begin artificially. Prostaglandins have been used intravenously, orally, sublingually, extra-amniotically, intravaginally, and intracervically to stimulate labor. The route of administration determines the frequency and severity of the side effects.

DIFFERENTIATE BETWEEN INDUCTION AND AUGMENTATION OF LABOR

Oxytocin is approved for induction of labor in women for a medical indication only. The most common medical and obstetrical indications are listed in Table 9-1. Contraindications to uterine stimulation are listed in Table 9-2.

Cervical ripeness is a very important variable in contemplating induction of labor. The probability for a successful induction is reduced when the cervix is unripe. Oxytocin (Pitocin) is administered by the intravenous route in a diluted solution for inductions. Inductions are no longer done solely for convenience.

Augmentation of labor is using amniotomy or intravenous administration of oxytocin to stimulate or regulate ineffective uterine contractions as in hypotonic inertia. Amniotomy for the purpose of augmenting labor is controversial.

Table 9-1. Induction of labor: common indications

Maternal indications
Hypertension
Premature rupture of membranes after the 36th week
Intrauterine fetal death
Deteriorating maternal illness
Hydramnios, fetal anomaly incompatible with life
Fetal indications
Diabetes
Rh sensitization
Intrauterine growth retardation (IUGR)
Prolonged pregnancy
Anomalies

Table 9-2. Contraindications to uterine stimulation

Absolute
Fetal distress
Central placenta previa
Unfavorable fetal position
Proven cephalopelvic disproportion
Scar in myometrium
Relative
Overdistended uterus
Grand multiparity (more than 5 pregnancies)
Breech presentation
Previous low transverse cesarean section
Prematurity
Maternal cardiac disease

DISCUSS THE NURSING CARE OF A WOMAN UNDERGOING INDUCTION OF LABOR

Oxytocin causes rhythmic uterine contractions by stimulating uterine muscle. The cervix should be soft ("ripe") before an induction is begun. A double-bottle set-up (the first bottle containing a plain intravenous solution and the second bottle containing intravenous solution with oxytocin added) and an infusion pump are mandatory when induction is by intravenous administration of Pitocin (Fig. 9-4). The oxytocin solution is infused at an initial dosage of 1 to 2 milliunits per minute, with the rate doubled every 15 to 20 minutes until mimicking of a normal labor pattern occurs.

If intense, sustained contractions occur, the resting period between contractions decreases or disappears, or fetal distress occurs, the intravenous drip containing the oxytocin should be stopped immediately and the plain bottle infused. Oxytocin is broken down in the kidney and liver and has a circulatory half-life of 3 to 4 minutes, whereas the uterine effects last 20 to 30 minutes. For most women the duration of action of the oxytocin is related to its half-life, and thus the stimulus is gone quickly. However, for those few women who are maximally sensitive, the effects of the oxytocin can last longer.

Other ways to start or stimulate labor include nipple or breast stimulation, as discussed in Unit V. Ambulation has also been found to help augment labor.

Nursing care. During induction constant observation is essential and continuous electronic fetal monitoring is recommended. Fetal heart tones, blood pressure, pulse, and the frequency, duration, and strength of contractions should be checked and recorded at least every 15 minutes. If it is ever necessary to shut off the oxytocin, the physician or midwife should be notified promptly.

Cesarean birth

A cesarean birth is the delivery of a baby through an incision made in the abdominal and uterine walls. Cesarean birth rates have increased dramatically in recent years. Some

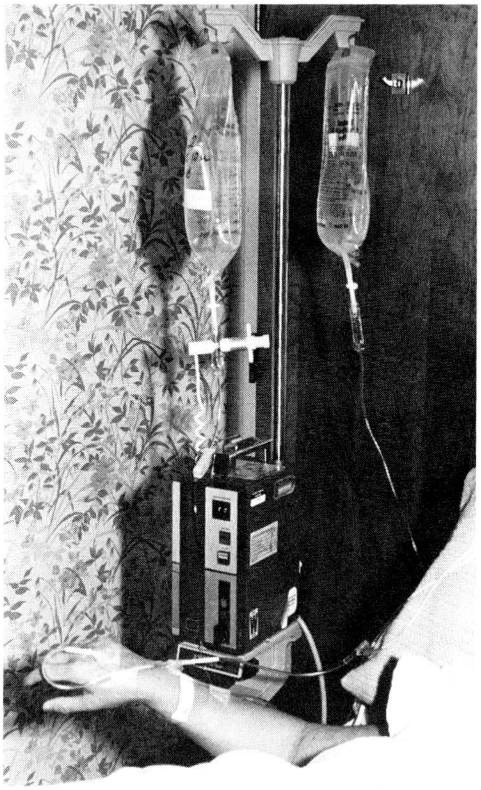

Fig. 9-4. Double-bottle set-up. Bottle on left contains intravenous solution with oxytocin added. Bottle closest to mother contains a plain intravenous solution.

hospitals in the United States currently have cesarean rates of 30%. A few factors leading to an increased cesarean rate include (1) changing attitudes in the management of breech presentation in primigravidas, (2) better antenatal screening techniques to assess the fetus in utero, (3) an increase in fetal heart rate monitoring, which can detect fetal distress in labor, and (4) a change in attitude of obstetricians concerning treatment of nonprogressive labor so that it is not prolonged unnecessarily. The indications for a cesarean birth are cephalopelvic disproportion, malpresentation (some breeches or transverse lie), fetal distress, uterine dysfunction, prolapsed cord, abruptio placentae, and placenta previa. Maternal disease and the need for a repeat cesarean are other indications.

IDENTIFY MATERNAL AND FETAL INDICATIONS FOR CESAREAN BIRTH

Types. There are three basic types of cesarean birth. (1) The *classic* cesarean is quick and easy to perform. The incision is made in the midline of the abdomen and in the midline of the thick fundus. However, a normal labor is contraindicated with any subsequent pregnancy because this incision can rupture easily. (2) A *low cervical* cesarean is preferred because the incision is made transversely in the lower uterine segment. This uterine scar is less apt to rupture with the next pregnancy. (3) In an *extraperitoneal* cesarean the bladder is dissected downward and the peritoneal cavity is not entered. A transverse incision is then made into the lower uterine segment (Fig. 9-5). Maternal morbidity with cesarean deliveries is two to four times that of vaginal birth. This increased maternal morbidity is largely due to infectious complications.

TYPES OF CESAREAN BIRTHS

Nursing care. The woman must be prepared for major surgery and given emotional support. Today many families are sharing the cesarean birth experience, with the father present at the cesarean birth. After all, a cesarean is a birth and the beginning of a new family unit just as a vaginal delivery is. To enhance parent-child attachment after the birth, the parents and infant should spend time together if the infant is not compromised.

If the family has prepared for a vaginal delivery, an unexpected cesarean may provoke

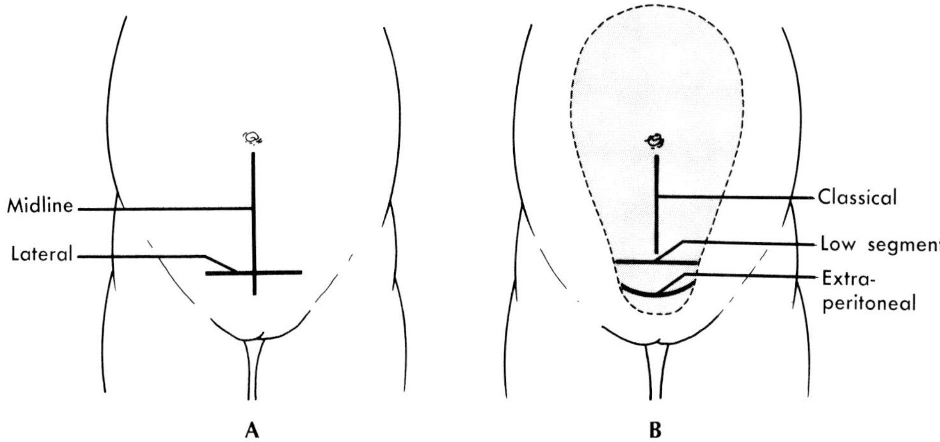

Fig. 9-5. Cesarean incisions. **A,** Skin incisions. **B,** Uterine incisions.

OPTIONS TO FACILITATE FAMILY-CENTERED CESAREAN BIRTHS*

1. Admission to the hospital on the morning of the birth for elective cesareans so that parents can spend the previous night together (provided they have had previous orientation).
2. Father to remain with the mother during the physical preparation, for example, shave, catheterization.
3. The choice of regional anesthesia where possible, and explanation of the differences between regional and general anesthesia.
4. Father in the delivery room when either regional or general anesthesia is the choice.
5. Mirror and/or ongoing commentary from a staff member for mother and/or father.
6. Photographs or video taken in the delivery room—if even one parent is unable to witness the birth.
7. Mother's hand freed from restraint for contact with husband and baby.
8. Opportunity for both parents to interact with the baby in the delivery room and/or postanesthetic recovery room.
9. Opportunity for breast-feeding in the delivery room or postanesthetic recovery room.
10. Modified Leboyer practices, for example, father to submerge baby in warm water until relaxed and alert in the delivery room or in the nursery, if available for vaginal delivery.
11. Delayed antimicrobials in baby's eyes.
12. If father chooses not to be in the delivery room:
    a) a support person should replace him at the mother's side
    b) father to be given baby to hold en route to nursery
    c) father to have the birth experience relayed to him by a staff member
13. Father to accompany baby to the nursery and remain with infant until both are reunited with the mother.
14. Family reunited in postanesthetic recovery room if possible.
15. Father to be in postanesthetic recovery room to tell his wife about the birth if she has had a general anesthetic.
16. If it is difficult to reunite the family in postanesthetic delivery room, the mother's condition should be judged individually to allow the family to be reunited as soon as possible.
17. Baby's condition to be judged individually so that time alone in an incubator in the nursery can be avoided if possible.
18. Provision of time alone for the family in those first critical hours.
19. Mother-baby nursing as soon as possible, that is, if mother feels well enough she may be able to have mother-baby nursing on the first day.
20. Father to be included in the teaching of caretaking skills.
21. Siblings to be included where possible.

*In an effort to make the cesarean delivery more family centered, the following options should be available where safety permits.

(Adapted from JOGN Nursing: Leach, Lynette, and Sproule, Valerie, Meeting the challenge of cesarean births, JOGN Nurs. **13**(3):193, 1984.)

feelings of anger, denial, and guilt in the family members. These feelings should not be ignored or minimized. By empathetic listening, a nurse can allow the parents to verbalize their feelings and then work through them. The accompanying box is a listing of options to facilitate family-centered cesarean births. In many communities there are cesarean birth support groups and preparation classes for couples scheduled for cesarean birth.

Vaginal delivery after cesarean

It has been shown that careful selection of expectant women and use of proper protocols can make vaginal delivery after cesarean as safe as repeated cesarean delivery. Vaginal delivery offers less maternal morbidity, better bonding, and more successful breast-feeding. According to guidelines published by the American College of Obstetricians and Gynecologists (ACOG) in 1985, cesarean delivery remains the proper course of action when there is: evidence of more than one previous cesarean, absolute cephalopelvic disproportion, a classic uterine incision, multiple pregnancy, or fetal weight of 4000 grams or more. But in the majority of cases, a vaginal trial of labor would be encouraged under the 1985 guidelines.

Nursing care. Women planning to undergo a trial of labor have special needs. They must understand the risks and possible complications involved and realize that a trial of labor could end in a cesarean. Preparation for labor with knowledge, relaxation, and breathing techniques is important. Many women who had previous cesareans for nonrecurring problems can experience normal births. Explaining the risks while providing encouragement and support can help to make the difference.

Forceps delivery

Forceps, skillfully applied, can aid in the safe delivery of a baby. When forceps are applied after the fetal head is crowning, the delivery is termed a *low forceps* or *outlet delivery*. This is the most common forceps application and is chosen by the physician to better control the delivery. When forceps are applied after the head is engaged but has not yet reached the perineal floor, the delivery is termed a *midforceps delivery*. Forceps may be applied in this case because of the mother's inability to push effectively resulting from exhaustion or regional or general anesthesia. Fetal distress requiring prompt delivery, abnormal presentations, failure to rotate, and arrested fetal descent are other reasons for a midforceps delivery. Application of forceps (*high forceps*) at any time prior to full engagement of the fetal head is not justified in modern obstetrical practice. Types of forceps are illustrated in Figure 9-6. To assure relaxation and prevent pain during midforceps delivery, anesthesia is given to the mother.

Vacuum extraction delivery

DIFFERENTIATE BETWEEN FORCEPS AND VACUUM EXTRACTION DELIVERY

Although in the United States forceps delivery is used most of the time when assistance is needed, vacuum extraction has been popular in much of the world for years. Vacuum extraction involves a disk-shaped cup being applied to the fetal head. A vacuum is then created by a pump that withdraws air between the fetal head and the cup. Traction is applied synchronized with uterine contractions (Fig. 9-7) when the mother needs assistance in the second stage.

There are no known risks to the mother associated with vacuum extraction. In fact, advantages include reduction in injuries to the mother's vaginal walls, bladder, uterus, and bowel. Also, the mother is able to push with her contractions, since little or no anesthesia is needed for vacuum extraction.

A major disadvantage of vacuum extraction is the swelling of the fetal head tissue *(caput succedaneum)* that develops from the suction cup. This caput will generally diminish in size within a few hours after birth and is not known to cause long-term problems. However, other possible risks to the fetus include cephalhematomas and scalp

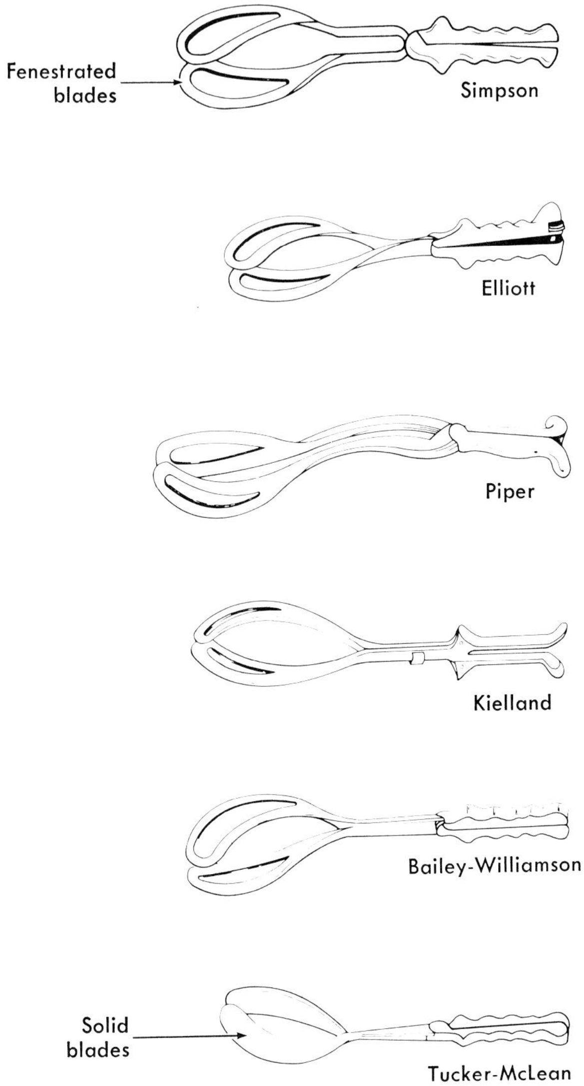

Fig. 9-6. Types of forceps. (From Jensen, M., Benson, R.C., and Bobak, I.M.: Maternity care: the nurse and the family, St. Louis, 1977, The C.V. Mosby Co.)

lacerations. Vacuum extraction is contraindicated with preterm deliveries because of the increased possibility of bleeding in the immature fetal head.

Because practitioners in the United States have been showing an increased interest in vacuum extraction, nurses must be prepared to discuss the advantages, disadvantages, and contraindications with families.

Uterine rupture

RECOGNIZE THE SIGNS OF RUPTURE OF UTERUS

Rupture of the uterus may occur: if a woman with a previous classic cesarean incision is allowed to go into labor, if labor is long and difficult, if a woman has had more than six deliveries, or if oxytocin is given injudiciously. The signs of uterine rupture are sudden, sharp abdominal pain, cessation of uterine contractions and fetal heart tones, and signs and symptoms of shock. The mother may complain of feeling a tearing sensation in her abdomen. This is a serious emergency and requires immediate surgical intervention. Often the hemorrhage is into the peritoneal cavity rather than out the vagina. The maternal mortality rate can be as high as 10%, and the perinatal mortality rate can be as high as 50%.

Treatment consists of oxygen therapy, blood transfusions, and the intravenous admin-

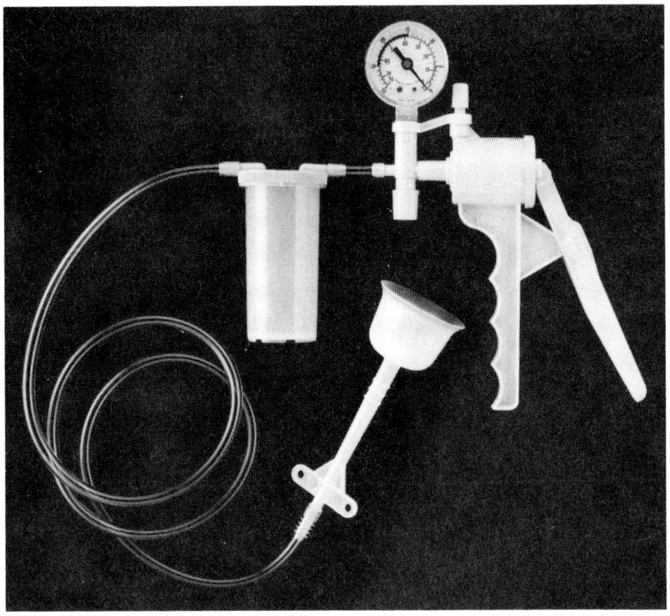

Fig. 9-7. Vacuum extraction. The Mityvac Vacuum Delivery System. (Courtesy Columbia Medical and Surgical, Inc., P.O. Box 5877, Bend, Oreg.)

istration of substances to restore the normal clotting mechanism. The baby may be saved if delivered immediately, but, as indicated, the mother may die. Although this complication is very rare, it is important to be aware of it and alert to its signs and symptoms.

Amniotic fluid embolism

The accidental infusion of amniotic fluid into the mother's endocervical veins or into the venous sinuses of the placental site causes an almost invariably fatal maternal death within 1 or 2 hours. This complication, amniotic fluid embolism, is very rare, occurring only once in many thousands of labors. Although it may occur at any time after the membranes have ruptured, it is most often reported near the end of the first stage of labor. Because the amniotic fluid contains small particles of matter, such as vernix, lanugo, and meconium, multiple tiny emboli may be drawn into the general circulation and in this way reach the pulmonary capillaries, causing occlusion.

Signs and symptoms appear suddenly. The woman experiences sudden dyspnea, cyanosis, chest pain, and may cough up blood-tinged mucus. Uterine relaxation with hemorrhage and profound shock occur. An important complication of amniotic fluid embolism is reduced fibrinogen blood levels and subsequent disseminated intravascular coagulation (DIC).

ANALGESIA AND ANESTHESIA

In unit V we discussed methods of preventing or relieving pain in childbirth without medication. Discomfort in labor can also be relieved by analgesics and anesthesia. *Analgesia* is absence of a normal sense of pain. *Anesthesia* is partial or complete loss of sensation with or without loss of consciousness resulting from administration of a drug. The nurse's understanding of the actions and effects of medication on both the mother and the fetus is very important. Women's responses to drugs are as variable as their responses to labor. Therefore, drug therapy should be flexible and individualized. Although any medication used during labor should not endanger the mother or the fetus, every drug has that potential. There is no drug that stops the discomfort of labor completely and at the same time is absolutely safe for both the mother and the baby. At the same time, despite the risks involved, drugs can reduce the anxiety and pain of labor and delivery and enhance the birth experience for some women. In considering the possible risks involved in using obstetrical drugs, one must also consider the benefits. For some women the stress of doing without medication in labor may do more harm than the drugs used. Therefore, the nurse must know how and when each medication should be used, the advantages and disadvantages, and possible complications related to the drugs.

There are six groups of medication given for labor and/or birth:

1. Sedatives and tranquilizers, which relieve anxiety and tension in early labor
2. Amnesics, which erase memories of pain and the labor
3. Regional analgesia, which interrupts pain pathways
4. General analgesia, which increases the tolerance of pain
5. General anesthesia, which prevents central perception of pain
6. Local anesthesia, which blocks pain sensations to a particular area

Table 9-3. Pain-relieving drugs for labor

Drug	Usual dosage	Route	When given in labor	Effects
Sedatives (barbiturates)				
Secobarbital sodium (Seconal)	100 to 200 mg (1.50 to 3 grains)	p.o., IM, rectally	Early in labor	Lowers perception of stimuli
Pentobarbital sodium (Nembutal)	30 to 100 mg (1.5 to 3 grains)	p.o., IM, rectally	Early in labor	Relieves tension Provides rest Produces sleep
Tranquilizers Promethazine (Phenergan) Hydroxyzine HCL (Vistaril) Propiomazine (Largon) Diazepam (Valium)	25 to 50 mg 25 to 100 mg 10 to 20 mg 2, 5 mg	IM, p.o. IM, p.o. IM, p.o. IV, IM, or p.o.	With narcotic or barbiturate or alone, in early labor	Sedative Relieves anxiety Tranquilizes Enhances physical mental relaxation
Promazine (Sparine)	50 mg	IM		Narcotic effects potentiated antiemetic
Amnesic				
Scopolamine (Hyoscine)	0.3 to 0.4 mg (1/200 to 1/150 grains)	IM	Early in labor	Amnesia Produces drowsiness and sleep
Narcotic analgesic				
Meperidine (Demerol)	50 to 100 mg	IM, IV	After cervix is 3 to 4 cm dilated	Relieves pain
Narcotic antagonist				
Naloxone hydrochloride (Narcan)	Neonate: 0.01 mg/kg of baby's weight Adult: 0.4 mg	IV or sub Q IM or IV	Immediately before, during, after delivery	Reverses effect of narcotic
Nalorphine (Nalline)	Neonate: 0.5 mg Adult: 5 mg	IM or IV IM or IV	Same as above	Same as above

p.o. = by mouth; IM = intramuscularly; IV = intravenously.

Sedatives and tranquilizers

Sedative drugs such as the barbiturates secobarbital (Seconal) and pentobarbital (Nembutal) can be very useful in relaxing an anxious woman during the early or beginning latent phase of labor.

Tranquilizers such as promethazine (Phenergan), hydroxyzine (Vistaril), propiomazine (Largon), and diazepam (Valium) are used in early labor either alone or with barbiturates or analgesics. When given alone these drugs do not affect the pain threshold; however, they potentiate the action of barbiturates and analgesics so that the doses of the barbiturates and analgesics can be reduced when tranquilizers are given with them.

Sedatives and tranquilizers are never given close to the time of delivery or when preterm deliveries are probable (Table 9-3).

Amnesics

Scopolamine used to be given to produce amnesia for laboring women. It was frequently combined with morphine sulphate and called "twilight sleep." The laboring woman still had pain but no memory of it or of the birth. Scopolamine given alone causes

DOSF, EFFECTS, AND SIDE EFFECTS OF DRUGS GIVEN DURING LABOR

Possible side effects		
Mother	**Fetus and newborn**	**Nursing care after administration**
May slow or prolong labor Can cause restlessness, excitement, disorientation	Drowsiness for 24 to 48 hours after birth Respiratory distress; decreased sucking ability	Inform the woman of what she will experience. Use power of positive thinking. Give reassurance and suggestions that drug will relieve pain and cause relaxation. Woman must remain in bed. Put side rails up on bed, and instruct woman not to get out of bed. Provide quiet environment. Observe progress of labor closely. Watch for signs of restlessness and excitement. Check fetal heart tones, respirations frequently.
Maternal hypotension May slow labor May cause dizziness, blurred vision, confusion	Delayed onset of respirations Altered attention span in first 24 to 48 hours after birth Slow adaptation to feeding	Inform the woman of what she will experience. Use power of positive thinking. Give reassurance and suggestions that drug will relieve pain and cause relaxation. Woman must remain in bed. Put side rails up on bed, and instruct woman not to get out of bed. Provide quiet environment. Check fetal heart tones, respirations, blood pressure frequently. Observe closely for changes in progress of labor.
Extreme restlessness, excitement, disorientation	Respiratory depression; drowsiness	Constant attendance to the woman. Watch for signs of extreme restlessness and excitement. Check fetal heart tones, blood pressure, respirations frequently.
Hypotension, facial flushing, oral dryness, nausea and vomiting, restlessness Can slow labor if given too early	Respiratory depression; changes in infant behavior first 24 to 72 hours of life (most serious neonatal depressions occur if meperidine is given 2 hours before delivery)	Inform the woman of what she will experience. Woman must remain in bed. Put side rails up. Check fetal heart tones, blood pressure, respirations frequently. Watch progress of labor closely. Remember meperidine does not become completely effective for 60 to 90 minutes.
	Baby can be depressed again after drug is metabolized	Continuous observation
	Same as above	

restlessness and bizarre behavior. When scopolamine is given with analgesia, the restlessness is less severe, but constant attendance is required so that the woman will not harm herself (Table 9-3).

Narcotic Analgesics

Meperidine (Demerol) is the analgesic used most often during labor to relieve pain. The best time to give Demerol is after the cervix is 3 to 4 centimeters dilated (active phase of labor). It is important to understand that the peak action of this analgesic occurs within 60 to 90 minutes of intramuscular administration, and it is effective for 2 to 3 hours. Given intravenously, peak effects occur within 10 to 60 minutes of administration of Demerol. Demerol can cause severe respiratory depression in 12% to 18% of neonates. Neurobehavioral scores show lower levels of activity in such neonates for up to 3 days, although these are subtle changes.

Research indicates that analgesic drugs may be linked with "adverse infant outcome" in behavioral and gross motor development. Although the long-term effect of analgesia and anesthesia used in labor on infant learning responses is not known, drugs for labor and birth should not be used indiscriminately (Table 9-3).

Inhalant analgesia

Methoxyflurane (Penthrane) and trichloroethylene (Trilene) are inhalants the mother can give to herself in first or second stage labor by means of a mask attached to her wrist. If she holds the mask herself, she will drop it when she begins to lose consciousness. Once a very popular form of self-administered analgesia during labor, this method is rapidly disappearing in the United States. Penthrane and Trilene are quite lipid soluble; therefore, placental transfer is prompt and sleepy infants are common (Table 9-4).

Regional anesthesia-analgesia

Regional anesthesia-analgesia provides complete or near-complete pain relief for the mother, allowing her to be awake during the birth, without significant side effects for the fetus, provided no complications occur. Drugs used for regional anesthesia-analgesia include procaine (Novocain), dibucaine (Nupercaine), lidocaine (Xylocaine), tetracaine (Pontocaine), mepivacaine (Carbocaine), chloroprocaine (Nesacaine), and bupivacaine (Marcaine) (Table 9-4).

REGIONAL ANESTHESIA

Paracervical block. *Paracervical block* is a type of regional anesthesia. Approximately 10 milliliters of local anesthetic is injected into the nerve plexus on each side of the cervix (corresponding to the 3 and 9 o'clock positions) when the cervix is 4 centimeters or more dilated. This injection interrupts the sensory impulses traveling from the uterus to the spinal cord in the paracervical area. Anesthesia relieving the discomfort of uterine contractions develops in 3 to 5 minutes and may last approximately 1 to 2 hours. However, the procedure does not anesthetize the perineum. Most women report considerable benefit. Injections may be repeated depending on the duration of labor. Temporary slowing of the fetal heart rate has been reported. Fetal heart tones should be checked frequently. Maternal blood pressure should also be taken regularly to detect possible medication reactions.

The risk of fetal bradycardia, hypoxia, and acidosis has caused the paracervical block to all but vanish in modern obstetrical practice (see Fig. 9-8).

Local infiltration. *Local infiltration* of the episiotomy site will provide anesthesia for performing the procedure and the repair but little else. A more extensive perineal infiltration has been described but is infrequently used today.

Pudendal block. *Pudendal block* is local anesthesia into the pudendal nerve centers on the right and left sides of the perineal area (Fig. 9-9). It is probably the safest anesthesia available today for both mother and baby. The injection is made through the vaginal

Table 9-4. Anesthesia for labor and delivery

Type of anesthesia	Usual dosage	Administration	Area anesthetized or effects	Possible side effects: Mother	Possible side effects: Baby	Nursing care after administration
Regional						
Paracervical block	5-10 ml of 1% solution of a "caine" drug	Injection, either side of cervix at 4 cm dilation	Cervix and uterus	Can slow labor	30% incidence of temporary slowing of fetal heart	Close monitoring of fetal heart tones and maternal vital signs and contractions
Pudendal block	5-10 ml of 1% solution of a "caine" drug	Injection into area of pudendal nerves for birth	Perineum	None unless allergic to drug	None	Reassurance and explanation; monitor fetal heart tones and maternal vital signs closely
Caudal and lumbar epidural	5-15 ml of 1%, 1.5%, or 2% solution of a "caine" drug	Caudal canal Epidural space at 4 cm dilation	Pelvic region	Hypotension; cannot "push" for delivery May slow labor if started too early	Slowing of fetal heart and fetal heart decelerates	Monitor fetal heart tones and maternal vital signs closely; use excellent aseptic techniques
Saddle block (low spinal)	1-1.5 ml of solution, concentration depends on "caine" drug used	Injection under dura of spinal cord for birth	Pelvic region	Postspinal headache Hypotension	None	Intravenous and O_2 usually used
General						
inhalation	Nitrous oxide Ethylene Cyclopropane Ether Or other similar agents	Inhaled through mask	Complete body	Could aspirate if vomits	Respiratory depression; hypoxia	Be alert and prepared for vomiting (with aspiration of food) and excessive uterine bleeding owing to uterine relaxation
Inhalant analgesia						
Methoxyflurane (Penthrane)	0.3% to 0.5% in first stage or at time of delivery	Volatile inhalant	Relieves pain	Hypotension; slow, shallow respirations	Hypoxia and central nervous system depression	Inform woman of what she will experience. Allow her to administer as needed. Do not hold mask for her. Check vital signs frequently.
Trichloroethylene (Trilene)	0.5% in first stage or at time of delivery			Irregular pulse; rapid respirations		

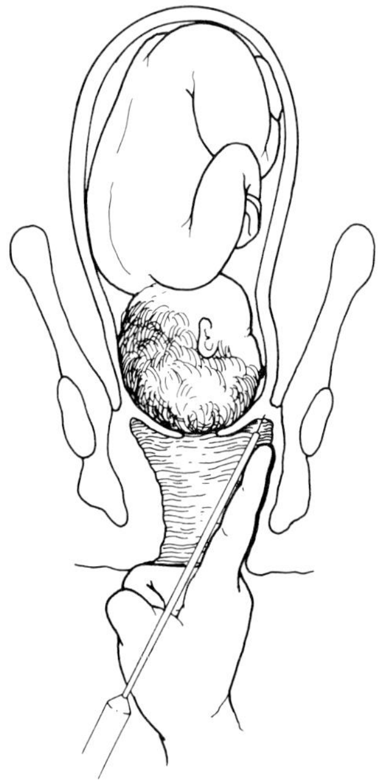

Fig. 9-8. Paracervical block.

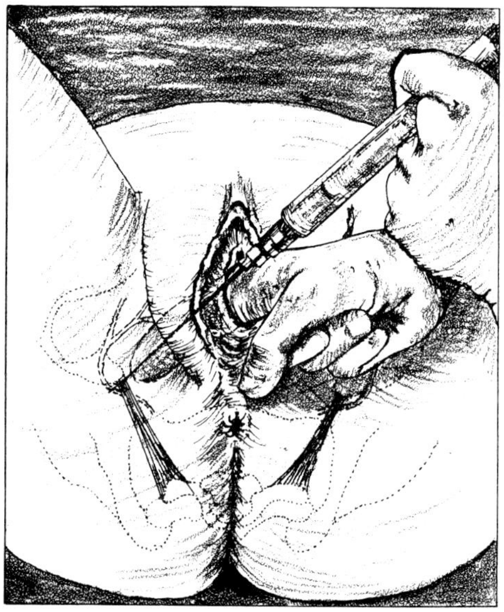

Fig. 9-9. Pudendal block. (From Ingalls, A.J., and Salerno, M.C.: Maternal and child health nursing, ed. 3, St. Louis, 1975, The C.V. Mosby Co.)

mucosa directly over the ischial spines. With its use, an episiotomy may be performed or outlet forceps applied. Although the perineum is blocked, the woman still feels contractions.

Caudal and lumbar epidural. *Caudal anesthesia* is achieved by "blocking" the nerves in the epidural space. It is a type of regional anesthesia achieved by injecting an anesthetic agent into the caudal space of the sacrum. This produces a loss of sensation from the waist down (Fig. 9-10). When a plastic catheter is inserted above the dural sac, additional anesthetic solution can be added at appropriate intervals. This continuous administration is called a continuous caudal epidural.

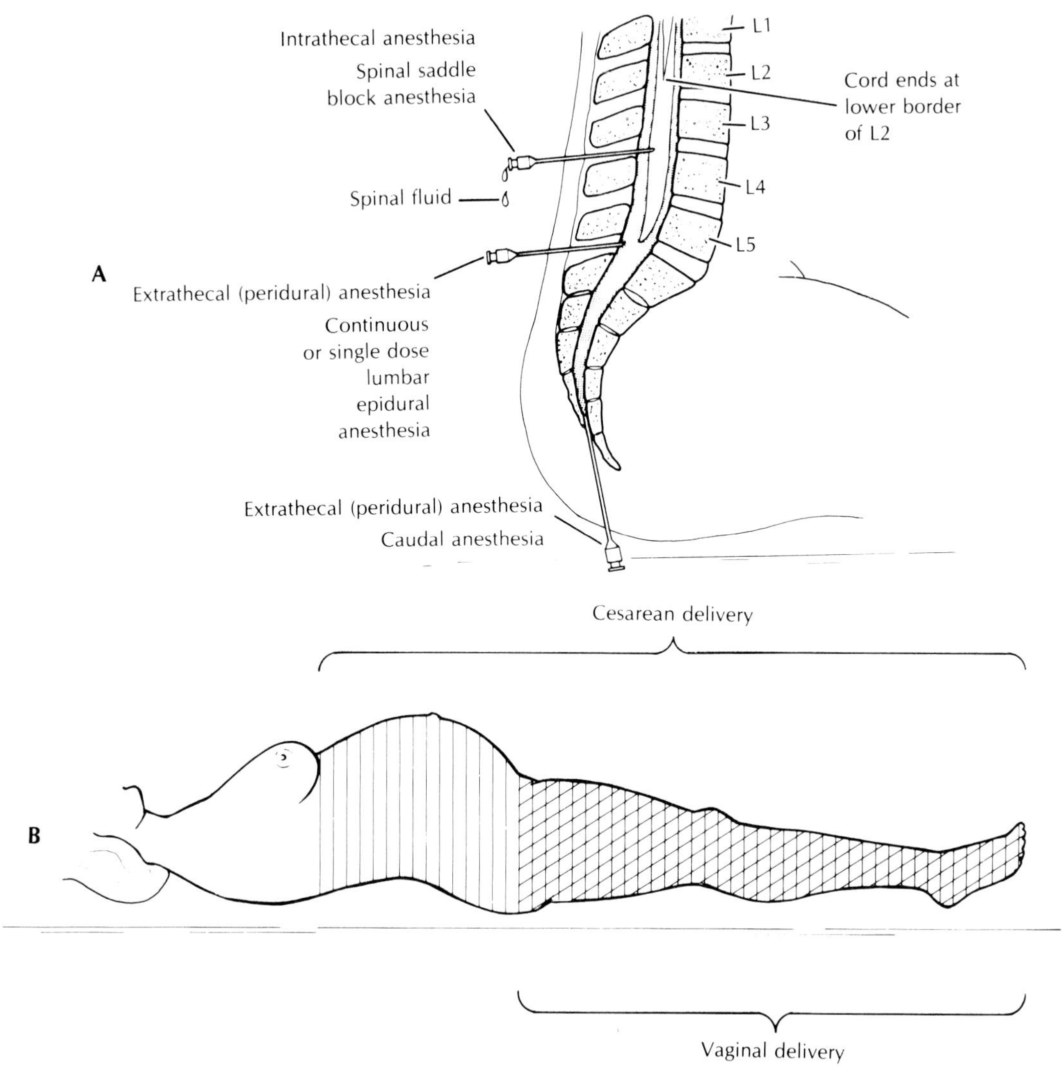

Fig. 9-10. A, Regional anesthesia in obstetrics. **B,** Level of anesthesia necessary for cesarean delivery and for vaginal delivery. (Courtesy Ross Laboratories, Columbus, Ohio.)

Lumbar epidural anesthesia is another regional anesthesia achieved by injecting the anesthetic agent outside of the dura into the extradural space. The space is approached between the third and fourth lumbar vertebrae rather than the caudal area (Fig. 9-10). As with caudal anesthesia, a single injection may be made or a plastic catheter may be threaded into the space to allow continuous anesthesia for labor and delivery.

Lumbar epidural is currently the most favored because the catheter is placed very close to the nerve roots conducting the pain of the first stage of labor, thus minimizing the required dosage of drug. Caudal epidural requires a larger volume of local anesthetic during the first stage of labor, although it may provide faster and more intense perineal anesthesia during the second stage of labor.

Spinal anesthesia. Spinal anesthesia is sometimes referred to as a *saddle block* because the anesthetized area is the area that would touch a saddle when riding a horse. This is a regional anesthesia achieved by injecting the anesthetic agent under the dura of the spinal cord (Fig. 9-10). This provides for a pain-free delivery and does not interfere with uterine contractions. When this type of anesthesia is used for cesarean section, a higher dose of medication is used. The woman must sit for the injection and remain seated for approximately 30 seconds after the injection so that the drug will move downward rather than upward, which could interfere with her ability to breathe.

Complications

Because one of the most common complications of regional analgesia for labor is maternal hypotension, it is important for the nurse to keep constant check on the patient's blood pressure. If the mother becomes hypotensive, immediate action should be taken to restore blood volume to the central circulation. Shifting the woman on her side or elevating and displacing the uterus to the left and administering oxygen may restore the blood pressure to normal. Also, if an intravenous infusion is running, the rate should be increased.

Nausea and vomiting are usually the first signs of hypotension and will subside when the woman's blood pressure returns to normal. Administration of oxygen and reassurance of the mother and her family are often very effective in relieving nausea.

There are studies available today correlating newborn behaviors with the administration of regional anesthesia during delivery. The findings report that as long as 3 days after birth, infants whose mothers received regional anesthesia were more irritable than infants whose mothers were not medicated. Also, the infants of medicated mothers showed decreased motor maturity. Many more studies need to be done on the relation-

Table 9-5. Nonpharmaceutical pain-relief methods

	Advantages	Disadvantages	Cost
Biofeedback	Wide applicability outside obstetrics No physician's order needed No devices needed after training	Difficulty in training time is variable Finding a certified biofeedback trainer	Equipment for training costs several thousand dollars. Individual cost is determined by training time.
Transcutaneous electrical nerve stimulation (TENS)	Wide applicability outside obstetrics	Constantly need the device Need physician's order Most effective if introduced before crisis or operation May interfere with continuous electronic fetal monitoring	TENS unit costs approximately $200 to $500
Acupuncture	Widely used in the Orient for years	Invasive Needles may cause infection Difficulty in finding a qualified professional	Variable, depending on treatments
Acupressure	Widely used in the Orient for years	Difficulty in finding a qualified professional	Variable, depending on treatments. Could be integrated into nursing treatments
Therapeutic touch	No devices needed No physician's order needed Noninvasive Nursing background in research and application Self-healing	Not studied well in obstetrics Unknown effect of energy transfer on fetus (two fields involved).	Essentially no cost because it usually is incorporated into nursing care
Bathing	Low cost High satisfaction No physician's order needed	May cause hyperthermia Continuous electronic fetal monitoring is impossible	Cost of tub and water

From Brucker, M.C., Nonpharmaceutical methods for relieving pain and discomfort during pregnancy, MCN **2**:390-394, 1984.

ship of anesthesia administration during childbirth to the functioning of the newborn infant.

General anesthesia. General anesthesia is avoided in the delivery room and used only for specific obstetrical indications, such as breech with entrapped head or shoulder dystocia, with no other anesthesia in place. There is significant risk of regurgitation of gastric contents with pulmonary aspiration.

Alternatives to medication

Nonpharmaceutical approaches to pain relief include biofeedback, transcutaneous electrical nerve stimulation (TENS), acupuncture, acupressure, therapeutic touch, and bathing (see Table 9-5 for the advantages and disadvantages of these methods).

With the support of others, a prepared woman who has learned to rely on herself can reduce the need for medical intervention with drugs. Prepared childbirth techniques, ambulation, different positions, loving support, and a comfortable environment for birth are low-risk and low-cost alternatives to medication.

SUMMARY

When emergencies occur during the intrapartum period, they are often life threatening; consequently, prompt recognition and response are essential. When the nurse has a firm understanding of the normal labor process, deviations from the process are easy to recognize. Unit X will help you apply your knowledge of the intrapartum period to the actual nursing care of the postpartum family.

BIBLIOGRAPHY

Affonso, D.D., and Harris, T.R.: Postterm pregnancy implications for mother and infant, challenge for the nurse, JOGN Nurs. **9**(3):139-145, 1980.

Aumann, G.M.E., and Blake, G.D.: Ritodrine hydrochloride in the control of premature labor implications for use, JOGN Nurs. **11**(2):75-79, 1982.

Brackbill, Y., and others: Obstetrical meperidine usage and assessment of neonatal status, Anesthesiology **40**:117-120, 1974.

Brengman, S.L., and Burns, M.K.: Vaginal delivery after c-section, Am. J. Nurs. **83**(11):1544-1547, 1983.

Brengman, S.L., and Burns, M.K.: Ritodrine hydrochloride and preterm labor, Am. J. Nurs. **83**(4):537-539, 1983.

Brucker, M.C.: Nonpharmaceutical methods for relieving pain and discomfort during pregnancy, MCN **2**:390-394, 1984.

Butterworth, M.H.: Automated incremental oxytocin infusion in the induction of labor, Obstet. Gynecol. **44**(2):238-245, 1974.

Chung, H.J.: Arresting premature labor, Am. J. Nurs. **76**(5):810-812, 1976.

Confino, E., and others: The breech dilemma. A review, Obstet. Gynec. Survey **40**(6):330-337, 1985.

Fuchs, F.: The sensitivity of the uterus to oxytocin: oxytocin-induced labor, Greenwich, Conn., 1976, CPC Communications, Inc.

Grad, R.K., and Woodside, J.: Obstetrical analgesics and anesthesia: methods of relief for the patient in labor. Am. J. Nurs. **77**(2):242-245, 1977.

Maloney, J.M.: Titrating with intravenous oxytocins, JOGN Nurs. **4**(3): 42-44, 1975.

Marshall, C.: The art of induction/augmentation of labor, JOGN Nurs. **14**(1):22-28, 1985.

Mevs, L.: The current status of cesarean section and today's maternity patient, JOGN Nurs. **6**(4):44-47, 1977.

Moore, M.L.: Realities in childbearing, ed. 2, Philadelphia, 1983, W.B. Saunders Co.

Nichols, C.W.: Postdate pregnancy, part I. A literature review, J. Nurs.-Midwif. **30**(4): 222-239, 1985.

Nichols, C.W.: Postdate pregnancy, part II. Clinical implications, J. Nurs.-Midwif. **30**(5): 259-268, 1985.

Pain-killers in labor: caution flag is up, Medical World News, Feb. 5, 1979.

Porreco, R.P.: High cesarean section rate: a new perspective, Obstet. Gynecol. **65**(3): 307-315, 1985.

Shearer, M.H., and Estes, M.: A critical review of the recent literature of postterm pregnancy and a look at women's experiences, Birth **12**(2):95-111, 1985.

Standley, K., and others: Local-regional anesthesia during childbirth: effect on newborn behaviors, Science 186(4164):634-635, 1974.

DEFINITIONS

Define the following terms:

- acupuncture
- analgesia
- anesthesia
- augmentation
- biofeedback
- breech
- caudal
- cephalopelvic disproportion
- cesarean birth
- dystocia
- epidural
- fetopelvic disproportion
- induction
- inertia
- labor curve
- oxytocin
- paracervical block
- passage
- passenger
- Pitocin
- posterior
- postmaturity syndrome
- powers
- preterm labor
- prolapsed cord
- pudendal block
- saddle block
- sedatives
- TENS
- therapeutic touch
- tocolytic agent
- tranquilizers
- VBAC
- version

LEARNING ACTIVITIES AND EXPERIENCES

1. Group discussions.
2. Guest speakers: a midwife or obstetrician to discuss their experiences with variations from normal labor; a couple who have experienced a cesarean birth.
3. View audiovisual aids and discuss.
4. Discover what organizations and/or groups exist in your community for cesarean birth teaching and support.

ENRICHMENT/IN-DEPTH STUDY

1. Draw and label normal labor curves for a primigravida and a multipara.
2. Draw and label abnormal labor curves for a primigravida and a multipara.
3. Working with a fellow student, position that student as you would a woman with a prolapsed cord in the first stage of labor.

SELF-ASSESSMENT

For questions 1 through 3, circle the best answer.

1. Some causes of uterine dysfunction include:
   a. abnormal fetal positions
   b. cephalopelvic disproportion
   c. prolapsed cord
   d. contracted pelvis
   Answer (circle one): 1. a and b
   2. c
   3. a, b, and d
   4. all of the above
2. Induction of labor is:
   a. causing labor to begin artificially
   b. causing a prolonged second stage
   c. stimulating labor
3. Signs that the uterus has ruptured include:
   a. sudden, sharp abdominal pain
   b. shock
   c. no fetal heart tones
   d. frequent, intense uterine contractions
   Answer (circle one): 1. a and d
   2. a, b, and c
   3. d
   4. all of the above

Supply the correct answer(s) for the following items:

4. Dystocia means ____ ____.
5. The main cause of uterine dysfunction in the latent phase of labor is ________ ____________________.
6. When uterine dysfunction occurs, there is a danger of fetal distress; consequently, it is very important for the nurse to ____________________.
7. A fetal indication for cesarean birth would be ______________________________ ____.
8. The cesarean incision most likely to rupture with subsequent labors is __________ ____________.
9. For what reasons may the nurse have to stop intravenous administration of the oxytocin?
10. Five maternal indications for cesarean birth are:
    a.
    b.
    c.
    d.
    e.

11. Discuss nursing care of a woman in preterm labor.

12. Below are schematic drawings of the three types of breech presentation. Write the correct name for each one.
A ____________________ B ____________________ C ____________________

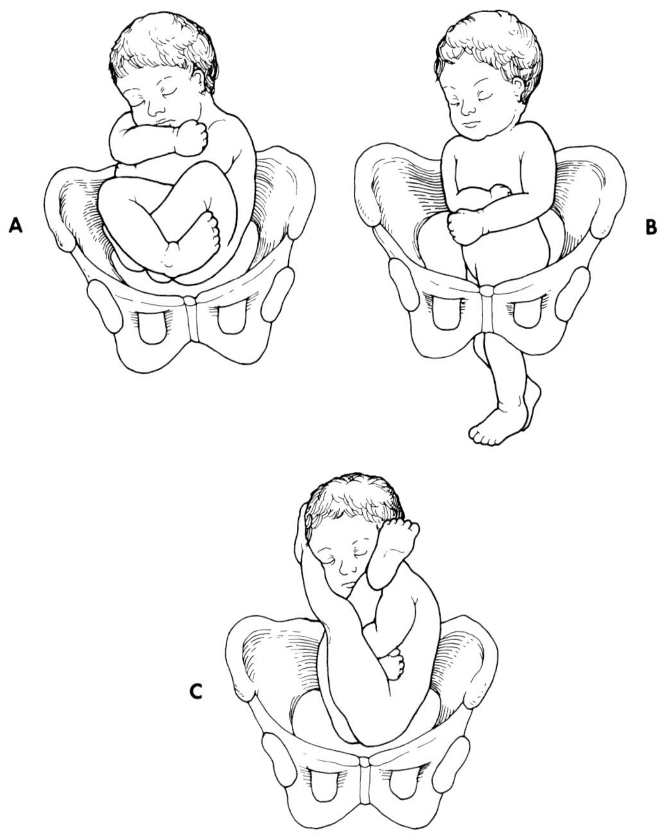

13. The majority of breech presentations are of which type?
14. What are the dangers involved in a breech presentation?
a.
b.
c.
15. Should the umbilical cord drop down alongside and below the presenting part after the membranes have ruptured, the appropriate emergency nursing measures are:

16. When abruptio placentae occurs in labor, the signs are:
a.
b.
c.

17. When providing nursing care to a laboring woman with placenta previa, the nurse would:

18. There are three basic types of cesarean births. They are:

a.

b.

c.

19. Match Column A with Column B.

	Column A	Column B
_____ _____	1. hypotonic contractions (primary inertia)	a. treatment is usually sedation
_____ _____	2. hypertonic contractions (secondary inertia)	b. happens in latent phase
		c. happens in active phase
		d. treatment is oxytocin

20. Complete the following chart of analgesics, sedatives, and tranquilizers used in labor:

Drugs	Effects	Possible side effects		Nursing care
		Mother	Fetus	
Meperidine (Demerol)				
Pentobarbital sodium (Nembutal)				
Promethazine (Phenergan)				

21. Complete the following chart of regional anesthetics used in labor:

	Areas anesthesized	Possible side effects		Nursing care
		Mother	Fetus	
Paracervical block				
Caudal				
Epidural				
Saddle block				

UNIT X
The postpartum family

GOALS

This unit is designed to provide the reader with information that will:

□ promote awareness of the physical and psychological needs of the newly delivered mother, her infant, and family.
□ develop an understanding of the bonding process.
□ introduce the concept of family planning.

STUDENT OBJECTIVES

After studying this unit, you should be able to:

1. Describe taking-in, taking-hold, and letting-go behavior in a new mother.
2. Compare the changes that occur in the postpartum mother in each of the following: (a) uterus, (b) lochia, (c) urinary system, and (d) perineum.
3. Differentiate between rooming-in and mother-baby nursing.
4. Plan how you would help a new mother cope with the following postpartum discomfort: (a) afterpains, (b) hemorrhoids, (c) episiotomy pain, and (d) constipation.
5. Identify the components, dosage, and method of administration of (a) chlorotrianisene (Tace) (b) combination of testosterone, enanthate, and estradiol valerate (Deladumone), and (c) bromocryptine mesylate (Parlodel).
6. Differentiate between the time periods when menstruation usually reappears in breast-feeding and nonnursing mothers.
7. Discuss the sexual feelings a breast-feeding mother may experience when nursing.
8. Identify the mode of action, effectiveness, contraindications, and side effects of the following temporary methods of birth control: (a) oral contraception, (b) intrauterine contraceptive devices, (c) foam, (d) diaphragm, (e) cervical cap, (f) vaginal suppositories, (g) vaginal sponges, (h) condom, and (i) rhythm.
9. Describe the optimal time, procedure, and risks for the following methods of induced abortion: (a) suction curettage, (b) dilation and evacuation using vacuum aspiration, (c) amniocentesis and injection of salt solution or prostaglandins, and (d) hysterotomy.

DEFINITIONS

The *puerperium* (L. *puer*, child; *parare*, to bring forth), or postpartum period, begins with the fourth stage of labor and lasts approximately 6 weeks. During the puerperium, the reproductive organs return to their approximate prepregnant state by a process known as *involution*. Also, during this time period, the woman undergoes significant role changes as she becomes a mother. The man also undergoes role changes in becoming a father, and because of the societal and cultural stereotypes, the fathering role is sometimes the more difficult transition of the two. Of course, other family members, such as siblings and grandparents, also undergo identity changes, which are often complicated by hospital rules and regulations that separate these family members from the mother and baby for several days. The length of the hospital stay postpartum differs greatly from one community to the next—from 6 hours to 5 days. The care this new family receives during the postpartum period is extremely important.

In Unit I we discussed the warm, affectionate tie that can develop between parents and infant during pregnancy and birth. This parent-infant love relationship (attachment) is facilitated by the shared birth experience (Unit VII) and when the family is given as much private time as possible during the third and fourth stages of labor. However, as explained earlier, attachment does not occur instantaneously; it is a process occurring over a period of time. Understanding the phases new parents go through in the postpartum period while developing their new roles will help you to make a positive influence on the parent-infant relationship (Fig. 10-1).

POSTPARTUM PHASES

The postpartum phases, as described by Reva Rubin, include the "taking-in," the "taking-hold," and the "letting-go" phases.

RECOGNIZING TAKING-IN, TAKING-HOLD, AND LETTING-GO BEHAVIOR IN A NEW MOTHER

The *taking-in phase* occurs in the first few days after delivery while physical recovery is also occurring. During this time, the mother is passive and dependent, needing to be mothered herself. She is fatigued after the hard work of labor and needs rest and sleep. However, she also needs her new baby so that the acquaintance process can continue. In the first part of this phase, women often relive the delivery to assimilate it. They want to talk about their experience and resolve any questions or feelings. New fathers and other family members who share the labor and birth have needs to relive their experiences also. Communication that occurred between the couple during the experience may need discussion, clarification, and resolution. If the new baby is not the sex they wanted, they need to work through disappointment together. It is very seldom that the real baby meets the parents' expectations for their perfect fantasized baby. In the taking-in phase the woman is usually passive, doing what she is told, and awaiting invitations from others to begin her own physical care and that of the baby.

During this phase, the nurse can be very helpful to the new mother in meeting her needs by offering supportive care, performing mothering tasks, and explaining this phase to her family and friends. When the mother's needs are met, she will be able to move

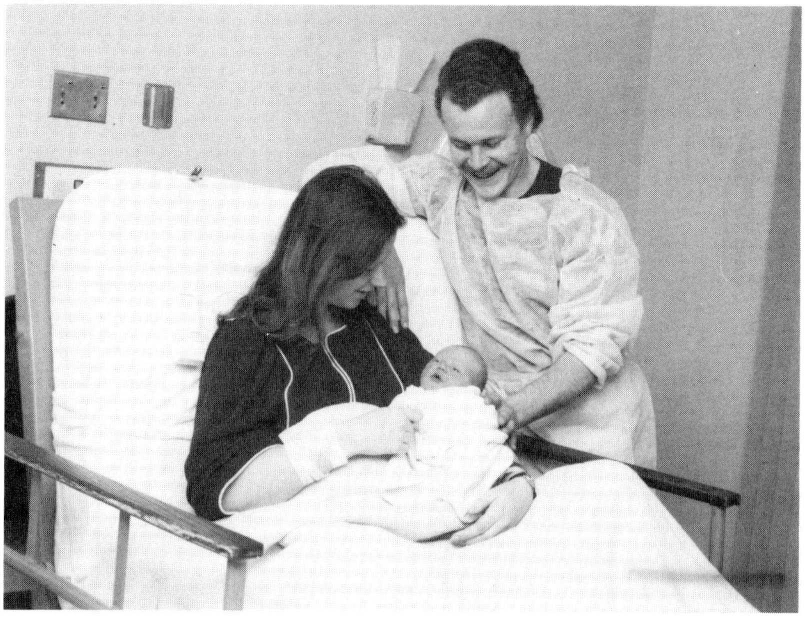

Fig. 10-1. Developing new roles. (Courtesy Valley Hospital and Medical Center, Spokane, Wash.)

on to the next phase in her maternal role change. Encouraging the father to talk about the birth experience and including him in infant care instruction will help him to feel comfortable in his new role also. Sex-role stereotyping in our culture has led us to believe that men are not capable of being nuturing and gentle with newborns. Nothing could be further from the truth.

Following the taking-in phase, women go through the taking-hold and letting-go phases. It has been generally accepted that these phases last 3 to 7 days each; however, these time periods can vary greatly. Women and men who have been well prepared for birth and experience normal labor and birth with a minimum of interference and medical intervention frequently move through all three phases in a matter of a few days. In the *taking-hold phase*, the woman regains control over her body and assumes the mothering role. She has recovered her energy and again asserts her independence and autonomy. In the *letting-go phase* the woman establishes new maternal role patterns, incorporating the necessary changes in personal and family life. While centering on her baby and the baby's needs, she begins to return to her nonpregnant state.

DESCRIBE THE NURSING ROLE IN ENHANCEMENT OF BONDING

In adapting to the fathering role, men experience the taking-in phase (passive and dependent) and other phases similar to the woman's taking-hold and letting-go phases. These male phases might be termed the *adjustment* and the *acceptance* phases. In the adjustment phase, men resume their day-to-day responsibilities with a new seriousness, aware of the dependency of their new family. This new awareness can be invigorating, causing them to shift career plans or revitalize their current career or job status. However, for some men, this new awareness can be very frightening, causing them anxiety and apprehension. Following the adjustment phase is the acceptance phase, in which men accept the intense intimate relationship between the mother and infant and their new role as fathers.

Couples who have experienced a long and difficult labor and traumatic birth may have a prolonged taking-in phase. These new parents would profit from group sessions in which they can share their experience and feelings with other couples. In groups there are always one or two others with similar experiences or feelings who can share and offer empathy. All parents who have had a traumatic experience for which they were unprepared need to resolve their feelings about that experience before they can move on to the role changes necessary to parenting.

PARENT-INFANT INTERACTION

How well and rapidly the parents go through the postpartum phases is influenced greatly by their interactions with the new baby. The baby's response to the parents' attempts at communication is very important. New parents first touch their babies with fingertips, then palms of the hands, then total hands, and then total body in hand to arm embrace. They frequently hold the infant on the left side with the baby close to the chest, near the parent's heart. Eye-to-eye contact is important in this "en face" positioning. Parents talk instinctively to their babies in high-pitched voices, cooing and oohing. Rhythm-reciprocity patterns are often developed: the parent "oohs" and the baby "oohs," the parent smiles and the baby smiles. When parental-infant bonding is occurring, the behaviors just identified are observable.

DISTINGUISH AMONG TAKING-IN, ADJUSTMENT, AND ACCEPTANCE PHASES NEW FATHERS MAY EXPERIENCE

The nurse can help the parents in the bonding process by explaining to them that their infant is a unique, distinct individual with a separate personality. Many parents do not understand that their infant can see, hear, and respond to stimuli and is not as fragile as they may believe. The infant's ability to exhibit purposeful movements and to imitate more adult movements never fails to amaze new parents. The nurse can also help parents to understand the phases a newborn goes through and the newborn's states of awareness so that they can truly know their new baby. The normal behavior of the newborn is discussed in Unit XII.

Assessment of bonding and attachment during all phases of the childbearing experience should be included in the maternity data base because parents who consistently manifest a lack of these behaviors may require additional care, support, and intervention.

ROOMING-IN

DIFFERENTIATE BETWEEN ROOMING-IN AND MOTHER-BABY NURSING

In conventional postpartum care the mother is separated from her baby, who is placed in a separate nursery and brought to her at designated periods. This practice of separating babies in hospital nurseries began at the turn of the century in this country. Reasons for the introduction of nurseries included a high incidence of maternal sepsis and the frequency of infections in the newborn that could be traced to this source. Also, many mothers received general anesthesia, "twilight sleep," and obstetrical intervention during labor and birth and were too incapacitated to care for their babies.

Rooming-in is the term used to designate a hospital arrangement whereby a mother may have her newborn baby in a crib by her bedside whenever she wishes (Fig. 10-2). In the late 1940s some hospitals started rooming-in units in the United Sates to establish more natural mother-baby relationships. An interesting reason for starting a rooming-in program at Duke University Hospital in Durham, North Carolina, was to avoid the possibility of a nursery epidemic of diarrhea. (It is fascinating to note that nurseries that began to prevent infection had become sources of cross-infection themselves). Major advantages cited from these rooming-in programs included reduced hospital costs, improved parenting skills, and reports of parent satisfaction. However, despite these advantages, rooming-in programs have not flourished in the United States.

Although rooming-in was started in an effort to foster development of the parent-child relationship, the actual implementation process often discouraged bonding and attachment. In the institutionalization and development of procedures and routines, the infant was often literally dumped on the new mother in her taking-in phase of postpartum adjustment. Often the mother was expected to assume primary responsibility for infant

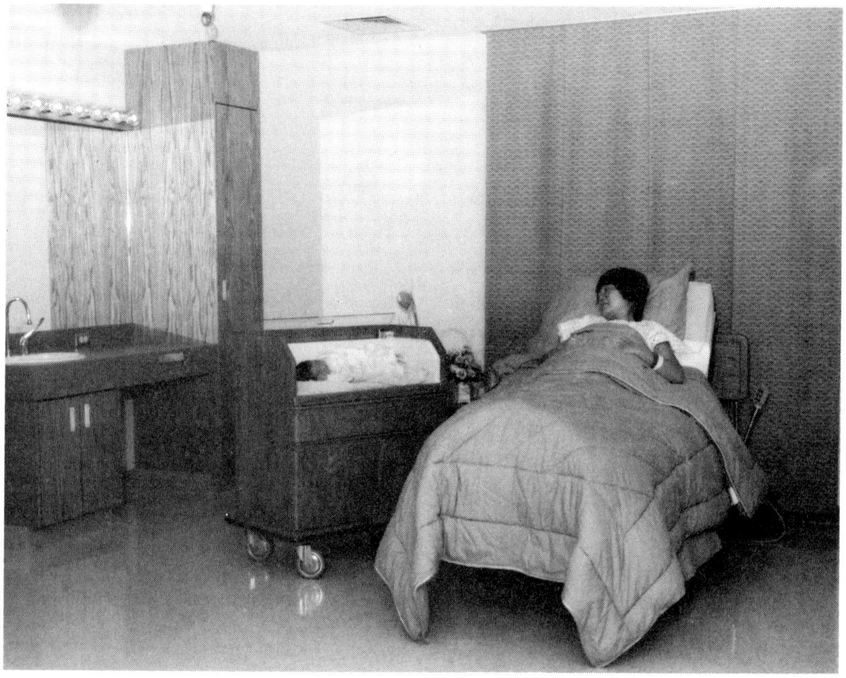

Fig. 10-2. Rooming-in. (Courtesy Valley Hospital and Medical Center, Spokane, Wash.)

care, with nurses available for assistance or teaching. Because the baby was assigned to the nursery nurse and the mother was assigned to the postpartum nurse, there was often confusion in messages and in lines of authority. Some hospital rooming-in protocols would not permit visitors or even allow the baby to be returned to the central nursery at night. Often, parents were not prepared for the rooming-in experience and were incapable of basic infant care.

Fatigue in the postpartum period can be extreme. Sleep disruption superimposed on profound fatigue can contribute to feelings of being overburdened. *Real* babies who cry at night and demand feeding every 2 to 3 hours are not like the fantasized babies of the pregnancy. To expect new mothers to assume responsibility for infant care in rooming-in violates everything we know about the postpartum phases, parent-infant interaction, and family beginnings.

MOTHER-BABY NURSING

Mother-baby nursing is not rooming-in. Instead, it is provision of primary mother and baby care by one nurse providing total care to both the mother and her infant. All policies and procedures are geared toward the new mother as a member of a family unit. This type of nursing care requires cross-education of nursery and postpartum nurses so that they can give complete care to the mother-baby couplet (Fig. 10-3).

Mother-baby nurses provide infant care at the mother's bedside, guide and teach parenting skills, attend to the mother's physiological and psychological needs, and integrate other family members into this care.

It is often necessary to maintain a newborn nursery staff for transitional observations,

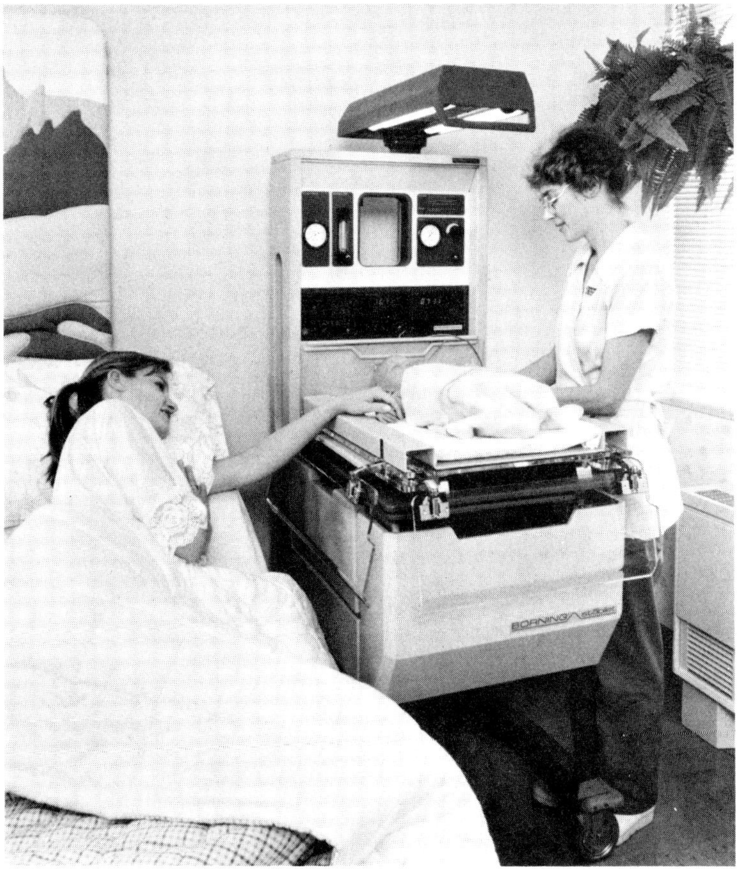

Fig. 10-3. Mother-baby nursing. (Courtesy The Borning Corporation, Spokane, Wash.)

special procedures, and care of babies who cannot remain with their mothers. However, these nurses rotate out of the nursery into mother-baby nursing so that mother-baby skills are maintained. Cost savings, parent satisfaction, and improved parent-infant relationships have been reported with mother-baby nursing.

Families need preparation for mother-baby nursing during the prenatal period. It is important to discuss the significance of the postpartum period to parent-infant relationships. Sibling involvement and ways to enhance family adjustment require anticipatory guidance.

FAMILY CARE UNITS

Postpartum programs in self-care, self-administration of medications, early hospital discharge, and home visits by nurses are options that can promote successful adjustment to parenting (Fig. 10-4).

Postpartum care begins prenatally and extends through the labor and birth process. Maternity nursing is concerned with each family's unique adjustment to the new roles needed in becoming a family.

PHYSICAL ADJUSTMENTS

The physical adjustments of postpartum involve all of the woman's body systems and require a significant expenditure of energy. Some women feel excited, uplifted, and energetic immediately after birth. Others feel exhausted and want to sleep.

Uterus

CHANGES THAT OCCUR IN THE POSTPARTUM MOTHER

Involution is the return of the uterus to its prepregnant state. Immediately after delivery, the uterus weighs about 2 pounds and is usually the size and consistency of a small, firm grapefruit. It can be felt through the abdominal wall at or below the level of the umbilicus, in the center of the abdomen. Within 12 hours of delivery, the fundal height rises to one finger-breadth (1 centimeter) above the umbilicus. On each succeed-

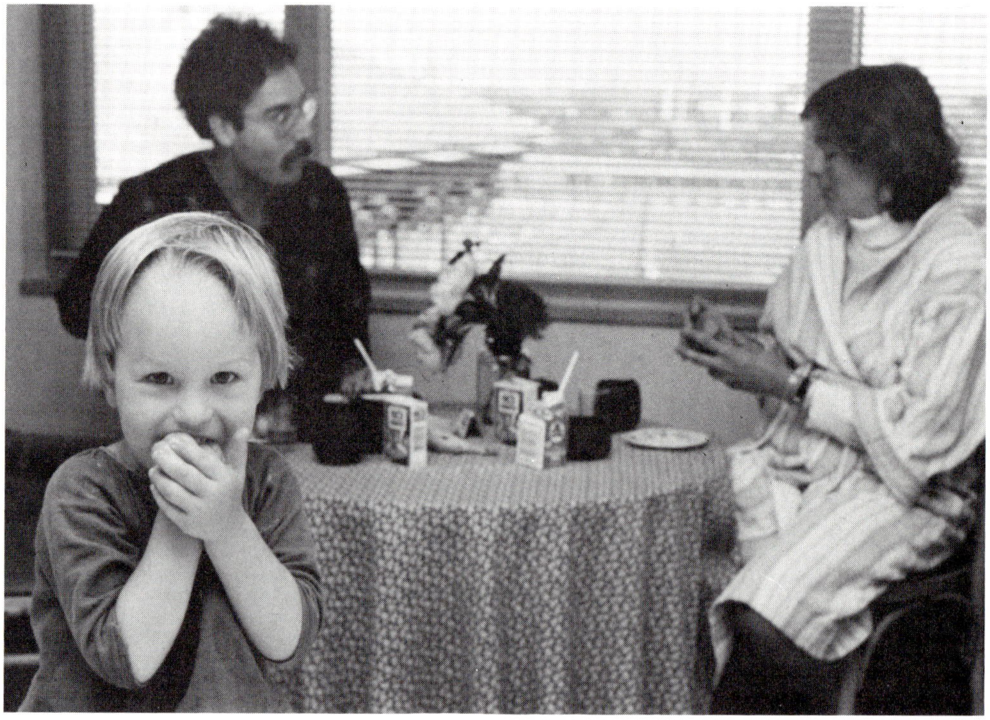

Fig. 10-4. Family care unit. (Courtesy Fairview-Riverside Hospital, Minneapolis, Minn.)

ing postpartum day, the uterus gradually becomes smaller and descends downward into the pelvic cavity (Fig. 10-5). By the tenth day, it is at or below the level of the symphysis pubis and can no longer be felt through the abdominal wall. As the uterus descends, it should remain firm and contracted to prevent hemorrhage. The height of the fundus indicates the rate of involution. The fundus should be about one finger-width lower each day and should always be located in the center of the abdomen. The nurse should palpate the uterus for fundal height and firmness and record these findings several times during each postpartum day so that any deviation from normal can be recognized immediately (see Fig. 10-6).

So that daily measurements are consistent, the mother should empty her bladder

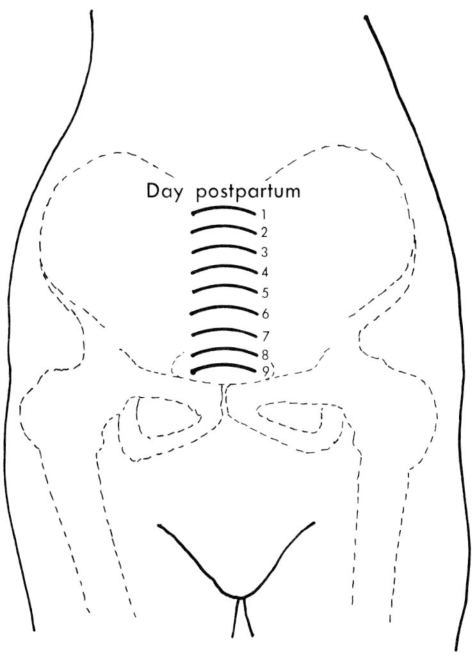

Fig. 10-5. Involution of the uterus.

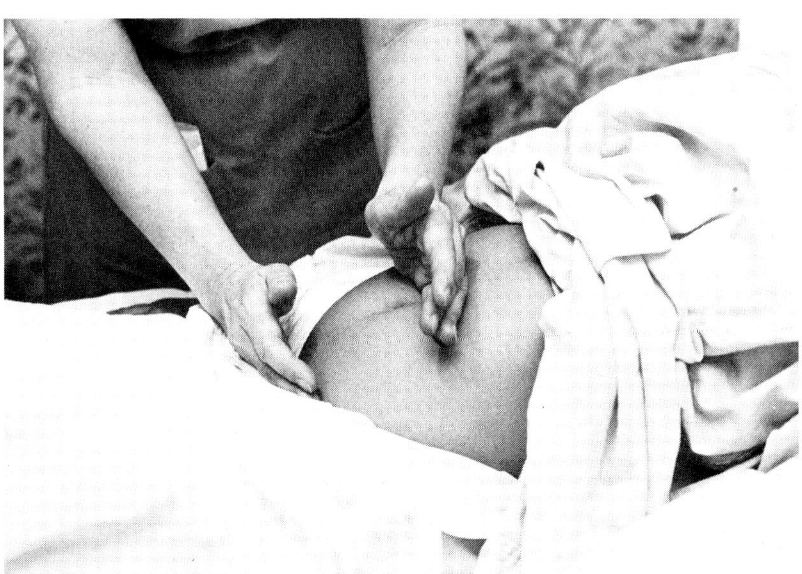

Fig. 10-6. Palpating the uterus.

before the uterus is palpated and should lie on her back with her knees bent and her feet flat on the bed. It is important that the new mother understands the process of involution and is taught how to massage her uterus to contract it.

Contractions of the uterus as it descends are often called *afterpains* and are more pronounced in multiparas than in primiparas. Afterpains are more prominent during breast-feeding. Also, oxytocic drugs are often given to new mothers to contract uterine muscles during the postpartum period. Medication may be ordered for the discomfort. The new mother needs to understand the physiological basis of the afterpains. Lying on the abdomen, relaxation, and slow breathing techniques are helpful in relieving pain. Extreme tenderness of the uterus should be reported immediately because it can indicate intrauterine infection.

Lochia

DIFFERENTIATE BETWEEN LOCHIA RUBRA, SEROSA, AND ALBA

Lochia is the normal uterine and vaginal discharge in the early postpartum period. Lochia consists of blood, shreds of decidual tissue, mucus, bacteria, and epithelial cells from the vagina. Occasionally, lochia also contains small clots. Lochia goes through the following three stages as the placental site heals. *Lochia rubra* is the first stage, wherein the lochia is red and bloody for 3 to 4 days. Gradually, as the lining of the rest of the uterus sloughs off, the discharge becomes brownish to pinkish in color and is called *lochia serosa*. By the tenth day, the lochia turns yellowish-white and is called *lochia alba*. Lochia has a fleshy odor, suggestive of fresh blood. It should not smell foul. Foul-smelling lochia is usually a sign of infection and should be reported immediately. Lochia is less in quantity in mothers who are breast-feeding and following a cesarean birth.

Nursing care. The nurse assesses the lochia for color, amount, consistency, and odor and records findings. Teaching the new mother about the normal amount, color, consistency, odor, and progression of lochia is very important. When she is aware of the normal lochia, a new mother can report any deviations from normal. Thus an infection could be treated before it becomes serious.

Perineum

If the new mother has had an episiotomy, she will experience some discomfort. The tissue around the episiotomy may be edematous, causing pressure on the sutures. Slight separation of the wound edges may occur; however, this is superficial and not serious. The perineum should be kept clean and as dry as possible to prevent infection. Although procedures for perineal care differ from hospital to hospital, the following basic procedures are common:

1. Remove the perineal pad from front to back to prevent contamination of the vaginal opening from rectal microorganisms. After the perineum is cleansed, apply the clean perineal pad tightly from front to back.
2. Cleanse the perineum from front to back by flushing the area with warm water or a mild antiseptic solution after each elimination.
3. Pat the perineum dry with gauze, soft tissue, or wipes.
4. When bathing, use a clean cloth to cleanse the perineal area. Wash the anal area last.

Measures that are very soothing and also facilitate healing of an episiotomy include warm sitz baths for 15 to 20 minutes twice a day, followed by exposure of the incision to warm, dry heat from a lamp. Emotional support and reassurance that the discomfort will decrease are also necessary. As with any pain, medication may be helpful.

It is important to inspect the perineum at least once each day to detect any unusual redness, swelling, or discharge around the episiotomy. Any of these signs should be reported. It may be necessary to use a flashlight to visualize the area well, or the woman can turn on her left side and bend her right leg to expose the suture line.

Women who have had an episiotomy find it helpful to contract their buttocks muscles before sitting on a hard surface. This muscular contraction lifts the perineal floor up off the hard surface. Also, the Kegel exercises discussed in Unit VI are very helpful in the immediate postpartum period.

Vital signs

NORMAL VITAL SIGNS IN FIRST FEW DAYS POSTPARTUM

The new mother's pulse may be from 40 to 70 beats per minute on the first and second days postpartum. This slowing of the pulse results from a decrease in cardiac output without a reduction in stroke volume. A rapid pulse may indicate hemorrhage and should be reported.

The temperature should remain within normal limits. A slight temperature elevation may be caused by inadequate intake and/or excessive output of fluid. If this is the case, the fluid intake should be increased. Any elevation over 100.4° F in any two consecutive 24-hour periods (excluding the first day) is considered significant and potentially serious. Any temperature elevation should be reported becuase it may be indicative of infection.

Respiration may be easier and slower because the smaller uterus is no longer pressing on the lungs and diaphragm. Blood pressure may drop slightly as the amount of circulating blood volume decreases. Of course, any abnormal findings in these vital signs should be reported immediately.

Hemorrhoids

Hemorrhoids may appear for the first time as the mother pushes to deliver the baby. These hemorrhoids will usually disappear in several weeks following delivery. Warm sitz baths, cold witch hazel compresses, and elevation of the buttocks on several pillows during rest are helpful remedies. Sometimes topical anesthetic ointments are ordered. The woman should avoid straining when defecating. Stool softeners, increased fluid intake, and addition of roughage to the diet are helpful.

Urinary system

INTERPRET NORMAL FINDINGS IN URINE POSTPARTUM

After the birth the 50% increase in extracellular fluid that was necessary in the pregnancy is no longer needed. Consequently, there is a significant diuresis in the early postpartum period (usually between the second and fifth postpartum days). The urinary output is up to 3000 milliliters per day. Also, the capacity of the bladder increases because of the decreased intra-abdominal pressure and the relaxed, stretched abdominal muscles. Overdistention of the bladder can occur along with incomplete emptying and retention of some residual urine. It is important for the new mother to excrete at least 150 milliliters of urine each time she voids. The first three voidings should be measured.

The first voiding may be difficult because of trauma on the bladder and urethra during the birth process, causing tenderness, edema, and reflex spasm of the urethra. If the woman has not urinated within 6 hours of delivery, catheterization may be necessary. The physician may also order a urine culture and sensitivity test. To encourage voiding, the nurse can provide fluids to drink, be sure the woman has privacy, and encourage her to walk to the bathroom if possible. Walking is very helpful, and the squatting position over a toilet helps to release pressure on the bladder. Sometimes the sound of water running or the actual flow of warm water over the perineum encourages voiding.

Laboratory findings on urinalysis in the first few days and weeks postpartum normally disclose the presence of protein and/or sugar. The proteinuria results from the increased nitrogen content of urine caused by protein destruction in the walls of the uterus as the uterine muscle cells become smaller. The sugar is present in the urine because of lactose absorption from the mammary glands (breasts) into the bloodstream.

Nursing care. It is important to explain to the mother the possible causes and limited nature of discomfort with voiding. Instruct the mother on the importance of frequent voiding, ambulation, and fluid intake. A full bladder is obvious because it is visible as a soft swelling above the symphysis pubis and feels like a soft balloon full of fluid when palpated. The bladder should be examined for distention at each postpartum check because a full bladder can displace the uterus, thus predisposing to uterine hemorrhage (Fig. 10-7). Pain and frequency of urination are also signs of a urinary tract infection. It is important to differentiate between the normal frequent urination postpartum that is associated with increased urinary output and urinary tract infection. Symptoms of urinary tract infection include suprapubic and costovertebral angle pain, fever, hematuria, and pain on urination.

Bowels

COPING WITH POSTPARTUM DISCOMFORTS

Constipation is a common problem in the postpartum period because of the relaxed abdominal walls and inactivity. Increased levels of progesterone relax smooth muscles and may contribute to bowel hypoactivity. Also, women who have had episiotomies often fear that they may have pain when defecating and consequently hold back their feces. The physician may order stool softeners, laxatives, suppositories, or enemas. However, if the new mother is breast-feeding, laxatives may be excreted in breast milk. Early ambulation, a diet that includes roughage and plenty of fluids, and exercise to tone stretched abdominal muscles are all helpful in re-establishing proper bowel functioning.

Diaphoresis

Hormonal changes and the body's attempt to rid itself of extra fluid can cause the woman to perspire profusely. Often this happens at night, and the woman may wake up drenched in perspiration. It is important that she be told that this is a normal body response.

Personal hygiene

Douching is not necessary in the postpartum period and has actually been declared medically unsound by the American College of Obstetricians and Gynecologists.

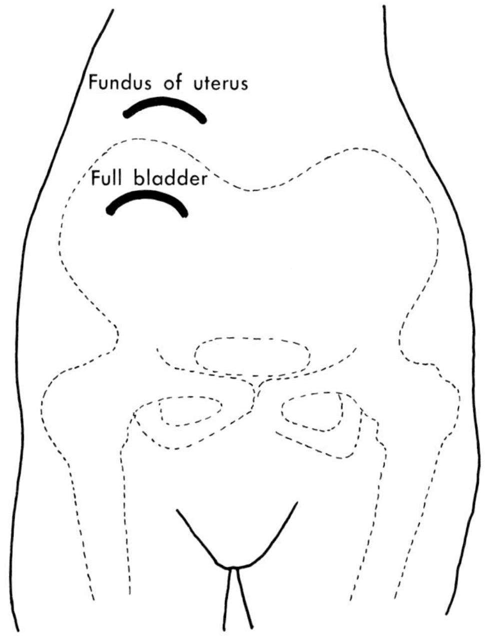

Fig. 10-7. Full bladder, uterus displaced.

Showers are preferred over tub baths until the lochia stops. The mother may soak in a tub of warm water for suture healing but should not bathe first in the same water.

When bathing, the woman should wash her hands first with soap and water and then wash her breasts. The nipples should be washed with plain water, no soap, because soap is drying. She should then wash the rest of her body in the usual manner. After washing her body, the woman should use a clean washcloth to cleanse the perineal area, washing the anal area last.

Extremities

Frequently new mothers have varying degrees of varicosities of the lower extremities, thighs, and vulva. It is important to check the extremities for red, hot, painful areas, which could be signs of acute thrombophlebitis and should be reported immediately. When examining the woman's legs, press down gently on her knee (with the legs flat on the bed) and ask her to point her toes toward her face. Pain or tenderness in the calf is a positive *Homans' sign* and an indication of thrombophlebitis. Report this immediately.

Laboratory findings

The blood volume and hemoglobin and hematocrit levels usually return to normal within 1 week postpartum. The white blood cell count is elevated in the first few days postpartum because leukocytosis occurs as the placental site heals. The white count usually returns to normal in 7 days.

Weight

IDENTIFY NORMAL WEIGHT LOSS FOR NEW MOTHER

At delivery the woman loses about 12 to 13 pounds (baby, placenta, amniotic fluid, membranes, and blood). Further loss of body weight during the puerperium may be approximately 5 pounds, although this loss does not occur until diuresis begins. Explain to the mother the process of gradual return to prepregnant weight.

Abdomen

The woman's abdominal walls tend to be soft and flabby in the first few weeks after birth because they were stretched during pregnancy. This can be very depressing for the new mother, and she needs reassurance that she will be able to wear her favorite clothing again. She determines to a great deal how soon and how well her muscles will return to their original condition. Exercises to improve the muscle tone of the abdomen may be started as soon as the lochia has stopped.

Postpartum exercises

For best results, exercises appropriate for the new mother should begin within 24 hours of delivery. The exercise program should begin with deep diaphragmatic breathing, diastasis recti correction, and the Kegel exercise. The woman should begin gradually and be careful not to overexert herself (Fig. 10-8).

Postpartum blues

DISTINGUISH BETWEEN POSTPARTUM BLUES AND POSTPARTUM DEPRESSION

"Baby blues," or maternity blues, are experienced by 80% of postpartum women. The main symptoms are mild depression, anxiety, preoccupation, and forgetfulness. These symptoms are usually transient, peak a few days after childbirth, last 1 to 10 days, and then disappear.

Women with *postpartum blues* frequently do not know why they feel depressed, will talk of feeling "silly," and will laugh through their tears. This phenomenon may be caused by the extreme drop in hormones that occurs about 72 hours postpartum. Also, many women experience disappointment that they have a large, flabby belly, feel tired, and generally do not look like the gorgeous, well-groomed new mothers on television or

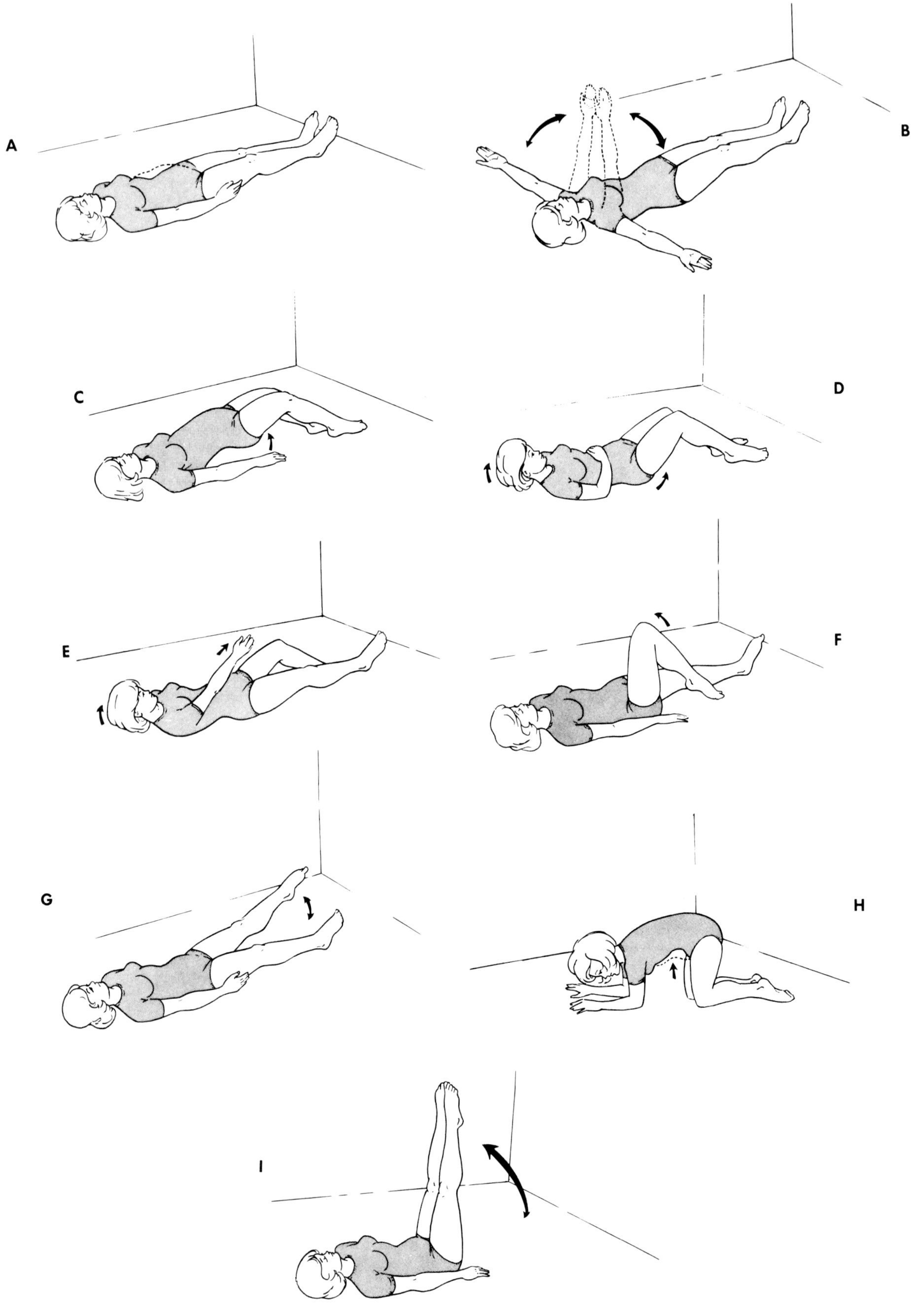

Fig. 10-8. Postpartum exercises. (Modified from Jensen, M., and Bobak, I.M.: Maternity and gynecologic care: the nurse and the family, ed. 3, St. Louis, 1985, The C.V. Mosby Co.)

in the movies. These women think that they must be failures because they are not perfect. Some women feel extreme disappointment if their labors and births did not go as planned. Others perceive inadequate emotional support from their partners or extreme stress caused by new mothering responsibilities. It is important to let these women talk, cry, and work through their feelings, to explain possible causes for "the blues," and to reassure the new mother. It is essential that she understand that other women experience the blues too—and perfect mothers exist only in fairy tales.

The family members can be very helpful by giving the mother attention. It is not unusual to find them all admiring the baby while the mother is left alone. Also, most gifts are for the baby and not for the mother.

Postpartum depression

As many as 10% of postpartum women are estimated to develop significant depressions that last for weeks or months and require medication, psychotherapy, or both. Periods of excessive crying, despondency, feelings of inadequacy and inability to cope, insomnia, anorexia, and social withdrawal may signal more than postpartum blues. Identification systems to determine women at risk for *postpartum depression* are needed. Many women take great pains to conceal their postpartum depression from families and friends because they feel it is not "womanly" or "motherly" or socially acceptable. Until postpartum depression is recognized and accepted as a legitimate entity, just as premenstrual syndrome (PMS) has been, future research will continue to be limited.

BREASTS

The breasts are enlarged and heavy after delivery as they change rapidly to prepare for nourishing the baby. The breasts may secrete small amounts of a thin, yellowish premilk fluid called *colostrum* during pregnancy, particularly in the last few months. Colostrum is rich in vitamins A and E, protein, and antibodies, and it is thought to have mild laxative properties. Colostrum continues to be secreted for the first 3 to 5 days after delivery, gradually changing to milk.

Frequent and early feeding of this colostrum encourages the milk supply *(lactation)* by the third to fifth day after birth. Lactation is believed to be caused by the pituitary hormone prolactin. During pregnancy, the breasts developed to prepare for lactation by the influence of high levels of estrogen and progesterone. It is believed that these high hormone levels inhibited the pituitary gland from producing prolactin during pregnancy. After the placenta is expelled, the woman's blood levels of estrogen and progesterone drop; consequently, the pituitary can produce prolactin to initiate lactation.

Prolactin stimulates the alveolar cells (acini cells) of the breasts and thus promotes milk production (see Unit II, Fig. 2-8). Under the influence of prolactin, milk is secreted continuously into the alveoli of the breasts and remains there until it is ejected or "let down" from the alveoli, through the milk ducts, to the lactiferous sinuses, and then to the baby. This process works on a supply-and-demand basis; the more the mother's breasts are stimulated, the more prolactin she will have. In the nonnursing mother, prolactin drops to prepregnant levels in about 14 days. When the baby sucks at the mother's breast, sensory impulses are transmitted through the mother's nervous system to her brain, causing the release of oxytocin from her pituitary gland. Within 30 seconds after the baby begins to suck, milk is available. The release of oxytocin from the pituitary causes the myoepithelial cells that surround the outer walls of the alveoli to contract and express the milk. If the breasts are not stimulated regularly, milk production ceases. (See Fig. 10-9 for a diagrammatical outline of the ejection reflex arc.)

As the breasts fill up, they become larger and firmer to the touch. The veins in the breasts become apparent, and the mother will say that her breasts are heavier, more

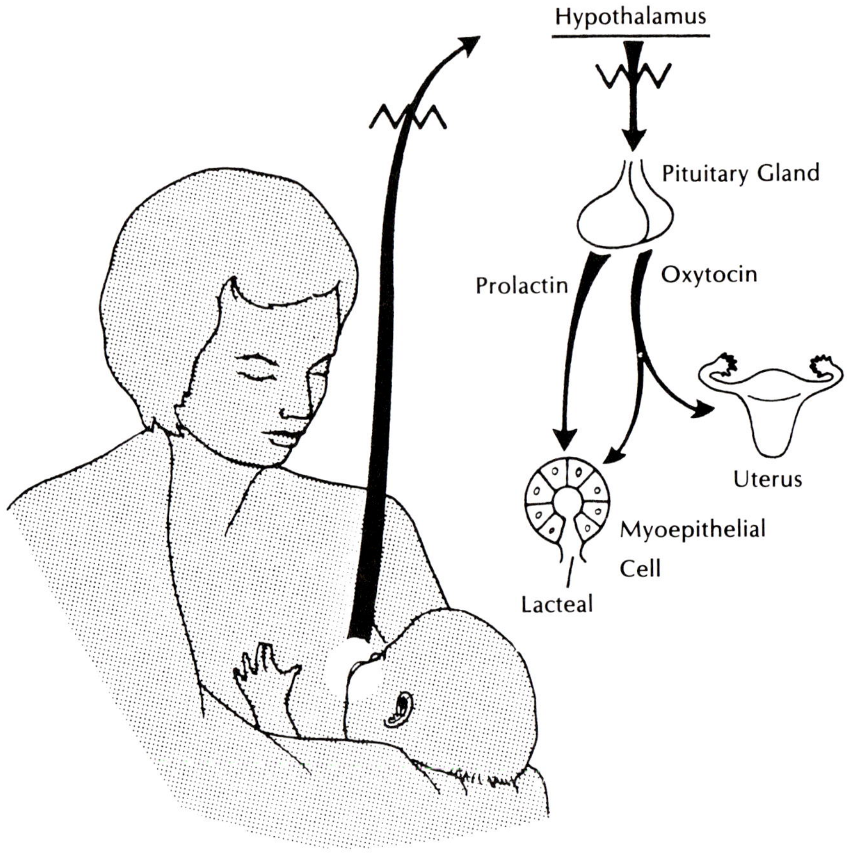

Fig. 10-9. Diagrammatical outline of ejection reflex arc. (Courtesy Ruth A. Lawrence, M.D.: Breast-feeding: a Guide for the Medical Profession, ed. 2, St. Louis, 1985, The C.V. Mosby Co.)

RECOGNIZE THE AVERAGE PERIOD OF TIME FOR ENGORGEMENT

DIAGRAM THE LET-DOWN REFLEX

tender, and warmer to the touch. *Engorgement* is the term given to this swelling of breast tissue and increased blood flow and congestion (Fig. 10-10). At the same time the secretion from the breasts changes from the thin, yellowish colostrum to the thin, bluish consistency of skim milk. Engorgement usually occurs by the third or fourth day postpartum and lasts only 24 to 48 hours. Comfort measures for engorgement include adequate support for the breasts by a supportive brassiere or breast binder. A warm shower (or hot towels placed over the breasts) is often helpful for relaxation and for the promotion of the *let-down reflex,* thus softening the breasts. This reflex is involuntary and is stimulated by the anticipation of a feeding, by hearing the baby cry, or by relaxation. The let-down reflex causes a tingling sensation accompanied by the leaking of milk from the nipples. Particularly when the breasts are large and hard, bringing the milk from the glands in the breast to the nipple helps the baby drink it more easily. Massaging the breasts between breast-feedings can also help to keep the ducts open. Engorged breasts can cause flattening of the nipple, making it difficult for the baby to grasp. Softening the breast by the let-down reflex or manual expression of milk relieves the hardness around the areola (Fig 10-11).

Breast care

To reduce the risk of breast infection, it is very important that anyone touching the breasts have clean hands and that the breasts and nipples be kept clean and free of dried secretions. The breasts should be washed with a clean cloth daily during shower or bath. It is not necessary to use soap because it removes the natural oils that protect the skin from drying and cracking, nor is it necessary to wash the nipples before or after breast-

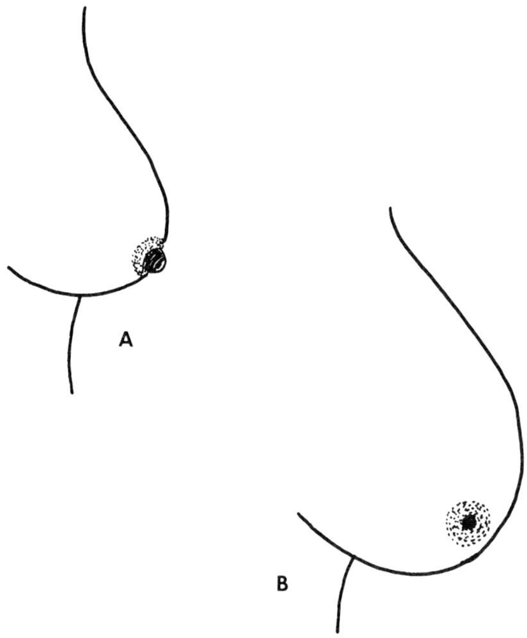

Fig. 10-10. Engorgement. **A,** Not engorged. **B,** Engorged.

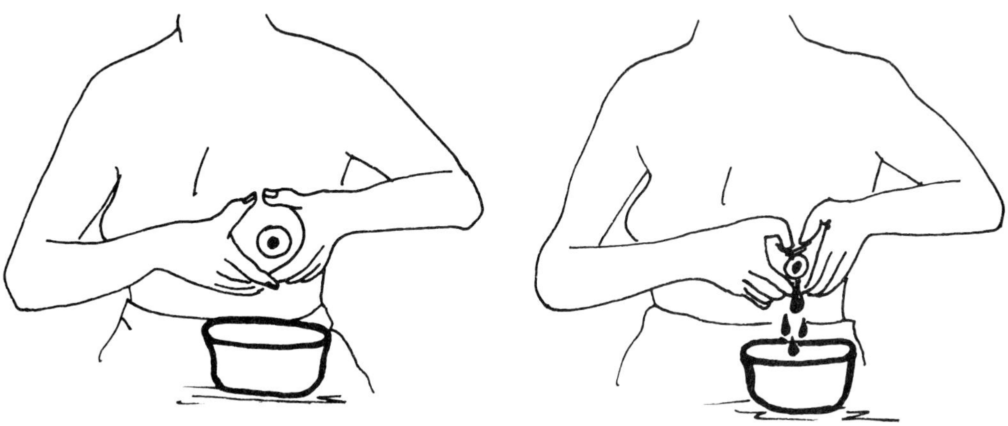

Fig. 10-11. Manual expression of milk.

IDENTIFY TWO NURSING MEASURES TO ELIMINATE DISCOMFORT OF SORE NIPPLES

feeding. However, it is important to air dry the nipples after feeding and before covering again with the bra. Because any damp material against the skin for a period of time can cause skin breakdown, the mother should not wear bras or pads with plastic liners. If leaking occurs and she wants to protect her clothing from milk stains, the mother may use nonplastic nursing pads, a gauze pad, clean perineal pads cut to fit, clean handkerchiefs, or milk cups as illustrated in Fig. 4-13. She should also change to a clean bra daily. After the nipples are dry, creams or ointments can be applied to help prevent soreness and cracking. The following preparations are helpful: aloe, A & D ointment, lanolin, cocoa butter, and vitamin E oil.

The nurse should inspect the breast-feeding mother's breasts and nipples and teach her how to inspect her own breasts for signs of nipple irritation or skin breakdown. The breasts should also be checked daily for signs of *mastitis* (breast infection), such as redness, swelling, tenderness, and fever. All observations should be recorded, and anything unusual should be reported immediately.

Breast-feeding

Each year scientific evidence provides increasing justification for breast-feeding. Among the key factors influencing the prevalence and duration of breast-feeding are the attitudes and behaviors of health care personnel and the hospital practices. (See Table 10-1 for a listing of hospital practices that influence breast-feeding initiation.)

Breast-feeding should be discussed during the prenatal period and dialogue established on the process, advantages, and disadvantages with the expectant mother and

Table 10-1. Hospital practices that influence breast-feeding initiation

Strongly encouraging	Encouraging	Discouraging	Strongly discouraging
Physical contact			
Baby put to breast immediately in delivery room.			Mother-infant separation at birth.
Baby not taken from mother after delivery.	Staff sensitivity to cultural norms and expectations of woman.	Scheduled feedings regardless of mother's breast-feeding wishes.	Mother-infant housed on separate floors in postpartum period.
Woman helped by staff to suckle baby in recovery room.			Mother separated from baby because of bilirubin problem.
Rooming-in, staff help with baby care *in* room; not only in nursery.			No rooming-in policy.
Verbal communication			
Staff initiates discussion regarding woman's intention to breast-feed pre- and intrapartum.	Appropriate language skills of staff, teaching how to handle breast engorgement and nipple problem.	Staff instructs woman "to get good night's rest and miss the feed."	Woman told to "take it easy," get your rest—impression that breast-feeding is effortful and tiring.
Staff encourages and reinforces breast-feeding immediately on labor and delivery.	Staff's own skills and comfort regarding art of breast-feeding and time to teach woman on one-to-one basis.	Strict times allotted for breast-feeding regardless of mother and baby's feeding "cycle."	Woman told she doesn't "do it right," staff interrupts her efforts; corrects her regarding positions and other matters.
Staff discusses use of breast pump and realities of separation from baby regarding breast-feeding.			
Non-verbal communication			
Pictures of woman breast-feeding. Literature on breast-feeding in understandable terms.		Pictures of woman bottle-feeding.	Woman given infant formula kit and infant food literature.
Staff (doctors as well as nurses) give reinforcement for breast-feeding (respect, smiles, affirmation).		Staff interrupts her breast-feeding session for laboratory tests and other matters.	
Nurse (or any attendant) making mother comfortable and helping to arrange baby at breast for nursing.		Woman does not see others breast-feeding.	Sees official-looking nurses authoritatively caring for babies by bottle-feeding (leads to woman's insecurities regarding own capability of care).
Woman sees others breast-feeding in hospital.	Closed-circuit TV show in hospital on breast-feeding.		
Experiential			
If breast-feeding not *immediately* successful, staff continues to be supportive.			
Previous success with breast-feeding experience in hospital.			Previous failure with breast-feeding experience in hospital.

From Scrimshaw, Susan C.M.: The cultural context of breast-feeding in the U.S. In report of the Surgeon General's Workshop on Breast-feeding and Human Lactation, U.S. Department of Health and Human Services, June 11, 12, 1984.

family members. Mothers should be encouraged to cuddle and put their infants to breast as soon as possible after birth. Thinking of the mother and baby as a unit and caring for the couple in mother-baby nursing allow the mother to learn about and care for her baby in a supportive environment (Fig. 10-12).

DESCRIBE THE ROOTING REFLEX OF NEWBORN

When helping a new mother breast-feed, encourage her to hold her baby so that the baby's cheek touches her breast. This stimulates the *rooting reflex* in which the baby's head moves from side to side in an attempt to locate the nipple. The entire nipple and some of the surrounding dark tissue (areola) should be inserted into the baby's mouth. If the breast is very full and firm, it will have to be compressed slightly beneath the baby's nose. The baby should suck at each breast for each feeding. One pattern of feeding that some mothers use is to nurse "on demand" for about 5 minutes on each breast on the day of delivery and first day of life. The idea is to start slowly and increase feeding time gradually to prevent sore and cracked nipples. It is important to begin each feeding with the last breast used so that at least one breast will be emptied each time.

To remove the baby from the breast, the mother should break the baby's suction by pressing the breast away from the corner of the baby's mouth or by inserting a clean finger into the corner of the baby's mouth. The baby should be burped, or "bubbled," when changing breasts or after the feeding is completed. "Over-the-shoulder," sitting the baby up on the mother's lap and patting the baby's back, or resting the baby on the mother's legs face down and patting the baby's back are all "bubbling" methods (see Fig. 12-15). Breast-fed babies may not burp at all because they swallow less air than bottle-fed babies.

Breast-fed babies do not require supplemental formula or glucose water under normal circumstances. If the infant is wetting six or eight diapers per day, the skin turgor is good, and the anterior fontanel is not sunken, the infant is receiving adequate nutrition.

The La Leche League International is a national organization dedicated to helping breast-feeding mothers. The address is given in Appendix B.

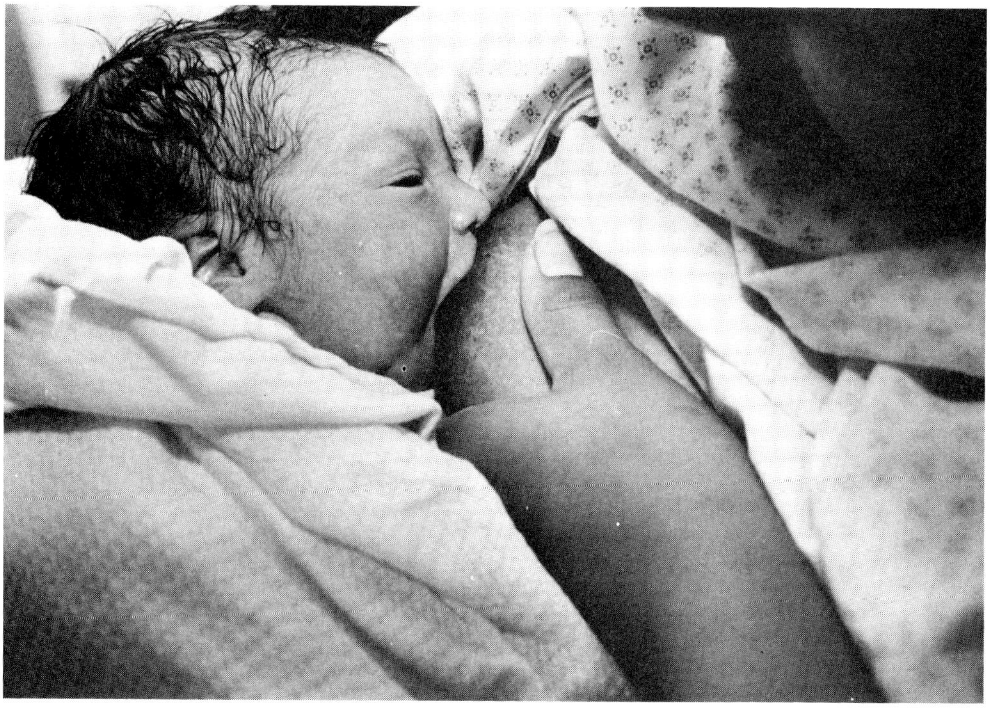

Fig. 10-12. Breast-feeding as soon as possible after birth. (Photo by Jacqueline Capra, from Phillips, C.R., and Anzalone, J.T.: Fathering, ed. 2, St. Louis, 1982, The C.V. Mosby Co.)

Breast-feeding women should be given the name and number of a community resource person before leaving the hospital. Follow-up phone calls and home visits by nurses can continue support and teaching that promote successful breast-feeding.

Working women

If the breast-feeding mother is returning to work outside the home after the baby's birth, she should be encouraged to hand express her milk or use a breast pump after feedings to increase her milk supply.

Returning to work outside the home does not mean that the mother cannot breast-feed. Breast milk can be frozen and the container dated for later feeding.

Drugs in human milk

Any drug taken by a breast-feeding mother has the potential to enter and be excreted in her milk. The following drugs in breast milk are most likely to produce problems for the infant: certain sulfonamides, aspirin, Coumadin anticoagulants, reserpine, phenytoin, bromides, and benzodiazepine tranquilizers. Appendix D has table of potential problems from drugs known to be excreted in human milk.

Nonnursing mother

EXPLAIN NURSING CARE FOR NONNURSING MOTHERS

If the mother is not nursing her baby and her breasts are full, it is important to have the breasts adequately supported with a properly fitted brassiere or a breast binder. Ice packs to each breast for an hour three or four times a day can reduce discomfort while discouraging lactation. Also, analgesics are somctimes prescribed to reduce discomfort. It is important that the woman not remove any breast milk by manual expression because this encourages further milk production. Occasionally, milk may reappear in the breasts in 10 to 12 days, and the same comfort measures are indicated.

TACE, DELADUMONE, AND PARLODEL

If a woman chooses not to breast-feed her baby, the physician may prescribe hormones to suppress the milk supply. Oral hormone medications used in the first 2 or 3 days are diethylstilbestrol, quinestrol, and chlorotrianisene (Tace). Deladumone is a long-acting hormone combination given intramuscularly immediately before delivery. These hormones are estrogen-androgen combinations or oral progestins, estrogens, or androgens alone. It is believed that these hormones discourage the release of prolactin by the pituitary gland. Several estrogens that have been used to suppress lactation have been shown to predispose to venous thrombosis and thromboembolism. Because there is much debate over the long-term effects of these hormones, their use varies greatly. These hormones do not help the engorgement that sometimes occurs 10 to 12 days postpartum. Before these drugs are given, the woman should be informed of their potential side effects, and her informed consent should be obtained.

Lactation also may be suppressed by bromocryptine mesylate (Parlodel). Bromocriptine is a dopamine receptor agonist. It stimulates the production of a prolactin inhibitory factor, which inhibits the secretion of prolactin and thus suppresses lactation. The recommended duration of treatment is by oral administration for 2 to 3 weeks, and the drug is costly. Common side effects include nasal congestion, headache, and nausea (all occur occasionally).

MENSTRUATION AND OVULATION

WHEN MENSTRUATION USUALLY REAPPEARS

When a woman does not breast-feed, any secretion of milk usually stops in 10 to 14 days and menstrual periods usually return in 6 to 8 weeks. Ovulation may occur in this time period as well. For breast-feeding mothers, menstruation may not return until the third or fourth month postpartum or until breast-feeding is stopped. The continued production of prolactin may inhibit the release of the follicle-stimulating hormone (FSH) from the pituitary gland, thus delaying ovulation. However, because the woman may ovulate while she is breast-feeding even though she is not menstruating, breast-feeding cannot be counted on as a contraceptive. If pregnancy is not desired, some form of birth control should be used.

Sexual intercourse can be resumed after the lochia has stopped, the perineum is healed, and the woman and her partner feel ready once again. If the woman is breast-feeding, there can be a milk let-down with sexual activity and particularly with orgasm. This may be perceived as erotic by some couples and as objectionable by others. Because of lowered estrogen levels, the woman may find that her vagina does not lubricate as well as usual, and for comfortable intercourse, some extra lubricant jelly may be helpful. Some women report experiencing feelings of sexual arousal when breast-feeding. The couple needs explanations of these changes and opportunities to discuss their feelings.

DISCUSS TIME FOR RESUMPTION OF VAGINAL INTERCOURSE POSTPARTUM

SEXUAL FEELINGS MOTHER MAY EXPERIENCE WHEN NURSING

TEACHING

The postpartum period is a prime time to teach the mother how to care for herself and the baby. The father and other family members should be included in this teaching whenever possible. Because most new mothers are not sick and require relatively little physical care, the nurse can devote a lot of time to teaching. The postpartum period can be a very rewarding time for both the family and the nurse who accepts this challenge of maternity nursing. The rewards of this teaching can extend for a lifetime.

The nurse can teach individually while providing the mother-baby care discussed in this unit. In addition, group discussions and even classes can be organized in the hospital. All mothers need to be included in teaching even though primiparas usually have the greatest need. It may be several years since a woman had a baby, or she may have a boy this time instead of a girl. When teaching, first find out what the woman already knows and begin at that point.

DEVELOP A PLAN OF PERSONAL HYGIENE FOR A NEW MOTHER

Anticipatory guidance

When teaching, it is always important to help the mother understand what she can expect in the 6-week postpartum period. During this "anticipatory guidance," stress the importance of adequate rest to maintain and build up her strength. Morning and afternoon rest periods and 8 hours of sleep at night are very helpful. It may be necessary for her to have help with the work at home or to have help in planning how she will manage so that she will not overwork. Referrals to public health nursing or home care may be necessary, or hospital staff nurses can phone and visit the new family in their home in the first few weeks of the baby's life. This follow-up checks not only on the recovery of the mother but also on the adaptation and development of the baby. Nursing follow-up also provides an opportunity to discuss feelings and any problems.

An appointment with the physician or midwife is usually recommended for 2 to 6 weeks postpartum. At this time, the pelvic organs and breasts are checked for any abnormalities.

Family planning

An important part of teaching in the postpartum period is teaching the woman and her mate about family planning methods. (A summary of the various birth control methods is given in Table 10-2.) As the population of the world increases rapidly, there has been a deepening concern about the quality of life. In an advanced society such as ours, birth control is often seen as enhancing family life. Effectiveness and safety are the major considerations in choosing a method of birth control. For a birth control method to be optimally effective, the method should be acceptable to both partners. In the postpartum period, the nurse can initiate discussion with both partners concerning all available methods, their action, description, advantages, and disadvantages. Figure 10-13 illustrates methods of contraception. Figure 10-14 shows a basal temperature record needed for the

TEMPORARY METHODS OF BIRTH CONTROL

Table 10-2. Birth control methods

Method	Description	How it works	Advantages	Disadvantages
Oral contraceptives	Oral tablet containing synthetic hormones, estrogen, and progesterone. Usually taken on 20 consecutive days beginning 5 days after menstruation starts. (Exact instructions vary according to type of pill given.) Must be prescribed.	Prevents release of egg from ovary Progestin-only tablet ("mini-pill") creates unfavorable environment for conception.	Virtually 100% effective when taken according to instructions. Convenient and allows for spontaneity in lovemaking. Reversible; can stop if pregnancy desired.	Not safe for everyone. Possible side effects include nausea, weight gain, headache, depression, blood and circulatory problems (high blood pressure and blood clots). Should be discontinued 3 months before a pregnancy to avoid potential birth defects.
Intrauterine device (IUD)	Small objects (coils, rings, loops, bows), usually of plastic, sometimes wrapped with fine copper wire, inserted into the uterus by physician or nurse-practitioner.	Action not completely known, but theory is that it prevents implantation of the fertilized egg in walls of uterus.	Highly effective. Allows for spontaneity in lovemaking. Can be removed if pregnancy is desired. Usually tolerated well by multiparous women.	May be expelled spontaneously without woman's knowledge. Possible side effects: pain, bleeding, vaginal discharge, pelvic inflammatory disease (PID) and subsequent increased chance of infertility. IUD may perforate wall of uterus. Insertion is difficult in nulliparas. Most IUDs withdrawn from sale in 1986.
Diaphragm	Circular rubber device placed over cervix before intercourse; spermicidal jelly or cream placed inside diaphragm to immobilize and kill sperm. Must be fitted by physician or nurse-practitioner.	Acts as a receptical for spermicidal preparations that immobilize and kill sperm.	Highly effective if used properly. Very safe; no systemic effects. When no longer used, pregnancy can occur if desired.	Requires highly motivated couple. Some people may find it somewhat "messy" to use. Could be displaced during intercourse. Must be removed, cleaned, and reapplied every 24 hours.
Contraceptive foams, creams, and suppositories	Chemicals kill or immobilize sperm. Inserted into vagina before intercourse.	Coat vaginal surfaces and cervical opening and destroy sperm. Suppositories must be inserted in sufficient time to melt before intercourse. Foams also produce mechanical barrier around cervix.	Easy to use. No prescription needed. No harmful side effects. No long-term effects on ability to conceive.	Risks of pregnancy higher than with pill or IUD. Must be used before each act of intercourse. Some couples find this method "messy."
Cervical cap	A small barrier device that can be filled with spermicidal agent and placed snugly over the cervix. Typically made of soft, pliable rubber or plastic.	Cap is applied to the exterior of the cervix. Can be left in place up to 7 days provided it retains contraceptive cream.	Highly effective. Nonhormonal and noninvasive. Does not require daily insertion. Little leakage of spermicide.	Not all women can be safely fitted at present. An extensive learning program is required for the user. May cause an undesirable odor.
Contraceptive sponge	2-inch circular sponge, made of soft polyurethane, presaturated with a spermicide.	Sponge is moistened with water, folded, and inserted into the vagina.	Does not require fitting. Spermicide is self-contained in the sponge and released during the wear time.	Possibility that the absorbency of sponge could lead to toxic shock syndrome if used during menstruation.

Condom	Thin rubber sheath placed over erect penis before intercourse.	Acts as mechanical barrier preventing sperm from entering vagina. May be used with vaginal creams or jellies for added protection.	No prescription needed. Easy to use. Inexpensive. Provides protection against venereal diseases and common vaginal infections. Completely reversible form of contraception.	May tear or slip off during intercourse. May diminish pleasurable sensations.
Rhythm (calendar-basal body temperature method)	Woman has intercourse only during her "safe" periods, which never include approximately 3 days before and 3 days after ovulation.	By avoiding intercourse during the fertile period. Woman takes her temperature every morning before rising to establish pattern of ovulation. Basal body temperature rises following ovulation and stays up until menstruation.	Accepted by the Catholic church. No physical side effects.	Not very reliable if menstrual cycles are irregular. Restriction of sexual relations could cause tension in the couple relationship.
Coitus interruptus (withdrawal)	Man withdraws penis from vagina before ejaculation occurs.	Semen does not enter vagina.	Probably better than nothing.	Requires great self-control. Sperm can be present in lubricating fluid of male before ejaculation. Can limit sexual gratification for both partners.
Ovulation method (cervical mucus method)	Basic changes in cervical mucus occur prior to ovulation.	Slippery mucus usually discharged from vagina 3 days before ovulation; following ovulation mucus becomes sticky.	No mechanical devices needed. Helps woman "tune into" her body.	Requires high level of motivation.
Sterilization Tubal ligation (female)	Surgical procedure, cutting and tying off or placing a clip on the fallopian tubes. Hospital procedure under anesthesia.	Ovum cannot get to uterus for fertilization.	Almost 100% effective. No need to use other methods of contraception.	Risk of anesthesia complications and infections (as with all surgery). Permanent in most cases.
Vasectomy (male)	Surgical procedure involving cutting and tying off tubes (vas deferens) that carry sperm to semen. Minor surgical procedure performed in doctor's office under local anesthesia.	Sperm absorbed by body rather than released.	Almost 100% effective. No deaths have been reported following vasectomy. Possible to store sperm in frozen semen banks preserving viable sperm of men who have had vasectomies.	Permanent in most cases.

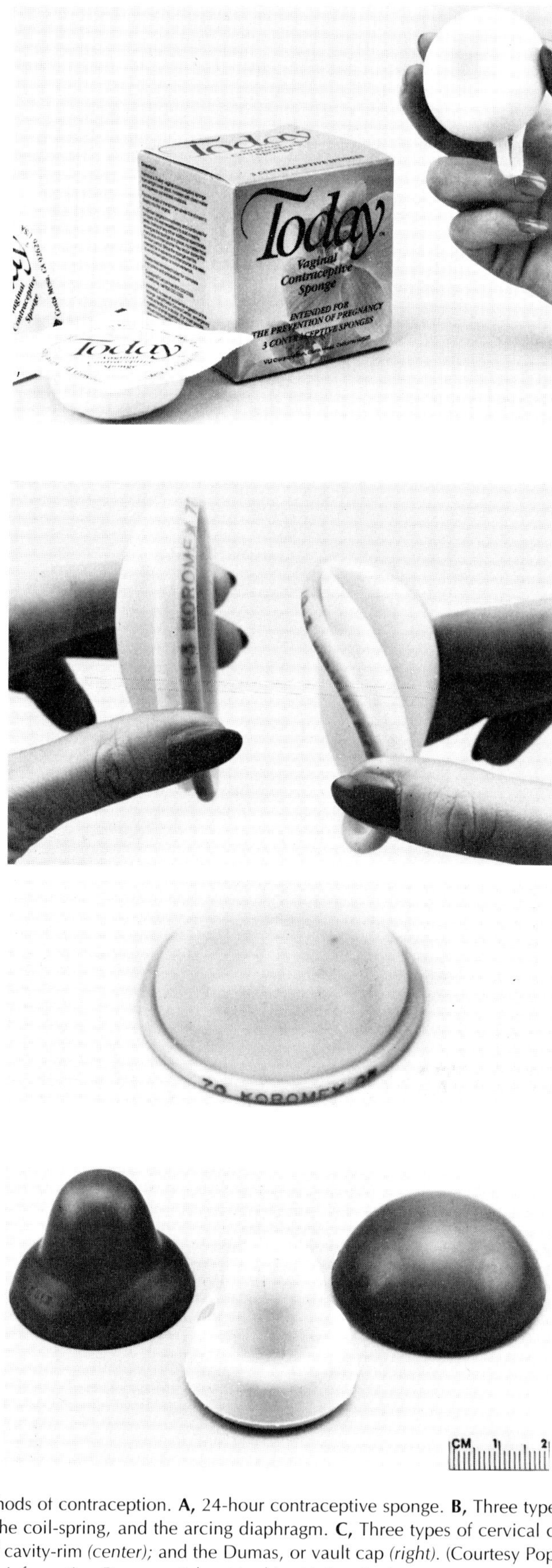

Fig. 10-13. Methods of contraception. **A,** 24-hour contraceptive sponge. **B,** Three types of diaphragm: the flat-spring, the coil-spring, and the arcing diaphragm. **C,** Three types of cervical caps: the Vimule *(left);* the Prentif cavity-rim *(center);* and the Dumas, or vault cap *(right).* (Courtesy Population Reports, H-7, Population Information Program, Johns Hopkins University.)

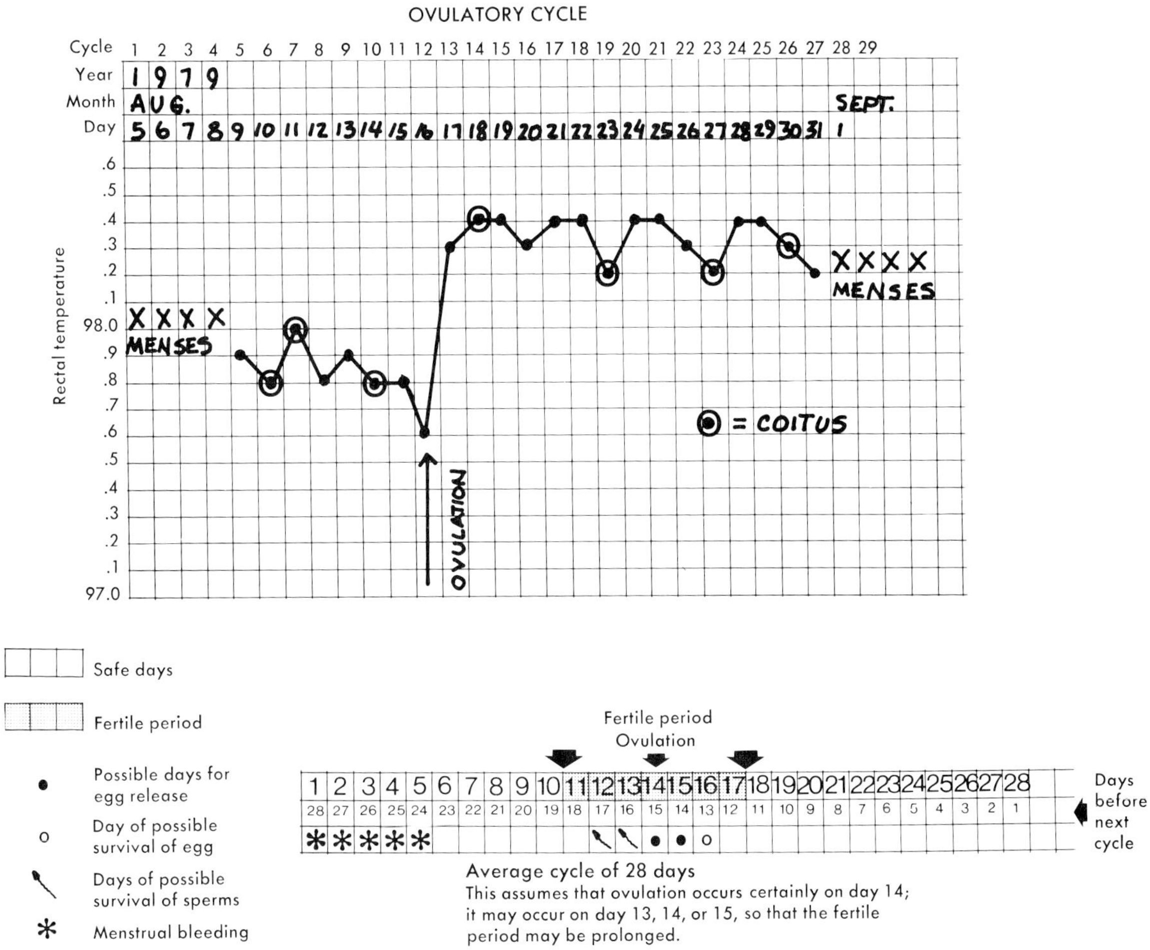

Fig. 10-14. Basal temperature method.

rhythm or calendar basal body temperature method. Figure 10-15 illustrates the placement of the diaphragm. Figure 10-16 illustrates the placement of a cervical cap.

Dangers of birth control methods. The intrauterine device (IUD), oral contraceptives, sterilization procedures (tubal ligations), and abortion all carry a definite risk of illness or death. The IUD can cause serious increased menstrual bleeding, severe and chronic cramping, and pelvic infections, many of which result in permanent sterility. The IUD user particularly at risk for developing pelvic inflammatory disease (PID) is young, nulliparous, sexually active, and from the lower socioeconomic classes. Women using IUDs should be warned to be alert for and promptly report the following symptoms: abnormal vaginal discharge, fever, abdominal or pelvic pain, new and different menstrual problems, and painful intercourse (dyspareunia). Most IUDs were withdrawn from sale in the U.S. in 1986.

Oral contraceptives should not ordinarily be prescribed for women with liver disease or diabetes or with a history of thrombophlebitis, hypertension, or suspected estrogen-dependent malignancies. Pregnancy is also a contraindication, of course. The main problem with oral contraceptives is that they increase the risk of blood clotting within the arteries and veins. Women should be carefully screened to determine their risks for complications before contraceptive pills are prescribed. In addition, periodic follow-up to detect any developing problems is essential.

As with all surgery, there is a risk of complications from anesthesia and infection with

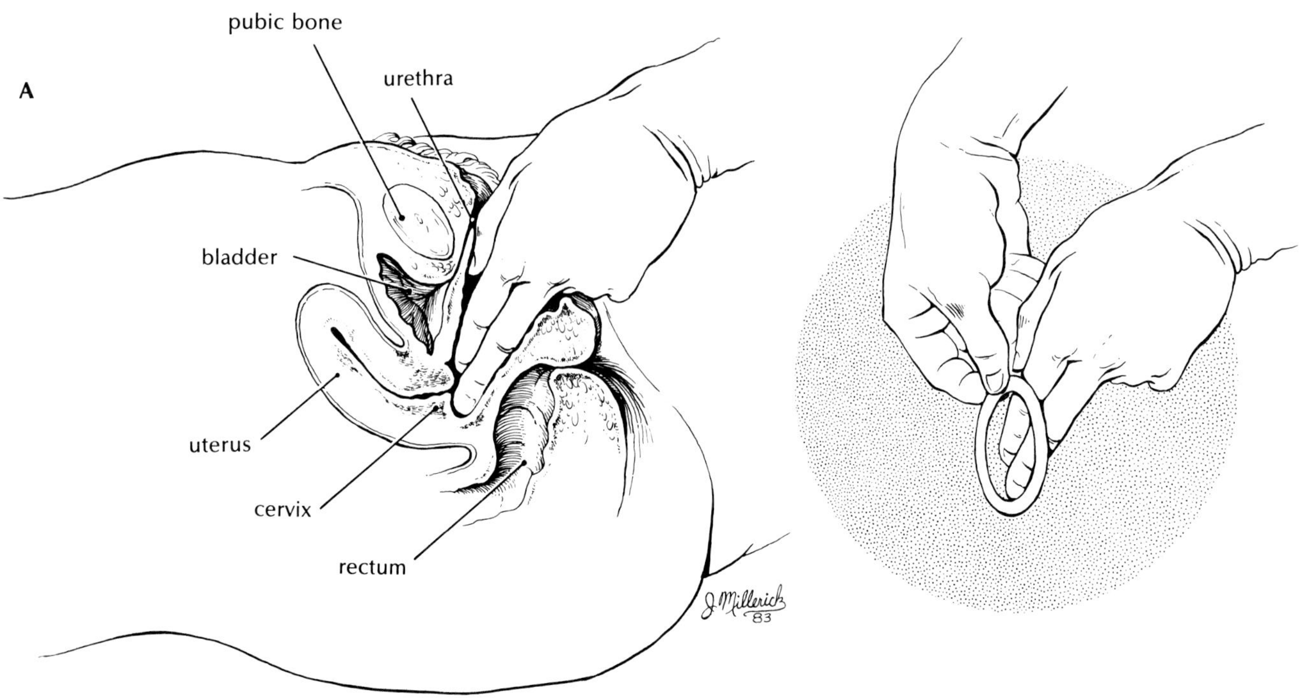

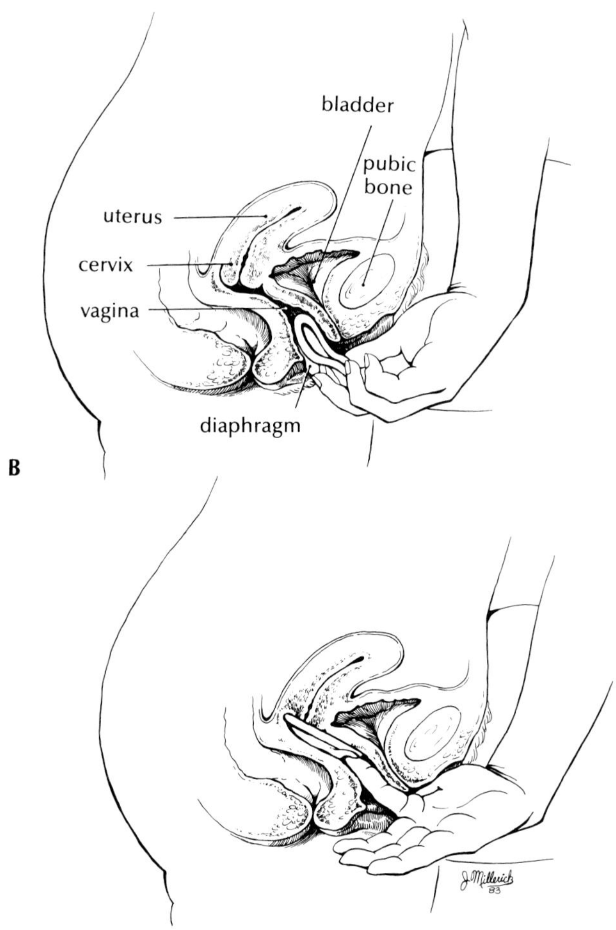

Fig. 10-15. A, Fitting a diaphragm. **B,** Inserting a diaphragm. (Courtesy Population Reports, H-7, Population Information Program, Johns Hopkins University.)

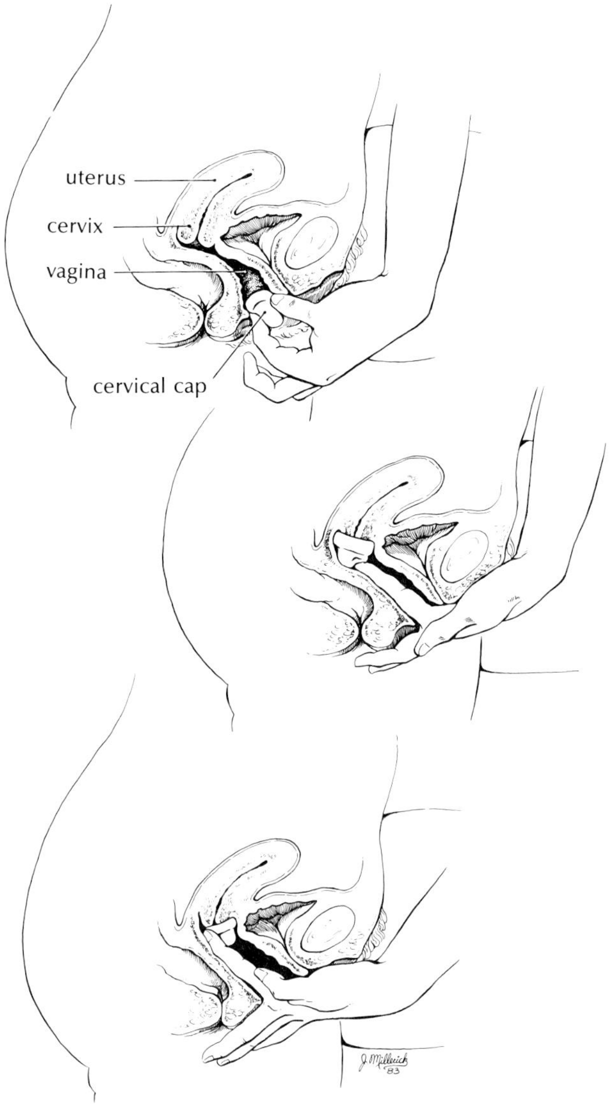

Fig. 10-16. Inserting a cervical cap. (Courtesy Population Reports, H-7, Population Information Program, Johns Hopkins University.)

both sterilization (tubal ligation) and abortion. Additional risks associated with abortion depend on the type of procedure as well as the length of gestation and general health of the woman. In general, morbidity and mortality risks increase after the twelfth week of gestation. Systemic reactions with prostaglandins include nausea, vomiting, and diarrhea. With saline injection, there is a risk of intravascular injection, peritoneal spill of the saline, bladder injection, and water intoxification resulting from the antidiuretic effect of the oxytocic drug used intravenously. With both saline and prostaglandin injections there is a risk of retention of the placenta and subsequent infection.

Induced abortion. Removal of the products of conception from the uterus before the fetus is able to survive at the choice of the woman is termed an induced abortion. Abortion raises the fundamental question about the extent to which the state may interfere with an individual's decision regarding one's own body. Abortion itself is probably older than written history.

METHODS OF ABORTION

The accepted procedures for performing an abortion are suction curettage, dilation and evacuation using vacuum aspiration, amniocentesis and injection of a salt solution or prostaglandins into the amniotic sac, and hysterotomy. Suction curettage is the preferred technique for abortion of pregnancies up to 12 weeks of gestation. Under anesthesia (usually paracervical block with intravenous sedation), the cervix is dilated and a vacuum tip is inserted into the uterus. The intense suction at the opening of the cannula separates the products of conception, which are then drawn out through the connecting tubing. The average time for the procedure is 10 minutes.

In the period between the twelfth and sixteenth weeks of pregnancy, the cervix can be dilated using metal dilators or laminaria (dried sterilized seaweed that expands on contact with moisture) inserted into the cervix 18 to 24 hours before the abortion. Under anesthesia (usually paracervical block with intravenous sedation), vacuum aspiration of the uterine contents is followed by scraping with a sharp curette for any missed fragments.

Starting at the sixteenth week of pregnancy amniocentesis and amnioinfusion procedures are recommended. With saline solution the physician inserts a needle into the intra-amniotic sac, withdraws 200 milliliters of amniotic fluid, and injects 200 milliliters of hypertonic salt solution. Uterine contractions usually begin about 12 hours after the salt solution is injected. In 12 to 24 hours the abortion is completed with the passage of the products of conception. Labor is assisted by a continuous intravenous drip containing oxytocin. The hypertonic saline solution causes water to diffuse into the amniotic sac from surrounding fetal and placental tissues, resulting in fetal death. With prostaglandin injection neither aspiration nor amniotic fluid is necessary; intravenous administration of oxytocin is usually not necessary. The physician injects prostaglandin into the amniotic sac, and contractions usually begin in 30 minutes. Within 24 hours the abortion is completed by the passage of the products of conception. Prostaglandin suppositories can also be inserted into the posterior vaginal fornix to cause abortion.

Hysterotomy is performed under spinal or general anesthesia and is comparable to a cesarean delivery. Hysterotomy is rarely performed in the United States.

Nursing support

Nurses whose religious, moral, or ethical beliefs do not condone abortion should not be required to care for women undergoing abortion. However, when giving nursing care to these women the primary objective is to give high-quality nursing care, and the nurse must take an active role. Remember that the woman is goal oriented—termination of the pregnancy. The nurse will have to take the initiative in making assessments and acting on them. Give the woman a realistic description of the procedure, the hospital surroundings, and the hospital stay. Touching and supportive care are vital. Before discharge, the woman needs to understand signs and symptoms of possible complications and the importance of follow-up care. Also, she may want to discuss contraceptive methods and their use. Often the questions the nurse asks help the woman to face reality. As an example: "Now that your abortion is over, what are you planning to do for contraception?" Remember also that accepting a woman's values and decisions does not mean you must agree with them. Try to understand and be caring. In abortion care nurses can make a unique contribution to the total care of women.

SUMMARY

In this unit we have discussed the postpartum family and briefly looked at the subject of family planning. For the first time in this book we have deviated from concern for saving lives to the issue of abortion (terminating life). This is a difficult subject for maternity personnel whose energies are often concentrated on preserving life at any cost. In the next unit, we will explore complications of the postpartum period.

BIBLIOGRAPHY

Affonso, D.D., and Domino, G.: Postpartum depression: a review, Birth **11**(4):231-235, 1984.

Arizmandi, T.G., and Affonso, D.D.: Research on psychosocial factors and postpartum depression: a critique, Birth **11**(4):237-240, 1984.

Auerbach, K.G.: Employed breastfeeding mothers: problems they encounter, Birth **11**(1):17-20, 1984.

Canavan, P.A., and Lewis, C.A.: The cervical cap: an alternative contraceptive, JOGN Nurs. **10**(4):271-273, 1981.

Cannon, R.B.: The development of maternal touch during early mother-infant interaction, JOGN Nurs. **6**(2):28-33, 1977.

Davis, J.E.: Vasectomy, Am. J. Nurs. **72**(3):509-513, 1972.

Deibel, P.: Natural family planning: different methods, MCN **3**(3):171-177, 1978.

Donaldson, N.E.: Fourth trimester follow-up, Am. J. Nurs. **77**(7):1176-1178, 1977.

Ellis, D.J., and Hewat, R.J.: Mother's postpartum perceptions of spousal relationships, JOGN Nurs. **14**(2):140-146, 1985.

Erickson, M.P.: Trends in assessing the newborn and his parents, MCN **3**(2):99-103, 1978.

FDA Drug Bulletin, vol. 8, no. 3, May-July 1978.

Gaginella, T.S.: Drugs and the nursing mother → infant, U.S. Pharm. **3**(3):40-50, March 1978.

Julick, E.E.: Informational correlates of successful breast-feeding, MCN **7**(6):370-375, 1982.

Ketter, D.E., and Shelton, B.J.: In-hospital exercises for the postpartal woman, MCN **8**(2):120-124, 1983.

Klaus, M.H., and Kennell, J.H.: Parent-infant bonding, ed. 2, St. Louis, 1982, The C.V. Mosby Co.

Ludington-Hoe, S.M.: Postpartum: development of maternicity, Am. J. Nurs. **77**(7):1171-1174, 1977.

Malinowski, J.: Bladder assessment in the postpartum patient, JOGN Nurs. **4**:14-16, July, 1978.

Marmet, C., and Shell, E.: Training neonates to suck correctly, MCN 9(6):401-407, 1984.

McBryde, A.: Compulsory rooming-in in the ward and private newborn service at Duke Hospital, J.A.M.A. **145**(9):625-628, 1951.

Mercer, R.T.: Postpartum: illness and acquaintance—attachment process, Am. J. Nurs. **77**(7):1174-1178, 1977.

Moore, M.L.: Realities in childbearing, ed. 2, Philadelphia, 1983, W.B. Saunders Co.

Petrick, J.M.: Postpartum depression identification of high-risk mothers, JOGN Nurs. **13**(1):37-40, 1984.

Population Reports: Law and policy, Series E, no. 3, March 1976; Pregnancy termination, Series F, no. 5, Sept. 1976; Prostaglandins, Series G, no. 7, Sept. 1976, Washington, D.C., The George Washington University Medical Center, Department of Medication and Public Affairs.

Rahwan, R.G.: Pharmacological approaches to birth control: contraceptives, interceptives, abortifacients, U.S. Pharm. **2**(10):31-42, Oct. 1977.

Rubin, R.: Cognitive style in pregnancy, Am. J. Nurs. **70**(3):502-508, 1970.

Rubin, R.: Maternal identity and the maternal experience, New York, 1984, Springer Publishing Co.

Schlegel, A.M.: Observations on breast-feeding technique: facts and fallacies, MCN **8**(3):204-208, 1983.

Sheehan, F.: Assessing postpartum adjustment: a pilot study, JOGN Nurs. **10**(1):19-23, 1981.

Stranik, M.K., and Hogberg, B.L.L.: Transition into parenthood, Am. J. Nurs. **89**:90-93, 1979.

Tanis, J.L.: Issues in contraception: recognizing the reasons for contraceptive non-use and abuse, MCN 2(6):364-369, 1977.

Wiedenbach, E.: Family-centered maternity nursing, ed. 2, New York, 1977, G.P. Putnam's Sons.

DEFINITIONS

Define the following terms:

alveoli	lochia alba
anticipatory guidance	lochia rubra
colostrum	lochia serosa
engorgement	mastitis
Homans' sign	mother-baby nursing
hypertonic	PID
induced abortion	prolactin
involution	prostaglandin
lactation	puerperium
leukocytosis	rooming-in
"let-down reflex"	rooting reflex
	sibling

LEARNING ACTIVITIES AND EXPERIENCES

1. Group discussions.
2. Visit local agencies concerned with family planning. Report on their facilities, policies, and fees charged.
3. View audiovisual aids and discuss.

ENRICHMENT/IN-DEPTH STUDY

1. If there is a postpartum support group in your community, seek permission to visit the group.
2. Interview new parents. Determine if caring for a new baby is what they thought it would be.
3. You might ask a new mother or new father to cut pictures out of a magazine depicting the baby they thought they would have ("before") and pictures descriptive of their new baby ("after"). Compare the "before" and "after" and discuss.

SELF-ASSESSMENT

1. Match Column A with Column B.

Column A	Column B
_____1. "taking-in" phase	a. regains control over body
_____2. "taking-hold" phase	b. establishes new maternal role patterns
_____3. "letting-go" phase	c. passive and dependent

For questions 2 through 12, choose the best answers and indicate your choice by circling the answer.

2. What would you suggest for a woman whose episiotomy hurts her?
   a. sitz baths
   b. reassurance
   c. heat lamp
   d. all of above
3. "Afterpains" are caused by:
   a. contractions of the uterus as it gets smaller again
   b. drugs
   c. mental depression
4. Comfort measures for hemorrhoids include:
   a. warm sitz baths
   b. walking
   c. cold witch hazel compresses
   d. elevating buttocks on several pillows

   Answer (circle one). 1. a and b
   2. a, b, and d
   3. b
   4. a, c, and d
5. To re-establish proper bowel functioning postpartum, the physician may order:
   a. stool softeners
   b. laxatives
   c. enemas
   d. vitamins

   Answer (circle one): 1. a and d
   2. all of the above
   3. a, b, and c
6. Immediate weight loss of the mother after delivery is:
   a. 20 pounds
   b. 13 pounds
   c. 7 pounds
7. The "let-down reflex" is involuntary and is stimulated by:
   a. hearing the baby cry
   b. anticipation of a feeding
   c. a and b
8. Breast engorgement usually occurs by
   a. 1 week
   b. 3 to 4 days
   c. 10 days

9. Menstruation usually reappears in the nonnursing mother:
   a. 2 weeks postpartum
   b. 4 months postpartum
   c. 6 to 8 weeks postpartum
10. Menstruation usually reappears in the breast-feeding mother:
   a. 4 weeks postpartum
   b. 3 to 4 months postpartum or when she stops breast-feeding
   c. 2 weeks postpartum
11. The clean perineal pad is applied from:
   a. back to front
   b. side to side
   c. front to back
12. Douching is contraindicated postpartum until:
   a. the lochia stops
   b. the 6 week check-up
   c. 6 months postpartum
13. Match Column A with Column B. Each item in Column B may be used once or more than once.

	Column A	Column B
_____	1. normal uterine and vaginal discharge postpartum	a. uterus
_____	2. goes through three stages	b. lochia
_____	3. involutes in the puerperium	c. urinary system
_____	4. by tenth postpartum day should be no longer palpable	d. perineum
_____	5. soothing measures include warm sitz baths	e. lochia rubra
_____	6. should be kept clean and dry	f. lochia serosa
_____	7. overdistention of bladder can occur	g. lochia alba
_____	8. significant diuresis early postpartum	
_____	9. brownish in color	
_____	10. red and bloody	
_____	11. yellowish white	

14. The new mother's pulse may be _____ or _____ beats per minute on the first and second days postpartum.
15. A normal postpartum temperature is _____.
16. Blood pressure may _____ slightly in the postpartum period.
17. Respiration may be _____ in the postpartum period.
18. Parent-infant attachment is influenced by the infant's ____________________.
19. As men adjust to their role as father, they also go through phases. In the adjustment phase men are aware of the ____________________ of their new family. In the acceptance phase men have to ____________________ the intense intimate relationship between the mother and ____________________.
20. What is the difference between sterilization and contraception?
____
____
____
____.

For questions 21 and 22, circle the best answer.

21. Disadvantages of the IUD include:
   a. depression

b. pelvic inflammatory disease
c. swelling of uterus

22. Use of the pill is contraindicated for women who:
    a. have a family history of Parkinson's disease
    b. have never delivered a baby
    c. have a history of blood clotting problems

UNIT XI
The postpartum family with complications

GOALS

This unit is designed to provide the reader with information that will:

□ promote awareness of deviations from normal in the postpartum period.
□ explore the role of support persons for grieving families.

STUDENT OBJECTIVES

After studying this unit, you should be able to:

1. Identify the woman at risk for developing a postpartum infection.
2. Explain the bonding needs of a mother who has been separated from her baby because of a postpartum infection.
3. Explain how a nurse can detect a uterus that is not involuting properly.
4. List the observations a nurse would make when caring for a woman following a cesarean birth.
5. Design a plan to meet the bonding needs of parents who have been separated from their babies immediately after birth.
6. In lay terms, describe how you would counsel the family concerning the expectations for both physical and emotional recovery following a cesarean birth.
7. Formulate a plan of support for a new family whose baby (1) is dead or (2) has a birth defect.

POSTPARTUM HEMORRHAGE

As emphasized in Unit VIII, the uterus must be kept firm to minimize bleeding. Because of the increased blood supply during pregnancy, a woman can lose from 250 to 350 milliliters of blood at birth without undesirable effects. However, excessive bleeding contributes to postpartum morbidity and can lead to maternal death, the leading cause of which is hemorrhage. Therefore, very careful and close evaluation of the uterine fundus height, vital signs, and amount of vaginal bleeding postpartum is extremely important.

Postpartum hemorrhage is defined as blood loss of 500 milliliters or more following separation and expulsion of the placenta. When the bleeding occurs within the first 24 hours following birth, it is considered *early* postpartum hemorrhage. *Late* postpartum hemorrhage occurs 24 hours to 6 weeks following delivery.

DIFFERENTIATE BETWEEN EARLY AND LATE POSTPARTUM HEMORRHAGE

Causes of early postpartum hemorrhage

The causes of early postpartum hemorrhage are (1) uterine atony, (2) placental complications (placenta accreta or retained placenta), (3) lacerations and hematoma of the genital tract, (4) ruptured uterus, and (5) inversion of the uterus. Early postpartum hemorrhage occurs in 2% to 5% of new mothers.

Uterine atony. In *uterine atony* the uterus does not have good muscle tone and consequently relaxes. Because the large blood vessels are not compressed by tight uterine muscle fibers, the blood vessels bleed freely. Common causes of uterine atony include prolonged labor, an overdistended uterus (multiple pregnancy, polyhydramnios), a uterus displaced by a full bladder, and general anesthesia. As discussed in Unit VIII, treatment of uterine atony is vigorous (but not rough) massage of the relaxed and enlarged fundus, firm expression of accumulated blood clots, and administration of oxytocics over an extended period.

Placental complications. Retention of placental fragments is also a common cause of delayed or late postpartum hemorrhage. Dilation and curettage (D & C) may have to be done to remove the placental fragments.

Lacerations and hematoma. If the uterus is firm at the umbilicus and in the midline but bright red bleeding persists, a laceration is probably the cause. When a new mother with a normal temperature complains of severe perineal or pelvic pain that is not relieved by analgesics, suspect a vaginal or retroperitoneal *hematoma.* Small hematomas can be watched to be sure they are not enlarging. Large hematomas may be evacuated through an incision in the vaginal wall.

RECOGNIZE SIGNS AND SYMPTOMS OF RUPTURED UTERUS

Ruptured uterus. The signs and symptoms of a *ruptured uterus* include localized abdominal pain and tenderness, a tearing feeling, and then hypovolemic shock. The causes of uterine rupture include a difficult vaginal delivery, a weak uterine operative scar, injudicious use of oxytocin, an obstructed labor, and residual damage from past trauma to the uterus. Emergency surgery to suture the laceration and blood replacement are essential. A hysterectomy may have to be done when a uterus has ruptured.

Inversion. *Inversion* of the uterus occurs when the uterus is turned inside out. This may be caused by pulling on the umbilical cord before the placenta is separated or by extreme pushing on the uterine fundus in an attempt to assist the delivery. Should this happen, the uterus is replaced manually and oxytocic drugs are given to cause it to contract. Antibiotics are also given to prevent infection. If manual replacement of the uterus is inadequate, surgery may be necessary to reposition or remove the uterus.

Causes of late postpartum hemorrhage

Late postpartum hemorrhage is less common than early hemorrhage. It occurs in 0.1% to 1.0% of new mothers. Causes of late postpartum hemorrhage are retained placenta or membranes, subinvolution of the uterus, and *endometritis* (infection of the uterine lining).

SUBINVOLUTION

Subinvolution is a failure of the uterus to return to its normal size following delivery. Two common causes are retention of pieces of placenta and infection of the endometrium *(endometritis).*

DETECTING THAT UTERUS IS NOT INVOLUTING PROPERLY

When checking the height of the uterine fundus and the firmness of the uterus daily, the nurse can detect a uterus that is not involuting properly. In addition to finding the uterus too large for the appropriate day postpartum, the nurse will notice the lochia to be more profuse and redder than it should be. Once lochia rubra is gone, it should not return.

If late postpartum hemorrhage occurs while the new mother is still hospitalized, treatment may include oxytocin, intravenous fluids, and curettage. Antibiotics are also prescribed for infection.

If the mother is at home and bleeding is minimal, bed rest and an oral oxytocic such as methylergonovine maleate (Methergine) may resolve the bleeding. Once again, antibiotics will be prescribed if there is evidence of infection. If the mother is at home and bleeding is heavy, she will be readmitted to the hospital and treated with intravenous fluids, oxytocin, curettage, and antibiotics. Mother-baby care to minimize separation is essential if the mother has to be readmitted to the hospital.

Nursing care

Blood loss of over 1000 milliliters can lead to severe postpartum infection, extensive pelvic thrombophlebitis, and hypovolemic shock with its side effects. The signs of shock are a drop in blood pressure, pallor, cold clammy skin, an increased pulse rate (rapid and weak), anxiety, apprehension, and air hunger.

In severe postpartum hemorrhage, transfusions may be given to replace blood lost, and antibiotics are given to prevent infection. In addition to monitoring the administration of blood, the nurse should keep close records of the woman's intake and output and blood loss. Perineal pad counts and weights (1 gram = 1 cubic centimeter) are helpful in measuring blood loss. If there is an adequate volume of circulating blood, the urinary output should be from 30 to 60 milliliters per hour (monitored with a Foley's catheter). Administration of oxygen and placement of the woman in a modified Trendelenburg's position may also be instituted.

Postpartum hemorrhage is frightening to the woman and her family, and they need constant support. The nurse should explain to the woman the necessity for uterine massage, since it can be very painful. It is important that the family be continually informed of what is happening at the same time they are being reassured.

DISSEMINATED INTRAVASCULAR COAGULATION

NAME AT LEAST FOUR OBSTETRICAL COMPLICATIONS THAT MAY CAUSE DISSEMINATED INTRAVASCULAR COAGULATION (DIC)

Deficiencies in the blood clotting mechanisms can complicate postpartum hemorrhage. When the elements necessary for homeostasis are depleted, the process is referred to as disseminated intravascular coagulation (DIC). Obstetrical complications that may cause a DIC are abruptio placentae, pre-eclampsia, eclampsia, incomplete abortion, septic abortion, induced saline abortion, prolonged retention of a dead fetus, amniotic fluid embolism, and sepsis.

DIC results when some factor (massive tissue injury, cell lysis, bacteremia, etc.) triggers the coagulation cascade. This uses up fibrinogen. Thus, low fibrinogen levels are an effect, not a cause. The woman's fibrinogen levels can be checked to determine if her clotting mechanism is abnormal. Treatment focuses on resolving the underlying cause. After the source of the DIC condition is removed, further intervention is usually unnecessary. However, when further intervention is necessary, administration of blood and blood products is considered. In rare cases, the administration of heparin is considered. Heparin therapy works by enhancing the effects of antithrombin III, a protein that combines with thrombin to break it down.

Nursing care

Closely monitoring bleeding, measuring and documenting blood loss, and preventing or minimizing blood loss are important facets of nursing care for the woman with DIC. Gentle handling and frequent turning and positioning with pillows will help minimize blood vessel and skin breakdown. Gentle mouth care and medications given intravenously or orally will also decrease unnecessary bruising and hematoma formation. Because these women are at risk of developing shock, they must be monitored closely for the signs of shock. Overwhelming fear and anxiety may be experienced by the woman with DIC as well as by family members. Understanding and accepting these emotional reactions are essential when providing care. The woman and her family need information about DIC and its treatment, plus information on all tests and procedures performed. Whenever possible, involving the woman and her family in nursing care is helpful because it gives them a measure of control over a very threatening situation.

PUERPERAL INFECTION

IDENTIFY SYMPTOMS AND COMMON CAUSES OF POSTPARTUM INFECTION

A *puerperal infection* is any infection of the genital tract during the puerperium. The identification of the puerperal infection is generally accepted to be a temperature elevation to 100.4° F (38° C) or more for any two successive days during the first 10 days postpartum (excluding the first 24 hours). However, because antibiotic therapy can mask symptoms, the criterion of an elevated temperature may no longer be valid for all women.

During labor and delivery the reproductive tract is particularly susceptible to infections. Invasive techniques used in monitoring the progress of labor can introduce new pathogenic organisms into the reproductive tract. Untreated local infections; long, difficult, traumatic labor and delivery; hemorrhage; anemia; and cesarean delivery can also increase the risk of infection. These infections can be caused by bacteria already present in the woman's genital tract or by organisms introduced from other individuals.

Whatever the cause, puerperal infection is a serious postpartum complication. Infections are classified by site. Sites and terms are (1) uterine lining *(endometritis)*, (2) connective tissue around the uterus *(parametritis)*, (3) pelvic cavity *(peritonitis)*, (4) vulva *(vulvitis)*, and (5) vagina *(vaginitis)*. Local infections may invade the lymph channels and the bloodstream, causing *septicemia* (infection of the bloodstream) and thrombophlebitis (inflammation of pelvic or femoral veins).

Causes and symptoms

Common causes are Streptococcus organisms, the colon bacillus Escherichia coli and other coliform bacteria, Staphylococcus and Bacteroides.

Symptoms of local infection include elevated temperature, edema, inflammation, and tenderness of the infected part. Signs and symptoms of a more serious infection include fever above 100.4° F (38° C), chills, rapid pulse, abdominal tenderness or pain, malaise, foul-smelling lochia, and an abnormally large uterus that is not involuting properly *(subinvolution)*. Any of these signs or symptoms should be recorded and reported immediately so that medical treatment can be started.

BONDING NEEDS OF MOTHER SEPARATED FROM BABY

Because many of the organisms that cause these postpartum infections can be dangerous for babies, the mother with a postpartum infection may not be able to take care of her baby until she is well. Careful handwashing and isolation precautions should be carried out by the staff on the maternity unit. The mother will need to be kept informed of her baby's progress, especially when they are separated, to facilitate bonding in spite of the physical separation. If the mother is breast-feeding and has to discontinue the feeding temporarily, manually expressing the milk or pumping the breasts should maintain the milk supply. The presence of infectious organisms and heavy doses of antibiotics would be contraindications to breast-feeding during the acute phase of the infection. The mother may be depressed because of her separation from the baby and will need skillful supportive care and constant reassurance.

Treatment

Treatment includes rest, a high fluid intake, administration of antibiotics to which the causative organisms have been determined to be sensitive, and administration of oxytocics to keep the uterus contracted to prevent spread of bacteria.

Nursing care

DESCRIBE NURSING CARE FOR MOTHER WITH POSTPARTUM INFECTION

Bed rest, increased fluid intake, and elevating the head of the bed to promote uterine drainage are important nursing care measures for the mother with puerperal infection. The nurse should be constantly vigilant for signs of extension of the infection, such as abdominal distention, vomiting, and diarrhea, in addition to the previously listed symptoms.

THROMBOPHLEBITIS

Thrombophlebitis in the postpartum period is usually caused by inflammation in the deep pelvic and femoral veins. If the original source of the infection is infected thrombi at the placental site, the thrombophlebitis may not appear until a week after delivery. The affected leg and thigh may gradually begin to swell and feel tender and warm. Temperature elevation and chills may be noted. Treatment consists of bed rest, application of Ace bandage or support stocking, and elevation of the leg and feet 30 to 45 degrees. Moist or dry heat to the leg may be prescribed. If a portion of a thrombus is dislodged, it is called an *embolus*. An embolus can travel through the bloodstream to the heart and lungs and cause death. Because of the possibility of causing an embolism, the affected leg should never be massaged. Anticoagulants, such as heparin, and antibiotics will be prescribed by the physician.

RECOGNIZE SIGNS AND SYMPTOMS OF THROMBOPHLEBITIS IN POSTPARTUM PERIOD

MASTITIS

Mastitis is an infection of breast tissue, usually by the bacterium Staphylococcus aureus. Predisposing factors are cracked or fissured nipples, bruising of the breast, and clogged ducts. Thorough cleanliness when handling the breasts has already been emphasized. Dirty hands of hospital personnel or the mother can introduce bacteria through a cracked or fissured nipple. Also, a baby who has acquired the Staphylococcus organism in the nursery may carry it to the mother's breasts when nursing. Symptoms of mastitis include fever, malaise, rapid pulse, and pain, tenderness, and swelling of the affected breast. The affected breast may feel very hard and hot to the touch.

Treatment includes rest, breast support, warm wet heat to the affected breast, keeping the breast as empty as possible, analgesics, and antibiotics, usually dicloxacillin or oxacillin. The mother does not have to discontinue breast-feeding, since the causative organism is possibly already in the baby's nose and mouth. In fact, a breast-feeding mother should nurse her baby frequently to keep the infected breast as empty as possible.

DISCUSS BREAST-FEEDING WHEN MOTHER DEVELOPED MASTITIS

CYSTITIS

Cystitis, or inflammation of the bladder, is an occasional postpartum complication. It can be caused by inadequate emptying of the bladder or by trauma from birth or catheterization. The woman should empty her bladder regularly and completely to prevent cystitis. Symptoms of cystitis include painful, frequent emptying of the bladder, pain over the bladder, and a slight temperature elevation (100° to 101° F) (37.8° to 38.3° C). Upon microscopic examination, pus, blood, and bacteria are found in the urine.

Treatment includes an antibiotic drug specific for the causative organisms, forcing fluids, and frequent emptying of the bladder.

RECOGNIZE SIGNS AND SYMPTOMS OF CYSTITIS

CESAREAN BIRTH

Mothers and families who have experienced a cesarean birth as an emergency or after a long and difficult labor have special needs. Mothers and families who undergo planned, scheduled cesareans can sometimes utilize coping mechanisms in preparation for the surgery. Reasons for a cesarean, the basic types, and emergency preparations were discussed in Unit IX. In this unit we will discuss the physical and emotional care needed following a cesarean birth. The term *cesarean birth* should be used rather than *cesarean section* (only grapefruits are sectioned; women give birth). Whenever possible, therefore, the term *cesarean birth* is used in this text.

Physical care

Following cesarean birth the mother's vital signs should be monitored every 15 minutes for the first 2 hours. Perineal pads and abdominal dressings should be checked frequently for bleeding. The mother usually has less lochia than the mother who experi-

CARING FOR WOMAN FOLLOWING CESAREAN BIRTH

enced a vaginal birth because the placenta and decidua have been manually removed. (More than two perineal pads saturated in 1 hour following a cesarean birth indicate excessive bleeding.) The uterus must be kept firm; if it should relax, gentle massage and increasing the amount of intravenous oxytocic may correct the problem. Until the woman is able to ambulate, she should turn, cough, and deep breathe every 2 hours to reduce the chance of respiratory compromise. Careful intake and output recording is essential to be sure the urinary system is functioning adequately. A Foley's catheter may be used for 24 to 48 hours until the bladder resumes normal function.

Because chills are a common postpartum problem, the mother should be covered with a warm blanket.

It is essential to keep the perineum as clean and dry as possible to reduce the risk of pathogenic organisms traveling up the vagina to the uterus. Of course, intravenous fluids must be carefully monitored and regulated; they are usually discontinued when the woman's oral intake is adequate and bowel sounds are present. Medication for pain is prescribed and given judiciously one half-hour prior to activities that increase discomfort.

Early ambulation is important in preventing thrombophlebitis and in facilitating normal bowel and bladder function. Intestinal gas (flatus) is common after abdominal surgery. Ambulation will help to minimize this gas and thus also minimize the pain that accompanies it. Teaching the woman to splint her abdomen by pressing a pillow against it to cushion the operative area and incision will make moving about and coughing less uncomfortable. Rectal suppositories, a rectal tube, or an enema may be prescribed to alleviate the discomfort. After the initial recovery days, most mothers need only oral analgesics for pain and are able to ambulate well.

For the entire hospital stay, in addition to postsurgical care, a daily postpartum assessment is done: checking breast and nipple condition, amount and character of lochia, height and consistency of the fundus, the abdominal incision, and extremities. By the third to fourth day, sutures are removed and the mother is discharged from the hospital.

Breast-feeding

In the first few days following a cesarean birth mothers may need extra help with breast-feeding. It is helpful for the woman to lie on her side in a fetal position, splinting her abdomen with a pillow. In this position she can tuck the baby into her body curve and minimize the stretch and any pressure on her incision. When abdominal discomfort is intense, the mother can use the football hold with the infant while breast-feeding in an upright position. Mother-baby nursing is ideal for this mother because it permits her to feed the baby on demand, thus stimulating lactation. During the first few days the mother will need help lifting, positioning, and changing the baby from one breast to another. The father may be the ideal person to help, if his work and home situations permit him to stay in the hospital.

Separation

BONDING NEEDS OF PARENTS SEPARATED FROM BABIES IMMEDIATELY AFTER BIRTH

If the baby born by cesarean is kept in a special care nursery, the mother and father should go to the nursery to interact with their baby whenever possible. If the baby is to be transferred, the mother should at least touch the baby before transport. Early mother-father-infant contact is very important. Information can be provided about the infant through telephone calls and photos.

Morbidity

Maternal morbidity associated with cesarean birth is higher than that for vaginal delivery, especially for those women who were in labor before the surgery. The main cause of maternal morbidity is postoperative endometritis. Serious infections of the uterus are likely to occur following a long labor with ruptured membranes, numerous vaginal examinations during labor, and postoperative anemia.

Recovery

PHYSICAL AND EMOTIONAL RECOVERY FOLLOWING A CESAREAN BIRTH

It is vital that these new mothers and families understand what to expect in the recovery period. Women who have undergone major abdominal surgery instead of vaginal delivery may have a need to "prove" they are good mothers by doing all the chores and giving all baby care. They need to understand the importance of rest, fluids, and adequate diet for recovery. It will be a minimum of 6 weeks before total recovery. The cesarean mother should refrain from lifting, housework, and driving for several weeks.

Sexual activity can usually be resumed when the vaginal discharge has stopped, the abdominal incision is healed, and the couple is ready. As with vaginal delivery, vaginal lubrication may be inadequate and lubricating jellies or creams will be helpful for comfortable intercourse. The woman's sexual partner may be afraid of hurting her or of rupturing the incision and should be reassured that there is no danger.

Some parents who have experienced cesarean births have organized groups that provide information and help others understand cesarean births (see Appendix B).

Emotional care

When a woman or a couple have prepared for a vaginal birth, their feelings after an unplanned cesarean can range from disappointment, frustration, and guilt to simply relief that the baby is all right. Fathers who have not been present in the operating suite often feel left out and cheated out of an experience for which they had prepared diligently. If the mother has had a general anesthetic and the father was excluded from the cesarean, they may both have difficulty relating to their baby. In fact, studies of abused children show that a proportionately high number were born either prematurely or by cesarean. It is theorized that separation from the newborn in the period immediately following the birth coupled with the surprise and unresolved feelings about the need for a cesarean can interfere with the bonding process. It is not unusual to have a new cesarean-birth mother tell the nurse in the 24 hours following delivery that she is not ready to hold her baby yet.

The nurse can help this new mother by pacing care to help her through the "taking-in" phase. She will have to work through and resolve her own and her partner's feelings about the unplanned surgery. The parents should be encouraged to share their feelings with each other and with the nurse. Reconstructing the events surrounding the labor and delivery will help the couple assimilate them. Talking about the surgery and explaining the surgery and healing process will help the mother accept the bodily changes she is experiencing. The new mother must also adjust to the shock of a surgical incision and the pain that accompanies it.

Unplanned separation from siblings remaining at home can be traumatic for both mother and siblings. Siblings should be encouraged to visit mother and new baby in the first hours and days postpartum. The parents can send Polaroid pictures of the mother and new baby home to the siblings. Daily phone calls and notes or small gifts from mother can all be used to involve the siblings in the birth event.

GRIEF AND MOURNING

Although most hospital postpartum units are happy places filled with congratulating families and friends, loss and grief, as well as death and mourning, do invade the happiness of the unit. For a hospital unit and personnel prepared for birth and life, death can be extremely unwelcome. Maternity personnel often feel a sense of failure, helplessness, and even guilt following a stillbirth or the death of a newborn. To be helpful to the parents experiencing the loss of a baby, the nurse must have a basic understanding of grief and mourning.

Bereavement signifies that someone important to a person has died. It is a fact and signifies a fact of loss.

Grief is how the person feels in response to bereavement. Grief is both physical and emotional distress. Grief is an expression.

Mourning refers to the culturally patterned expressions of a bereaved person's thoughts and feelings. Mourning is a process. Maternal-infant, paternal-infant, and family-infant attachment begins during pregnancy. With perinatal death, a mother and her family lose the "inside baby" of their hopes and dreams. Instead of having someone they remember to mourn, the family has to mourn someone they have not really known.

IDENTIFY FIVE STAGES OF GRIEF AND MOURNING AS DESCRIBED BY KÜBLER-ROSS

According to Dr. Elisabeth Kübler-Ross, it is possible to identify five stages of grief and mourning that people experience in coping with death. These are:

1. Shock with denial ("No, not me.")
2. Anger ("Why me?")
3. Bargaining ("If I . . . ")
4. Depression and anticipatory grief ("How can I?")
5. Acceptance ("I can, I must.")

According to Dr. Ross, the coping mechanisms that people use to deal with death last for different periods of time, replace each other, or coexist. It is her conclusion that hope persists through all these stages.

Major manifestations of normal acute grief reactions in the working phase include:

1. Somatic distress
2. Preoccupation with the image and memories of the dead person
3. Guilt and self-blame while searching for a cause
4. Irritability, impatience, and social withdrawal
5. Inability to maintain normal patterns of conduct and functioning, with insomnia, overactivity, or restlessness

PLAN OF SUPPORT FOR PARENTS EXPERIENCING GRIEF AND MOURNING

Parents who have grieved have spoken of feeling pain, guilt, anger, and loneliness. Whether parents weep or sob or scream when grieving depends on their cultural background. Weeping and wailing and pounding one's chest may be quite natural in some cultures when experiencing grief, whereas in other cultures, quiet crying and even silence may be quite natural. Although the reactions can be extremely different, everyone has some response to grief. Be alert for the parents who appear inappropriately cheerful and seem to focus on external events having nothing to do with the unfortunate events that would normally cause a grief reaction. It is possible that these parents need intervention to help them deal with the reality of the loss.

Remember, nurses often go through the same stages of grief and mourning that the mother and family do. Be aware of what you feel and identify where you are in the grief process. Do not be afraid to cry. Being human is not being "unprofessional." Once you have come to grips with what you feel, you will be ready to be supportive to the mother and the family.

Death of an infant

To lose a baby in death is to grieve over someone that parents never had a chance to know, except in fantasy. In the case of stillbirths and neonatal deaths there is often a need for "closure" (to complete the cycle). To accomplish this, many parents request to see and touch and even hold their dead infant. The choice should be theirs. Parents' fantasies about what the baby looks like can be much worse than reality.

If the mother and family wish to see their baby, prepare them first for what the baby looks like. Give them a verbal description of body temperature, color, and any marks or discolorations on the body. Present the mother with her baby, washed and nicely wrapped in a colorful blanket. It is very helpful to point out to the mother the family characteristics and unique characteristics of her baby. Take the time to listen and encourage the mother and her family to verbalize their feelings.

Wanting to have a dead infant baptized, naming the baby (even a stillborn infant), taking photos, and making arrangements for burial are important steps for many parents as they seek closure. It is often very helpful for these parents to talk with others who have lost a baby. Many communities have support groups for parents who experience perinatal loss (see Appendix G). Avoid cliches such as "You can always have another baby," "You're still young," or "Everything always works out for the best." The mother and her family need from the nurse a demonstration of caring about what has happened in the here and now and not unrealistic promises.

How the mother and father resolve their feelings in this time of crisis may very well determine the future of their relationship. Many relationships do not weather a crisis such as the death of a baby, particularly when the grief is unresolved.

Fathers can have a particularly difficult time resolving the death of an infant. Many cultures place a heavy burden on men, requiring them to be "manly" and not to cry. They are frequently expected to maintain family stability during the crisis, while they are in great need of compassionate support themselves. Fathers should be able to share the grief experience without limitations on visiting hours. In fact, the most difficult time for a grieving father may be the nighttime hours when he is home alone. He should be encouraged to spend the night with his wife should he need her support—and she his.

Siblings and other family members must also be included in the grief process. Siblings sometimes react to the death of a baby brother or sister with nightmares, depression, withdrawal, and guilt feelings. Some siblings feel they have caused the baby to die by feeling jealousy or resentment about the new baby entering the family.

Parents should be encouraged to remain in an area where nurses are skilled in postpartum care and able to help parents experiencing perinatal loss. However, for many women who have lost a baby the adjustment is more difficult if they remain on the maternity unit. If possible, offer these women a quiet private room away from happy mothers with their babies. This does not mean that the mother wants to be isolated and alone. Indeed, the opposite is true: she wants and needs human contact. It is simply that the obvious happy interactions of new mothers and babies may be more than she can handle at this time in the grief process.

Infant with a birth defect

When faced with the birth of a baby with a defect, the parents are confronted with the loss of their hopes for a perfect baby, plus the prospect of coping with a life-long disability. These parents also go through the stages of grief and mourning. They also can exhibit pathological reactions, which can range from extreme guilt, leading to overprotection and dedication, to extreme intolerance, leading to denial of the infant.

Once again, as a nurse you must acknowledge what you feel and then you can help the parents. When helping these parents respond to the infant, point out the good features about the baby, such as pretty eyes, cute nose, and round arms. You can act as a role model, feeding and changing the baby, touching the baby's defect, and cuddling the baby as you would any baby while encouraging the parents to interact with their infant. Often the parents of a baby with a defect express guilt and self-doubt and consequently need much support and positive reinforcement. Encourage them to provide the care for their baby and reassure them about how well they are doing.

In making decisions about the long-term care of the infant, the parents need to have all alternatives presented and possible outcomes explored. The final decision must be theirs and not the decision of a physician, midwife, or nurse. Always remember the baby belongs to the parents and not to the hospital or the health care providers. The parents have a right to make their own decision. It is hoped that their decision will be one that will allow them to function and to cope with their situation.

Genetic counseling is very helpful to parents who want to avoid having another baby with a defect. The nurse can explain genetic counseling and recommend a referral to a counseling center.

Often in their anxiety when first learning of the defect, the parents do not comprehend the explanations given. They may need more thorough explanations later and photographs or descriptive written explanations. If the defect is one that can be corrected surgically, photographs of other babies before and after surgery can be useful. Realistic plans for long-term care plus referral to public health or home nurses and social workers may be needed.

Adoption

DESCRIBE SUPPORTIVE MEASURES FOR A WOMAN RELINQUISHING HER BABY

Mothers who relinquish their babies also experience grief and mourning for they, too, are experiencing a loss. It is hoped that in prenatal care this mother has received help from the physicians, midwives, nurses, social workers, and her family. If she has had this help, by the time of delivery she may have worked through anticipatory grief and be prepared for the loss. However, prepared or not, the actual event of the birth is a crisis for this mother and her family. This mother will have to decide how much contact, if any, she wishes with her baby. It is thought that interacting with the baby facilitates the grieving process and may be advisable. Just as in coping with the death of a baby, it is difficult to move past the denial phase if the baby is never real. However, the mother needs advance preparation for how she may feel when holding her baby. Feelings of warmth, tenderness, and love for the baby are natural and to be expected. The mother needs to understand that having these feelings does not mean that she has made the wrong decision. If the baby looks like a family member, the mother may be profoundly affected. She needs supportive, nonjudgmental care to help her express her emotions, and she also needs counseling about any guilt feelings.

After the baby's birth, most women who are relinquishing their babies prefer not to be with new mothers and babies who are going home together. However, if this mother moves to another unit in the hospital, she still needs follow-up care from the maternity nurses who cared for her during labor and delivery. It is important for her to talk about the labor and delivery to resolve the experience and facilitate the grieving process. She will also need help in planning her future: going home empty-handed, anniversary depressions, follow-up care, the baby's future, and her own sexuality and birth control.

A woman who gives up her baby can come out of the experience with self-respect and dignity when she is given respect and sympathetic care.

SUMMARY

In this unit we have discussed complications in the postpartum period. For many women cesarean birth is not a complication but just another way to give birth; it was included in this unit for those times when cesarean birth follows a complication in labor. A brief look at grief and mourning completed this unit with a discussion of coping with death of a newborn, a newborn with a birth defect, and relinquishing a baby. The next unit will introduce you to the newborn, a truly marvelous being.

BIBLIOGRAPHY

Christensen, A.Z.: Coping with the crisis of a premature birth—one couple's story, MCN **2**(1):33-37, 1977.

Conklin, M.M.: Discussion groups as preparation for cesarean section, JOGN Nurs. **6**(4):52-54, 1977.

Estok, P., and Lehman, A.: Perinatal death: grief support for families, Birth **10**(1):17-25, 1983.

Frink, B.B., and Chally, P.: Managing pain responses to cesarean childbirth, MCN **9**(4):270-272, 1984.

Harvey, K.: Caring perceptively for the relinquishing mother, MCN **2**(1):24-28, 1977.

Hasson, N.M.: The role of enzymes in disseminated intravascular coagulation: an overview, JOGN Nurs. **3**:27-29, May/June 1974.

Kowalski, K., and Osborn, M.R.: Helping mothers of stillborn infants to grieve, MCN **2**(1):29-32, 1977.

Kübler-Ross, E.: On death and dying, London, 1969, The Macmillan Co.

Marut, J.S.: The special needs of the cesarean mother, MCN **3**(4):202-206, 1978.

Mayberry, L.J., and Forte, A.B.: Pregnancy-related disseminated intravascular coagulation (DIC), MCN **10**(3):168-173, 1985.

Mercer, R.T.: Crisis: a baby is born with a defect, Nursing 1977 **7**(11):45-47, 1977.

Mevs, L.: The current status of cesarean section and today's maternity patient, JOGN Nurs. **6**(4):44-47, 1977.

Moore, M.L.: Realities in childbearing, ed. 2, Philadelphia, 1983, W.B. Saunders Co.

O'Brian, B.S., and Woods, S.: The paradox of DIC, Am. J. Nurs. **78**(11):1878-1889, 1978.

Revocation of fibrinogen licenses, FDA Drug Bulletin, vol. 8, no. 2, Department of Health, Education, and Welfare, March–April 1978.

Reynolds, C.B.: Updating care of cesarean section patients, JOGN Nurs. **6**(4):48-51, 1977.

Schlosser, S.: The emergency C-section patient. Why she needs help—what you can do, RN, 53-57, Sept. 1978.

Stichler, J.F., and Affonso, D.D.: Cesarean birth, Am. J. Nurs. **80**(3):466-472, 1980.

Young, R.K.: Chronic sorrow: parent's response to the birth of a child with a defect, MCN **2**(1):38-42, 1977.

Zahourek, R., and Jensen, J.S.: Grieving and the loss of the newborn, Am. J. Nurs. **73**(5):836-839, 1973.

DEFINITIONS

Define the following terms:

anticoagulants	mastitis
atony	morbidity
bereavement	mourning
closure	parametritis
cystitis	peritonitis
D & C	placenta accreta
disseminated intravascular coagulation (DIC)	puerperal infection
	septicemia
	sibling
embolism	somatic
endometritis	subinvolution
fibrinogen	thrombin
grief	thrombophlebitis
hemostasis	thrombus
hypovolemic shock	vaginitis
inversion	vulvitis

LEARNING ACTIVITIES AND EXPERIENCES

1. Group discussion.
2. Review isolation procedures in your hospital.
3. View audiovisual aids and discuss.

ENRICHMENT/IN-DEPTH STUDY

1. Research DIC and write a summary paper for class discussion.
2. Draw a temperature graph representative of a postpartum infection in a woman who has not received antibiotic therapy.
3. Investigate whether a cesarean birth support group exists in your community. If there is such a group, attend a meeting and share your observations with classmates.
4. Interview parents who were separated from their newborns immediately after birth. What were their feelings?
5. Is there a support group for parents experiencing perinatal death in your community?

SELF-ASSESSMENT

For questions 1 through 6, circle the best answer.

1. If a new mother complains of tenderness and warmth in her leg and has a fever, you would suspect that she may have:
   a. thrombophlebitis
   b. leg cramps
   c. dehydration and stiffness
2. When checking the height of the uterine fundus on the second postpartum day, the nurse should find the fundus:
   a. at the umbilicus
   b. two finger-widths below the umbilicus
   c. two finger-widths above the umbilicus
3. The signs and symptoms of a ruptured uterus include all of the following *except:*
   a. localized abdominal pain and tenderness
   b. a tearing feeling
   c. elevated blood pressure
   d. hypovolemic shock
4. Which of the following are major factors leading to postpartum infection?
   a. prolonged rupture of the membranes
   b. long, difficult labors
   c. hemorrhage
   d. invasive techniques in labor
   e. nothing by mouth during labor
   Answer (circle one): 1. a and b
   2. a, b, and c
   3. a, b, c, and d
   4. all of above
5. Signs and symptoms of cystitis include:
   a. frequent urination
   b. painful urination
   c. slight temperature elevation
   d. copious amounts of urine
   Answer (circle one): 1. a and b
   2. all of above
   3. a, b, and c
   4. b
6. If a woman has had an abruptio placentae, the following complication might occur:
   a. DIC
   b. distended bladder
   c. infection

Supply the correct answer(s) for items 7 through 17.

7. If a breast-feeding mother develops mastitis, will she have to discontinue breast-feeding? Why or why not?

8. Obstetrical complications that may predispose a mother to DIC include:
   a.

b.
c.
d.

9. If parents must be separated from their infant in the immediate postpartum period because of complications, what can the nurse do to encourage bonding?

10. What kinds of activities are contraindicated for the cesarean mother during her recovery period at home?

11. What are some possible emotional reactions the parents may have following a cesarean birth?

12. According to Dr. Elisabeth Kübler-Ross, it is possible to identify five stages of grief and mourning that people experience when coping with death. These are:
    a.
    b.
    c.
    d.
    e.

13. Mourning is defined as:

14. Describe ways in which the nurse can be supportive of a new family whose baby (1) is dead or (2) has a birth defect.

15. What are the observations you would make when giving nursing care to a new mother following a cesarean birth?
    a.
    b.
    c.
    d.
    e.
    f.
    g.
    h.
    i.

16. What are the bonding needs of a mother who has been separated from her baby because of a postpartum infection?

17. The physician's orders for a new mother with a postpartum infection include bed rest. How would you position this mother to promote uterine drainage?

Fill in the blanks for questions 18 through 21.

18. The organisms most often responsible for the development of postpartum infections are ____________________, ____________________, ____________________, and ____________________.

19. The cesarean mother usually has ____________________ lochia than the woman who experiences a vaginal birth.

20. Early postpartum hemorrhage is defined as blood loss of 500 milliliters or more in the __________ __________ hours following delivery.

21. Late postpartum hemorrhage occurs after __________ hours to __________ weeks following delivery.

UNIT XII
The newborn

GOALS

This unit is designed to provide the reader with information that will:

□ promote awareness of the newborn's potential for interaction.
□ develop a basic understanding of the normal newborn.

STUDENT OBJECTIVES

After studying this unit, you should be able to:

1. Briefly describe normal behavior of a newborn, emphasizing (a) the four phases of newborn activity in the first 24 hours after birth and (b) the first six "state" cycles.
2. Identify and describe the characteristics of the normal newborn related to the following criteria: average temperature, pulse, and respiration.
3. Define the following terms used when discussing gestational age: (a) AGA, (b) SGA, (c) LGA, (d) preterm, (e) term, and (f) postterm.
4. Describe the physical criteria for determining gestational age (using the clinical form in this book).
5. Demonstrate how to determine gestational age.
6. Identify and describe the characteristics of the normal newborn related to the following criteria: average measurements: weight, length, chest, head.
7. Identify and describe the characteristics of the normal newborn related to the following criteria: (a) skin: color, texture; (b) ears: lobe, hearing; (c) face: chin, marks; (d) eyes: color, discharge; (e) nose: smell; (f) mouth: palates; (g) neck: size; (h) breasts: tissue size; (i) chest: breathing; (j) abdomen: shape; (k) cord: condition; (l) genitourinary system (testes or labia); and (m) anus: patency.
8. Describe the following reflexes, their importance, how stimulated, and the approximate time of disappearance: (a) Moro's, (b) rooting, (c) grasp, (d) step, (e) tonic neck, (f) sucking.
9. Given the following list of common variations in the neonate, (a) define these variations, (b) explain reasons for their occurrence, and (c) state how long they last: caput succedaneum, cephalhematoma, erythema toxicum, "stork bites," milia, subconjunctival hemorrhage, and "epithelial pearls."

In the United States many newborn babies are cared for in a hospital nursery by hospital personnel for the first hours or days of life. Policies concerning length of nursery stay, type of nursery, and infant feeding schedule may differ from hospital to hospital. Many hospitals have a transition or observation nursery where newly born babies are observed closely for the first 12 to 24 hours after birth. When stabilized, and if special care is not required, infants are moved from this transition nursery to traditional nursery care or to rooming-in units. Traditional nursery care may involve a schedule for infant feeding in which the babies are taken to their mothers every 4 hours or "on-demand," in which case the babies are taken to their mothers when hungry. An area of the hospital maternity department may be designated as a rooming-in area where mothers and fathers can keep their babies in their room. Policies for rooming-in can vary from keeping the baby in the mother's room at all times to returning the baby to the nursery whenever the mother wants to sleep.

When a hospital does not have a special nursery set aside for a transition or observation nursery, one particular area of the nursery will usually be designated as the receiving area for newly born babies. This grouping of infants in a nursery according to the type of care they require has been termed *area care*. In area care, certain spaces of the nursery are designated for special types of care depending on the needs of the babies. The nursery may be divided into a recovery area, routine observation area, intermediate area, and intensive care area.

In some hospitals there are small, multiple nurseries, housing four to six infants. In this type of care, no new infants are admitted to a nursery untill all previous babies are discharged and the nursery has been thoroughly cleaned. This type of care is called a "cohort" system.

In developing family-centered care, many hospitals are designing procedures whereby newborns can be observed closely by nurses without separating the babies from their parents. Some hospitals have a list of "on-call" nurses who will provide special one-on-one nursing care for the new family in their own hospital room in the first 6 to 8 hours of life. In this way, the baby can be closely observed and cared for without separation from parents. Other hospitals offer this same nursing care as routine with mother-baby nursing. Close observation and care of the newborn in a room with the parents require nurses skilled in all aspects of maternity care. The nurse who has supported the mother and family through labor and birth may be the same nurse who assesses the newborn and provides necessary care. This is indeed a challenge to nurses who have functioned in only one area (labor and delivery, nursery, or postpartum) for many years. Keeping the baby with the new parents does not negate the fact that the first 12 to 24 hours of life are very special transition hours. In fact, the parents can be valuable team members contributing to the observation and care of the infant. These parents need to be prepared before the birth for what to expect in the way of normal transition of their newborn. The prenatal classes discussed earlier in Unit V should prepare parents to assume some of the responsibility in the immediate care of their baby.

TRANSITION TO EXTRAUTERINE LIFE

The newborn emerges from a warm, dark, liquid environment to a cool, bright, dry environment filled with noise (Fig. 12-1). As the fetus passes through the birth canal, its chest is compressed and thus some of the fluid that had filled its lungs in utero is expelled from its mouth. After delivery of the thorax, as the chest cage re-expands, air is sucked into the airways. Some childbirth researchers believe that this stimulates the first breath of life. Others believe it is the newborn's reaction to sudden changes in pressure and temperature. Whatever the case may be, the first breath is really a "gasp." The resistant forces of the lung tissue and of the remaining lung fluid are reduced by *surfactant*, a chemical substance within lung air spaces responsible for aiding in lung expansion. Most of the *alveoli* (gas-exchanging areas of the lung) are expanded within 1 hour after birth. Most lung fluid is removed by absorption and lymphatic drainage within 6 to 12 hours. Thus even with the best delivery the baby will be slightly acidotic immediately after birth but will "blow off" the excess carbon dioxide in 1 to 2 hours.

When the umbilical cord is severed at delivery, closure of the fetal circulatory structures begins. The umbilical arteries and then the umbilical vein contract within a short time after birth. This constriction is initially due to cold temperature and stretching of the umbilical cord but is probably maintained by exposure to rising levels of blood O_2.

The ductus venosus closes within 3 to 7 days after birth, probably passively as a result of reduced blood flow and pressure due to the absence of umbilical vein blood. As the

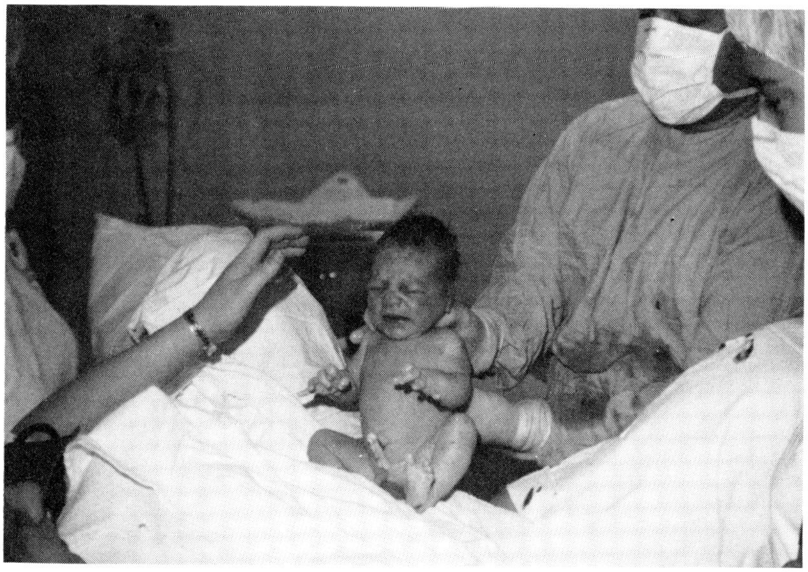

Fig. 12-1. The newborn.

newborn begins to breathe and its blood oxygen levels begin to rise, its lung vessels respond by relaxing their muscular walls and allowing an increase in pulmonary blood flow. More blood flows through the lungs to the pulmonary veins and thus to the left atrium. Left atrial pressure increases as right atrial pressure decreases (because of decreased blood return from the loss of umbilical venous flow), and thus a valvelike fold of tissue snaps shut over the foramen ovale. This tissue fuses with the wall between the atria within 6 to 8 weeks. In many infants the foramen ovale closes incompletely and a small amount of blood is shunted between atria for 1 to 2 months. The ductus arteriosus closes usually within 10 to 15 hours, probably as a reaction to increasing blood oxygen tension and prostaglandin interactions.

Normal laboratory values for blood for a term infant are:

STATE THE RANGE OF NEWBORNS AT BIRTH FOR Hgb, Hct, AND WHITE BLOOD COUNT

	Birth	*7 days of age*	*3 months*
Hemoglobin (Hgb) (grams/100 milliliters):			
Average	19.0	17.9	11.3
Range	16.8 to 21.2	53.6 to 68.4	10.4 to 12.2
Hematocrit (Hct) (%):			
Average	61	56	33
Range	53.6 to 68.4	46.6 to 65.4	29.7 to 36.3
Leukocytes:			
Average	18,000	12,000	12,000
Range	9000 to 30,000	5000 to 21,000	6000 to 18,000

The normal fall in total hemoglobin and hematocrit values, the so-called "physiological anemia of the newborn," is usually fully corrected by the age of 6 months, as the infant begins to produce more and more red blood cells.

EXPLAIN THE USE OF VITAMIN K FOR NEWBORN

The newborn's immature liver and gastrointestinal system sometimes cannot provide adequate amounts of vitamin K because their formation is dependent on the presence of bacteria in the intestine. Vitamin K aids in the formation of prothrombin, which is necessary for blood coagulation. In many nurseries vitamin K is given to most newborns intramuscularly in the anterior lateral aspect of the thigh shortly after birth (Fig. 12-2). When the newborn begins to ingest food, normal bacteria will grow in the intestinal tract and vitamin K will be manufactured by the second week of life.

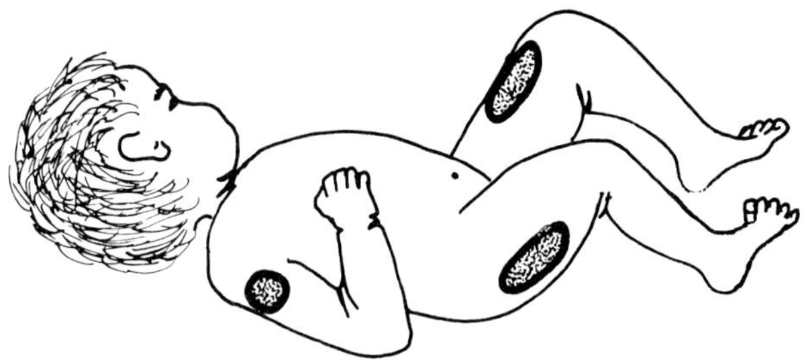

Fig. 12-2. Newborn injection sites.

The number of red blood cells decreases during the first week after birth (see preceding discussion). Cell breakdown occurs in the spleen and liver; hemoglobin is converted in the liver to bilirubin. Bilirubin is eliminated through the gastrointestinal tract. If the immature liver cannot eliminate all the bilirubin, it will be reabsorbed into the circulation as unmetabolized bilirubin (indirect, unconjugated bilirubin). This usually happens after the second day of life, and the infant appears jaundiced. This jaundice is known as physiological jaundice *(icterus neonatorum)*. Any jaundice during the first 24 hours of life should be recorded and reported promptly because it is probably not normal physiological jaundice (see p. 318).

Normal laboratory values are:

STATE THE RANGE OF NORMAL BILIRUBIN LEVELS AT BIRTH, 1 DAY, AND 5 DAYS OF LIFE

	Age	*Normal range*
Bilirubin (milligrams per 100 milliliters [deciliters])	Cord	Under 2 milligrams per deciliter
	0 to 1 day	Under 6 milligrams per deciliter
	3 to 5 days	Under 12 milligrams per deciliter
	After 5 days	Under 1 milligram per deciliter

The digestive system and the kidneys begin to function immediately after birth. In the uterus the fetus drank amniotic fluid and urinated normally but did not have a bowel movement.

CAPABILITIES OF THE NEWBORN

Research is now available concerning the amazing capabilities of the newborn. The newborn is a socially responsive human being who can probably learn better on the first day of life than ever again. A baby, immediately after birth, will stare intently at the parents' faces and see them. In fact, newborns prefer looking at the mother's face, especially the eyes, rather than at other objects. Other capabilities of the newborn include the ability to recognize an approaching object as a threat and to turn away to avoid it and the ability to reach for an object and usually come close to touching it. The newborn also seems to realize that he or she is a human being and will imitate another person's facial expressions such as sticking out the tongue, opening the mouth, and pursing the lips. Newborn babies are active stimulus seekers where repetition and the level of stimulation are important. The baby is actually capable of shutting out stimuli and can even learn to respond by turning its head at the sound of a bell.

Indeed, babies are not passive and unresponsive creatures to be hurried off to the hospital nursery after birth. The affectionate bond between mother and child and between father and child begins at the moment of birth (Fig. 12-3). As long as the newborn is responding normally, immediate skin-to-skin contact with the parents is very important

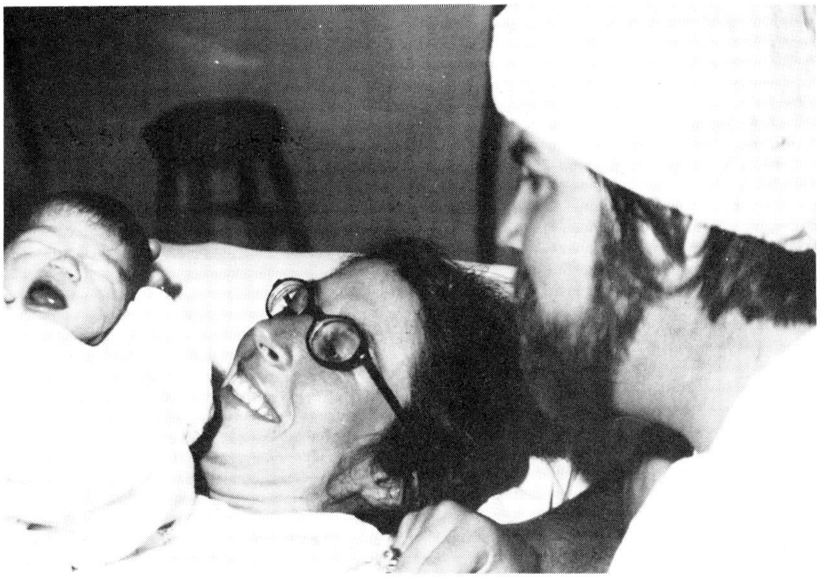

Fig. 12-3. A bond forming.

in bonding. The newborn will have difficulty opening its eyes under bright spotlights but will look around if the lights are dimmed. (It is possible to dim the main lights in the delivery area and still have light focused over the perineum for episiotomy repair or other necessary procedures.) Also, shielding the infant's face with the one's hands or a blanket will provide enough protection from the light to encourage the baby to open its eyes. Refraining from using prophylactic eyedrops and weighing and measuring the baby for 30 minutes to 1 hour after birth will allow the parents time alone with their baby so that the attachment process can proceed without interruption.

The mother may wish to breast-feed in the first hour after birth; the nurse or the father can assist her.

NEWBORN BEHAVIOR

NORMAL BEHAVIOR OF NEWBORN

Newborns experience *phases of activity* as they adjust to life outside the uterus. These phases can be measured in timespans as follows:

first reactive phase (from birth to 30 minutes of life). In this phase the newborn is alert and responsive to stimuli, searching and inquiring about the new world. Respirations are 60 to 90 per minute; heart rate is 180 or more.

sleep phase (from 30 to 60 minutes to 2 hours of life). During this phase the newborn goes into a deep sleep and may secrete large amounts of mucus from the mouth. The infant may also pass a meconium stool. During this phase it is not unusual for the infant to have periods of apnea. Heart rate declines to 120 to 140 beats per minute.

second reactive phase (from 2 to 6 hours of life). During this phase the newborn is again awake and alert. The baby may still be secreting mucus. Body temperature should be normal. Rapid color changes may occur.

stability phase (6 to 24 hours of life). During this phase the newborn is successfully making the adjustment to the extrauterine world. The newborn's vital signs should be stable now and its color normal. Following this stability phase the newborn sleeps from 18 to 20 hours a day for the first few weeks.

There will be variations in these phases from baby to baby according to the difficulty of the labor and birth and the amount and types of analgesia or anesthesia the mother received.

Crying

LIST THE REASONS WHY A NEWBORN CRIES

The newborn operates with an urgent sense of "now" and is not able to delay physiological needs. The most common causes of crying are (1) fatigue, (2) hunger, (3) loneliness, (4) colic pain, and (5) irritability. A normal cry is loud and gusty and neither high pitched nor weak. It is important for a baby to be fed when hungry and not be kept waiting because of an arbitrary feeding schedule. Contrary to the myth that picking up a crying newborn "spoils" the baby, consistent response to the baby's cries for help establishes trust in the caretakers. Research indicates that babies whose mothers responded promptly to their crying cried less when they were a year old. The babies who were allowed to cry for a while (15 to 20 minutes) were likely to be the "crybabies" at 1 year of age. This research would indicate that it is best to respond consistently to a newborn's cry and attempt to meet the baby's needs. Responding to the baby's cry helps to establish trust. Most authorities agree that it is impossible to "spoil" a baby by too much rocking or holding during the first few months of life. However, even when responding consistently and meeting the baby's physical and emotional needs, there will still be times when the baby will cry and fret for no apparent reason. When all attempts at comfort no longer work, the baby may just have to cry awhile.

State cycles

Each baby also has an individual pattern of reactivity in which separate states of awareness can be identified. These are:

quiet sleep state. Respirations are slow and regular, and the infant rarely moves.
REM sleep state (rapid eye movement sleep). Respirations are irregular and grimaces and other facial expressions are frequent. Rapid eye movements can be seen through the eyelids.
active alert state. There is diffuse motor activity involving the whole body. The face may be relaxed or in a cry expression.
quiet alert state. The infant is alert and relaxed, and the eyes are open wide and focusing. It is in this state that the infant is most apt to mimic facial expressions.
crying state. Vigorous diffuse motor activity accompanies crying.
transitional state. In this state the infant may be between any of the preceding states (moving from one to the other).

It is important for the new parents to know about these phases and states of awareness so that they can understand their own babies. Each baby is a separate individual and responds in a unique way. Parents are usually fascinated to learn this, because they may have grown up with the myths that babies cannot see or smile or react to stimuli. Meaningful interaction between infants and parents helps to facilitate bonding.

At the first contact with the newborn after birth, the nurse can reassure the parents that the baby can and wants to see them.

IMMEDIATE NEEDS

EXPLAIN THE IMMEDIATE NEEDS OF NEWBORN FOLLOWING DELIVERY

The immediate needs of the newborn include establishing and maintaining an open airway for unobstructed breathing and maintenance of a normal body temperature. Apgar scoring at 1 and 5 minutes is essential, as is identification of the newborn before leaving the delivery area (see Unit VIII). Initial physical and gestational age assessments are vital to recognizing any problems immediately. If the parents are holding the baby, the nurse can make these initial observations without disturbing the parent-infant interaction.

Respirations

Spontaneous respirations should begin within a few seconds to 1 minute after birth. For most babies gentle aspiration of mucus with a bulb syringe and the help of gravity with the baby in a head-down position are all that is necessary to facilitate respirations.

If the infant does not breathe at birth, the stimulation of a nasal suction catheter or a few breaths of positive pressure by oxygen mask will usually initiate spontaneous respiration. In the severely depressed newborn, resuscitation may be necessary (see Unit XIII). For the average baby, holding the baby upside down by the feet and "spanking" on the back are not necessary. Tactile stimuli should be gentle.

Dr. Frederick LeBoyer has added an interesting dimension to the childbirth experience with his book, *Birth Without Violence*. In this book he emphasizes the "humanness" of the newborn and advocates that this new person be handled with sensitivity and gentleness. The transition from womb to world is indeed harsh, and gentleness is something we can add to that experience. Unfortunately, hospital personnel often get caught up in discussing the safety or validity of immersing a newborn in warm water (the LeBoyer bath) and fail to see the sensitivity to the newborn that LeBoyer advocates.

Temperature

A *neutral thermal environment* is one in which an infant's metabolic rate and oxygen consumption are minimal and body temperature remains within normal limits. A newborn of average size maintains a body temperature between 36.5° and 37° C (97.7° and 99° F) with a minimum use of energy. DEFINE A NEUTRAL THERMAL ENVIRONMENT

Adults produce heat by voluntary muscle activity, such as shivering, but newborns do not. Newborns produce heat by chemical or nonshivering thermogenesis. In chemical thermogenesis, norepinephrine is released, which initiates a chemical reaction in the brown fat stores of the infant. From 2% to 6% of the body weight of full-term babies consists of brown fat, which is a type of adipose tissue capable of unusual thermogenic activity. This brown fat is found between the scapulae, around muscles and blood vessels in the neck, behind the sternum, and around the kidneys and adrenals. The brown fat contains triglycerides, which break down and oxidize to produce heat. Thermogenesis through this means is limited and requires energy expenditures on the part of the newborn, thus causing an increase in oxygen consumption. If the baby is unable to meet oxygen needs from room air, it may be necessary to convert to anaerobic metabolism and thus cause an increase in lactic acid production. Metabolic acidosis can then develop. Another consequence of a baby being cold (neonatal cold stress) may be weight loss or failure to gain weight because of increased metabolic consumption of calories. Also, the increased glucose consumption may lead to hypoglycemia. EXPLAIN HOW NEWBORNS PRODUCE HEAT

Whereas nonshivering thermogenesis is the principal means of heat production in the newborn, vasoconstriction is the principal means of heat retention. If the mother has been treated with magnesium sulfate for pre-eclampsia or eclampsia, the baby's vasoconstrictive mechanisms may not be functioning well. EXPLAIN HOW NEWBORNS RETAIN HEAT

Insulation is not a significant means of heat conservation for the newborn because of the limited supply of subcutaneous fat and large surface area in relation to body mass.

Premature and low-birth-weight babies have less body fat than normal infants and consequently are at much greater risk for cold stress. Because of all the problems cold stress may cause, it is important to keep the newborn warm and to provide a neutral thermal environment as quickly as possible after birth.

To provide this thermoneutral environment, it is important to understand the four major mechanisms by which heat is transferred between the neonate and the environment. Body heat is lost from the skin surface chiefly by (1) radiation, (2) evaporation, (3) convection, and (4) conduction. Loss by *radiation* occurs when heat transfers from the body surface to cooler surfaces or surrounding objects: that is, incubator wall, room wall, and windows cooled by air conditioners. To minimize heat loss by radiation, bassinets, radiant warmers, and incubators should not be placed near cold outside walls and windows. DISTINGUISH AMONG FOUR MECHANISMS OF HEAT LOSS IN NEWBORN

Evaporative heat loss occurs when moisture evaporates from wet skin in a relatively dry atmosphere. A baby wet with amniotic fluid in an air-conditioned room loses body heat rapidly. To minimize heat loss by evaporation, the baby should be dried immediately after delivery with a warm blanket; it is especially important to dry and cover the baby's head. The baby is then wrapped in a second warm, dry blanket before being handed to the parents. If it is necessary to place the baby in an incubator, it should be prewarmed. Any oxygen as well as any solution applied to the infant's skin should be warmed also. The baby should not be bathed until the temperature has stabilized.

EXPLAIN WAYS TO PREVENT OR MINIMIZE HEAT LOSS IN NEWBORN

Heat loss by *convection* is enhanced by surrounding air currents, cold oxygen, and cold air blown by air conditioners. To prevent convective heat loss, the temperature in delivery rooms and nurseries should be adequate and drafts avoided. Also oxygen should be warmed prior to administration.

Heat loss by *conduction* occurs by transfer of heat from a warm object to a cooler object by direct contact. To minimize heat loss by conduction, a warm blanket is placed between the infant's body and the cold surface of a scale, X-ray table, or other object.

There is also evidence that babies can be overprotected and kept too warm (hyperthermia), so that they have to increase their metabolic work to cool down. This could also lead to hypoglycemia. Careful regulation of incubator temperatures, not overdressing, and not placing infants too near sunshine or heating ducts will minimize the risk of hyperthermia.

It is possible, simply by minimizing or eliminating heat loss, to keep the average well newborn warm without placing the baby in a heated bed or incubator. Research has shown that term newborns who were thoroughly dried and covered with warm, dry blankets could be held by their mothers for 15 minutes in the delivery room without significant temperature loss.

COMPARE A WARM INCUBATOR AND RADIANT WARMER FOR MAINTAINING NEWBORN'S BODY WARMTH

If for some reason the baby needs resuscitation or other medical attention, it will be necessary to place the baby in a warm incubator or radiant warmer. Overhead radiant warmers use the principle of radiation. These warmers may have automatic or manual control or both. Infants under manually controlled radiant warmers should be observed continually because it is possible to overheat an infant in a short time if the unit is on full-powered output. At the same time the low-powered output may be insufficient to warm a cold baby. With an automatic warmer a thermistor (probe) is attached to the infant's abdominal skin to sense the baby's skin temperature (Fig. 12-4). If the baby's skin temperature goes below or above set points, warning systems will be activated. These warning systems may be auditory and/or visual. When using a probe, the nurse must be sure that it remains attached to the baby's skin; if it becomes detached, the warmer may continue to heat the baby. Because radiant heat can cause significant water loss, an infant who remains under a radiant warmer more than a few hours will need increased fluid intake. Overhead radiant warmers are valuable because they provide direct and free access to an infant. However, the nurse must remember that a baby under a radiant warmer needs close observation and frequent axillary temperature checks (every 30 minutes) with a thermometer. Because temperature probes can become defective and inaccurate, the nurse should not rely on the skin probe temperature readout alone.

Prewarmed incubators can maintain the baby's temperature very well; however, they do limit access to the baby. Heat is lost whenever the incubator doors or portholes are opened, and radiant heat loss to incubator walls is a potential problem (Fig. 12-5).

EXAMINATION AND OBSERVATION OF INFANT

Within a few minutes after birth, careful observation of the infant for obvious anomalies is important. The infant should be observed carefully for general appearance. The infant's *muscle* tone should be firm and strong, *skin* smooth, and *posture* flexed with symmetrical movements of all extremities. The *cry* should be strong and vigorous. The

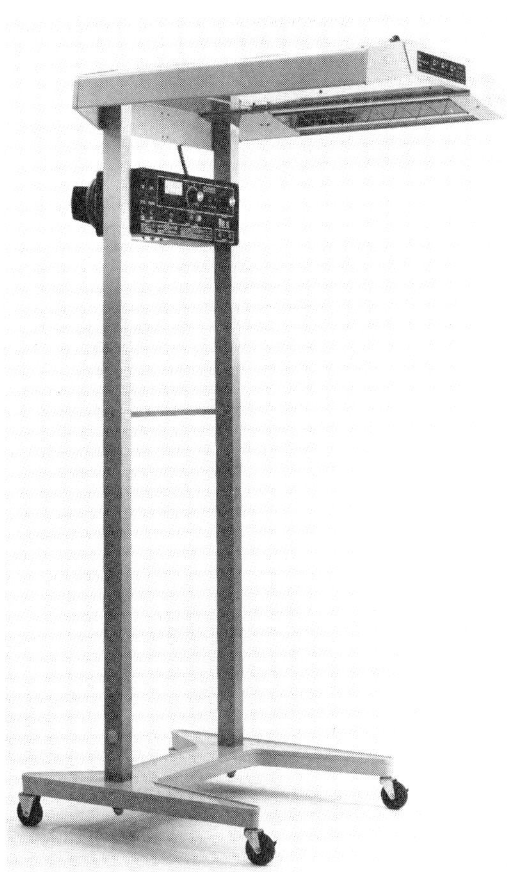

Fig. 12-4. Ohio Free-Standing Radiant Heater. (Courtesy Ohio Medical Products, Madison, Wis.)

Moro's reflex should be elicited easily, and the white newborn's color should be pink or red. Cyanotic hands and feet are common and, in fact, are a healthy response to extrauterine life. The mucosal lining of the mouth of a black baby should be pink or red.

Vital signs

CHARACTERISTICS OF NORMAL NEWBORN

Vital signs should be checked and recorded. Initial temperature should be taken rectally to check on patency of the anus. A temperature range from 97.7° to 99° F (36.5° to 37° C) (axillary) is within the normal range. The respiratory rate and pattern will often range from 40 to 70 or more in the first hour or so. Most important is noting signs of difficulty: retractions, grunting, flaring of nares, and generalized cyanosis. Any of these signs should be reported to the physician. The preceding vital signs should be checked at least every hour for the first 3 hours or longer if necessary. Initial voiding and meconium should be noted and recorded.

Estimation of gestational age

TERMS USED WHEN DISCUSSING GESTATIONAL AGE

PHYSICAL CRITERIA FOR DETERMINING GESTATIONAL AGE

If the infant is in good condition, an estimate should be made of the infant's maturity. These findings fall into three major categories: (1) *Preterm*—prior to 38 weeks of gestation; (2) *term*—38 to 42 weeks of gestation; and (3) *postterm*—more than 42 weeks of gestation. Within these categories the baby can be classified as AGA (appropriate for gestational age), LGA (large for gestational age), or SGA (small for gestational age). An accurate gestational age assessment helps to differentiate the premature from the small-for-gestational-age baby and the term from the preterm large-for-gestational-age baby. Gestational age can be determined after birth by physical characteristics, neurological examination, and plotting of length, weight, and head circumference on appropriate growth charts.

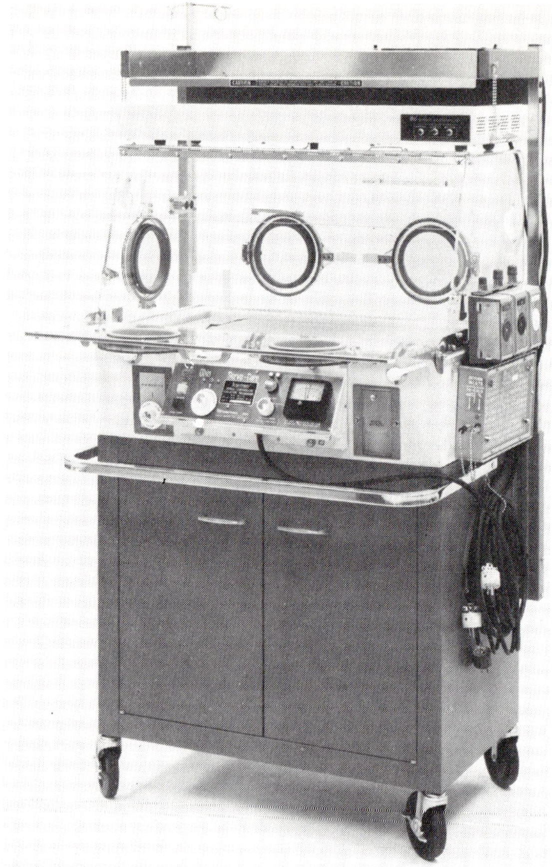

Fig. 12-5. Ohio Servo-Care Incubator. (Courtesy Ohio Medical Products, Madison, Wis.)

The physical signs checked are vernix, lanugo, abdominal skin, ear pinna, breast tissue, plantar creases on the feet, and male and female genitalia. The neuromuscular system is checked by estimating the maturity of the following: (1) posture, (2) square window (wrist or ankle), (3) arm recoil, (4) popliteal angle, (5) scarf sign, and (6) heel to ear. Scores are obtained for both physical and neurological examinations conducted within minutes to an hour after birth. A score of 40 indicates a gestational age of 40 weeks. A score of 30 indicates a gestational age of 36 weeks (Fig. 12-6).

HOW TO DETERMINE GESTATIONAL AGE

The baby's weight, length, and head circumference are measured and charted on the growth charts according to gestational age by examination. The baby's measurements can then be compared with the norms of the chart. Babies whose weight, length, and head circumference fall between the tenth and ninetieth percentiles are classifed as appropriate for the gestational age. Those above the ninetieth percentile are classified LGA, and those below the tenth percentile are classified SGA (Fig. 12-6). Babies who are AGA have a better chance for survival than those who are small or large for gestational age. Classification of infants by birth weight and gestational age allows the identification of general risks of a group of infants who would benefit from admission to a special care nursery. The special problems of infants who are large or small for gestational age will be discussed in Unit XIII.

Physical examination

After the initial observation of the newborn and a quick assessment of gestational age, the parents can safely have their time alone with the newborn. Usually, within the first 2 hours after birth, the newborn is transferred either to a nursery or to the mother's room. A physical examination by the nurse at this time is important to detect any abnormalities missed in the initial general observations. This examination does not replace but

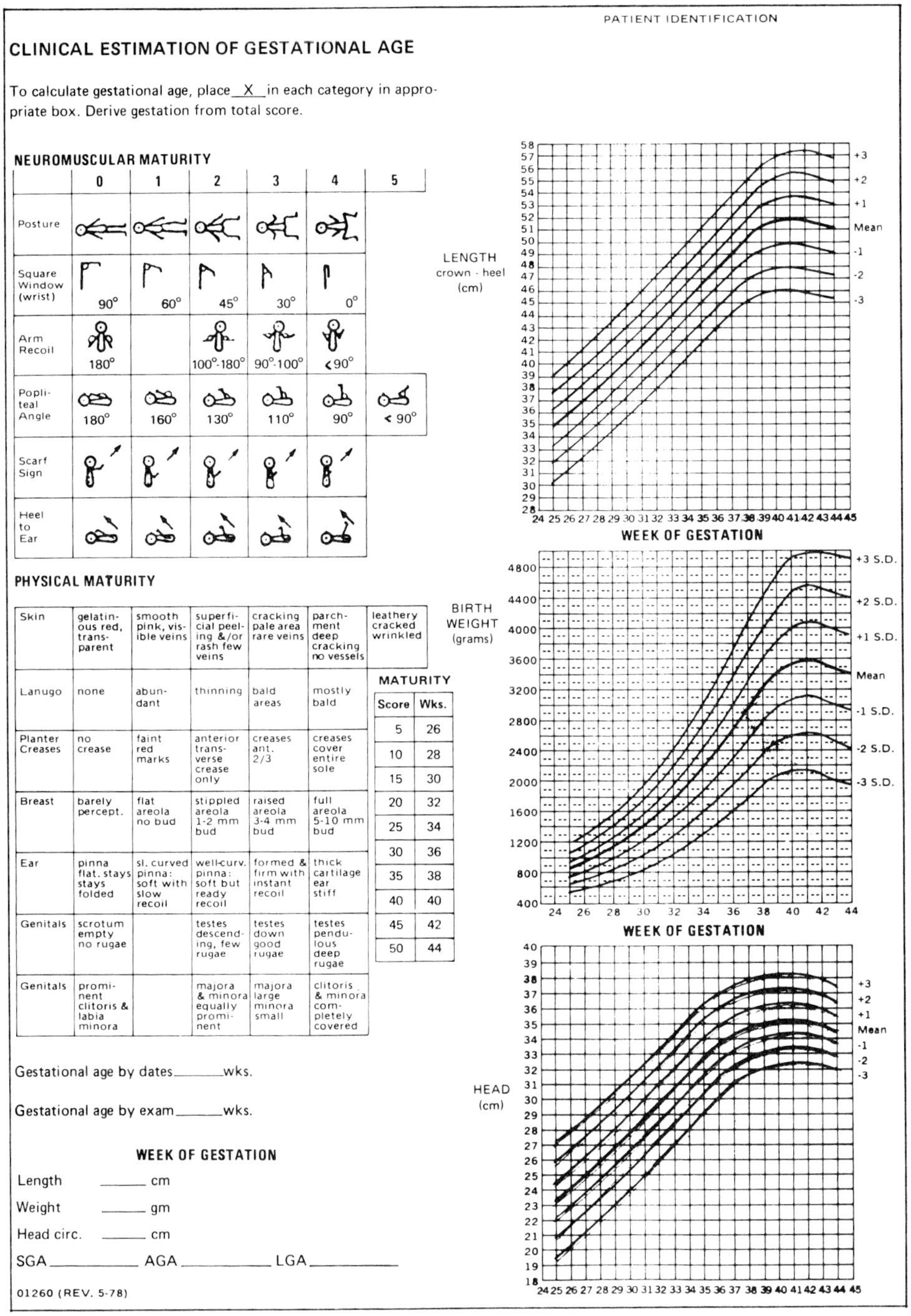

PATIENT IDENTIFICATION

CLINICAL ESTIMATION OF GESTATIONAL AGE

To calculate gestational age, place __X__ in each category in appropriate box. Derive gestation from total score.

NEUROMUSCULAR MATURITY

	0	1	2	3	4	5
Posture						
Square Window (wrist)	90°	60°	45°	30°	0°	
Arm Recoil	180°		100°-180°	90°-100°	<90°	
Popliteal Angle	180°	160°	130°	110°	90°	< 90°
Scarf Sign						
Heel to Ear						

PHYSICAL MATURITY

Skin	gelatinous red, transparent	smooth pink, visible veins	superficial peeling &/or rash few veins	cracking pale area rare veins	parchment deep cracking no vessels	leathery cracked wrinkled
Lanugo	none	abundant	thinning	bald areas	mostly bald	
Planter Creases	no crease	faint red marks	anterior transverse crease only	creases ant. 2/3	creases cover entire sole	
Breast	barely percept.	flat areola no bud	stippled areola 1-2 mm bud	raised areola 3-4 mm bud	full areola 5-10 mm bud	
Ear	pinna flat, stays folded	sl. curved pinna; soft with slow recoil	well-curv. pinna; soft but ready recoil	formed & firm with instant recoil	thick cartilage ear stiff	
Genitals	scrotum empty no rugae		testes descending, few rugae	testes down good rugae	testes pendulous deep rugae	
Genitals	prominent clitoris & labia minora		majora & minora equally prominent	majora large minora small	clitoris & minora completely covered	

MATURITY

Score	Wks.
5	26
10	28
15	30
20	32
25	34
30	36
35	38
40	40
45	42
50	44

Gestational age by dates______wks.

Gestational age by exam______wks.

WEEK OF GESTATION

Length ______ cm

Weight ______ gm

Head circ. ______ cm

SGA __________ AGA __________ LGA __________

01260 (REV. 5-78)

Fig. 12-6. Clinical estimation of gestational age. (Courtesy Ross Laboratories, Columbus, Ohio, Rev. May 1978.)

complements the physician's physical examination. The examination should be done while keeping the infant warm and with adequate lighting.

CHARACTERISTICS OF NORMAL NEWBORN

Characteristics of a normal neonate. If the infant is AGA, the nurse should expect to find the following.

Weight. The weight is approximately 7½ pounds (males are slightly heavier than females).*

Length. The average length is 20 inches (18 to 22 inches is a normal range).*

Chest circumference. The chest circumference is 12 to 13 inches (33 centimeters).

*These measurements are based on white infants in the United States.

Head circumference. The head circumference is 13.8 inches (35 centimeters).

Temperature. The rectal or axillary temperature is 36.5° to 37° C (97.7° to 99° F).

Respirations. Respirations are regular to irregular, abdominally and synchronous 30 to 60 per minute (Fig. 12-6), varying according to the baby's activity. It is normal for newborns to have apneic spells lasting 5 to 10 seconds during sleep.

Pulse. The pulse is 120 to 160 beats per minute, varying according to the baby's activity. For a sleeping baby a heart rate of 80 to 90 beats per minute may be normal.

Blood pressure. The average systolic pressure for a baby weighing 3 kilograms is 60 mm Hg. Average systolic pressure for a baby weighing 2 kilograms is 50 mm Hg. Average systolic pressure for a baby weighing 1 kilogram is 40 mm Hg.

Head. The head is larger in proportion to the rest of the body and is approximately one third its adult size. In fact, the infant's head at birth is one quarter the total length of the body.

The bones of the head are joined together by narrow spaces called *sutures.* Because these bones have not grown together they can overlap, and thus the head can mold to the birth canal. If molding has occurred during labor and birth, the head may be elongated instead of round. This molding will be gone within a few hours after birth (Fig. 12-7).

COMMON VARIATIONS IN NEWBORN

In contrast, the *caput succedaneum* (often called simply caput) is somewhat more firm and ill defined in outline, representing edema of the scalp. It pits on pressure and subsides within 24 to 48 hours after birth (see Figure 12-8, **A**).

A *cephalhematoma* may be present after several hours. This subperiosteal hemorrhage results from trauma during delivery. It will be a localized swelling limited to the boundaries of one cranial bone and may enlarge during the first 2 to 3 days. The cephalhematoma will be absorbed within 6 weeks (Fig. 12-8, **B**,) but can cause a rapid increase in the level of bilirubin in the first hours of life.

The *anterior fontanel* is diamond shaped and opened 4 to 6 centimeters (closes by 18 months of age); it feels flat and soft.

The *posterior fontanel* is triangular shaped and opened 0.5 to 1 centimeters or closed (closes by 3 months of age); it feels flat and soft.

A sunken fontanel may indicate dehydration or decreased intracranial pressure; a bulging fontanel may indicate increased intracranial pressure. A fontanel may bulge slightly while the infant cries or strains. This is normal. Washing an infant's head and rubbing the fontanels are not harmful.

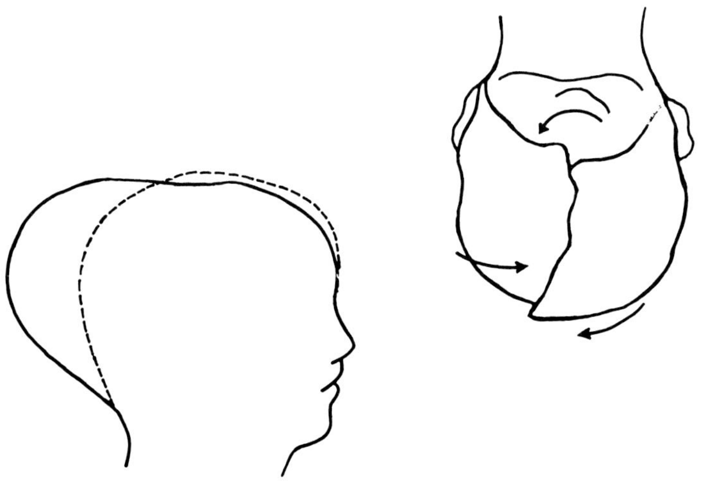

Fig. 12-7. Molding. (From Hamilton, M,P.: Basic maternity nursing, ed. 5, St. Louis, 1985, The C.V. Mosby Co.)

Skin. In the full-term baby at birth vernix may be found in the axilla and groin only. This may be washed off or allowed to remain until it is absorbed or dries and flakes off. The baby's skin is thin, delicate, and velvety smooth and veins may be seen through it. The skin of most babies appears reddish for 6 hours after birth and gradually fades over the next 24 hours. This reddish color is due to the excessive amount of hemoglobin needed to transport oxygen during fetal life. It is normal for a baby's hands and feet to be slightly blue because of poor peripheral perfusion.

The infant may have fine downy hair *(lanugo)* on the shoulders and forehead. Lanugo is more common on preterm infants or dark-haired babies.

A newborn may have a fine rash that appears like wheals surrounded by erythema *(erythema toxicum)*. This is noncontagious and needs no treatment. Small hemangiomas, *"stork bites,"* are common on the eyelids and back of the neck and disappear in 6 to 12 months.

Ears. Earlobes of a full-term baby are stiffened by thick cartilage and tend to stand out slightly from the head. The baby should respond to sounds. Malformation or misplacement of the ears may indicate an abnormality.

Face. The forehead appears to bulge, and the chin appears to recede. There may be tiny white spots called *milia* (which look like "whiteheads") across the baby's nose and forehead. Red marks may appear on the cheeks in front of the ears if forceps were used in delivery. They will disappear without treatment. Any breaks in the skin should be recorded and reported.

Eyes. The structure is normal, although the baby's eyelids may be swollen if silver nitrate has been used for eye care. If pus is present the physician should be notified. The tear ducts may not secrete tears for 2 to 4 weeks. Most newborns have bluish-gray eyes at birth. Permanent eye color is not present until 3 months of age. Subconjunctival hemorrhages may be present. They are caused by pressure during delivery and will disappear within a few weeks. The newborn baby can see, track a moving object, discriminate patterns, and focus on objects at a distance of about 18 inches.

Nose. The newborn breathes through the nose rather than the mouth. There is evidence that the baby can smell breast milk. Drainage from the nose may indicate infection.

Mouth. The mouth should be pink, and the tongue should move freely at the frenulum and should not protrude. The baby should be able to suck strongly. The hard and soft palates should be intact. Large white spots or plaques on the tongue or mucosa of the mouth may indicate *thrush* and should be reported to the physician. Thrush is not to be confused with the normal "epithelial pearls" (also called Epstein's pearls), which

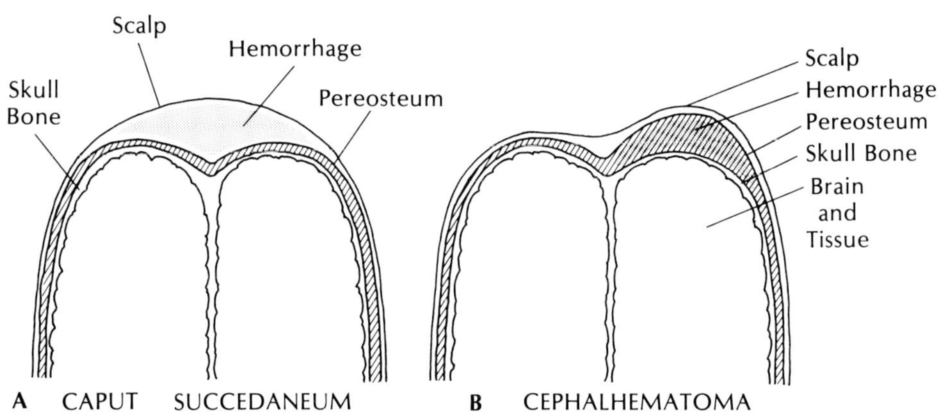

Fig. 12-8. A, Caput succedaneum. **B,** A cephalhematoma.

appear in the mouth on the hard palate or gums. These "pearls" are small, white, ricelike epidermal plaques.

Neck. The baby's neck is short and can be flexed. The head seems to settle on the shoulders.

Breasts. In both girls and boys mammary glands may appear swollen because of absorption of hormones from the mother prior to delivery. This swelling should subside in 2 weeks. The breast tissue should be 1 centimeter or more in diameter.

Chest. The chest is smaller than the head by up to 2 centimeters and wider than it is long. Movement of the chest and abdomen should be synchronized. Some abnormal respirations and abdominal breathing are normal; however, retractions, grunting, and nasal flaring may indicate respiratory distress. The clavicles should be checked to be sure they are intact and not fractured.

Abdomen. The abdomen appears rounded and large in relation to hips and pelvis. The abdomen should usually move with breathing. Bowel sounds should be present a few hours after delivery.

Umbilicus. There should be two arteries and one vein. The cord is whitish and soft immediately after birth and begins drying until it dries and falls off in 7 to 10 days. Alcohol can be applied three to four times a day to facilitate drying the cord. The diaper should be kept below the umbilicus to expose it to air. Sponge baths should be given until the cord falls off. Any drainage or inflammation around the cord may indicate infection and should be noted and reported.

Genitourinary system. Genitals of both sexes will seem large. In the female the labia minora and clitoris are more developed than the labia majora. In the male both testes should be palpable in the scrotum. In the female white caseous discharge, sometimes blood tinged, is normal. This slight bloody vaginal discharge for 2 to 3 days after birth is the result of hormone action on the lining of the uterus before birth. It will not recur.

Passage of urine is often not noticed for 24 hours because the infant usually urinates at birth. Occasionally the urine appears reddish-tan or "bloody" on the diaper until feeding is well established. This is caused by presence of uric acid crystals and is harmless.

The urethral meatus in the male should be easily visualized at the tip of the penis. The foreskin of the penis may be adherent to the glans.

Anus and bowels. The anus should be open. The infant passes meconium within 24 to 48 hours. The initial meconium stool is dark greenish-black, tarry, and odorless.

The infant may have only one *transitional stool,* beginning with meconium and ending with yellow stool, or the infant may pass greenish-yellowish material two or three times.

The stools of a breast-fed infant are usually very loose at first, golden yellow, with only a faint sour odor. In 5 to 7 days, stools of a breast-fed infant may become pasty and soft but still remain almost odorless. The stools of formula-fed infants are a paler yellow, are semiformed or contain curds, and have a foul odor. The infant may pass four to six stools a day during the first week or two; following this, the number of stools gradually decreases. However, breast-fed babies may not have stools for several days. Greenish, watery, foamy, mucous, or bloody stools are abnormal and should be reported.

Extremities. The newborn's legs are shorter than the arms at birth. Both arms and legs are flexed when the baby is quiet. Hips are checked by abducting the thighs to the bed and rotating the hips through full range of motion. If a thigh cannot be readily abducted to touch the bed, the hip may be dislocated. When the infant is lying on the abdomen, the buttocks and leg crease should be equal and symmetrical. When the thigh is being moved downward and inward with the index finger on the hip, a "click" may also indicate dislocation. In a prone position a preterm infant lies in a "frog" position, whereas a term infant lies with legs flexed (see Fig. 12-9).

Mongolian spots (darkened pigmented areas) may be present on the buttocks or lower

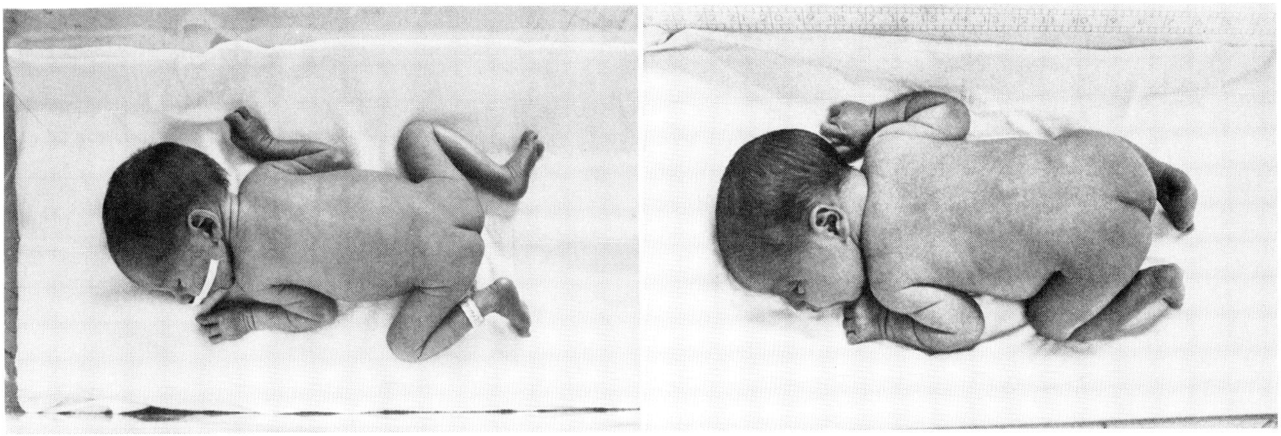

A B

Fig. 12-9. Prone position. A, Preterm infant lies in a "frog" position. B, Term infant lies with legs flexed. (Courtesy Mead Johnson Laboratories, Evansville, Ind.)

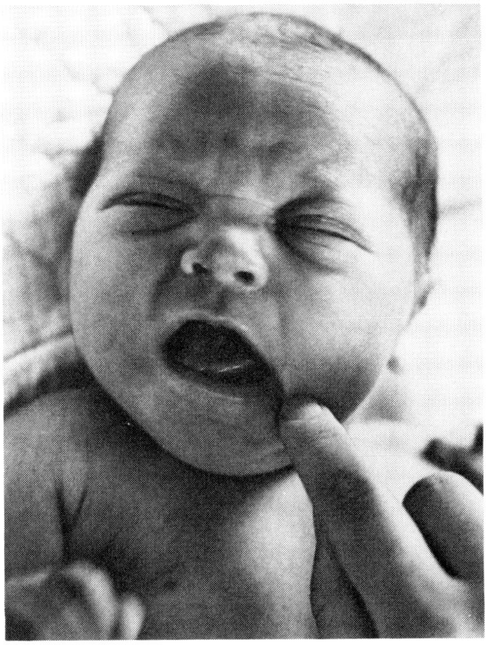

Fig. 12-10. Rooting reflex. (Courtesy Mead Johnson Laboratories, Evansville, Ind.)

back. These are most commonly found on dark-complexioned babies and appear like bruises. They will disappear by the time the baby is 3 years old.

Nervous system. Numerous reflex reactions can be obtained on examination of the newborn. A crying infant will not provide accurate responses.

The *grasp reflex* is present and strong. The infant will tightly grasp an object placed in its hand. The grasp reflex usually disappears by the age of 3 months.

The *rooting reflex* is present and can be stimulated by gently stroking or touching one of the infant's cheeks. The infant will turn toward the touch with open mouth. This reflex is useful when helping a new mother and infant to breast-feed (Fig. 12-10).

The *sucking reflex* is present, and the infant will suck any object placed in the mouth. The sucking reflex is usually accompanied by the swallowing and gag reflexes, which persist throughout life.

The *step reflex* (Fig. 12-11) is present and can be elicited by holding the infant up-

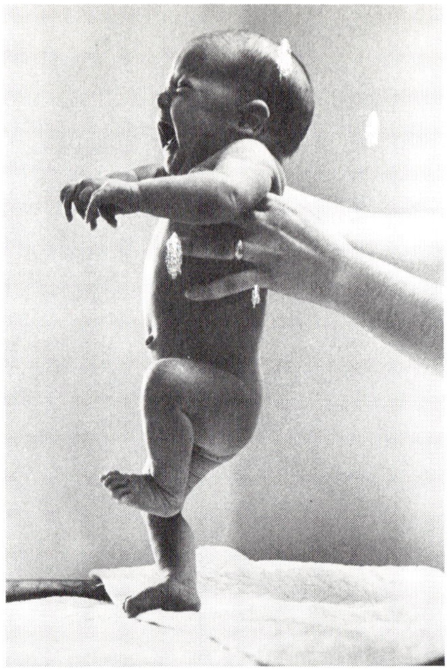

Fig. 12-11. Walking reflex. (Courtesy Mead Johnson Laboratories, Evansville, Ind.)

A

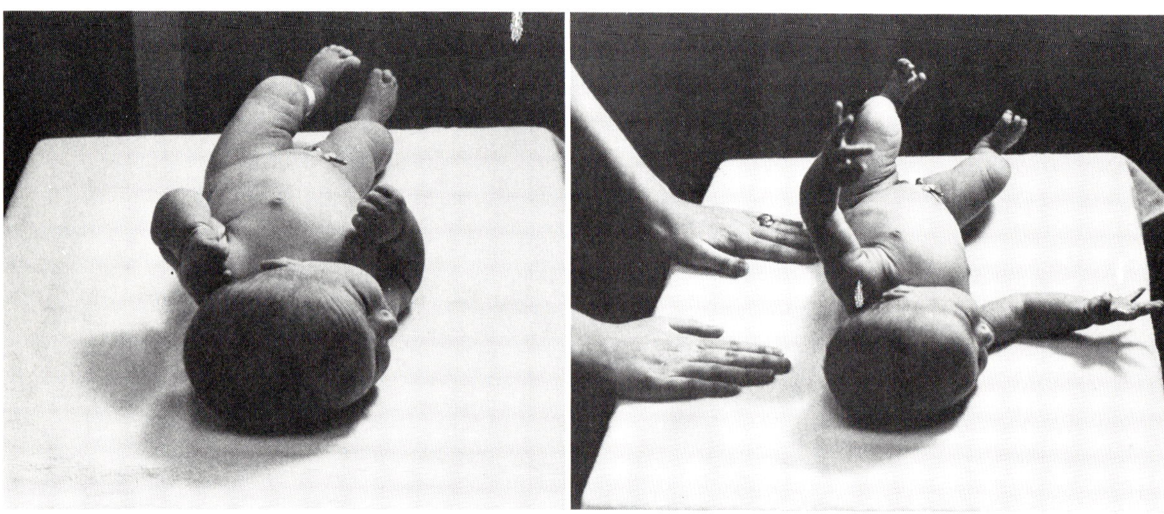

B

Fig. 12-12. Moro's reflex. (Courtesy Mead Johnson Laboratories, Evansville, Ind.)

right with the feet barely touching a hard surface. The infant will alternate feet as though walking. This step reflex usually disappears by 4 weeks.

The *Moro's reflex* ("startle" reflex) can be elicited by making a sudden, loud noise or a sudden motion. In response the infant throws both arms outward, then brings them together in quivering, embracing movement. The Moro's reflex disappears by the age of 3 months (Fig. 12-12).

The *tonic neck reflex* (Fig. 12-13) is a position that most infants usually assume for sleeping. The infant's head turns to one side, and the arm on that side extends while the opposite arm flexes. This resembles a fencing position. The tonic neck reflex disappears at 6 or 7 months of age.

Reflexes vary from baby to baby and also in the same baby at different times. For instance, immediately after feeding, the rooting and sucking reflexes may not be easy to

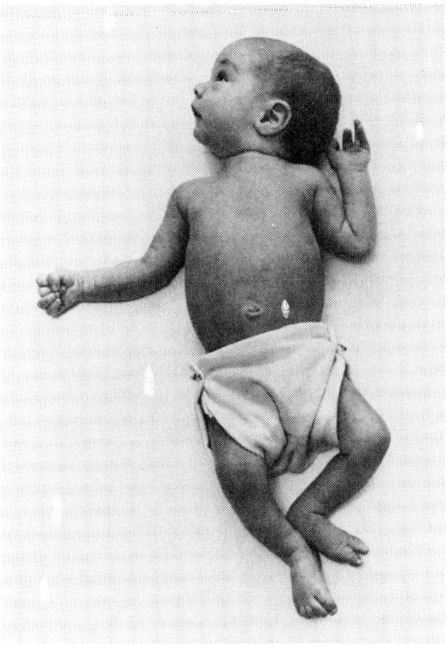

Fig. 12-13. Tonic neck reflex. (Courtesy Mead Johnson Laboratories, Evansville, Ind.)

elicit. Absent or poor reflexes should be reported immediately. The persistence of a primitive reflex after the first year or so of life may indicate a neurological problem.

Very important in an evaluation of the nervous system is observation of the infant's behavior. Limpness, poor muscle tone, and decreased activity suggest central nervous system disturbance.

Back. When the infant is turned over and held in the palm of the hand, the back will flex slightly. A deep dimple and palpable spinal bone defect should be reported promptly. The spine should be straight and vertebrae symmetrical. Careful documentation of all the preceding observations is very important to give a baseline for continuing care of the infant. Continued daily observations are also very important. Daily observations should include vital signs, weight (evaluated according to birth weight), color and activity, feeding status, elimination, parent-infant interaction, and health education needs of the parents. If anything abnormal is observed, it should be recorded and reported immediately.

INFANT CARE

RECOGNIZE APPROPRIATE TEMPERATURE AND HUMIDITY FOR NEWBORN NURSERY

Because the baby's temperature-regulating mechanisms will not be functioning for at least a few days after birth, heat conservation is important. The baby's room or nursery temperature should be kept at approximately 75.0° F (24.0° C) with humidity at 50%; the room should be kept free from drafts. Although the baby's initial temperature was taken rectally to check for a patent anus, subsequent temperatures should be taken in the axilla. Axillary temperatures eliminate the danger of irritating or perforating the rectum.

Skin care

DESCRIBE THE TECHNIQUE OF DRY SKIN CARE

The policies and procedures for bathing a newborn vary greatly. Nursing care of the newborn skin should use a technique referred to as dry skin care. The reasons for this recommendation include (1) the infant is subjected to less heat loss by exposure, (2) skin trauma is diminished, (3) less time is required, and (4) it does not expose the infant to agents with known or unknown side effects. The "dry technique" consists of the following points: (1) Cleansing of the newly born infant should be delayed until the infant's temperature has stabilized after the cold stress of delivery. (2) Only the face, head, and infant's body folds should be cleansed with cotton sponges moistened with sterile water. (3) The remainder of the skin should be untouched unless grossly soiled. There is evidence to indicate that vernix caseosa may serve a protective function, some evidence to indicate it has no effect, and no evidence to indicate it is harmful. (4) For the remainder of the infant's stay in the hospital nursery, the buttocks and perianal regions should be cleansed with sterile water and cotton. As an alternative, a mild soap with water rinsing may be used as required at diaper changes and more often if indicated. The use of creams, lotions, and emollients should be avoided. There is no single method of cord care that has been proved to limit bacterial colonization and disease. Methods currently in use include local application of alcohol, triple dye, and antimicrobial agents.

If the dry technique is not used and newborns are bathed with soap and water, the initial bath should not be given until the baby's temperature has stabilized. Do not bathe a baby immediately after a feeding because the handling may cause vomiting of the feeding and the possibility of aspiration. When bathing a baby, conserve the baby's heat by uncovering only that part of the body that is being washed. When that body part is washed, promptly cover it again. Wash the cleanest parts first and then proceed to the most soiled areas. Particular care should be given to the cleansing, rinsing, and drying of the scalp, creases of the neck, axillae, hands, under the knees, feet, buttocks, and perineum.

During the bath or during dry skin care, the baby can be observed for any abnormalities. Any deviation from normal should be reported. A tub bath for the baby should be delayed until the cord drops off and the navel has healed (usually 10 days to 2 weeks).

Instructing the new parents in infant care centers on a bath demonstration in most hospitals. While demonstrating a sponge bath, the nurse can also explain the procedure for a tub bath. Emphasize to the parents the importance of the bath time as a social time. Point out to them the unique characteristics of their infant. Encourage interaction: siblings can help with bath time and enjoy the family togetherness at home. Talk with the parents about ways in which they can include other siblings in infant care.

Basic principles of tub bathing

After the cord drops off, the skin should be cleansed every other day with a soft, clean washcloth, warm water, and a mild soap. All bathing supplies, equipment, and clothing should be assembled and ready for use in the work area. A large pan or basin can be used for bathing; however, it should be kept *only* for the baby's bath. The bath water should be warm (98° to 100° F). The environment should also be warm (75° to 80° F) and free from drafts.

Bath supplies	
Pan, basin, or tub	Pad or receiving blanket
Mild soap	Warm water
Soft towel and washcloth	Waste container
Cotton balls	Clean clothing (shirt, diaper, gown)

Always wash your hands before handling the baby. *Never* leave the baby alone when bathing. Wash each eye from the nose outward, using a clean portion of the washcloth for the second eye. Soap the baby's head. Hold the baby securely in a football position (Fig. 12-14), and rinse the head with water. Dry well. Soap the trunk, arms, axillae, and abdomen. Turn the baby over to wash the back. Wash the genitals last. Immerse the baby in the tub to rinse; pat the baby dry. Check all skin creases to be sure they are dry and clean. Dress the baby and brush the hair.

Cotton balls moistened with warm water can be used to clean the genitals if the baby has a diaper soiled with feces. This cleaning should be done if necessary when undressing the baby for the bath.

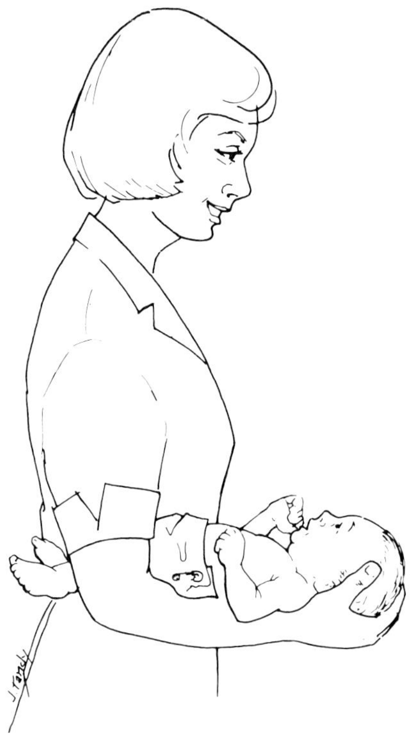

Fig. 12-14. Football hold. (From Jensen, M., and Bobak, I.M.: Maternity and gynecologic care: the nurse and the family, ed. 3, St. Louis, 1985, The C.V. Mosby Co.)

Prevention of infection

DESCRIBE GOOD TECHNIQUE TO PREVENT INFECTION

The infant's immature immune system leaves the newborn susceptible to infection, particularly to those organisms with which the newborn has had no previous contact. The most important nursing measure to prevent infection is careful handwashing. Upon entering the nursery at the beginning of the working day and when returning from lunch or dinner, the nurse should scrub hands and arms up to the elbows for 3 minutes with a hexachlorophene or iodophor preparation. After caring for each baby, the hands should be washed again. Also, nurses should wash their hands after touching any equipment considered "contaminated," such as pens, pencils, telephones, charts—anything not specifically used on the baby. The nurse should wear a clean scrub gown or suit each day. Removing all jewelry from the hands and arms and keeping fingernails short and polish-free are also important in preventing infection.

Of course, any person (staff or family) with an infectious disease should not enter the nursery, and any infant suspected of infection should be isolated from the other babies. A space of 2 feet should be kept between infant cribs to separate babies from each other. It is advisable to wash the nursery and all nursery equipment with disinfectant each day. All nursery linens are handled separately from the regular hospital linens. Everyone working in the nursery should be familiar with the American Academy of Pediatrics' recommended standards.

Family members should be instructed to wash their hands well before handling their baby.

Family-centered care practices do not increase newborn infection rates. Well siblings may visit and hold their new baby brother or sister without increasing bacterial colonization in newborns.

Nutritional needs

EXPLAIN AVERAGE WEIGHT LOSS IN NEWBORN

A weight loss of 5% to 10% of the original birth weight can be considered normal for the newborn in the first days of life, although some babies do not lose weight. The newborn loses this weight because of the meconium, the use of calories to meet metabolic needs, and the loss of more body fluids than taken in. Within 3 to 5 days after birth the baby will begin gaining weight and will reach birth weight by 10 days to 2 weeks of age. By 4 months of life, the baby will double the birth weight.

A newborn infant is regulating its internal environment at birth and should be fed within 4 hours of birth to keep blood glucose levels up.

IDENTIFY NUTRITIONAL REQUIREMENTS OF NEWBORN

A newborn needs water, calories, protein, carbohydrate, fat, vitamins, and minerals. The amount of fluid a newborn needs is in proportion to body weight; that is, the larger the baby, the greater the fluid need. A newborn cannot conserve water and loses it quickly. Water replacement is particularly important for newborns in hot weather or when they are placed under lights that increase their body temperature. By the third to fourth day of life, the term baby needs approximately 140 to 160 milliliters of fluid per kilogram of body weight in 24 hours. (A baby weighing 5 kilograms [10.5 pounds] requires 750 milliliters of fluid intake in 24 hours, providing 150 milliliters per kilogram.) With eight feedings in a 24-hour period, this would translate into 93 milliliters per feeding, or about 3 ounces.

During the first few weeks of life the average baby probably needs about 112 calories per kilogram of body weight. (A 3-kilogram [6.6-pound] baby would require 336 calories per day.) Most infant formulas contain 20 calories per ounce. Because of the baby's rapid growth, protein is very important in infant nutrition. The newborn needs at least 9 grams of protein per day, although 14 grams per day in the first month is the usual recommendation. This recommendation increases to 15 grams per day in the second month and 16 grams per day from 4 months to 1 year of age. The infant receives its principal protein from lactalbumin in human milk or casein in cow's milk. The carbohydrate of milk is lactose.

Fat is the main source of calories in human milk and is more easily digested than the fat in cow's milk. Because the newborn needs the fat in milk as an important energy source, skim milk is not advised for infants or children under 2 years of age. Skim milk also contains too much salt, ash, potassium, and calcium for infants and young children.

Formula-fed infants require vitamin supplementation. Breast milk contains all the vitamins but vitamin D, which must be supplemented. Many formula-fed infants are given formulas fortified with iron; however, iron supplements are given if a nonfortified formula is used. Well babies who are being breast-fed have adequate amounts of iron stores for up to 3 to 4 months past delivery. After that initial 3 to 4 months, many physicians recommend adding 1 to 2 milligrams per kilogram of the baby's body weight per day to the breast-fed baby's intake, or iron supplements may be prescribed for the mother's diet. Some physicians prescribe a fluoride supplement for newborns to aid in prevention of dental caries.

Breast-feeding and the pros and cons of both breast and bottle feeding were discussed earlier. Helping the mother who chooses to bottle feed will be discussed here.

Bottle feeding

On discharge from the hospital, the new mother is given instructions on the formula to be used for her baby. Often sample formulas and a supply of formula for 2 to 3 days are provided by the pharmaceutical firm that manufactures the formula. The mother and her family need a thorough understanding of these instructions before going home.

Ready-to-feed formulas and *disposable bottles* are convenient but often add considerable expense. Disposable plastic liners can be inserted in thoroughly washed bottles. The nipples and caps need to be sterile (boiled 5 minutes) to protect the baby from illness.

One method for home preparation is *terminal sterilization*. The formula is prepared under a clean technique: nipples, nipple caps, and bottles are washed thoroughly. Next, formula is prepared and poured into bottles, and the nipples and caps are applied loosely. The filled bottles are then placed in a sterilizer (pan with lid) and sterilized with boiling water for 25 minutes. After this the lids are screwed on tightly and the bottles are cooled and refrigerated until use. Enough formula should be made daily for one 24-hour period.

COMPARE METHODS OF STERILIZATION FOR BOTTLE-FED BABIES

Perhaps the easiest method to prepare formula is the *single-bottle method*. One bottle at a time is thoroughly washed in hot soapy water, rinsed, and filled with formula. The liquid formula or powder is mixed from fresh tap water. This bottle is given to the baby after preparation, and all unused formula in the bottle is discarded. The nipple is also thoroughly washed in hot soapy water and rinsed both before and after use.

Feeding is done in the semiupright position. Holding the baby is the preferred method of feeding because of the infant's need for emotional warmth during the feeding time. Babies should never be fed lying flat with bottles "propped" because of the danger of aspiration.

Burping, or "bubbling," the infant is done after the first 5 minutes of feeding, in the middle of feeding, and at the end of the feeding to help the baby release the accumulation of air. The infant is held in an upright position and the back is gently patted or stroked (Fig. 12-15).

DEMONSTRATE METHODS OF "BUBBLING" BABY

After feeding, the infant should be placed on the stomach or side and not on the back. In these positions, if the baby should spit up, the vomitus will run out of the mouth and lessen the chance of aspiration.

There are various types of nipples used: firm and resistant for babies who suck vigorously and soft, pliable nipples for premature babies who tire easily (Fig. 12-16). The rate of flow through the nipple will vary according to the size and shape of the nipple hole. Large holes are needed for cereals.

Giving water to a baby may be helpful during hot weather or if the baby is constipated. However, never mix honey in the baby's water or formula. Giving either cooked or uncooked honey to a baby under 1 year of age has been associated with infant botulism.

Diaper care

Mild laundry soap such as Ivory soap or pure castile soap and moderately warm water should be used to wash the baby's clothing and diapers. Most detergent and clothing softeners should not be used because of the irritating effect on the baby's skin. It is important to rinse the clothing and diapers thoroughly.

Circumcision

Circumcision is the surgical removal of the foreskin on the penis. The operation is usually performed on the second or third day of life. Circumcision is a religious ritual in the Jewish religion and is performed on the eighth day of life. At that time the baby is officially named.

The American Academy of Pediatrics reports no medical justification for routine circumcision. Whether or not the infant is circumcised should be decided by the parents after a thorough explanation of the procedure and discussion of the pros and cons. Circumcision has been recommended to avoid the emotional distress of being the only uncircumcised boy in school or camp. Other reasons given for circumcision include avoiding the surgical and psychological risks should the operation be necessary at a later age and aesthetic considerations. Arguments against circumcision include the fact that it carries risks: hemorrhage, infection, and surgical mishaps. These risks can lead to sutures, transfusions, scarring, and deformity.

LIST THREE PROS AND CONS OF CIRCUMCISION

Another argument against circumcision is that it exposes the newborn to unnecessary

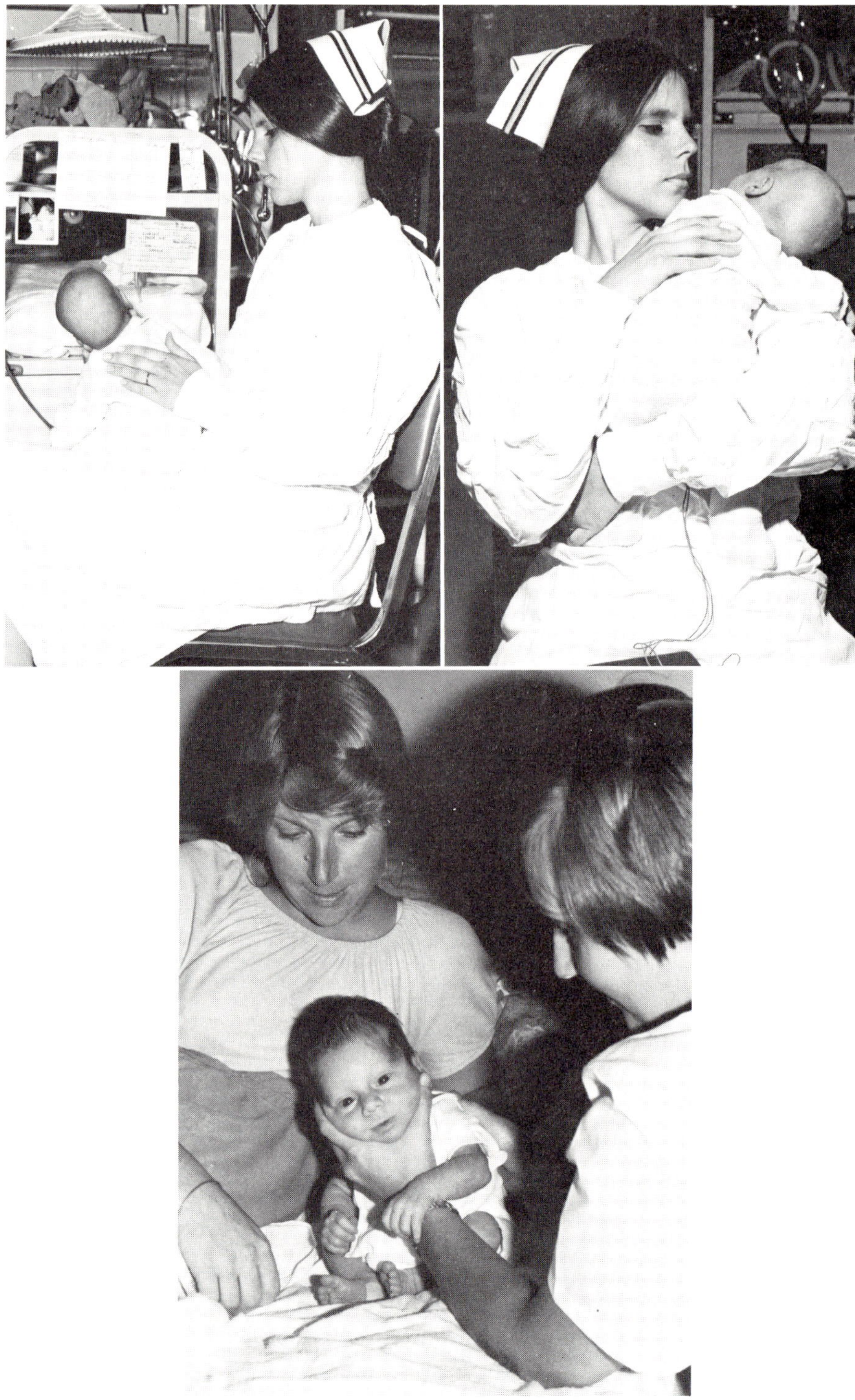

Fig. 12-15. Bubbling an infant. (From Lerch, C., and Bliss, V.J.: Maternity nursing, ed. 3, St. Louis, 1978, The C.V. Mosby Co.)

pain and trauma. For the operation the infant is restrained on a circumcision board, and the penis is cleansed with soap and water and an antiseptic solution. The baby is draped with a sterile drape that also serves to provide warmth. Sterile surgical instruments are used. Fig. 12-17 illustrates one device (Plastibell) used for circumcisions.

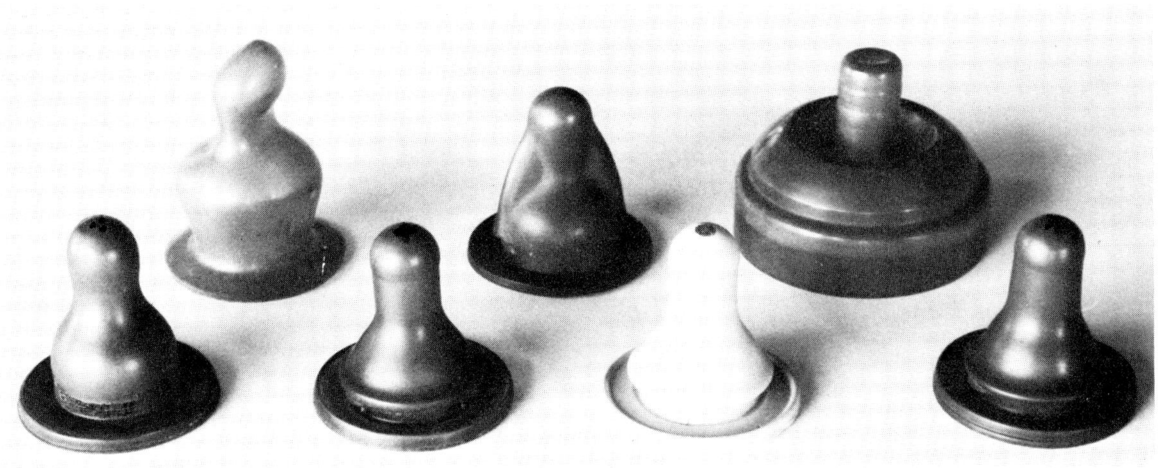

Fig. 12-16. Types of nipples. (From Ingalls, A.J., and Salerno, M.C.: Maternal and child health nursing, ed. 5, St. Louis, 1986, The C.V. Mosby Co.)

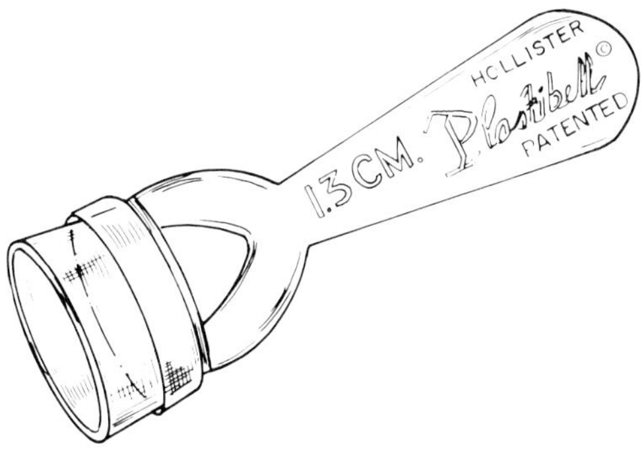

Fig. 12-17. Plastibell. (From Lerch, C., and Bliss, V.J.: Maternity nursing, ed. 3, St. Louis, 1978, The C.V. Mosby Co.)

EXPLAIN NURSING RESPONSIBILITIES BEFORE AND FOLLOWING CIRCUMCISION OF INFANT

Following the circumcision, the penis is covered with sterile gauze saturated with petrolatum. The nurse must observe the newly circumcised baby frequently for abnormal bleeding. Securing a red identification tag to the crib helps to remind the nurse to check that baby frequently.

If the baby is being discharged early, the parents need to learn how to observe and care for the newly circumcised baby at home. It will be helpful to observe any bleeding if only one layer of diaper fabric covers the penis. Cleansing the penis with cotton balls moistened in warm water must be gentle. A fresh sterile gauze with petrolatum dressing should be applied after each diaper change. The parents must understand how to apply gentle pressure to the penis to control bleeding and when to bring the baby back to the hospital for an examination by the physician.

Care of the uncircumcised penis

It is not necessary to retract any part of the infant's foreskin to wash under it. Daily external washing and rinsing are all that is necessary. The foreskin and glans develop as one tissue. Separation will evolve over time. It should never be forced. Instruct the parents to test foreskin retraction occasionally by gently trying to pull back the foreskin when bathing the baby at about 6 months. If there is any discomfort or resistance, they should stop and try again in a few months. There should be no rush to retract. By 3 years of age, about 90% of boys have retractable foreskins, and by age 17, 99% do. As the male child learns to bathe himself, he will learn how to clean his penis as well.

DISCHARGE TO HOME

DISCUSS SUCCESSFUL ADAPTATION OF PARENTS, SIBLINGS, AND GRANDPARENTS TO NEW BABY

Whether the infant and new family go home in 12 hours or after several days, health education for the new family is extremely important. Special referrals to public health or visiting nurses or other health care workers may be needed. Follow-up appointments with the physician for mother and baby should be made. In many hospitals today follow-up home visits by hospital nurses are also being made. Whatever the hospital policy, the new parents must learn how to care for their infant.

Parents will also need anticipatory guidance on how to handle sibling relationships and how to take advantage of support systems available. It is important to encourage parents to allow the siblings to share in infant care. A healthy relationship can be encouraged by giving the sibling special attention as an individual needing love and reinforcement of that love. Participation by the sibling in infant care is essential.

Support systems are vital to serve as an emotional sounding board and to release the parents of some of the responsibilities of the new family life. Responding to a new baby 24 hours a day can be very tiring very quickly. Parents need some support, too.

SUMMARY

This unit has offered an introduction to the newborn. Because the safe transition from the uterus to the world outside is so important, it is vital for the nurse to have the knowledge and skills needed to understand the normal newborn.

With a basic understanding of the normal newborn, recognition of deviations from normal becomes possible. Such early recognition can determine whether or not the infant survives or with what degree of wellness the infant grows and develops. The next unit will explore complications in the newborn period.

BIBLIOGRAPHY

Affonso, D.D.: The newborn's potential for interaction, JOGN Nurs. **5**(6):9-14, 1976.

American Academy of Pediatrics: Standards and recommendations for hospital care of newborn infants, Evanston, Ill., 1977, The Academy.

Benson, R.C., editor: Current obstetric and gynecologic diagnosis and treatment, ed. 4, Los Altos, Calif., 1982, Lange Medical Publications.

Binzley, V.: State: overlooked factor in newborn nursing, Am. J. Nurs. **77**(1):102-103, 1977.

Bower, T.G.R.: The perceptual world of the child, Cambridge, Mass., 1977, Harvard University Press.

Farrar, C.A.: Assessing individuality in the newborn, Nurs. Digest:16-19, July, 1975.

Freeman, M.H.: Giving family life a good start in the hospital, MCN **4**(1):51-54, 1979.

Grimes, D.A.: Routine circumcision of the newborn infant: a reappraisal, Am. J. Obstet. Gynecol. **130**(2):125-129, 1978.

LeBoyer, F.: Birth without violence, New York, 1975, Alfred A. Knopf, Inc.

McLean, F.H.: Significance of birthweight for gestational age in identifying infants at risk, JOGN Nurs. **3**(6):19-24, 1974.

Moore, M.L.: Realities in childbearing, ed. 2, Philadelphia, 1983, W.B.Saunders Co.

Newton, L.D.: Helping parents cope with infant crying, JOGN Nurs. **12**(3):199-204, 1983.

The Nurses Association of the American College of Obstetricians and Gynecologists: Neonatal skin care, OGN Nursing Practice Resource, 12, March 1985, The Association.

Phillips, C.R.: The essence of birth without violence, MCN **1**(3):162-163, 1976.

Phillips, C.R.: Neonatal heat loss in heated cribs vs. mother's arms, JOGN Nurs. **3**(6):11-15, 1974.

Porth, C.M., and Kaylor, L.E.: Temperature regulation in the newborn, Am. J. Nurs. **78**(10):1691-1693, 1978.

Preston, E.N.: Wither the foreskin? A consideration of routine neonatal circumcision, J.A.M.A. **213**(11):1853-1858, 1970.

Statement of the Committee on Fetus and Newborn, American Academy of Pediatrics: Skin care of newborns, Pediatrics **54**:(6), Dec. 1974.

Sullivan, R., Foster, J., and Schreiner, R.L.: Determining a newborn's gestational age, MCN **4**:38-45, Jan./Feb. 1979.

Thoman, E.B., and Trotter, S., editors: Social responsiveness of infants: a round table, 1978, Johnson & Johnson Baby Products.

Whiteside, D.: Proper use of radiant warmers, Am. J. Nurs. **78**:1694-1696, 1978.

Williams, J.K., and Lancaster, J.: Thermoregulation of the newborn, MCN **1**(6):355-360, 1976.

Wranesh, B.L.: The effect of sibling visitation on bacterial colonization rate in neonates, JOGN Nurs. **11**(4):211-213.

DEFINITIONS

Define the following terms:

acidotic	LGA
AGA	metabolic acidosis
area care	milia
bilirubin	mongolian spots
brown fat	Moro's reflex
caput succedaneum	neutral thermal environment
cephalhematoma	radiant warmer
cohort system	radiation
conduction	SGA
convection	single bottle method
dry skin care	surfactant
erythema toxicum	synchronous
hemangioma	thermogenesis
hyperthermia	thermogenic activity
icterus neonatorum	thrush
iodophor preparation	tonic neck reflex
lanugo	traditional stool
vernix	vitamin K

LEARNING ACTIVITIES AND EXPERIENCES

1. Group discussions.
2. Interview a new mother concerning her baby. Ask her if her baby can recognize her in a group of strangers. What does she see as unique about her baby?
3. View audiovisual aids and discuss.

ENRICHMENT/IN-DEPTH STUDY

1. Visit a local drugstore and inspect the prepared formulas for sale (composition? cost?). Price disposable paper diapers, bottles, nipples.
2. Visit a local department store and price diapers (cloth) and baby clothing.
3. Obtain and read the pamphlet, "Care of the Uncircumcised Penis." For copies, contact: American Academy of Pediatrics, Publications Department, P.O. Box 927, Elk Grove Village, IL 60007.

SELF-ASSESSMENT

1. Circle those laboratory values that suggest anemia on day 1 in the life of a newborn:
   a. Hct 60%
   b. Hct 55%
   c. Hct 40%
   d. Hgb 19.0 grams/100 milliliters
   e. Hgb 16.8 grams/100 milliliters
   f. Hgb 12.5 grams/100 milliliters
2. What is the normal leukocyte count on day 1 of life?
   a. 12,000
   b. 6,000
   c. 18,000
3. Normal bilirubin on day 1 of life is under ________ milligrams per deciliter, and on day 5 of life is under ________ milligrams per deciliter.
4. When would you expect physiological jaundice to become apparent?

5. Vitamin K aids in the formation of ________________, which is necessary for blood ________________.
6. What special precautions are necessary when using a manual mode of radiant warmer?

7. The nursery temperature should be kept at approximately ________, with humidity at ________%.

For questions 8 through 11, circle the best answer.

8. Average weight loss in the normal newborn in the first days of life is:
   a. 5% to 10% of birth weight
   b. 2% to 4% of birth weight
   c. 12% of birth weight
9. Newborn skin care recommended by the American Academy of Pediatrics is:
   a. hexachlorophene baths
   b. tub baths
   c. dry technique
10. Newborns cry because they are:
    a. lonely
    b. hungry
    c. in pain
    d. tired
    e. spoiled

    Answers (circle one): 1. a,b,c
    2. e
    3. a,b,c,d
    4. all of the above
11. A newborn's vital signs would be which of the following:
    a. axillary temperature, 99° F; pulse, 110 per minute; respiration, 20 per minute

b. axillary temperature, 98° F; pulse, 120 per minute; respiration, 40 per minute
c. axillary temperature, 100° F; pulse, 200 per minute; respiration, 80 per minute

12. Statistics for average American white baby include:
weight (female) __________ (male) __________
length __________
chest circumference __________
head circumference __________

13. In examination of the normal newborn, briefly note what you would expect to find for each of the following:
a. skin:

b. ears:

c. face (include nose and mouth):

d. eyes:

e. neck:

f. chest (include breasts):

g. abdomen (include cord):

h. genitals: male
female

14. Match Column A with Column B

Column A	Column B
______1. meconium	a. pale yellow and semiformed
______2. breast-fed stools	b. golden yellow and pasty
______3. formula-fed stools	c. black, tarry, and odorless

15. Complete the following chart:

Reflex	Appearance	How stimulated	Time of disappearance
Moro's			
Grasp			
Walking			
Sucking			

16. Match Column A with Column B.

Column A	Column B
______1. caput succedaneum	a. bleeding into conjunctiva caused by pressure of delivery
______2. cephalhematoma	b. edema of the scalp
______3. erythema toxicum	c. tiny white spots on face
______4. "stork bites"	d. fine rash of newborn
______5. milia	e. subperiosteal hemorrhage
______6. subconjunctival hemorrhage	f. small, white, ricelike epidermal plaques in mouth
______7. "epithelial pearls"	g. small hemangiomas
______8. molding	h. uneven and unsymmetrical shape of newborn's head

17. Describe the first reactive phase in the life of a newborn. How long does it last? What are the baby's respirations and heart rate?

18. During what phase of newborn activity does the baby's body temperature return to normal?

19. List the six "state" cycles of the newborn:
    a.
    b.
    c.
    d.
    e.
    f.

20. Match Column A with Column B.

Column A	Column B
______1. convection	a. transfer of heat from a warm object to a cool object
______2. conduction	b. newborn's method of producing heat
______3. evaporation	c. heat loss from wet skin in a dry atmosphere
______4. radiation	d. newborn's means of heat retention
______5. nonshivering thermogenesis	e. enhanced by surrounding air currents
______6. vasoconstriction	f. transfer of heat from body surfaces to cooler surfaces

21. Newborn heat loss by convection can be minimized by ____________________.
22. Newborn heat loss by evaporation can be prevented by ____________________.
23. Newborn heat loss by conduction can be minimized by ____________________.
24. If a newborn baby required extensive life-saving procedures, would you place the baby in a warm incubator or a radiant warmer? Why?

25. Match Column A with Column B.

Column A	Column B
______1. SGA	a. before 38 weeks gestation
______2. AGA	b. average for gestational age
______3. LGA	c. 38 to 42 weeks gestation
______4. preterm	d. large for gestational age
______5. term	e. 42 weeks or more gestation
______6. postterm	f. small for gestational age

26. When determining gestational age (using the clinical form in this book), the nurse checks the following physical characteristics:
    a.
    b.
    c.
    d.
    e.
    f.
    g.

UNIT XIII
The newborn with complications

GOALS

This unit is designed to provide the reader with information that will:

□ promote awareness of deviations from normal in the newborn period.

STUDENT OBJECTIVES

After studying this unit you should be able to:

1. Distinguish between the resuscitation needs of newborns with Apgar scores of 4 to 6, 0 to 3, and 7 to 10.
2. Describe the special needs for support of the parents of a low-birth-weight baby who is in a special care nursery.
3. Compare physiological jaundice and that appearing before the baby is 24 hours old.
4. Name the six major causes of hyperbilirubinemia in the newborn.
5. Design a plan of care for the newborn receiving phototherapy for hyperbilirubinemia.
6. Identify blood sugar (glucose) levels indicating low blood sugar (hypoglycemia) in full-term infants (both before and after 72 hours of age).
7. When given a description of the following conditions, be able to associate the description with the condition: cleft lip and/or palate, hydrocephalus, spina bifida, Down's syndrome, and phenylketonuria.

The average newborn is mildly hypoxic and acidotic at birth. Normal values at birth are pO_2, 20 to 30 mm Hg; pH, 7.25; and pCO_2, 45 to 50 mm Hg.

For the normal neonate at 24 hours of age, values are pO_2, 90 to 100 mm Hg; pH, 7.35 to 7.45; pCO_2, 35 to 45 mm Hg.

For most babies breathing begins immediately after birth; however, for some babies breathing is delayed. These babies require immediate assistance.

RESUSCITATION OF THE NEWBORN

Every delivery area should be equipped with newborn resuscitation equipment and staffed with personnel who know how to use it (Fig. 13-1).

Resuscitation equipment:
Source of heat for baby (preferably a radiant heater)
Adequate lighting
Infant stethoscope
Bulb syringe for suctioning
DeLee mucus trap with catheter for aspiration of mucus
Suction capabilities
Suction catheters Nos. 5, 8 and 10
Source of 100% oxygen
Oxygen tubing with and without masks (premature and newborn sizes)
Laryngoscope with spare batteries
Dextrostix (bottle)
Soluset
NS intravenous IV 250 cubic centimeters
D5/w 500 cubic centimeters
D10/w 1000 cubic centimeters
Stopcocks
Laryngoscope blades, sizes 1 and 0 with spare bulbs for laryngoscope
Feeding tubes with syringes
Endotracheal tubes of various sizes (2.5, 3.0, 3.5, 4.0 mm) with adaptors to fit all sizes

A

B

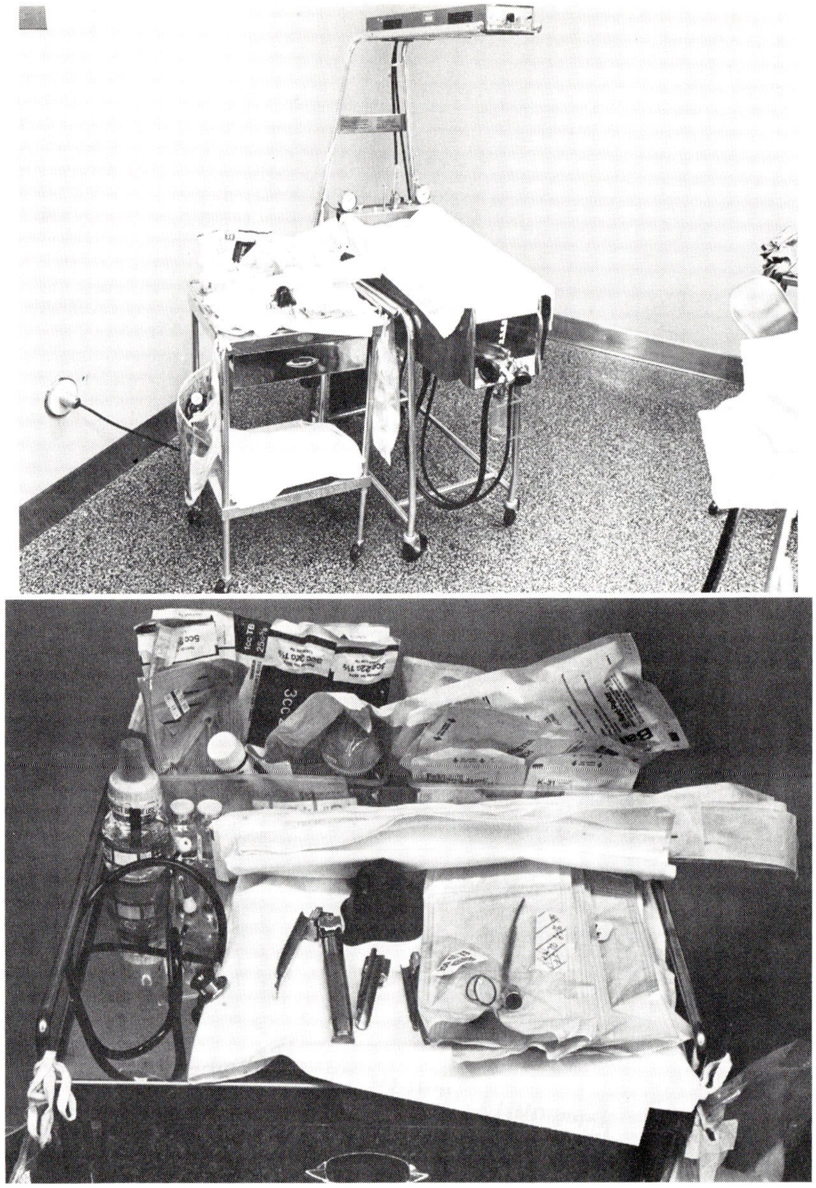

Fig. 13-1. A, Resuscitation area. **B,** Resuscitation equipment. (Courtesy Kaiser-Permanente Medical Center, Santa Clara, Calif.)

Infant airways
Adhesive tape
Warm blankets
Umbilical vein catheters with umbilical catheterization tray
Assorted sizes of syringes and needles
Drugs:
Epinephrine 1:10,000
Narcotic antagonists
Dextrose 10% in water
Sodium bicarbonate
Calcium gluconate
Heparin sodium 1000 per milliliter
Glucagon 1 unit per milliliter
Isoproteronol (Isuprel) 1:5000
Adrenaline 1/1000
Calcium chloride
Atropine

At the beginning of each shift, the emergency equipment should be checked to be sure it is all present and in working order.

It is usually possible to identify the fetus that will be in jeopardy even before delivery occurs. Intrapartum conditions such as meconium-stained fluid, maternal bleeding, heavy maternal sedation, prolapse of the cord, or fetal distress without identified cause predispose to the birth of an infant requiring resuscitation. Prematurity and labors associated with medical problems such as diabetes, chronic hypertensive states, and postterm gestation can result in both fetal and neonatal asphyxia. Also, cesarean birth frequently results in the need for resuscitation of the newborn.

RESUSCITATION OF NEWBORNS WITH VARIOUS APGAR SCORES

The Apgar score will give an estimation of a term infant's condition at birth. The infant with an Apgar score of 7 to 10 at 1 minute will not require resuscitation, but an infant scoring 0 to 3 will require resuscitation. The baby scoring 4 to 6 may need only suction, gentle stimulation, and a few whiffs of oxygen. It is important to remember that depressant drugs and anesthesia given to the mother may produce low Apgar scores even though the baby is not asphyxiated. (See Table 13-1 for neonatal resuscitation scores and procedures.)

When asphyxiated, the infant's oxygen level is low, carbon dioxide level is high, and there is sub-optimal ventilation. The infant who is cyanotic and gasping with good muscle tone and heart rate of 100 needs to be kept dry and warm, stimulated, and given oxygen. The infant who is born pale, limp, and severely depressed needs immediate resuscitation and intubation.

Technique for resuscitation of infant

EXPLAIN THE TECHNIQUE FOR RESUSCITATION OF INFANT

1. The baby should be placed under a radiant warmer with the head lower than thorax and should be dried immediately.
2. The airway must be cleared by gentle suction of the oropharynx to remove meco-

Table 13-1. Neonatal resuscitation

Apgar score	Baby's condition	Resuscitation procedure
7-10 Normal	Responsive Heart rate normal (>100 per minute) Respirations normal (40 per minute)	1. Clear airway by suctioning mouth and nose with a bulb syringe. Catheter suction may cause bradycardia; if used, do brief, gentle suctioning. 2. Maintain thermal neutrality by drying infant with warm, dry towel and placing infant under a radiant warmer. 3. Routine identification procedures. 4. Neonatal ophthalmic prophylaxis. 5. Brief physical examination.
4-6 Moderately depressed	Poor response Decreased or absent respirations Heart rate less than 100 or normal Decreased muscle tone	1. Routine drying, warming, and suctioning as above. 2. Stimulate to breathe by rubbing up and down spine or slapping soles of feet. 3. Administer warm humid oxygen over the nose and mouth. 4. If infant's condition fails to improve, ventilate with oxygen by bag and mask. 5. If condition improves, continue as for a normal infant. 6. If no response to bag and mask ventilation, proceed to endotracheal intubation as for severely depressed infant below.
0-3 Severely depressed	Unresponsive Depressed or absent respirations Decreased or absent heart rate Pale, flaccid	1. Suction, dry, warm, stimulate. 2. If no response to ventilation with 100% oxygen by bag and mask, intubate with endotracheal tube and ventilate by bag and mask at a rate of 30 to 40 per minute. 3. If heart rate less than 70, administer external cardiac massage. Compress to chest one half to three quarters of an inch at a rate of 100 to 120 compressions per minute. Maintain a ratio of three compressions per one ventilation. 4. If continued poor response, perform umbilical catheterization and infuse appropriate medication.

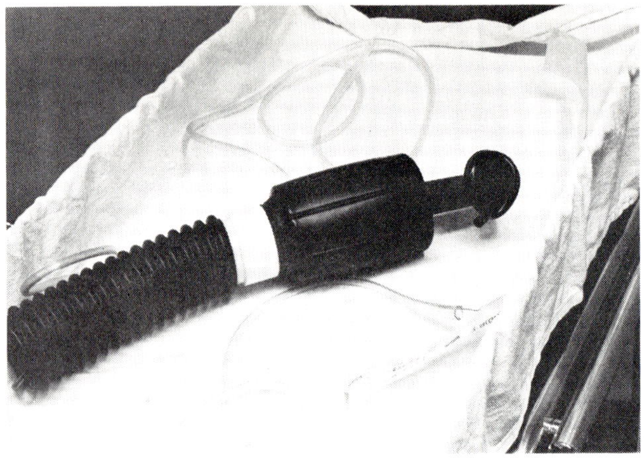

Fig. 13-2. Bag and mask.

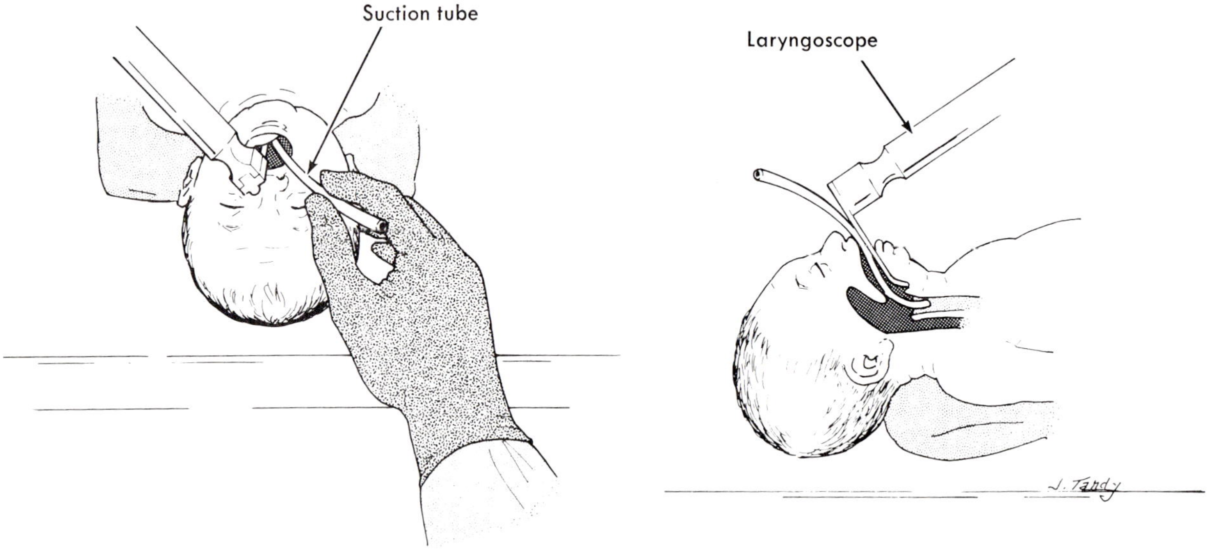

Fig. 13-3. Laryngoscope and tracheal suctioning. (From Jensen, M., and Bobak, I.M.: Maternity and gynecologic care: the nurse and the family, ed. 3, St. Louis, 1985, The C.V. Mosby Co.)

nium secretions. A bulb syringe is usually adequate. Too much suctioning with a long catheter in the first few minutes of life can cause laryngospasm.

3. Ventilation is assisted by giving oxygen by bag and mask at 20 to 30 breaths per minute (Fig. 13-2). To prevent overexpansion of the infant's lungs, the pressure on the bag should be light. If there is a possibility that meconium was aspirated, the baby should be intubated and suctioned before assisted ventilation is begun.
4. A member of the resuscitation team should monitor the infant's heartbeat during this time by tapping a finger in time to the beat. If the heart rate does not increase immediately, intubation will be needed.
5. Intubation should be done by someone experienced in the use of a laryngoscope. Secretions, blood, and meconium are quickly aspirated and an endotracheal tube inserted (Fig. 13-3). Mouth-to-tube or bag-to-tube ventilation is begun at a rate of 30 to 40 per minute. A team member continues to tap out the baby's heartbeat and observe the chest for movement.
6. If the baby's heartbeat should fall under 70 beats per minute, cardiac massage is instituted (Fig. 13-4). However, never perform cardiac massage and ventilate at the same time because simultaneous cardiac massage and ventilation can cause

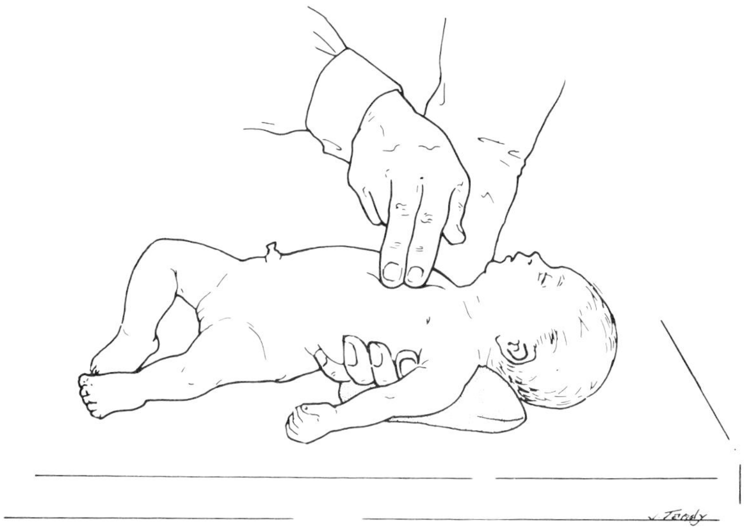

Fig. 13-4. Cardiac massage. (From Jensen, M., and Bobak, I.M.: Maternity and gynecologic care: the nurse and the family, ed. 3, St. Louis, 1985, The C.V. Mosby Co.)

pneumothorax. Compress chest one half to three quarters of an inch at a rate of 100 to 120 compressions per minute. The ratio of chest wall compression to ventilation is 3:1 (three compressions to one ventilation).

7. If the baby is still unresponsive at this point, sodium bicarbonate, 3 milliequivalents per kilogram, diluted with an equal volume of water, may be given through an umbilical catheter over a 2- to 5-minute period to combat acidosis.
8. Should the baby continue to be depressed, 0.5 milliliter of 1:10,000 epinephrine can be given through an umbilical catheter and 1 to 2 milliliters of 50% glucose started by slow infusion.

A baby who has been resuscitated will require close management and care and should be transferred to a neonatal intensive care unit. The possibility of brain damage in infants requiring resuscitation at birth is greater than for normal infants.

In Unit I levels of care were discussed (regionalization of perinatal care). Level III (tertiary care) was identified as that level at which neonatal intensive care could be provided. Neonatal intensive care nursing is a fascinating, rapidly changing specialty area of nursing that is beyond the scope of a basic text such as this. In this chapter we will present very basic information on the newborn with complications. Figs. 13-5 and 13-6 will give some idea of the equipment in an intensive care unit. One-to-one nursing is usually provided around the clock to the infants in intensive care.

DESCRIBE THE ESSENTIAL ELEMENTS IN HIGH-RISK NURSERY

CLASSIFICATION OF NEWBORNS

A *preterm* baby is a live infant whose gestation period is less than 38 weeks, regardless of the baby's weight. A *low-birth-weight infant* is a baby weighing less than 5.5 pounds (2,500 grams) at birth. A low-birth-weight infant may be either preterm or full-term but small for gestational age. A *small-for-gestational-age* (SGA) baby is one whose birth weight is below the tenth percentile. Some infants are both preterm and growth retarded. Maternal factors contributing to prematurity include multiple pregnancy, maternal disease, premature rupture of the membranes, placenta previa, abruptio placentae, incompetent cervix, low socioeconomic status, and maternal age. Maternal characteristics frequently associated with SGA babies include vascular insufficiencies, renal disease, pregnancy-induced hypertension, maternal age under 16 years, nutritional deficiency, cigarette smoking, alcoholism, narcotic addiction, and certain genetic disorders.

DIFFERENTIATE BETWEEN PRETERM AND SMALL-FOR-GESTATIONAL-AGE BABY

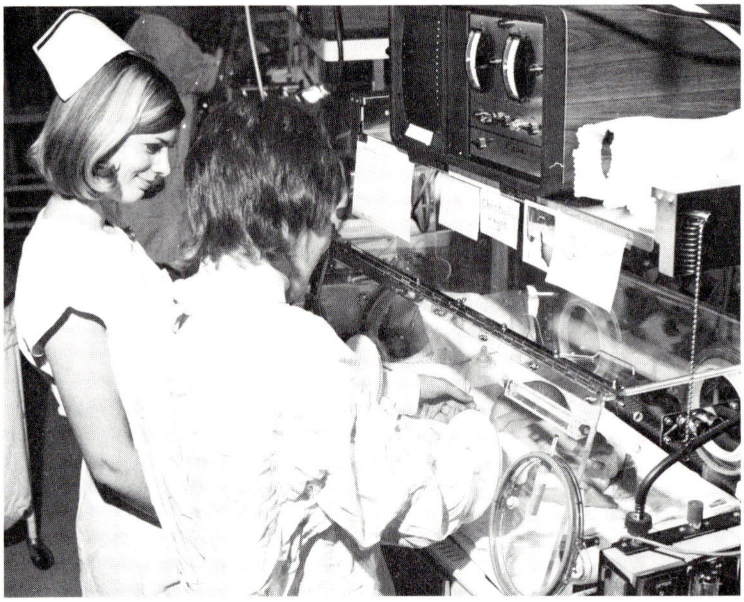

Fig. 13-5. Mother interacting with her infant. (From Lerch, C., and Bliss, V.J.: Maternity nursing, ed. 3, St. Louis, 1978, The C.V. Mosby Co.)

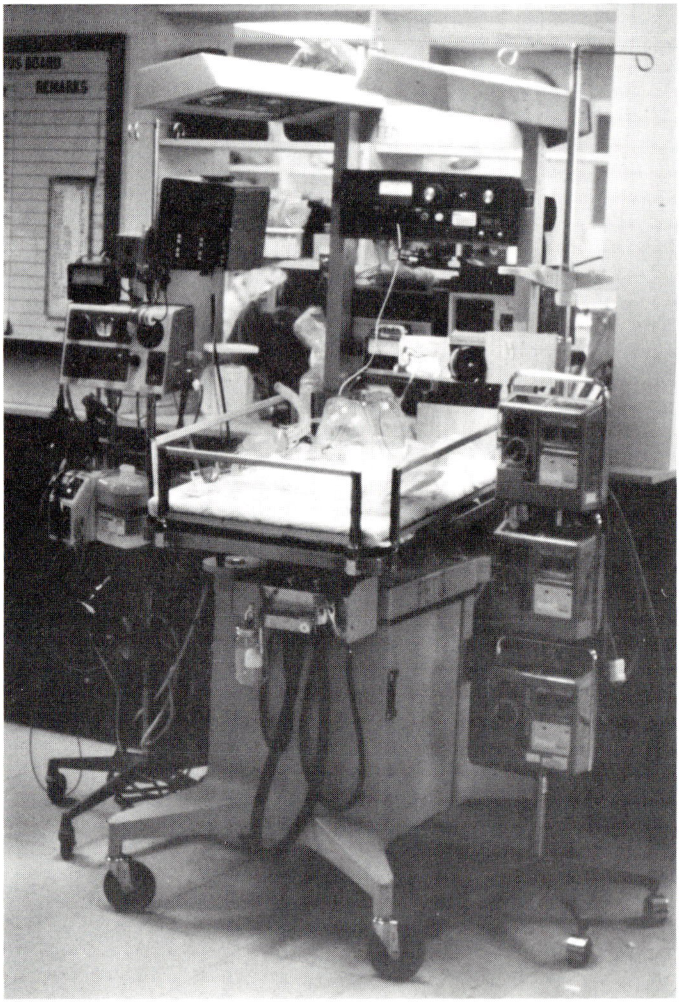

Fig. 13-6. Intensive care nursery.

The majority of infants in the United States who die during the first year of life are either preterm or SGA.

SGA babies are subject to metabolic, nutritional, and neurological disorders. Preterm babies are subject to respiratory, thermal, and neurological problems. (Neonatal risks in preterm and SGA babies can be found in the accompanying boxes.) The classification of a baby as either preterm or SGA is based on a number of criteria. Some of these criteria are included in Unit XII (p. 285).

NEONATAL RISKS IN PRETERM BABIES (REGARDLESS OF BIRTHWEIGHT)

Hyaline membrane disease
Recurrent apnea
Hypothermia and acidosis
Hypoglycemia
Hypocalcemia
Infection
Hyperbilirubinemia and kernicterus
Necrotizing enterocolitis
Intraventricular hemorrhage and pulmonary hemorrhage
Anemia
Patent ductus arteriosus

NEONATAL RISKS IN SMALL-FOR-GESTATIONAL-AGE INFANTS

Hypothermia
Hypoglycemia
Perinatal asphyxia and its sequelae
Polycythemia
Congenital malformations
Chronic intrauterine infection
Massive pulmonary hemorrhage

Preterm baby

The cry of a preterm baby is feeble and the sucking, gag, and swallowing reflexes are frequently poor or absent, necessitating *gavage feeding*. Tonic neck and Moro's reflexes may be absent or ill defined (Fig. 13-7).

Because of an immature temperature-regulating center and very little subcutaneous fat, the preterm baby has a very unstable body temperature. A controlled environment (radiant warmer or incubator) that will maintain the baby's optimal body temperature is essential.

IDENTIFY CRY, SKIN, AND ACTIVITY CHARACTERISTICS OF PRETERM AND FULL-TERM BABY

The preterm baby's skin may be covered by vernix caseosa. The hands and feet may be cyanotic (acrocyanosis). Lanugo (fine hair) is present on the sides of the face, extremities, and back. Generalized edema is present at birth but disappears in a few days, leaving the skin loose and wrinkled with very apparent blood vessels. The ears are soft and small, containing little cartilage. The nipples and areola are inconspicuous. Heel creases are absent, and the soles of the feet are almost smooth.

Immaturity of the neurological system results in uncoordinated jerky movements. The preterm infant lies in a prone position with the pelvis flat and legs splayed out sideways like a frog. Respirations are shallow and irregular, ranging from 40 to 60 per minute. Because the liver is immature, the preterm baby is likely to have hyperbilirubinemia. Because of an immature immunological system the preterm infant is extremely susceptible to infection, making extreme caution with handwashing and cleanliness vital.

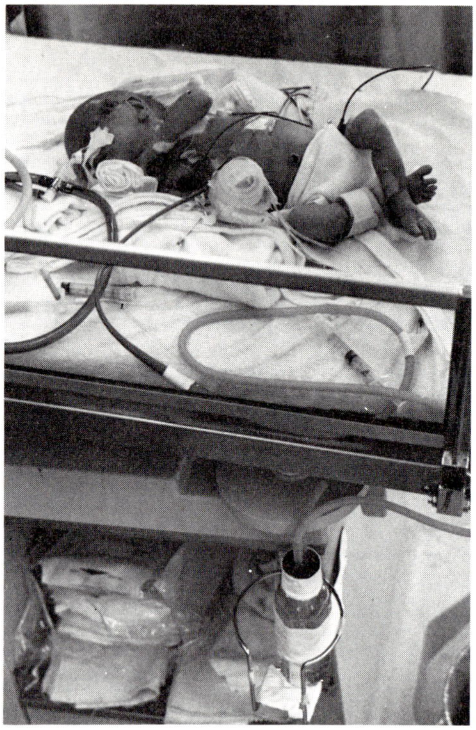

Fig. 13-7. Preterm baby. (From Chinn, P.: Child health maintenance concepts in family-centered care, ed. 2, St. Louis, 1979, The C.V. Mosby Co.)

EXPLAIN COMPLICATIONS OF PREMATURITY IN IMMEDIATE STABILIZATION OF NEWBORN

The preterm infant's body systems are too immature to maintain life without a specialized environment and care. An Isolette infant incubator or radiant warmer system should always be available to receive a preterm baby in any hospital where babies are born. In a warming unit, the baby wears only a diaper.

Oxygen is not always necessary for preterm babies and will be ordered as needed by the physician in the appropriate concentration. Excessive oxygen may cause retrolental fibroplasia resulting in blindness. If oxygen is required, an oxygen monitor or oxygen analyzer should be used to test the oxygen concentration and thus facilitate keeping it at the desired level. Arterial blood gas measurements accurately record the level of arterial oxygen. If blood gas measurements are not available and an infant has generalized cyanosis, it is usually safe to give just enough oxygen to correct the cyanosis.

Nursing care of the preterm infant includes:

1. Conserving the infant's energy
2. Maintaining safety
3. Preventing infections
4. Maintaining body temperature
5. Providing adequate fluid and calorie intake
6. Maintaining airway and adequate oxygen intake

Preterm babies who can suck and swallow are fed with a soft nipple and bottle. The mother can express her breast milk, which can be used to feed the infant if the physician so orders. Vitamins and iron supplements are given to preterm babies. Because the baby's growth rate parallels fetal growth rate, the protein and caloric needs are higher than those of the term newborn. However, because the baby's gastric capacity is limited, feedings must be frequent and small.

The infant who has no sucking or swallowing reflexes may be fed by a medicine dropper with a rubber tip or by gavage feeding. The physician prescribes the formula and amount for gavage feeding.

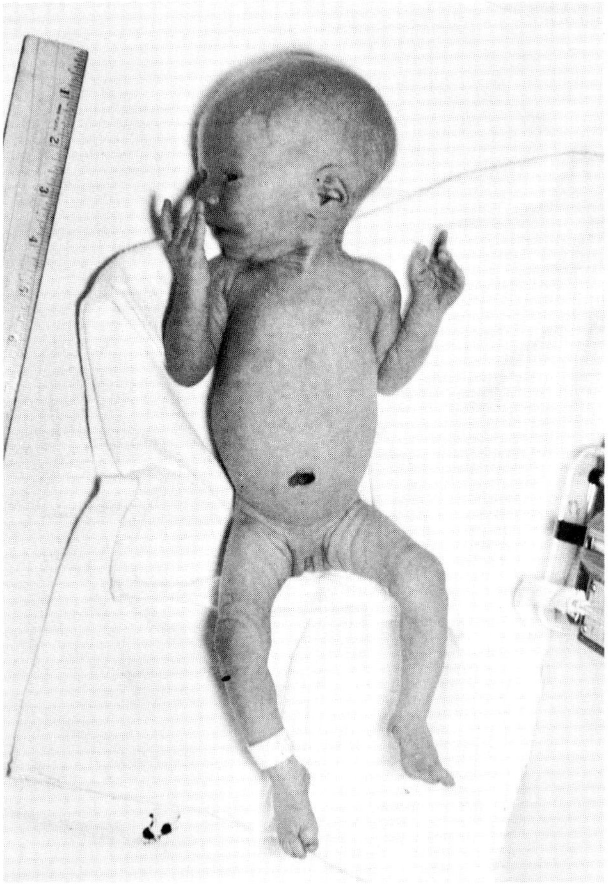

Fig. 13-8. Small-for-gestational-age baby. (From Babson, S.G., and Benson, R.C.: Management of high-risk pregnancy and intensive care of the neonate, ed. 3, St. Louis, 1975, The C.V. Mosby Co.)

Small-for-gestational-age babies

STATE POTENTIAL COMPLICATIONS FOR SGA AND POSTTERM BABIES

The baby who is small for gestational age frequently requires intensive care during the first 3 to 4 days of life. In contrast to the preterm baby, these babies are alert but give the appearance of being malnourished, with little subcutaneous fat and loose, dry skin (Fig. 13-8). Because the incidence of major congenital anomalies is high in these babies, close inspection and observation are necessary. These small babies are particularly susceptible to hypoglycemia and should not be without feeding for long periods of time. These babies are also predisposed to asphyxia resulting from hypoxic episodes in utero and to aspiration syndrome because of aspiration of meconium when hypoxic. Because of the lack of subcutaneous fat and a disproportionately large surface area, temperature regulation is often difficult in these infants.

The long-term outlook for normal function for premature and SGA babies has improved greatly with the application of intensive care techniques.

Postterm babies

In most pregnancies there is a progressive increase in placental dysfunction after 42 weeks of gestation. When this happens, the infant may appear wasted (Fig. 13-9). The postterm baby's skin becomes dry and cracked after birth and almost has the look of parchment paper. These babies may be stained with the meconium they discharged in utero in response to hypoxic periods. They are also at risk for aspirating meconium and asphyxia.

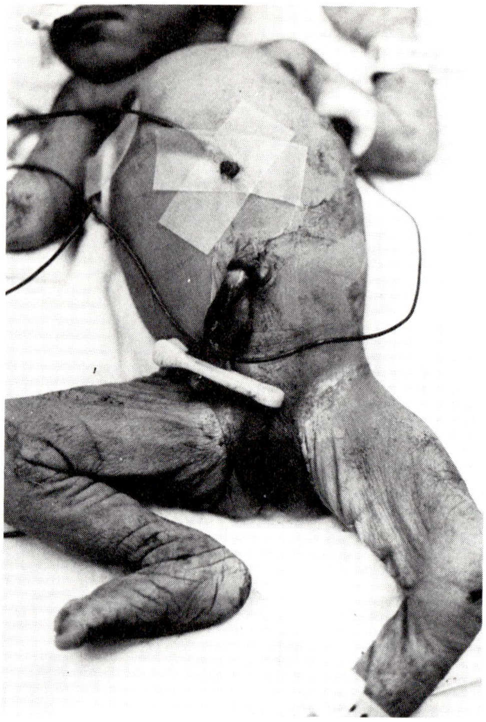

Fig. 13-9. Postterm baby. (From Korones, S.B.: High-risk newborn infants, ed. 3, St. Louis, 1985, The C.V. Mosby Co.)

Postterm babies do not tolerate the stress of labor very well and are candidates for continuous fetal monitoring.

Neonatal risks in postterm babies include perinatal asphyxia, meconium aspiration, pneumothorax, and polycythemia (which causes the hyperviscosity syndrome).

Large-for-gestational-age babies

A large-for-gestational-age baby is one whose birth weight is above the ninetieth percentile. Neonatal risks in LGA infants are listed in the accompanying box.

NEONATAL RISKS IN LARGE-FOR-GESTATIONAL-AGE INFANTS (REGARDLESS OF GESTATIONAL AGE)

Birth Injuries

- Cervical and brachial plexus palsy
- Phrenic nerve palsy
- Fractured clavicle or humerus
- Cephalhematoma
- Subdural hematoma

Infants of Diabetic Mothers (often LGA)

- Respiratory distress syndrome (RDS)
- Hypoglycemia, hypocalcemia
- Hyperbilirubinemia
- Congenital malformations
- Renal vein thrombosis
- Hyperviscosity syndrome

EMOTIONAL CARE

SUPPORT OF PARENTS

Assuming the role of parent can be very difficult for the parents of a low-birth-weight baby. The holding, touching, and eye-to-eye contact important in establishing a bond between parents and infant often have to be delayed to initiate immediate life-support measures. There is also a period of grieving by the parents for the perfect child they expected but did not have. Preterm labor and delivery happened when the parents were unprepared. If the preterm baby has to be transported to an intensive care nursery in another hospital or city, the separation can be very stressful for the parents. Because the parents may feel that the baby will probably die, they may protect themselves by delaying bonding.

Whenever a baby is in an intensive care unit (whatever the reason), the parents need special nursing care, too. It is very important for the parents to be encouraged to visit their baby in the nursery and to participate in the care. Because the responsibility for providing life-long physical and emotional care will be the parents, parents and infant must be treated as a unit from the very beginning. Before parents visit the intensive care nursery for the first time, they need preparation for the unfamiliar environment they are about to enter. The flashing lights and buzzers on the monitors and all of the equipment attached to the baby can be very frightening. Visual aids in the form of photographs of babies in the intensive care nursery plus photographs and descriptions of equipment are very helpful in preparing the parents for what they will see.

Flexible visiting hours in the nursery based on the specific needs of each family are vital. The parents should scrub their hands and arms with water and an antiseptic soap and cover their street clothes with clean gowns before entering the nursery. The same precautions concerning communicable disease that apply to staff also apply to parents.

Some parents may want to touch or hold the baby on the first visit to the nursery, and others may be reluctant to touch. When the outcome for the baby is very uncertain, some parents protect and prepare themselves for the possible death of the baby by withdrawing from contact with the baby. The nurse needs to recognize and accept negative feelings of the family while remaining realistic and not giving false assurances. Encouraging the family to express feelings, concerns, and expectations can be very helpful as they begin to adapt to the new situation. The family can be helped to see their baby as a unique individual if they are encouraged to touch and interact with the infant. The nurse can point out the baby's specific responses. Bringing baby clothes and toys for their baby and taking photographs to share with siblings are ways to facilitate the attachment process. The baby's first name should be used by all personnel in communicating with the parents. In caring for the family of a preterm or sick baby, the goal should be to send a well baby home as a family member and not as a stranger.

COMPLICATIONS

Careful observation of the newborn is a vital nursing responsibility. Such observation coupled with prompt recognition and reporting of variations from normal can assure early initiation of treatment. An introduction to common newborn disorders follows.

Respiratory distress problems

LIST SIGNS OF RESPIRATORY DISTRESS

Signs of respiratory distress include:

1. Nasal flaring
2. Cyanosis in room air
3. Expiratory grunt
4. Retractions (sternal, substernal, suprasternal, intercostal)
5. Tachypnea

Although there are numerous causes of respiratory distress in the newborn, only the most common problems will be introduced here.

RELATIONSHIP OF SURFACTANT TO RDS IN NEWBORN

Respiratory distress syndrome. Respiratory distress syndrome (RDS) is also known as idiopathic respiratory distress syndrome, hyaline membrane disease, surfactant deficiency syndrome, or neonatal atelectasis. RDS primarily involves preterm babies and accounts for about 25% of death in the neonatal period. In these babies there is a relative lack of surfactant in the alveoli in the lungs. This surfactant is a complex of phospholipids in which the phospholipids lecithin and sphingomyelin can be measured. Without this surfactant, the alveoli collapse and gases cannot be exchanged. It is possible to sample the amniotic fluid by amniocentesis to measure the surfactant levels before birth. Administration of corticosteroids to mothers 24 hours prior to delivery may reduce the severity and incidence of RDS. Corticosteroids (dexamethasone and betamethasone) accelerate the fetal production of surfactant. If possible, induction of labor and cesarean birth can be delayed until the ratio of lecithin to sphingomyelin (L/S) is 2.0 or greater (L/S ratio). An L/S ratio of 2.0 or greater indicates maturity of lung tissue. One of the constant features of respiratory distress syndrome is the early onset of symptoms. Infants who breathe normally the first 6 to 8 hours of life do not have RDS.

DISCUSS TREATMENT OF INFANT WITH RDS

The treatment of RDS includes respiratory support and correction of as many secondary factors as possible. Respirations must be immediately established and adequately maintained. Blood gas sampling is essential for managing a baby with RDS. The course of RDS has been dramatically altered by the use of respirators to prevent alveolar collapse. Continuous positive airway pressure (CPAP) is one of many beneficial techniques now being used in neonatal intensive care units to treat newborns with RDS.

Transient tachypnea. As its name indicates, transient tachypnea is a transient condition (affected babies recover), that sometimes follows cesarean or breech delivery. There are good air exchange, minimal retractions, and no grunting. Cyanosis is not prominent, but a small percentage of infants may require oxygen to remain pink. This condition is generally not considered pathological and passes within a few days.

Meconium aspiration. Meconium is present in the amniotic fluid in 10% of all births. Some fetuses aspirate the meconium, which is then inspired more deeply into the alveoli with the first breaths. When meconium is present in the amniotic fluid, it is recommended that the baby's airway be cleared by gentle suction as soon as the head is born. This can be accomplished before the chest is delivered to reduce the amount of meconium present in the baby's airway. As mentioned previously, positive pressure breathing should be avoided until most of the meconium has been removed from the infant's lung. A complication of meconium aspiration is pneumothorax.

DESCRIBE A COMPLICATION OF MECONIUM ASPIRATION

Pneumothorax. Pneumothorax is air outside the lungs and airways, but in the thoracic cavity. It may occur spontaneously, as a result of trauma, or as a result of some other pathological process. Sudden deterioration of the baby's clinical condition follows a pneumothorax. Dyspnea, irritability, and restlessness denoting air hunger are present. The breath sounds over the affected side or lobe diminish and signs of shock follow. This is an emergency situation requiring immediate medical care.

DISTINGUISH BETWEEN COMMON AND PATHOLOGICAL BREATHING PATTERNS IN NEWBORNS

Apnea. Irregular breathing patterns are common in newborn infants and particularly in preterm babies. Characteristically, these babies will have a cyclic breathing pattern with rapid respirations followed by 5- to 10-second episodes of no breathing (apneic pauses). However, if the periods of apnea are prolonged, they may be the first signs of hypoglycemia, infection, or neurological damage. Close observation and a thorough diagnostic work-up are indicated for apnea.

Gentle physical stimulation of the newborn's extremities can stimulate breathing when apneic pauses occur.

LIST FIVE CRITERIA OF SILVERMAN-ANDERSON INDEX

Silverman-Anderson index. The Silverman-Anderson index (Fig. 13-10) was designed to provide a continuous evaluation of the infant's respiratory status. An index of respiratory distress is determined by values assigned to five criteria: chest lag, intercostal retraction,

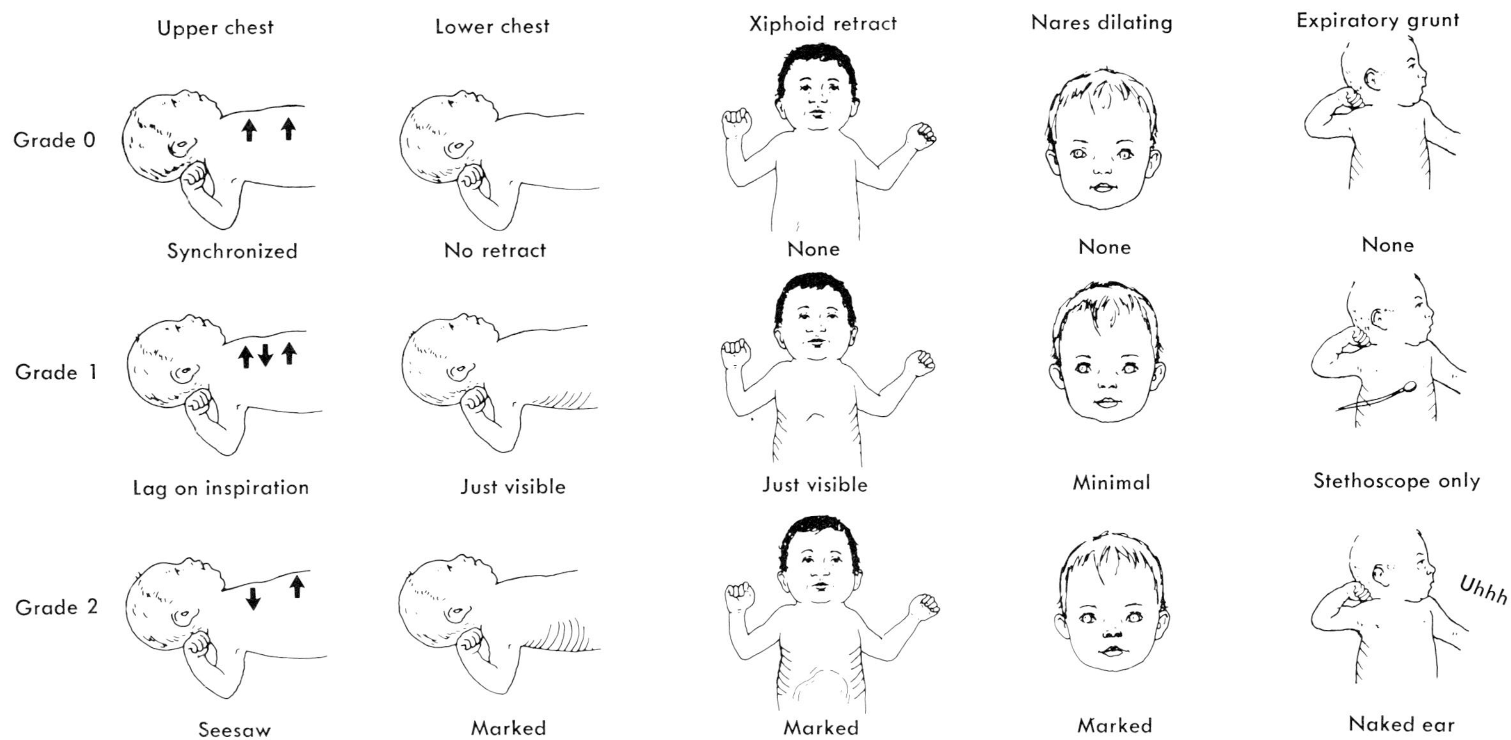

Fig. 13-10. Silverman-Anderson index of respiratory distress. (From Jensen, M., and Bobak, I.M.: Maternity and gynecologic care: the nurse and the family, ed. 3, St. Louis, 1985, The C.V. Mosby Co.)

xiphoid retraction, nares dilation, and expiratory grunt. A score of 0 indicates no respiratory distress; a score of 10 indicates severe respiratory distress.

Hyperbilirubinemia

Hyperbilirubinemia is present when serum bilirubin levels exceed 1.6 milligrams per deciliter at up to 1 day of age. Bilirubin is the end product of hemoglobin breakdown. There are two kinds of bilirubin, indirect and direct. Indirect (unconjugated) bilirubin is the by-product of red blood cell breakdown. Because indirect bilirubin is fat soluble, it cannot be easily excreted in bile or urine. To be excreted, indirect bilirubin must be converted (conjugated) to the direct (water-soluble) form of bilirubin by the liver. Because after birth the infant no longer needs the large amount of hemoglobin needed in utero, the red blood cells begin to break down. Often the infant's immature liver is not able to clear all the bilirubin, and thus the bilirubin is reabsorbed into the infant's circulatory system as unmetabolized bilirubin (indirect or unconjugated). As the circulatory system carries this bilirubin to all body tissues, dilute bilirubin is seen in the skin and sclera as jaundice. Visible jaundice usually occurs when serum bilirubin levels exceed 5 milligrams per 100 milliliters. Normal physiological jaundice occurs on the third or fourth day of life in 60% of term babies and 80% of preterm babies. Jaundice appearing before the baby is 24 hours old may be pathological and is usually caused by Rh and ABO incompatibilities. Prematurity, hemorrhage, infection, acidosis, low serum albumin levels, and certain drugs (see Appendices A and D) also predispose an infant to hyperbilirubinemia.

PHYSIOLOGICAL JAUNDICE AND THAT APPEARING BEFORE BABY IS 24 HOURS OLD

In rare instances an inhibitory steroid, pregnanediol, is secreted in human milk and interferes with the metabolism of bilirubin in the breast-fed infant. Recognition of breast milk jaundice should not discourage breast-feeding, since it can be treated by phototherapy and/or temporary weaning for a few days. Such jaundice usually starts on the third or fourth day of life and disappears, without harming the baby.

CAUSES OF HYPERBILIRUBINEMIA IN NEWBORN

Rh incompatibility. Rh incompatibility occurs when an Rh-negative mother gives birth to an Rh-positive fetus. If a small amount of the fetal blood has entered the mother's bloodstream during pregnancy or at birth, she may have formed Rh antibodies (sensitization). These Rh antibodies may have crossed the placenta, mixed with the blood of her fetus, and begun destroying the fetal red blood cells.

When an Rh-negative mother gives birth, a sample of umbilical cord blood is tested to determine (1) blood group, (2) Rh factor, (3) hemoglobin level, (4) results of a Coombs's test, and (5) bilirubin levels. The Coombs's test measures the amount of antibody present in the infant's circulation. A positive Coombs's test indicates that the baby's red blood cells are coated with antibodies. A positive Coombs's test, along with high bilirubin and low hemoglobin levels in the newborn, is an indication of erythroblastosis fetalis, a hemolytic disease of the newborn.

Erythroblastosis fetalis is destruction of the fetal red blood cells by maternal antibodies that cross the placenta and attack fetal red blood cell antigens. Mildly affected infants may have an enlarged liver or spleen at birth, but they look normal. Effects may range from mild hyperbilirubinemia to severe anemia to congestive heart failure and death.

Because the hemolytic process that began in utero continues after birth, replacing the baby's blood with an exchange transfusion may be necessary. Rh-negative blood is cross-matched with the infant's blood, or type O Rh-negative blood is used. Phototherapy may be used for treatment along with the exchange transfusions.

Erythroblastosis is not commonly found in first babies.

ABO incompatibility. When the mother's blood type is O and the baby's blood type is A or B, ABO incompatibility may develop. It is similar to Rh incompatibility but usually not severe because maternal anti-A and anti-B antibodies do not cross the placenta as readily or in as large amounts as the antibodies formed in Rh incompatibility.

In ABO incompatibility the first baby may be affected, since prior exposure and sensitization are not required.

Kernicterus. Clinical toxicity of bilirubin in the neonatal period is known as *kernicterus*. This is a syndrome of neurological damage resulting from deposits of bilirubin in brain cells. Kernicterus is a very rare disease, although it does occur in a few preterm babies. Although kernicterus has been associated with unconjugated or indirect serum bilirubin levels over 20 milligrams per 100 milliliters, the "dangerous" level of bilirubin in the infant's blood is dependent on each individual infant's condition.

Whether and how to treat jaundice in a newborn depend first on the cause of the jaundice. Sepsis (infection) requires prompt identification of the infecting organism and immediate treatment with antibiotics. Most cases of physiological jaundice and of breast milk jaundice require no treatment. However, jaundice in preterm babies or in Rh sensitization may require immediate treatment. The key to treatment is to individualize decision-making.

Babies must be observed closely for jaundice in the first days of life. For the most accurate color determination, it is best to get the infant into daylight. Blanching the infant's skin by pressing gently on the chest, forehead, or back of the neck and releasing pressure will reveal a yellow color if the baby is jaundiced.

In the screening procedure, called transcutaneous bilirubinometry, a hand-held screening device can estimate the amount of bilirubin in the baby's blood. This noninvasive procedure can quickly determine whether the newborn needs further laboratory determination of serum bilirubin levels. In transcutaneous bilirubinometry a spectrophotometric hand-held fiber-optic instrument is held for a few seconds against the baby's forehead. A white light flashes and a meter reads an estimation of the baby's bilirubin level from a window (the size of an adult fingertip). This instrument illuminates the skin and measures the intensity of the yellow color in the skin.

PLAN OF CARE FOR NEWBORN RECEIVING PHOTOTHERAPY FOR HYPERBILIRUBINEMIA

Phototherapy. Although exchange transfusion was formerly the most common treatment, today the most common treatment of hyperbilirubinemia is phototherapy. Exposure to the light's rays causes the unconjugated bilirubin in the infant's circulation to undergo chemical decomposition and to be changed into nontoxic products that are excreted in the urine and feces. The infant is exposed to fluorescent or incandescent lights that emit light at the appropriate wavelength. The effectiveness of phototherapy depends on the amount of radiant energy (not brightness) that strikes the infant's skin. This dose-response theory of phototherapy explains why the radiant flux of phototherapy lights should be measured frequently. Phototherapy lights should be changed when the irradiance falls below the level that is considered therapeutic for that particular light.

The infant's clothing is kept to a minimum, and preferably not even a diaper is worn. The eyes of the infant are shielded with patches during phototherapy. Vital signs must be checked every 2 hours and the infant turned frequently. Temperature control and adequate fluid intake are important because the infant's body temperature can rise in response to the heat of the lights. Complications of phototherapy include increased insensible water loss and dehydration, skin rash, and loose, green stools. Weight loss, lethargy, and tanning have also been reported. Parents should be informed about these side effects and supported when they occur. The lights should be turned off for eye care and blood samplings. Home phototherapy is an excellent alternative to hospitalization if the baby is well enough to be discharged to home care.

Sepsis neonatorum

RECOGNIZE SIGNS OF SEPSIS IN NEWBORN

Sepsis neonatorum is a disease of infants less than 1 month of age who are clinically ill and who have positive blood cultures. Generally, the incidence is only one in 1000 births of full-term infants but can be as high as 1 in 250 in preterm infants. The first evidence of sepsis may be vomiting, tachypnea, lethargy, failure to feed, inability to maintain body temperature, and gray or mottled skin color. The diagnosis of septicemia is made by recovery of the pathogen from blood cultures. The septic baby should be cared for in a high-risk nursery. Antibiotics specific for the cultured organisms are used in treatment.

Hypoglycemia

BLOOD SUGAR LEVELS INDICATING HYPOGLYCEMIA IN FULL-TERM INFANTS

IDENTIFY NEWBORNS AT RISK FOR DEVELOPING HYPOGLYCEMIA

For a term, normal-weight newborn the lower limit of blood glucose in the first 72 hours of life is 30 milligrams per 100 milliliters. After the first 3 days of life, the lower limit is 40 milligrams per 100 milliliters. Low-birth-weight infants are considered to be hypoglycemic if the blood sugar level is less than 20 milligrams per 100 milliliters within the first 72 hours of life, and 30 milligrams per 100 milliliters after 72 hours. Infants at risk for developing hypoglycemia are (1) small-for-gestational age infants, (2) infants of diabetic mothers, and (3) severely stressed infants. A low blood glucose level is reflected by central nervous system dysfunctions, such as tremors, convulsions, apnea, lethargy, limpness, jittery or tremulous movements, and irregular respirations.

Early recognition and treatment of hypoglycemia in the newborn are vital because neurological impairment may occur if the brain is deprived of glucose.

Most hospitals treat low glucose levels by administering glucose. Asymptomatic infants who can be fed should be breast-fed or given glucose or formula as early as it is safely possible. Symptomatic infants and babies too sick or unable to feed may require continuous intravenous infusions of glucose. The rate of intravenous glucose is adjusted and tapered over a period of time until blood glucose levels have been stable at 40 milligrams per 100 milliliters for 18 to 24 hours, and the oral intake is sufficient to meet caloric needs.

Screening for hypoglycemia can be done by obtaining a drop of blood from the infant's heel and testing it for glucose level with reagent strips. In some hospitals this screening is a routine nursing procedure for all infants classified at risk for developing hypoglycemia.

CONGENITAL PROBLEMS

Congenital problems are those malformations that occur during intrauterine life. These anomalies are present at and existing from the time of birth.

Cleft lip and/or cleft palate

DESCRIPTIONS OF CONDITIONS

Cleft lip and palate are conditions in which there is failure of growth and union of the bony or soft tissue structures on one (unilateral) or both (bilateral) sides of the midline of the palate and upper jaw. Occurrence of each is approximately 1 of 800 births. It is possible to have a normal lip and defective palate, a defective lip and normal palate, or both defects. These defects are obvious on gross examination and can be corrected by surgical repair. A cleft lip is usually repaired by 2 to 3 months of age. A cleft palate is usually repaired by 18 months of age. Several successive operations may be necessary.

Infants with a cleft lip or palate are difficult to feed. Feeding techniques include use of a palate prosthesis, a rubber-tipped medicine dropper, an Asepto syringe, or a special nipple. Because these babies swallow a lot of air, they need frequent bubbling and should be held in an upright position during feedings to prevent aspiration.

Hydrocephalus

Hydrocephalus is a condition characterized by abnormal accumulation of cerebrospinal fluid within the skull, with enlargement of the head. Hydrocephalus may be caused by an obstruction of the cerebrospinal fluid pathways or by overproduction or defective absorption of the cerebrospinal fluid.

Hydrocephalus may be recognized at birth, or it may not be evident until later.

When it is present before birth, the labor can be long and difficult because of cephalopelvic disproportion.

Surgical treatment consists of inserting a shunting device that bypasses the point of obstruction and drains the excess fluid into a body cavity. Many affected infants show brain damage at birth. The shunting procedure often prevents further damage.

Spina bifida

Spina bifida is a spinal malformation in which the bony part of the spinal canal fails to close, presenting an opening through which the spinal meninges and spinal cord may or may not protrude. This occurs in about 1 out of 1000 births. If the meninges do not protrude, the spina bifida may present no problems (spina bifida occulta). When the meninges bulge through the opening, they form a cystic sac known as *meningocele* (Fig. 13-11). Because no nerve roots are involved, there is no paralysis or lack of sphincter control below the lesion. A meningocele can be corrected by surgical removal of the sac with closure of the skin.

If nerve fibers as well as the meninges protrude, the condition is known as *meningomyelocele* (or myelomeningocele), in which there may be partial or total paralysis below the lesion. With surgical correction the neurological deficit can be improved. There is a danger of the sac rupturing and the baby developing meningitis in either of these cases.

Nursing care is mainly of protective routine until surgery can be done. Every effort must be made to protect the sac from pressure and the danger of infection from urine and feces.

Down's syndrome

Down's syndrome results from chromosomal abnormalities. Its most common cause is trisomy of the chromosome 21, making a total of 47 chromosomes instead of the normal 46. This abnormality is most likely to happen to a mother over the age of 40. The two other types of chromosomal abnormalities that cause Down's syndrome are less common: (1) In *translocation* of a chromosome during cell division, the chromosome count is still

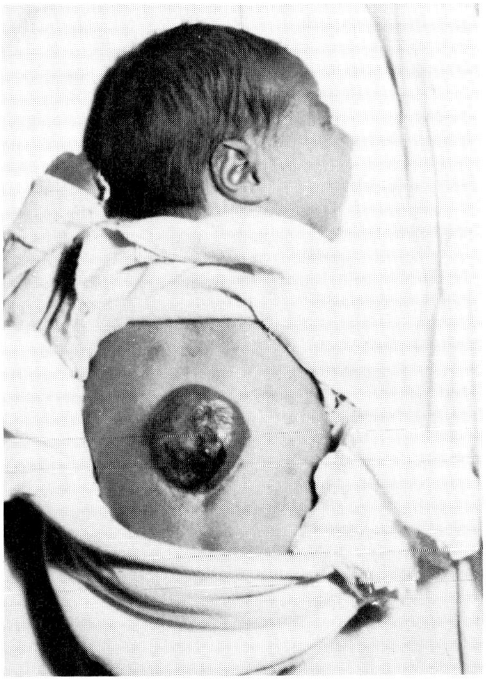

Fig. 13-11. Meningocele. (From Lerch, C., and Bliss, V.J.: Maternity nursing, ed. 3, St. Louis, 1978, The C.V. Mosby Co.)

46 but 2 chromosomes are misplaced. This can occur in infants born to young women. (2) In *mosaicism*, the least common cause of Down's syndrome, the affected infant has a different number of chromosomes in some cells than in others.

The infant with Down's syndrome may have physical defects. The level of mental retardation in these babies varies greatly.

Phenylketonuria

Phenylketonuria (PKU) is a congenital inborn error of metabolism that, if not diagnosed and treated within a month or two after birth, will result in permanent mental retardation. In PKU the baby is unable to metabolize the protein phenylalanine, permitting accumulation of phenylalanine and its metabolic products (phenylketones) in body fluids. PKU can be treated by a diet low in phenylalanine.

PKU can be detected within a few days after birth by means of a simple blood test. After 4 to 6 weeks of age, a urine test can be done to detect PKU. Most states have public health laws requiring that all newborns be tested for PKU by the age of 28 days.

SUMMARY

This unit has presented only a brief introduction to the newborn with complications. If you are interested in the care of the newborn with complications, the sources listed at the end of this unit will give you a place to begin your study.

BIBLIOGRAPHY

Affonso, D., and Harris, T.: CPAP, continuous positive airway pressure, Am. J. Nurs. **76**(4):570-573, 1976.

Brown, J., and Hepler, R.: Care of the critically ill newborn: stimulation a corollary to physical care, Am. J. Nurs. **76**(4):578-581, 1976.

Ennis, S., and Harris, T.R.: Positioning infants with hyaline membrane disease, Am. J. Nurs. **78**(3):398-401, 1978.

Evans, H.E., and Glass, L.: Perinatal medicine, Hagerstown, Md., 1976, Harper & Row.

Justice, P., and Smith, G.E.: Phenylketonuria, Am. J. Nurs. **75**(8):1303-1305, 1975.

Korones, S.B., and Lancaster, J.: High-risk newborn infants: the basis for intensive nursing care, St. Louis, 1976, The C.V. Mosby Co.

Miller, C.: Working with parents of high-risk infants, Am. J. Nurs. **78**(7):1228-1230, 1978.

Miner, H.: Problems and prognosis for the small-for-gestational-age and the premature infant, MCN **3**(4):221-226, 1978.

Moore, M.L.: Newborn, family and nurse, ed. 2, Philadelphia, 1981, W.B. Saunders Co.

Oehler, T.M.: Family-centered neonatal nursing care, Philadelphia, 1981, J.B. Lippincott Co.

Passo, S.D.: Positioning infants with myelomeningocele, Am. J. Nurs. **74**(9):1653-1660, 1974.

DEFINITIONS

Define the following terms:

acidosis	kernicterus
apnea	laryngoscope
breast milk jaundice	low-birth-weight baby
cleft lip and palate	meningocele
CPAP (continuous positive airway pressure)	phenylketonuria (PKU)
	phototherapy
Down's syndrome	pneumothorax
endotracheal tube	preterm baby
erythroblastosis	retrolental fibroplasia
gavage feeding	spina bifida
hydrocephalus	surfactant
hyperbilirubinemia	tachypnea
hypoglycemia	transcutaneous bilirubinometry
intubation	

LEARNING ACTIVITIES AND EXPERIENCES

1. Group discussions.
2. Visit a neonatal intensive care nursery for observation. What equipment is in use?
3. Is there a transport service available for sick newborns in your community?
4. View audiovisual aids and discuss.

ENRICHMENT/IN DEPTH STUDY

1. Interview a family whose baby received care in a neonatal intensive care unit. What are their feelings about the experience?
2. Do you know a child born with a congenital defect? Have there been changes in the family's life-style because of this birth?

SELF-ASSESSMENT

For questions 1 through 10, circle the best answer.

1. The infant with an Apgar's score of 4 to 6 at birth will:
   a. probably require resuscitation
   b. not require any assistance
   c. need only gentle stimulation
2. A preterm baby is a live born infant whose:
   a. weight is less than 5 pounds
   b. gestation period is less than 38 weeks
   c. mother is sick
3. A small-for-gestational-age baby is one whose:
   a. birth weight is below the tenth percentile
   b. weight is less than 5 pounds
   c. gestation period is less than 38 weeks
4. A preterm baby is extremely susceptible to infection because of:
   a. an immature liver
   b. immature temperature regulating mechanisms
   c. an immature immunological system
5. In stabilizing the preterm newborn, nursing care should include specialized care and environment because:
   a. the preterm infant has little chance of survival
   b. the preterm infant needs oxygen
   c. the preterm infant's body systems are immature
6. Signs of respiratory distress in the newborn include all but one of the following. Which of the following is *not* a sign of RDS?
   a. tachypnea
   b. nasal flaring
   c. elevated temperature
   d. expiratory grunt
   e. retractions
   f. cyanosis in room air
7. Babies with respiratory distress lack adequate surfactant in their lungs. Surfactant is needed to:
   a. clean the lungs
   b. produce amniotic fluid
   c. prevent alveolar collapse
8. Infants at risk for developing hypoglycemia are:
   a. full-term normal infants
   b. infants of diabetic mothers
   c. infants with PKU
9. The first evidence of sepsis in the newborn may be:
   a. flushing of the skin
   b. inability to maintain body temperature
   c. respiratory distress
10. Which one of the following breathing patterns in the newborn is pathological:
    a. transient tachypnea

b. irregular breathing
c. prolonged apneic spells

Supply the correct answer(s) for items 11 through 21.

11. The Silverman-Anderson index of respiratory distress is determined by values assigned to what five criteria?
    a.
    b.
    c.
    d.
    e.
12. Physiological jaundice is caused by ______________________.
13. Jaundice appearing before the baby is 24 hours old may be pathological and is usually caused by ______________ and ______________ incompatibilities.
14. List six causes of jaundice in the newborn:
    a.
    b.
    c.
    d.
    e.
    f.
15. The treatment of RDS includes ______________ support and correction of as many secondary factors as possible.
16. What is a complication of meconium aspiration? ______________________.
17. The cry of a full-term baby is lusty and loud, and the cry of the preterm baby is ______________ and ______________.
18. Nursing care of the infant receiving phototherapy for hyperbilirubinemia includes ______________, ______________, ______________, and ______________.
19. Explain what you would do for an infant who has an Apgar score of 3 at 1 minute of life. There was no meconium in the amniotic fluid.

20. A preterm baby has just been transported by ambulance to a high-risk nursery. Explain to the parents what the high-risk nursery looks like and what care their baby will receive there.

21. What could you do to offer support for these parents?

22. Match Column A with Column B.

Column A	Column B
_____1. cleft lip and/or palate	a. abnormal accumulation of cerebrospinal fluid
_____2. hydrocephalus	b. results from chromosome abnormalities
_____3. spina bifida	c. defective growth and union of bony and soft tissue structure
_____4. Down's syndrome	d. spinal malformation
_____5. phenylketonuria	e. inborn error of metabolism

23. Match Column A with Column B.

Column A	Column B
______1. postterm baby	a. hypoglycemia
______2. SGA baby	b. meconium aspiration

24. Match Column A with Column B.

Column A	Column B
	Lower limits of normal for blood glucose
______1. Term infants: before 72 hours of age	a. 30 milligrams per milliliter
______2. Term infants: after 72 hours of age	b. 20 milligrams per milliliter
	c. 40 milligrams per milliliter
	d. 50 milligrams per milliliter

UNIT XIV
Trends in childbearing

GOALS

This unit is designed to provide the reader with information that will:

- □ promote awareness of contemporary trends in maternity care.
- □ develop an understanding of the concept of team practice in maternity care.

STUDENT OBJECTIVES

Upon completion of this unit, the student should be able to:

1. Describe programs that seek to meet the needs of today's childbearing families.
2. Discuss home birth in the United States.
3. Differentiate between nurse-midwifery and lay midwifery.
4. Distinguish between the role of a nurse practitioner in maternal-child practice and pediatric practice.
5. Discuss the concept of team as applied to maternity care.
6. Design a plan for family-centered maternity/newborn care in your community.

The American health care system has been undergoing rapid and dramatic change since the introduction of a prospective payment system for Medicare recipients in October 1983. No longer working on a cost-plus basis, hospitals have had to reduce costs. This need for cost control has led to more efficiency, home health care programs, wellness and fitness programs, and innovative care options both outside and within hospitals.

The conventional multitransfer surgical system of hospital maternity care is not cost-effective. In addition, it is not marketable. The issue of marketability will become more important as the health care industry becomes competitive, price-sensitive, and economically driven. Much of the change that has occurred in maternity care in the last decade has been the result of consumer pressure for more humanized birth. Direct and indirect pressure by consumers of maternity care will continue. A combination of increased competition and pressure for cost reduction will also continue. At the same time more families will make conscious choices about their place of birth.

The components of family-centered care have proven to be both cost-effective and highly marketable. In this new era in maternity care, the chief beneficiaries will be childbearing families. This time of rapid change is especially exciting for maternity nursing because it offers the opportunity to develop truly comprehensive family-centered maternity care.

And this is only the beginning! Where will we go from here?

BIRTH CENTERS

PROGRAMS THAT SEEK TO MEET NEEDS OF TODAY'S CHILDBEARING FAMILIES

In many hospitals rigid rules, procedures, and attitudes are being re-evaluated and, when found to be without scientific basis, are being revised and adjusted to fit the concept of family-centered maternity/newborn care. Some institutions have pioneered family-centered care with family-care units designated as alternative birth units or simply as family birth centers or rooms. These units were originally designed to offer low-risk

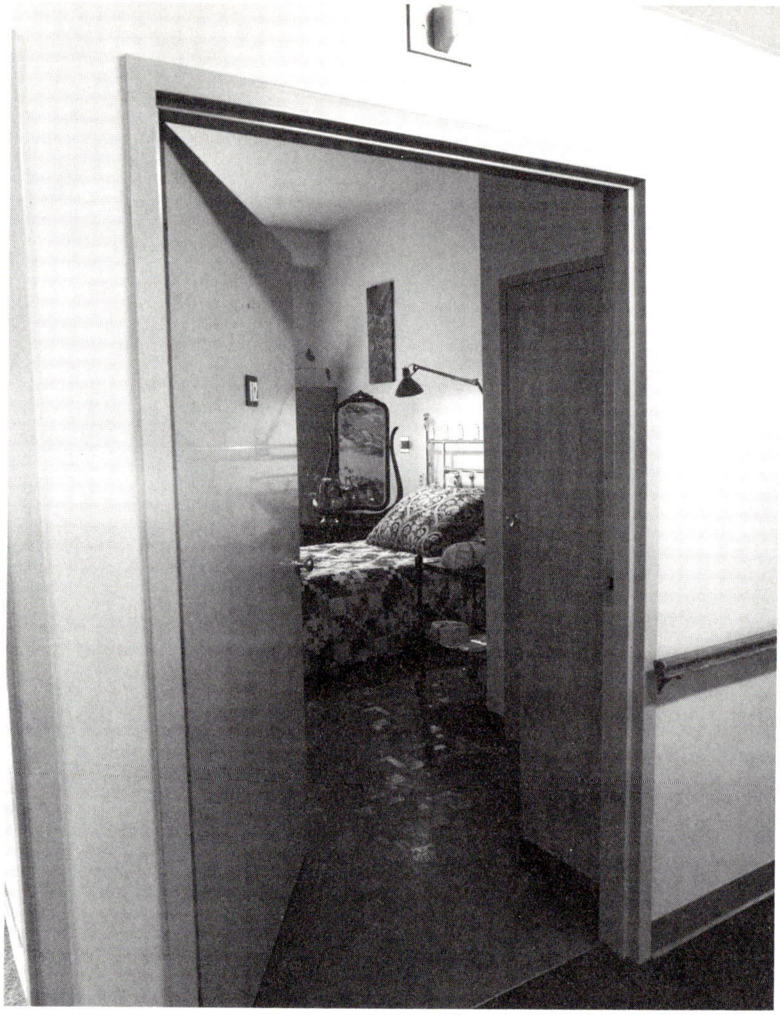

Fig. 14-1. An alternative birth center (ABC) in a hospital setting.

families an alternative to home birth, that is, a compromise between hospital and home. Their developers conceived of these units in response to a growing number of parents who chose to boycott the institutions they felt did not meet their childbirth needs and to deliver their babies at home, sometimes with skilled attendants and sometimes without.

An alternative birth center (ABC) or birth room offers a homelike environment in a hospital, usually on the maternity unit, with immediate access to emergency intervention and all of the tools that modern medicine has to offer (Fig. 14-1). These birthing rooms are cheerfully and comfortably furnished, in homelike fashion. The family is admitted to this room, labors there, gives birth there, and may be discharged from there if the time interval and requirements for room utilization permit. If the family chooses to remain in the hospital for more than 24 hours from the time of admission, they may be required to transfer to a standard postpartum room if the birthing room is needed by another family.

A birthing room is a private space designed for only low-risk childbearing families to stay throughout their birth experience and until they are ready to go home. All medicines and equipment that may be needed are stored out of sight in a cabinet in the room. The mother gives birth, positioning herself to meet her own comfort needs (Fig. 14-2). After the birth, the infant remains with the family (Fig. 14-3). Ideally, one nurse stays with the family throughout labor and birth and the immediate postpartum period, thus providing continuity of care. Within 24 to 72 hours after discharge, two home visits to

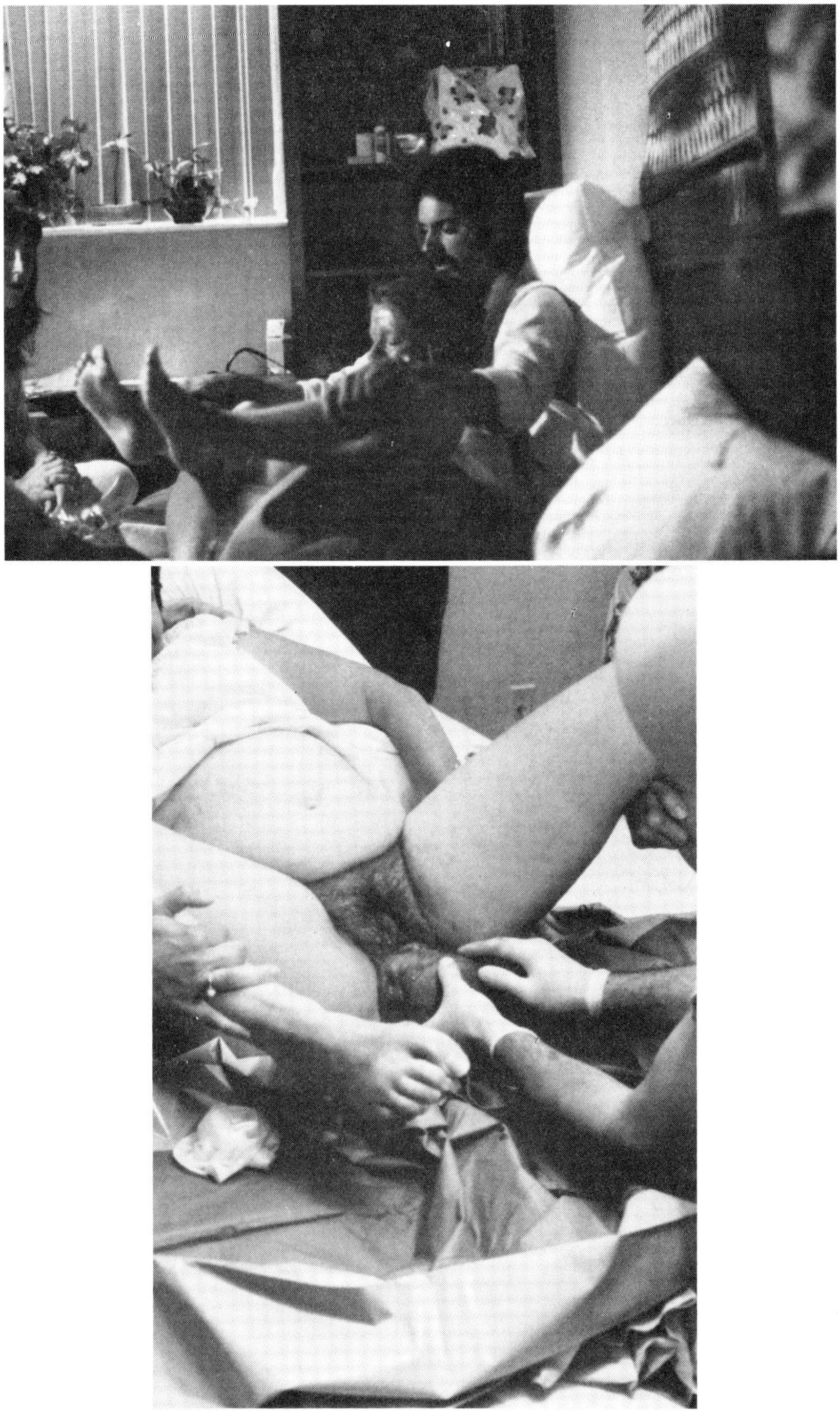

Fig. 14-2. Birth. (Top photo by Joan Mirov; bottom photo by Timothy McGarry.)

the family are made by this nurse to check the mother and baby and provide support for the family.

Utilization of ABCs varied dramatically because of diverse "risking out criteria" and because nurses often were busy in the conventional labor and delivery rooms and could not (or would not) be spared to staff an isolated ABC. Also, low room utilization rates, extra supplies, and staffing requirements to operate two parallel systems proved to be very costly.

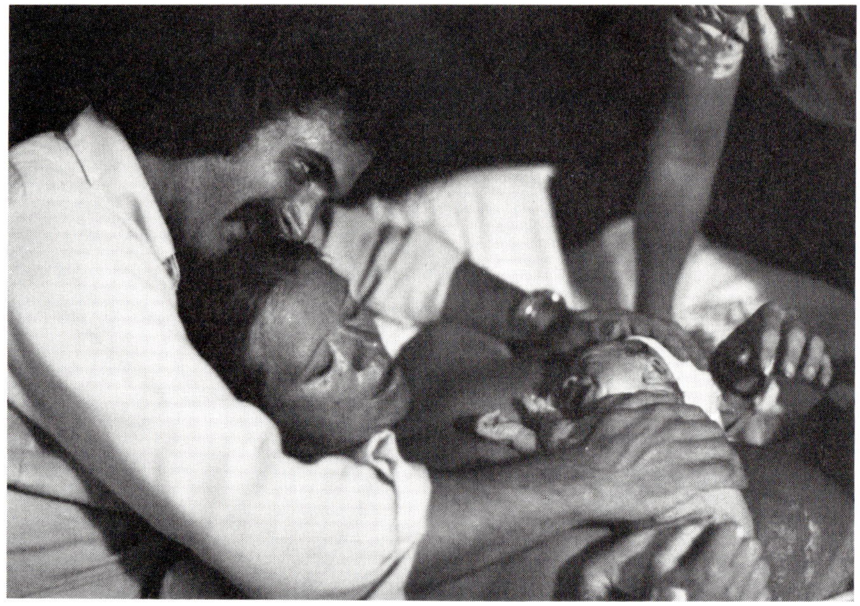

Fig. 14-3. A family. (Photo by Joan Mirov.)

However, parents liked birth rooms for the "intimate" birth experience possible, with partner and family sharing the event. Elimination of the transfer from the labor room to the delivery suite was often singled out as the best feature of the ABC.

Although costs of ABC births varied, they were usually less than costs for traditional care. In fact, in some ABCs, the cost of birth was one third the cost of a regular birth and a 3-day hospitalization.

Labor, delivery, and recovery room

As ABCs grew in number, clinical experience in alternative birth centers proved these settings to be safe and satisfactory for many health care providers and families. Evaluation of these changes in clinical practice led to new obstetrical unit designs. The combination labor, delivery, and recovery (LDR) room was designed by Ross Planning Associates (Fig. 14-4). This room was designed to eliminate transfer from labor to delivery to recovery. It is sized to accommodate up to eight persons during the birth process and equipped to provide care for all births other than cesarean births. There is no need for risk criteria or transfer to labor and delivery to cope with problems.

These LDR rooms provide many cost savings through reduction in space requirements, maintenance, and supplies. Women do not have to be moved to three different rooms for the childbirth experience. Nurses can spend less time in nonnursing transfer and housekeeping tasks and thus spend more time providing nursing care. As a result, nursing productivity increases and so does consumer satisfaction. Clinical care in LDRs has proved to be safe, satisfying, cost-effective, and marketable.

Labor, delivery, recovery, and pospartum room

Single-room maternity care (SRMC) in labor, delivery, recovery, and postpartum rooms (LDRPs) was designed by the Borning Corporation in 1977. LDRP rooms are designed to offer a clinically safe, satisfying, and cost-effective environment for both providers of care and families. These childbearing rooms are home for the family from the time of admission to the time of discharge, thus eliminating separate labor, delivery, postpartum, and nursing areas. Both low-risk and high-risk childbearing families are eligible to use these flexible family-centered settings (see Fig. 8-14, p. 190).

These LDRP rooms provide the maximum cost savings of new unit design. Eliminat-

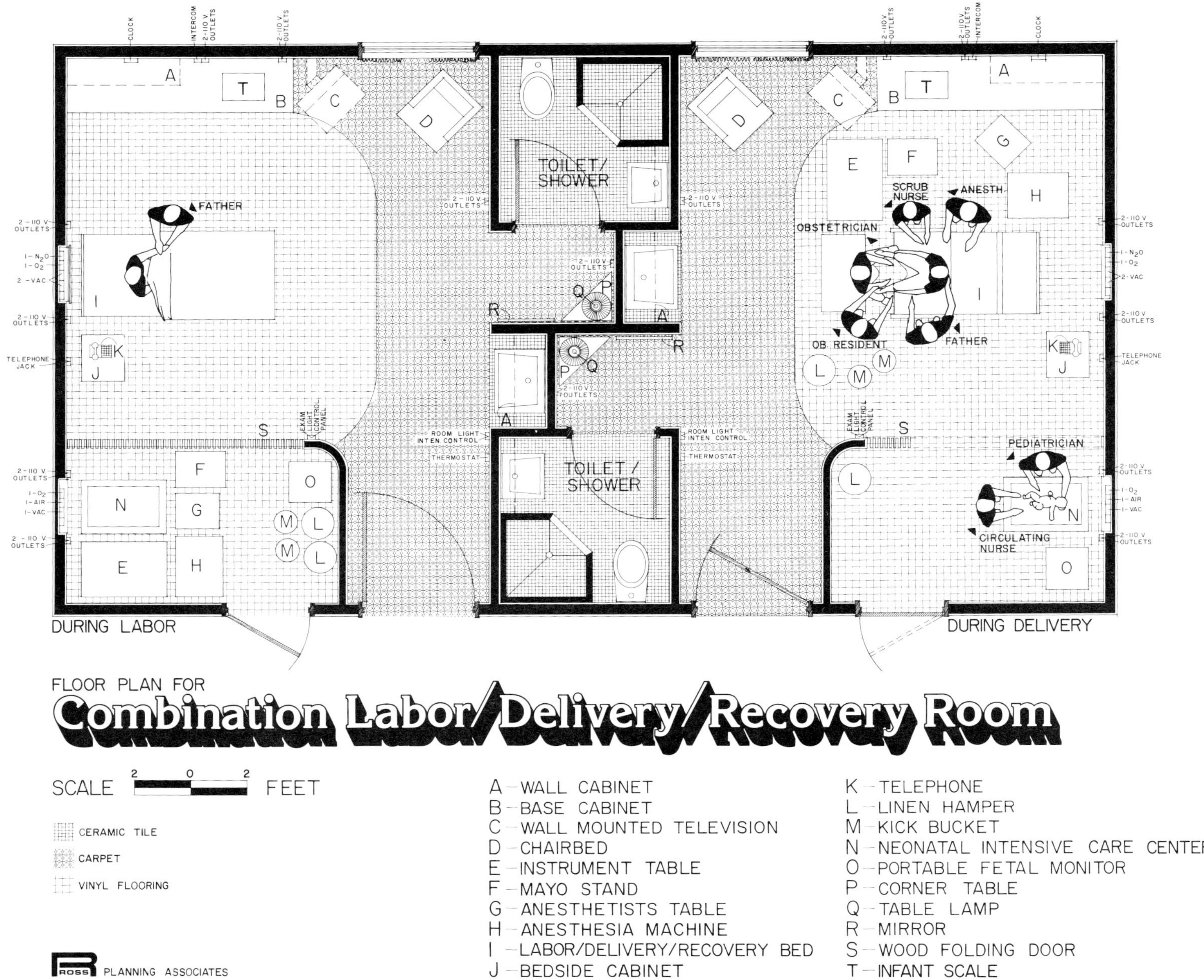

Fig. 14-4. The combination labor delivery recovery room (LDR). (Courtesy Ross Planning Associates, Columbus, Ohio.)

ing all transfers increases savings through reduction in space, maintenance, and supply requirements. In addition, more cost-effective staffing patterns are possible than in any other system.

Nursing care provided in LDRP rooms is truly family-centered and requires nurses capable of caring for families in all phases of the childbearing experience. These nurses are not limited in skills by functioning in only one subspecialty; that is, only the nursery, only postpartum, or only labor and delivery. They are prepared to provide care for mother and baby together in mother-baby nursing and often provide this mother-baby care to the same couple they supported during labor and birth on the previous day. Instead of providing the old impersonal, fragmented, and compartmentalized care, today's nurses can put the pieces of families together in comprehensive care. Obviously, rooms do not provide humanized care. People do. However, contemporary settings such as LDR and LDRP rooms provide the environment in which maternity care can become more humane, productive, cost-effective, and marketable.

FREESTANDING BIRTH CENTERS

Although most alternative birth centers or birthing rooms are located within existing hospitals, there are a growing number of freestanding birth centers. These units are outside of the hospital but are often close to a major hospital so that quick transport to that institution is possible if necessary. With well over 2000 births recorded, the Maternity Center Association in New York City pioneered operating a center in a homelike setting designed to serve families in the childbearing experience. Families are accommodated in the center for prenatal care, classes in preparation for childbirth and infant care, labor and delivery, pediatric examination, and postpartum care. The environment is personalized and homelike, emphasizing family involvement and parent responsibility. The mother and baby are discharged to home within 12 hours of delivery and follow-up care at home is provided by the Visiting Nurse Association of New York. As in hospital birth centers, careful prenatal screening is done and only well mothers without complications are accepted.

Statistics on maternal and infant morbidity and mortality differ in freestanding birth centers; however, they are consistently comparable with hospital statistics, indicating that birth in a birth center is probably very safe. Economic considerations have been the driving force behind the development of some freestanding birth centers. Maternity care in some birth centers is one third to one half the cost in a hospital. Reasons for this cost reduction include the provision of care in a residential rather than a hospital space. There is no need for cost shifting of other hospital services such as laboratories, laundries, and diet kitchens to the maternity fees. As a result, overhead is kept to a minimum and consists of only the costs of operating the birth center. An additional important factor is the provision of much of the care by nurse-midwives, and that means savings in staff salaries. However, increasing liability insurance costs and lack of availability of liability insurance for many nurse-midwives may negate the financial benefits of a nurse-midwifery staff. Studies dealing with questions such as economics, safety, personnel, quality control, and malpractice impact are currently being conducted by birth centers as well as by some state health departments and other government agencies.

HOME BIRTH

HOME BIRTH IN THE UNITED STATES

According to the California Health Department, reported home births in 1975 rose to 3516 from 2038 four years previously. This figure (3516) represented 1.1% of the total births in California in 1975, and these were only those home births that were reported. There were estimates in some communities in California that 10% of the births occurred at home.

This trend to home birth was reported in many other states in the early 1970s. However, with the emergence of alternative birth centers in hospitals, many families returned to hospitals for birth. Recent data on home births show a small drop from the preceding year in the number of home births. In fact, out-of-hospital births have remained almost constant at 1% of total births occurring in the United States since 1975.

National groups supporting home birth are HOME (Home Oriented Maternity Experience) and NAPSAC (National Association of Parents for Safe Alternatives in Childbirth). These groups support changes toward more humane childbearing practices at all levels, intergrating the alternatives for childbirth to meet the needs of the total population.

The literature on childbirth contains excellent statistics on medically directed home birth services with skilled nurse-midwives and medical backup. Two examples of such services are the Chicago Maternity Center with 12,000 home births from 1950 to 1960 without a single maternal death and the home delivery statistics of the Frontier Nursing Service in Appalachia with 23 years without a single maternal death. In the United States today there are reports of very low-risk home delivery populations who have very low levels of difficulty and consequently have excellent statistics. However, there is danger in taking these data on very select populations and applying them to the total population. It must be recognized that even though labor and delivery are normal physiological events, they do present potential hazards to the mother and fetus both before and after birth. These hazards require provisions for emergency intervention and medical backup that are available in hospitals and birthing homes or in independent birth centers.

People who choose home birth are often very sincere and concerned about their own safety and the health and safety of their unborn child. In fact, there are probably as many sincere and well-considered reasons for choosing home birth as there are home births. For many people birth is a very special, intensely personal event to be shared only with family and friends, and not with assorted hospital personnel who are strangers. For many other people birth is an intensely spiritual experience for which a hospital setting is totally inappropriate. Still others do not relish giving up responsibility for their births to hospital personnel. Most people choosing home birth understand fully the risk involved but understand that there are also risks in hospital birth.

In this time of rapid change, the day is probably coming when home birth will be provided with all the necessary emergency standards and medical backup. But in the meantime health professionals have the urgent and immediate responsibility to develop alternative methods within the hospital environment that provide the highest possible standards in maternity care.

MIDWIFERY

NURSE-MIDWIFERY AND LAY MIDWIFERY

The term midwife literally means "a helping woman." Every culture has had its midwives, with their work being recognized from time immemorial. American midwifery was given a professional status when the first school of nurse-midwifery was started in 1932. In 1983 there were 25 educational programs in the United States and approximately 2600 nurse-midwives, with almost one-half of these graduates since 1969. The "average" American nurse-midwife today is licensed as a registered nurse, has a master's degree, and is certified as a nurse-midwife (CNM) by the American College of Nurse Midwives (ACNM). The practice of nurse-midwifery has achieved separate legal recognition in a number of states, and nurse-midwives are practicing in all 50 state plus Washington, D.C.

Nurse-midwives practice true family-centered maternity/newborn care as interdependent health professionals, whether working in maternity centers, in hospitals and community agencies, or with obstetricians in private practice. Nurse-midwives focus on the complete maternity cycle: ensuring health and growth, preventing illness, fostering family life, and helping families to take responsibility for their health care while providing care for pregnancy, labor, and birth. In fact, nurse-midwives have provided many of the models for viable alternatives to conventional maternity care.

Despite an increasing awareness on the part of the consumer and the health professional that CNMs are valuable and often essential members of the health team, the number of lay midwives (empirical midwives) in this country is growing. A lay midwife may be exceptionally well prepared for practice through self-study, apprenticeship, formal study in the basic sciences, and teaching from sympathetic health professionals. In some states lay midwives may become licensed. Conversely, a lay midwife may have very little preparation or education. Because there is no formal licensing of lay midwifery practice, a wide range of skills can be found among lay midwives. In several states legislation has been proposed to combine lay and nurse-midwives and/or licensed lay midwives and/or to develop education programs for nonnurse midwifery. Just as the issue of home birth will eventually have to be addressed, so will the issue of lay midwifery.

NURSE PRACTITIONERS

ROLE OF NURSE PRACTITIONER IN MATERNAL-CHILD PRACTICE AND PEDIATRIC PRACTICE

Nursing today is dynamic—changing to include more sophisticated care requiring a substantial amount of knowledge or technical skill. Nurses are prodding the conscience of health professionals, legislatures, the government, and the public alike in their determination to improve health care. A nursing role designed to bridge the gap in the delivery of primary health care is the role of nurse practitioner, in which the nurse is prepared to practice in an expanded role. The term *nurse practitioner* originated in 1965 with the establishment of a Pediatric Nurse Practitioner program at the University of Colorado. Important functions of nurse practitioners as members of the health teams include health maintenance and preventive care. Depending on where nurse practitioners function, their duties may range from history taking and physical assessment to ordering laboratory tests and writing prescriptions for medications approved as appropriate by the physician in charge. More than half of the nurse practitioners are employed by private physicians, with the remainder being employed in clinics and community agencies.

Maternal-child nurse practitioner

Nurse practitioners prepared in the specialty area of maternal and child health provide continuity of care for the mother and child throughout pregnancy and then in child health and development. Although they may function during the prenatal period much like nurse-midwives, maternal-child nurse practitioners do not deliver the baby.

Pediatric nurse practitioner

Nurse practitioners prepared in the specialty area of pediatrics provide care for infants and children in clinic settings, physicians' offices, community agencies, and hospitals. They serve a very important function in well baby care and in teaching and counseling of families with infants and children.

CHILDBIRTH EDUCATORS

Persons who call themselves childbirth educators may range from registered nurses to paraprofessionals to laypersons. The International Childbirth Education Association (ICEA), the American Society for Psychoprophylaxis is Obstetrics (ASPO), and the Childbirth without Pain Education League (CWPEL) are examples of groups that have national teacher-training programs and national certification programs (see Appendix B for a list of childbirth education associations).

Currently standards for childbirth educators depend on the association to which they belong, and there are no generally accepted national standards. There are also no national standards for nurses practicing in expanding roles.

OTHER TEAM MEMBERS

CONCEPT OF TEAM APPLIED TO MATERNITY CARE

There are innovative programs in the country preparing valuable maternity team members in paraprofessional roles, that is, the obstetrical technician and home health aide. The obstetrical technician is a licensed vocational nurse (LVN) or a licensed practical nurse (LPN) with intensive preparation in maternity nursing over and above the basic education program. This team member is prepared to give supportive care to well families in the childbearing cycle within the hospital or birth centers. The home health aide is usually a high school graduate who receives special preparation in the home care of mothers and babies. This health care team member can provide valuable assistance to the new family as they make the transition from hospital to home when there is no extended family to help.

SUMMARY

This unit began with the statement that it is an exciting time to be involved in maternity care in this country, Indeed, it is! It is a time for team work, for many levels of personnel to cooperate to deliver maternity care to families. It is a time for each member of the team to develop self-esteem and recognize his or her potential. In nursing we have come a long way.

PLAN FOR FAMILY-CENTERED MATERNITY/NEWBORN CARE

Family-centered maternity/newborn care is flexible, safe, individualized care emphasizing family rights and responsibilities. In family-centered care the new family leaves the hospital prepared to care for their new baby (Fig. 14-5). Each family is helped to achieve their own goals within the context of their own culture. The major change in maternity care that is needed to make family-centered maternity care a reality is attitudinal. Family-centered maternity/newborn care is a philosophy whose time has come.

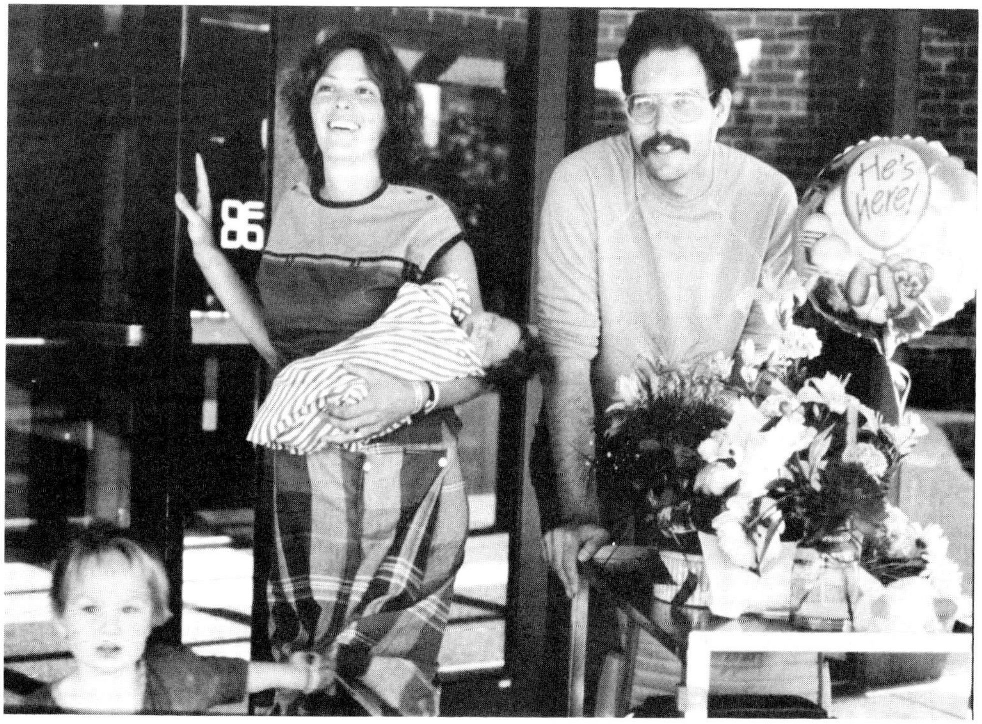

Fig. 14-5. The new family leaves the hospital. (Courtesy Fairview-Riverside Hospital, Minneapolis, Minn.)

BIBLIOGRAPHY

American College of Nurse-Midwives: Statement of qualifications, standards and functions; philosophy and definitions. Available from ACNM, 1012 Fourteenth Street, NW, Suite 801, Washington, D.C. 20005.

Averitt, S.S.: Adapting the birthing center concept to a traditional hospital setting, JOGN Nurs. **9**(2):103-104, 1980.

California: Furor over home births, Medical World News, April 4, 1977, p. 32.

Caplan, G.: Family support systems in a changing world. In Anthony, J., and Chiland, C., editors: The child and his family: children and their parents in a changing world, New York, 1978, John Wiley & Sons, Inc.

DeVries, R.G.: Image and reality: an evaluation of hospital alternative birth centers, J. Nurse Midwife **28**(3):3-9, 1983.

Diers, D., and Burst, H.V.: Effectiveness of policy related research: nurse-midwifery as case study, Image: The Journal of Nursing Scholarship, **XV**(3):68-74, 1983.

Edwards, M.E.: Unattended home birth, Am. J. Nurs. **73**:8, Aug. 1973.

Eiduson, B., Cohen, J., and Alexander, T.: Alternatives in child rearing in the late 1970s, Am J. Orthopsychiatry **43**:5, October 1973.

Fondiller, S.: Childbearing center—new approach to maternal care, Am. Nurs. **9**(5):9, 11, 1977.

Klein, M., and Westreich, R.: Birth room transfer and procedure rates—what do they tell about the setting? Birth **10**(2):93-97, 1983.

Lubic, R.W.: Nurse-midwifery in context, Briefs **39**:3, 36-39, March 1975.

Lubic, R.W., and Ernst, E.K.M.: The childbearing center, an alternative to conventional care, Nurs. Outlook **26**(12):754-760, 1978.

Maloni, J.A.: The birthing room: some insights into parents' experiences, MCN **5**(6):314-319, Sept./Oct. 1980.

McKay, S., and Phillips, C.: Family-centered maternity care: implementation strategies. Rockville, Md., 1984, Aspen Systems Corp.

Meglen, M.: Nurse-midwives and the maternity health care team, Bull. Am. Coll. Nurse Pract. **17**:3, Aug. 1972.

Mehl, L., and others: Complications of home birth, Birth Family J. **2**(2):123-129, 1975.

Nielsen, I.: Nurse-midwifery in an alternative birth center, Birth Family J. **4**:1, Spring 1977.

Phillips, C.R., and Anzalone, J.T.: Fathering: participation in labor and birth, St. Louis, 1978, the C. V. Mosby Co.

Rising, S.S.: A consumer oriented nurse-midwifery service, Nurs. Clin. North Am. **10**(2):251-263, 1975.

Rubin, R.: Maternity nursing stops too soon, Am. J. Nurs. **75**:10, October 1975.

Searles, C.: The impetus toward home birth. J. Nurse Midwife **26**(3):51-56, 1981.

Selavan, I.: Bobba Hannah, midwife. Am. J. Nurs. **73**:4, April 1973.

Sousa, M.: Childbirth at home, New York, 1977, Bantam Book, Inc.

Sumner, P.E.: The birthing room—safe, joyous childbirth, Speech presented at the 5th International Congress of Psychosomatic Obstetrics and Gynecology, Rome, Nov. 18, 1977.

Thiede, H.A.: The cooperative role of the physician and nurse in obstetric practice, J. Obstet. Gynecol. **1**:6, Nov./Dec. 1975.

DEFINITIONS

Define the following terms:

alternative birth center (ABC)
American College of Nurse-Midwives (ACNM)
American College of Obstetricians and Gynecologists (ACOG)
American Society of Psychoprophylaxis in Obstetrics (ASPO)
birth room
Childbirth without Pain Education League (CWPEL)
freestanding birth center
home health aide
International Childbirth Education Association (ICEA)
lay midwife
LDR room
LDRP room
maternal-child nurse practitioner
midwife
nurse-midwife
nurse practitioner
obstetrical technician
pediatric nurse practitioner
single-room maternity care

LEARNING ACTIVITIES AND EXPERIENCES

1. Check to see if there is an alternative birth center in your community. What are the ABC's policies? Cost? If possible, visit the center.
2. Are there LDR or LDRP rooms in your community? Evaluate their cost-effectiveness.
3. Guest speakers: certified nurse-midwife, lay midwife, nurse practitioner.
4. View audiovisual aids and discuss.
5. If you wrote a paper on "The Therapeutic Use of Self in Maternity Care" at the end

of Unit I, review that paper now. Do you still feel the same?

6. What duties would a maternal-child nurse practitioner perform?
7. What duties would a pediatric nurse practitioner perform?
8. List at least four team members in provision of maternity care.
9. Write a paragraph defining family-centered maternity/newborn care.

SELF-ASSESSMENT

1. How would you describe an alternative birth center within a hospital to an expectant couple?

2. What are the risks of home birth?

3. Why do people choose home birth?

4. Nurse-midwives are certified by a national organization known as:
   a. ACNM
   b. NAACOG
   c. ANA
5. Lay midwives are certified by a national organization known as:
   a. ACNM
   b. they are not certified
   c. ACLM

UNIT XV
Clinical application

The objectives that follow have been designed to help you use your clinical time effectively. Although the opportunity to complete these objectives will depend on the clinical experiences available, use all available resources to prepare yourself to meet these objectives whenever possible.

An excellent clinical reference for writing and using nursing care plans for childbearing families is *Nursing Care Plans for the Childbearing Family*, by Virginia Aukamp, R.N., M.S. This 1984 reference is published by Appleton-Century-Crofts, 25 Van Zant Street, East Norwalk, CT 06855.

ANTEPARTUM CLINICAL OBJECTIVES

Clinical objective	Discussed and/or demonstrated	Learning activities and comments
1. Demonstrate a broad and basic understanding of the female bony pelvis and external and internal genitalia.		Review Unit II. Diagram the female external and internal genitalia, identifying the basic structures. Inspect a female bony pelvis in an anatomy laboratory or locate a drawing of a female bony pelvis in a text. Compare the female and male bony pelvis.
2. In antepartum clinic or office, when examining an expectant mother, demonstrate the following skills: a. calculation of estimated date of delivery b. evaluation of fetal heart tone c. abdominal palpation and inspection using Leopold's maneuvers		Review Unit IV. Review Unit VIII. Review Unit VIII.
3. Interview an expectant mother and assess her need for instruction in the antepartum period in regard to: a. diet b. rest c. elimination d. exercise e. hygiene f. clothing g. smoking h. ingesting medications or alcohol i. sexuality in pregnancy		Review Unit IV. What instruction booklets are available in the prenatal clinic for use by childbearing families? What audiovisual aids are available? What classes are available?
4. Distinguish between the psychological and physiological changes in pregnancy.		Review Unit IV. Interview a pregnant woman during the third trimester of pregnancy and have her describe changes that occurred during the pregnancy. How did she know she was pregnant? How did she feel in each trimester: Physically? Emotionally?

Continued.

ANTEPARTUM CLINICAL OBJECTIVES—cont'd

Clinical objective	Discussed and/or demonstrated	Learning activities and comments
5. Analyze family's instructional needs for the following: a. preparation of baby's room and clothing b. sibling rivalry		Interview an expectant family. What are their plans for incorporating the new baby into their family?
6. Examine the adjustments involved in making the decision on whether to bottle feed or breast-feed.		Review Units II and IV. Describe the advice you would give to a young expectant mother who is debating between breast- and bottle feeding her infant. Evaluate a LaLeche League meeting in your community (group support, group strengths, group weaknesses).
7. Evaluate a prenatal class relative to: a. physical environment b. emotional environment (1) support (2) discussion c. use of audiovisual aids d. demonstrations e. group participation		Review Unit VI. What group strengths were observed? What group weaknesses were observed? How were anxieties manifested?
8. Facilitate decision-making for expectant parents who announce they plan to deliver at home.		Read Unit XIV. Ask them why; ask yourself why. Do not impose your value system. What are the pros and cons?
9. Discuss measures appropriate for the various minor discomforts of pregnancy.		Review Unit IV.
10. Plan a basis for nursing action in the following deviations from normal in the antepartum period: a. Rh incompatibility b. abortion c. ectopic pregnancy d. bleeding problems e. hyperemesis gravidarum f. diabetes g. heart disease h. pregnancy-induced hypertension		Review Unit V.
11. Design an information booklet for expectant parents, identifying the danger signs that could indicate complications of pregnancy.		Review Unit IV.

INTRAPARTUM CLINICAL OBJECTIVES

Clinical objective	Discussed and/or demonstrated	Learning activities
1. Demonstrate basic understanding of psychological, emotional, sexual, and sociocultural factors in labor.		Review Unit VII. Talk with families in early labor. Did they take any prenatal classes? What are their expectations? What are their past experiences?
2. Demonstrate basic understanding of pelvic floor musculature.		Review Unit II and VII. Watch an episiotomy repair. Identify the pelvic floor muscles.
3. Demonstrate basic understanding of fetopelvic relationships.		Review Unit VII. When admitting a woman in labor, try to palpate the baby's neck and small parts.
4. Admit a laboring woman to labor a. review history and all prenatal records b. complete admission assessment (1) vital signs: blood pressure; temperature, pulse, and respiration; fetal heart tone (2) urine specimen: sugar, albumin		Review Units VIII and VII. In addition to the information on the woman's history records, what other information do you need to proceed with care?
5. Demonstrate providing nursing care to laboring women and their families:		
a. enema if indicated		Review Unit VIII.
b. testing for ruptured membranes c. assisting with artificial rupture of membranes (ARM)		Review Unit VII.
d. evaluating contractions		
e. rectal and/or vaginal examinations		Review Units VII and IX.
f. administration of medication g. assistance with administration of anesthetic		Review Unit IX.
h. maintaining an empty urinary bladder i. maintaining hydration j. proper positioning		Review Unit VIII.
6. Demonstrate an understanding of and an ability to give supportive nursing care for a woman and her family who are using prepared childbirth techniques.		Review Unit VI. What type of prenatal class did this family attend (Lamaze, Bradly, Yoga, or other)? Did they read any books on birth?
7. On printouts of electronic fetal monitoring, evaluate: a. baseline fetal heart rate b. early decelerations c. late decelerations d. flattening of baseline (fetal heart tone) e. variable decelerations f. tachycardia g. bradycardia		Review Unit VIII. Examine old fetal monitoring records of patients who have been discharged. Compare and contrast the "strips" from three or four such records.
8. Demonstrate assisting with application of internal fetal monitor.		Observe a nurse assisting the physician first. Role play procedure with help of fellow student.
9. Demonstrate an understanding of medical and surgical asepsis.		Observe nurse or instructor set up delivery equipment. Check hospital procedure book on setup for delivery.

Continued.

INTRAPARTUM CLINICAL OBJECTIVES—cont'd

Clinical objective	Discussed and/or demonstrated	Learning activities
10. Design a plan for nursing action in each of the following unexpected deviations from normal:		Review Unit IX.
a. preterm labor		
b. prolapsed cord c. placenta previa d. abruptio placentae		Review Unit IX.
e. irregular fetal heart tone or fetal distress		Review Unit VIII. Review Unit V.
f. convulsions or eclampsia		Review Unit IX.
g. oxytocin induction or augmentation of labor.		
11. Prepare a woman for cesarean birth: a. abdominal preparation b. Foley catheter c. presurgical paper work d. necessary equipment for baby e. emotional support (mother, family, father)		Review Unit IX.
12. In preparation for delivery examine all equipment in delivery area.		How does the delivery table or bed operate? Can you use the resuscitator? suction? oxygen? Where is the infant resuscitation tray? What are the emergency codes?
13. Demonstrate giving appropriate nursing care during delivery:		Review Unit VIII.
a. support mother		
b. support father		Review Unit VII.
c. administer medications		Review Unit VIII.
14. Demonstrate general care of newborn following delivery:		Review Unit VIII.
a. receive newborn b. Apgar scoring		Watch a nurse assign an Apgar score to a newborn at birth and 5 minutes after birth. Do you agree with the score?
15. Provide for interaction that will facilitate bonding in immediate postdelivery period.		Review Units I and VIII.
16. Identify the needs of the woman and her family in the fourth stage of labor.		Review Unit VIII.
17. Provide recovery care for the new mother and family in the immediate postpartum period. a. vital signs b. bladder care c. fundus check d. express clots e. vaginal bleeding monitoring		Review Unit VIII.
18. Plan a basis for nursing action in the following deviations from normal:		Review Unit VIII.
a. perineal lacerations		
b. postpartum hemorrhage		Review Unit VIII.
c. resuscitation of a neonate with a low Apgar score		Review Unit XIII.

NEWBORN CLINICAL OBJECTIVES

Clinical objective	Discussed and/or demonstrated	Learning activities and comments
1. Demonstrate to your instructor the different nursing actions necessary in caring for the following infants: a. Apgar score 7 to 10 b. Apgar score 4 to 6 c. Apgar score 0 to 3		Review Unit XIII. Turn on and operate infant stabilization crib. At what pressure would you operate the suction? How would you suction a newborn? How does the DeLee's mucus trap work? How does the laryngoscope work? With a fellow student to assist you, role play resuscitation of a newborn. Do you know how to give cardiac massage to a newborn? Do you know how to use bulb suction? When do you compress rubber suction bulb?
2. Receive a newborn immediately after birth and make appropriate nursing observations and interventions.		Review Unit XII. Observe a nurse receiving a newborn immediately after birth. What does the nurse do? What can you do to conserve the newborn's body heat? When should the eye prophylaxis be administered?
3. Demonstrate caring for a newborn: a. vital signs (temperature, pulse, and respiration) b. weighing c. identification d. notification of physician e. measurements (length, head, chest) f. gestational age g. observations (color, cry, activity) h. charting		Review Unit XII. Observe a nurse admitting a newborn to the nursery or birth room. Complete *Observation of a newborn* form.
4. Demonstrate nursing actions in regard to safety and important daily care while bathing a newborn:		Observe a nurse giving daily care to a newborn.
a. eye care		Review Unit XII.
b. cord care		
c. skin care		
d. circumcision care		Review Unit XII.
e. elimination		Review Unit XII.
5. Administer medications to newborns as ordered.		Review Unit XII.
6. On a walking tour of a newborn nursery, explain to your instructor how you can differentiate among newborns when describing normal observations.		Review Unit XII. Always wash your hands before touching any baby. *Look* at three or more babies. What is their color when crying? Not crying? What are their respirations like? How are their heads shaped? What is the relationship of the head to body size? What is the average weight and length? How does the cry sound? How have you seen newborns express their individuality?
7. Demonstrate teaching and assisting a new mother to breast feed.		Review Units XII and X. Check the charts of breast-feeding mothers. How do you expect the medication given in labor and delivery to affect the babies? Notice the attitude of the mother, how she handles her infant and positions herself, and the ba-

Continued.

NEWBORN CLINICAL OBJECTIVES—cont'd

Clinical objective	Discussed and/or demonstrated	Learning activities and comments
		by's alertness, sucking ability, and interest.
8. Demonstrate teaching and assisting a new mother to bottle feed.		Review Unit XII. Does the mother understand formula preparation? What are the types of formula available commercially? Where? How much do they cost?
9. Demonstrate the ability to effectively communicate with families regarding their infant's health maintenance and well-being. Complete a demonstration baby bath.		Review Unit XII. Select a family whom you have assessed is in need of teaching (for example, first baby, no prenatal education). Ask them if they would like a demonstration baby bath.
10. Compare the preterm infant with the normal newborn in relation to: a. cry b. size c. weight d. skin e. activity		Review Unit XIII. Visit the neonatal intensive care unit to observe preterm babies. Read charts of preterm infants or infants with "problems." Note how their Apgar scores may vary. Note their progress.
11. Design a plan to assist the parents in coping with the death of a newborn.		Review Unit XI.
12. Design a plan to assist the parents in coping with the sick neonate.		Review Unit XI.
13. Interview families who have used rooming-in. Examine their feelings.		Review the hospital policies and procedures manual on rooming-in.
14. Interview families who have experienced birth in labor, delivery, recovery (LDR), or labor, delivery, recovery, postpartum (LDRP) rooms. Examine their feelings.		Review Unit XIV.
15. Design a plan for nursing action in each of the following deviations from normal: a. pathological jaundice b. infection (sepsis) c. respiratory distress syndrome d. hypoglycemia		Review Unit XIII.
16. Demonstrate discharging an infant with the family. a. identification process b. teaching c. support		Review Unit XII. Are they ready to go home?

POSTPARTUM CLINICAL OBJECTIVES

Clinical objective	Discussed and/or demonstrated	Learning activities and comments
1. Evaluate the condition of the fundus, lochia, breasts, extremities, episiotomy, voiding, and vital signs of a woman on the first postpartum day and report and record findings.		Review Unit X. Check postpartum charts. How are these findings recorded?
2. Demonstrate giving perineal care and/or teaching a new mother to care for herself.		Review Unit X. 1. Where is the sitz bath? How does it operate? 2. Where is the peri-lamp? How does it operate? 3. Tucks? Witch hazel? Peri compresses?
3. Examine the attitude of a new mother toward her new baby.		Review Unit X. Stay with a mother and her baby during a feeding. Look for maternal attitudes and interactions. Complete one *Mother-Infant Observation* form.
4. Examine the attitude of a new father toward his new baby.		Review Units I and X. Observe a father interacting with his baby. Complete one *Father-Infant Observation* form.
5. Demonstrate making three observations during your first visit to a postpartum mother following a cesarean birth that would be different from observations you would make for a mother following a vaginal delivery. a. breasts b. fundus c. incision d. lochia e. extremities f. abdomen g. pain h. vital signs i. voiding		Review Unit XI. A cesarean birth is major abdominal surgery. What observations would you make in the first hours after surgery? Remember this cesarean patient is also a new mother.
6. Demonstrate helpful postpartum exercises.		Visit hospital physiotherapist. What exercises do they recommend? Check handout on postpartum exercises on hospital unit and those given by physicians.
7. Describe the purpose of the postpartum checkup by the physician.		Ask physician what happens at postpartum checkup. Visit clinic; ask nurses what happens at postpartum checkup. Arrange a visit to a postpartum clinic and assist with postpartum checks, if possible.
8. Demonstrate helping a new mother recognize her change in emotional needs.		Ask multiparous mothers to identify what worried them after they went home (for example, baby's care, their own physical condition). Meet the husband and/or woman's family. Note the relationships. What is said and how is it said? Complete the *Postpartum Family Assessment Guide*.
9. Compare attitudes of mothers who have had vaginal deliveries with those of mothers who have had cesarean birth.		Visit mothers who have had both vaginal and cesarean births. Talk with the fathers. Were they present at the cesarean? Would they like to

Continued.

POSTPARTUM CLINICAL OBJECTIVES—cont'd

Clinical objective	Discussed and/or demonstrated	Learning activities and comments
		have been? Why? When did they hold their baby for the first time?
10. Discuss normal aspects of sexuality with postpartum parents. a. resumption of coitus b. sexual feelings about breast-feeding c. contraception		Review Unit X.
11. Design a plan for therapeutic nursing care for the mother of a preterm infant.		Review Unit XI. Visit the mother of a preterm infant. What are her special worries? Note the Apgar score of the baby.
12. Design a plan for nursing action in each of the following deviations from normal in the postpartum period: a. puerperal infection b. thrombophlebitis c. mastitis		How can you help this mother and family? Review Unit X. Review Unit XI.
13. Administer medications as ordered: a. RhoGAM b. rubella vaccine c. postpartum medicines		Review Unit X.
14. Demonstrate knowledge of grieving process of families with neonatal loss and appropriate intervention.		Review Unit XI.

MOTHER-INFANT OBSERVATION

DIRECTIONS

1. Obtain the following information from the chart before meeting the mother: age ________ para ________ gravida ________ abortions ________ ages of other children ________ postpartum day ________ bottle feeding ________ date and time last analgesic drug given ________
2. Ask the mother if you may observe her and her baby together. Be sure the mother understands that you are interested in their normal interactions and not in a "good show." Determine if the mother has any physical discomfort. ________ How is she feeling emotionally (happy, tense, worried, relaxed)? ________
3. Observe verbal and nonverbal actions and interactions of the mother and her baby. Also observe any other interaction that takes place in the room (for example, staff, other family members, roommate.) Focus on these interactions, keeping in mind the process of bonding and the postpartum phases: taking-in, taking-hold, and letting-go.
4. After 20 minutes, report to the conference area. Record your observations:
   a. Mother's nonverbal actions. How did she hold the baby?

   b. What did the mother say to the baby? What was her tone of voice?

   c. Baby's actions and responses:

   d. Mother's interactions with you or others in the room:

The conference will be designed to promote an understanding of the mother-infant interaction you have observed.

FATHER-INFANT OBSERVATION

This is a tool to help you assess fathering capabilities. Select a father to interview. First study the mother's chart. Review prenatal care, labor, and delivery.

1. Is this her first child with this man?
2. Are they married?
3. How long have they been together?
4. Is he a father for the first time? If not, what was his previous childbirth experience?
5. How old is he?
6. Is he employed?
7. If yes, where?
8. What is his education background?
9. What is his ethnic background?

Next, interview the father:

DATA GATHERING:

1. During pregnancy, did the father experience any physiological or psychological reactions or concerns similar to those the mother experienced?

2. What were the high points of the pregnancy for him?

3. Did the father attend prenatal classes? What did he learn there? Why did he attend?

4. Was the father present during labor? What was his role during labor (that is, passive observer, active participant)? Did he think the staff was helpful to *him* during labor?

5. Was the father present during birth? What does he remember of the actual delivery (that is, responses, feelings, touching, holding)? If answer to No. 5 is no, when did he first see and/or hold his infant?

6. Did he have a preference for a boy or girl?

7. What does he see as his role or responsibility in infant and child care?

OBSERVE THE BABY AND FATHER TOGETHER. LOOK FOR THE FATHER'S:

1. Visual awareness of the newborn and father's verbal response:
   a. Does he enjoy looking at his baby?

   b. Does he see his baby as pretty, beautiful, or ugly?

   c. What does he say?

   d. Does he call the baby by name?

2. Tactile awareness of the newborn:
   a. Does he want to pick up his baby?

   b. How does the baby's skin feel to him?

   c. Describe how he touches and holds his baby (for example, close to him, stiff, rough, gentle, hesitant, assured).

3. Awareness of distinct characteristics of newborn:
   a. Can he distinguish his own baby from others?

   b. Does he feel that his baby looks like him or the mother?

   c. Does he perceive his infant as "perfect"?

   d. What aspects of the infant's behavior have impact on the father (that is, baby opening eyes, grimacing, grasp reflex)? Write down what he answers.

   e. Do you feel that this father is forming a bond with his newborn? What leads you to feel this?

POSTPARTUM FAMILY ASSESSMENT GUIDE

Date ____________ Postpartum day ____________ Marital status ____________
Ethnic group ____________ Religion ____________ Age ____________
Gravida ____________ Para ____________ Abortions ____________
Weeks gestation ____________ Pregancy planned____________
Education/occupation: Mother____________
Father ____________

Antepartum:

Preparation classes? ________ Did both attend? ________ Reading?____________
Physical preparation (exercises, breasts)____________
Mother's blood type ____________ Rh ____________ Serology____________
Father's blood type ____________ Rh ____________ Serology____________
Medications taken during pregnancy____________
Significant family, personal, OB history____________

Labor:

Length of labor: stage 1 ________ stage 2 ________ stage 3 ________ stage 4 ________
Medications (drug, dose, route, and time)____________

Continuous fetal monitoring____________
Fetal distress ____________
Rupture of membranes (artificial or spontaneous)____________
Anesthesia or analgesia ____________
Labor complications ____________

Delivery:

Type of delivery ____________
Date and time of delivery ____________
Episiotomy or cesarean incision ____________

Estimated blood loss____________
Admission hematocrit ____________
Postpartum hematocrit ____________

Infant:

Apgar (1 minute) ____________ (5 minutes) ____________
Sex ____________ Weight ____________ Length ____________
Feeding: breast ____________ bottle ____________
Cry (frequent, strong, weak)____________
Activity level (alert, lethargic)____________
Complications ____________

Postpartum:

Maternal physical condition

	Day 1	Day 2	Day 3
Vital signs			
Bladder			
Fundus			
Breasts and nipples			
Lochia (color, odor, number of pads)			
Episiotomy or cesarean incision			
Hemorrhoids			
Legs			
Elimination Urinary			
Bowels			

Family-infant interaction:

Mother:

Appearance ______

Feelings about labor and delivery ______

Physical complaints ______

Activity level (passive, initiates activity, nervous, lethargic). Would you say she is in the taking-in, taking-hold, or letting-go phase? Why? ______

Father:

Appearance ______

Feelings about labor and delivery ______

Involvement in infant care (passive, active) ______

Siblings:

Appearance ______

Feelings about new baby ______

Interaction with parents ______

Grandparents:

Appearance ______

Involvement in infant care ______

Attitudes about birth experience and recovery ______

Interaction with new parents ______

Communication:

	Mother:	Father:
Calls baby by name		
Calls baby "it"		
Looks at baby		
Holds baby close to body		
Holds baby stiffly away from body		
Immediately meets baby's needs		
Explores baby		
Makes eye contact with baby		
Is satisfied with sex of baby		
Physically overstimulates baby (slaps, hits, shakes, pokes)		
Says baby stinks		
Focuses more on own needs		

Infant:

Behaviors in response to:
Mother ______________________________
____
Father ______________________________
____
Sleep patterns ______________________________
Breast feeding: Patterns ______________________________
Problems ______________________________
____

Information needs:

Knowledge of baby care:

	Mother:	Father:
Bath		
Cord care		
Circumcision care		
Diapering		
Temperature		
Diaper rash		
Pediatric follow-up		
Infant safety		

Knowledge of infant feeding:

	Mother:	Father:
Bottle:		
Rooting reflex		
Type of formula		
Amount per feeding		
Preparation		
Burping		
Vitamins and iron		
Introduction of solid foods		
Feeding schedules		
Breast:		
Rooting reflex		
Nipple care		
Let-down reflex		
Supportive bra		
Positioning		
Length of feeding		
Techniques for expressing milk		
Medications and breast-feeding		
Diet		
Smoking		

Nutrition:

Typical diet at home ______________________________
____
____
Approximate caloric intake ______________________________
Fluid intake ______________________________

Birth control:

Understands time for resumption of sexual activity ____________________

Type of contraception ____________________

Understanding ____________________

Exercise:

Type ____________________

Understanding ____________________

Personal hygiene:

Bathing ____________________

Showering ____________________

Douching ____________________

Help at home (grandparents, other children)? ____________________

____

Layette? ____________________

____

What follow-up would you recommend (family resources, community resources)? ____________________

____

____

____

____

OBSERVATION OF A NEWBORN

Select a newborn infant for observation. Before entering the nursery:

1. Review the mother's chart:
   Gravida ____________ Para ____________ Expected date of delivery ____________
   Estimated gestational age: ____________ Small for gestational age ____________
   Average for gestational age ____________ Large for gestational age ____________
   Rh ______________________________ Serology ______________________________
   Length of labor: first stage ____________________ second stage ____________________
   Type of delivery: vaginal ____________________ cesarean ____________________
   Analgesia and anesthesia: ____
2. Review the infant's chart:
   Apgar at 1 minute ____________________ 5 minutes ____________________
   Birth weight ____________________ loss or gain ____________________
   Type feeding ____
3. Complete Column 1 of the following guide with textbook information of the norms to be expected.
4. Using aseptic nursery technique and providing warmth for the infant, observe the infant. Complete Column 2.
5. Date: ____
6. Time of examination: ____

Observations	COLUMN 1 Textbook information	COLUMN 2 Observation of infant
General appearance:		
1. Posture, body alignment, and symmetry		
a. sleeping		
b. awake (quiet)		
c. crying (loud, strong, weak, high-pitched)		
2. Respirations		
3. Apical pulse rate		
4. Length		
5. Weight		
6. Axillary temperature		
Assessment of head and neck:		
7. Head		
a. circumference		
b. size in relation to rest of body		
c. size compared with adult		
d. symmetry		
e. molding		
f. cephalhematoma		
8. Fontanels (size, shape, consistency)		
a. anterior fontanel		
b. posterior fontanel		
9. Skin		
a. color		
b. rash		
10. Ears		
a. response to sound		
b. position and shape		
c. location of ears		
11. Face		
a. chin		
b. milia		
12. Eyes		
a. color		
b. condition (clear, discharge, swelling)		
c. eye movement		

13. Nose		
a. patent		
b. blocked		
c. drainage		
14. Mouth		
a. palate (intact or abnormal)		
b. mucosa (pink or white patches or cyanotic)		
15. Neck		
a. length		
b. mobility		
c. presence of webbing and/or fat pad		
16. Breasts		
a. size of areola		
b. fullness		
c. engorgement		
d. discharge		
17. Chest		
a. symmetry		
b. type of respiration (shallow, irregular, grunting)		
18. Abdomen		
a. condition (soft, hard, distended)		
19. Umbilicus		
a. color		
b. odor		
c. condition		
20. Genitourinary system		
a. first passage of urine		
b. female (condition of external genitalia)		
c. male (testes)		
21. Anus and bowels		
a. stool (first)		
b. daily stools (color, consistency)		
c. anus, patent		
22. Extremities		
a. symmetry		
b. number of fingers and toes		
c. rotation of hips		
d. buttocks and leg creases		
23. Nervous system		
a. grasp reflex		
b. rooting reflex		
c. sucking reflex		
d. walking reflex		
e. Moro's ("startle") reflex		
f. tonic neck reflex		
24. State of awareness		
a. deep sleep		
b. rapid eye movement sleep		
c. crying		
d. transitional		
e. quiet alert		
f. active awake		

Answers to self-assessments

UNIT 1

1. False
2. False
3. True
4. True
5. False
6. True
7. True
8. True
9. False
10. True
11. True
12. False
13. 2
14. b
15. b
16. 1
17. a. right to be informed
    b. right to access to hospital medical records
    c. right to have well baby at her bedside
    d. right to companionship in labor
    e. right to know name and qualifications of care providers
18. a. disinterest in infant
    b. not touching infant
    c. anger and noncommunication with partner
19. a. better prenatal care for *all* people
    b. emphasis on prevention
    c. regionalization
20. a. prematurity
    b. asphyxia and atelectasis
    c. congenital malformations
    d. birth injuries
21. a. late prenatal care
    b. inadequate nutrition
    c. inconsistency in following instructions about health care
22. a. sibling visiting
    b. fathers involved in labor and birth
    c. early discharge
23. attitudinal
24. preparing
25. respect
26. responsibilities
27. almost doubled

UNIT II

1. examine Fig. 2-1
2. examine Fig. 2-15
3. examine Fig. 2-2
4. examine Fig. 2-8
5. examine Fig. 2-9
6. examine Fig. 2-14
7. a. serves as sphincters to close openings
   b. serves as a hammock or sling
8. b, d, and e
9. c
10. d
11. c
12. a
13. a
14. middle layer
15. a. to provide sexual gratification
    b. to produce hormones
    c. to reproduce
16. a. coccyx
    b. sacrum
    c. innominate bone
    d. innominate bone
17. a. proliferative phase
    b. ovulatory phase
    c. secretory phase
    d. menstrual phase
18. a. follicular phase
    b. luteal phase
19. 1. c
    2. b
    3. a
    4. d
    5. d
20. 1. c
    2. b
    3. d
    4. a
    5. e
    6. f
21. estrogen, progesterone
22. proliferative
23. secretory
24. linea terminalis
25. examine Fig. 2-5, **A**
26. efferent (motor) and afferent (sensory)
27. examine Fig. 2-17, **B**
28. examine Fig. 2-17, **A**
29. a. tubules
    b. seminal vesicles
    c. prostate gland

UNIT III

1. True
2. False
3. True
4. False
5. True
6. True
7. True
8. False
9. True
10. False

11. True
12. False
13. False
14. True
15. True
16. d
17. I
18. a
19. b
20. c
21. c
22. a
23. 1. b
    2. c
    3. a
    4. c
    5. a
24. 1. c
    2. a
    3. b
25. Examine Figs. 3-8 and 3-9
26. age
27. Down's syndrome
28. 1. case-finding
    2. making referrals
    3. explaining procedure
29. congenital anomalies
30. embryo
31. birth
32. growth and development
33. a. respiratory
    b. metabolic
    c. excretory
34. T for toxoplasmosis
    O for "other" (syphilis)
    R for rubella
    C for cytomegalovirus
    H for herpes simplex
35. 10% to 15%

UNIT IV

1. False
2. True
3. False
4. True
5. c
6. c
7. b
8. a
9. c
10. d
11. d
12. d
13. b
14. c
15. b
16. b
17. 4
18. c
19. a. protect and support optimal health of unborn baby
    b. protect and promote physical and emotional health and well-being of expectant mother
    c. assist expectant father to adapt to new role
    d. assist siblings and other family members to adapt to new roles
20. a. easily digested
    b. offers immunity
    c. creates closeness
21. number of pregnancies
22. number of deliveries of infants a woman has had
23. a. Hematocrit > 36%, hemoglobin > 12 grams
    b. (1) negative
       (2) negative
24. a. what the mother sees when pregnant influences how the baby appears
    b. heartburn means curly hair
    c. by how mother carries baby
    d. activity of fetus in uterus indicates how well baby will sleep
25. assess the family's needs and attempt to meet them
26. elevate legs during rest periods
27. a. 4
    b. 4
    c. 1
    d. 1
    e. 1
    f. 2 animal and 2 vegetable
28. increase calcium intake
29. a. washing nipples daily without using soap
    b. nipple toughening exercises
30. a. can take oral contraceptives
    b. can return to work
    c. can be nutritionally adequate
31. a. bleeding from vagina
    b. swelling of face and fingers
    c. severe continuous headache
    d. blurring of vision
    e. pain in abdomen
    f. persistent vomiting
    g. chills and fever
    h. scant urine
    i. sudden escape of large amount of fluid from vagina
32. 1. h
    2. a
    3. d
    4. e
    5. c
    6. b
    7. g
    8. i
    9. f
33. backache
34. simple dependent edema
35. suspect pre-eclampsia

36. soap
37. increases, decreases
38. 5, 4, 1

UNIT V

1. a
2. c
3. b
4. a
5. fetal activity
6. full
7. ultrasonography
8. fetal death
9. amniocentesis
10. intrauterine transfusions
11. titer
12. blood transfusion
13. RhoGAM
14. inducing end of pregnancy
15. termination of pregnancy before fetus has become viable
16. rest
17. overdistention of uterus
18. 17, 35, 6
19. a. hemorrhage
    b. hypertension
20. diabetes, heart disease
21. after, before
22. to help the mother and family to work through the grief process of denial, anger, bargaining, depression, and acceptance
23. to carefully regulate insulin dosage and dietary management
24. gestational diabetis
25. a. recognition of fears about uncertain pregnancy outcome
    b. make sure each woman who should get RhoGAM is treated
    c. explain causes of Rh incompatibilities to families
26. a. abortion
    b. ectopic pregnancy
    c. hydatidiform mole
27. a. placenta previa
    b. abruptio placentae
28. a. inaccessibility
    b. high cost
    c. not understanding the value
29. a. encourage her to express her fears
    b. encourage her to control her own environment, that is, plan her daily care
    c. offer anticipatory guidance
30. it is possible
31. a. edema
    b. proteinuria
    c. elevated blood pressure
32. a. quiet room
    b. weigh daily
    c. intake and output
    d. medication
    e. eclamptic precautions
    f. check urine for albumin AM and PM
    g. collect laboratory specimens
    h. monitor fetus
    i. check patellar reflexes four times a day
33. a. marginal
    b. complete
    c. partial
34. 1. e
    2. a, b
    3. c, d
35. 1. b
    2. d
    3. c
    4. e
    5. a

UNIT VI

1. a. relaxation
   b. breathing
   c. focused concentration
   d. second-stage coping
   e. good posture and body mechanics
   f. genital and pelvic floor awareness
2. c
3. b
4. d
5. c
6. b
7. c
8. c
9. c
10. (demonstration to instructor)

UNIT VII

1. c
2. a
3. c
4. complete dilation
5. 13 hours; 7 hours
6. birth
7. 30 minutes to 2 hours; 5 to 30 minutes
8. placental
9. 5 to 30 minutes; 5 to 30 minutes
10. birth, until vital signs are stable
11. 1 to 2 hours
12. station
13. fear, happiness, increased anxiety, seriousness, heavy perspiration, restlessness, elation
14. true: regular and dilate cervix
    prelabor: irregular and do not dilate cervix
15. A
16. 10 centimeters
17. 1 centimeter
18. 10 centimeters
19. a. perspiration
    b. chills
    c. hiccups
    d. nausea and vomiting

20. this is a normal experience
21. because the pelvic inlet's widest diameter is transverse, and the widest diameter of the outlet is anterior-posterior
22. a. engagement
    b. descent
    c. flexion
    d. internal rotation
    e. extension
    f. restitution
    g. expulsion
23. a. cephalic
    b. breech
    c. shoulder
    d. face
24. 200 to 500 milliliters
25. a. to facilitate delivery when fetal distress occurs
    b. to relieve prolonged pressure on fetal head
    c. to enlarge vaginal outlet
26. second stage
27. firm
28. a
29. longitudinal
30. cephalic presentation
31. a. LOA
    b. LOT
    c. LOP
    d. ROA
    e. ROT
    f. ROP
32. 1. d
    2. b
    3. c

UNIT VIII

1. preference profile, identification, and financial arrangements
2. a. when contractions began, frequency, duration
   b. vaginal discharge
   c. membranes
   d. EDD
   e. time of last meal
   f. general condition of mother
3. 4, recorded, 2 hours
4. albumin, pre-eclampsia
5. 80
6. with strong uterine contractions the uterine wall cannot be indented by the examiner's fingers
7. head, fundus, back, symphysis, pubis, feet
8. 120 to 160
9. a. after any procedure
   b. after membranes rupture
   c. after medicating the mother
10. to pick up early warning signs of fetal distress
11. 1. b, d
    2. e, f
    3. a, c
12. baseline
13. 1, c, d
    2. a, b
14. b
15. a
16. b
17. a
18. a
19. a
20. b
21. 1. can slow down descent of fetus
    2. can cause supine-hypotensive syndrome
    3. may mean fetal distress
    4. may mean complete dilation
22. increased bloody show, urge to move bowels, vomiting
23. both legs, straining ligaments
24. silver nitrate
25. explain that it is required by law and why
26. a. skin and mucous membrane
    b. skin and muscles
    c. skin, muscles, and rectal sphincter
    d. skin, mucus, muscle, rectal sphincter, and anal wall
27. a. Ergotrate 0.2 milligrams by mouth or intramuscularly
    b. Methergine 0.2 milligrams by mouth or intramuscularly
    c. Pitocin 10 to 40 units intravenously by infusion in 500 to 1000 ml of intravenous solution
28. a. color
    b. reflex response
    c. heart rate
    d. respiratory effort
    e. muscle tone
29. warmth, open airway, identification
30. 15 minutes
31. massage the uterus
32. 500

UNIT IX

1. 3
2. a
3. 2
4. difficult labor
5. ill-timed, too much analgesia
6. monitor fetal heart tone closely
7. fetal distress
8. classical
9. hypertonic uterine contractions or fetal distress
10. a. failure to progress in labor
    b. previous cesarean birth
    c. uterine dysfunction
    d. abruptio placentae
    e. placenta previa

11. close observation and recording of vital signs, fetal heart tone, intake and output, and emotional status, plus constant and consistent emotional support
12. a. complete
    b. footling
    c. frank
13. frank
14. a. prolapsed cord
    b. cord compression
    c. head trapped
15. take the pressure off the cord and keep it pulsating
16. a. tense uterus
    b. uterus does not relax
    c. pain
17. be alert for any increase in bright red vaginal bleeding, a drop in blood pressure, and change in fetal heart tones
18. a. classic
    b. low cervical
    c. extraperitoneal
19. 1. a, b
    2. c, d
20. see Table 9-3
21. see Table 9-4

UNIT X

1. 1. c
   2. a
   3. b
2. d
3. a
4. 4
5. 3
6. b
7. c
8. b
9. c
10. b
11. c
12. a
13. 1. b
    2. b
    3. a
    4. a
    5. d
    6. d
    7. c
    8. c
    9. f
    10. e
    11. g
14. 40, 70
15. 98.6° F
16. drop
17. easier and slower
18. response to the parents
19. dependency
    accept
    baby
20. sterilization is final; contraception is temporary
21. b
22. c

UNIT XI

1. a
2. b
3. c
4. 3
5. 3
6. a
7. no, because it is important to drain the ducts
8. a. abruptio placentae
   b. eclampsia
   c. incomplete abortion
   d. sepsis
9. a. send photos of infant
   b. have parents name infant
   c. have parents send clothing for infant
   d. speak of infant by name
10. she should refrain from lifting, housework, and driving for several weeks
11. disappointment if they expected a vaginal delivery, or relief that baby is all right
12. a. shock and denial
    b. anger
    c. bargaining
    d. depression
    e. acceptance
13. a process that expresses bereaved persons' thoughts and feelings
14. allow them to grieve; be open and honest
15. a. check vaginal flow
    b. check fundus
    c. check dressings
    d. check chest; turn, cough, and deep breathe
    e. check intake and output
    f. check catheter
    g. check breasts
    h. check abdomen for distention
    i. check extremities
16. mother needs to know condition of her infant
17. elevate head of bed
18. *Streptococcus, Bacteroides,* colon bacillus, *Staphylococcus*
19. less
20. first 24
21. 24; 3

UNIT XII

1. c and f
2. c
3. 6 milligrams per deciliter; 12 milligrams per deciliter
4. after 24 hours of life

5. prothrombin coagulation
6. close observation because overheating is possible
7. 75.0° F (24.0° C), 50%
8. a
9. c
10. 3
11. b
12. 7 pounds; 7½ pounds; 20 inches; 12 to 13 inches; 13.8 inches (35 centimeters)
13. a. may have vernix in creases
    b. stand out slightly from head
    c. milia, nose breather, strong suck
    d. baby can see, focuses at 18 inches
    e. short and can be flexed
    f. smaller than head by up to 2 centimeters
    g. appears rounded and large in relation to hips and pelvis
    h. appear large
14. 1. c
    2. b
    3. a
15. See chart at bottom of page.
16. 1. b
    2. e
    3. d
    4. g
    5. c
    6. a
    7. f
    8. h
17. lasts from birth to 30 minutes of life; respirations are 60 to 90 per minute, heart rate is 180 or more; baby is alert
18. second reactive phase
19. a. quiet sleep
    b. REM sleep
    c. active alert
    d. quiet alert
    e. crying
    f. transitional
20. 1. e
    2. a
    3. c
    4. f
    5. b
    6. d
21. avoid drafts
22. drying baby
23. a warm blanket between baby and cold surface
24. radiant warmer because there is more room to work
25. 1. f
    2. b
    3. d
    4. a
    5. c
    6. e
26. a. skin
    b. lanugo
    c. plantar creases
    d. breast
    e. ear
    f. genitals (male)
    g. genitals (female)

UNIT XIII

1. c
2. b
3. a
4. c
5. c
6. c
7. c
8. b
9. b
10. c
11. a. chest lag
    b. intercostal retraction
    c. xiphoid retraction
    d. nares dilation
    e. expiratory grunt
12. hyperbilirubinemia
13. Rh and ABO
14. a. prematurity
    b. hemorrhage
    c. infection
    d. acidosis
    e. certain drugs
    f. low serum albumin levels
15. respiratory
16. pneumonia
17. soft, feeble
18. vital signs every 2 hours; turning infant

Reflex	Appearance	How stimulated	Time of disappearance
Moro's	Present at birth	Sudden noise or motion	3 months
Grasp	Strong at birth	Object to hand	3 months
Step	Present at birth	Feet barely touching surface	4 weeks
Sucking	Strong at birth	Object to mouth	Never

frequently; adequate fluid intake; temperature control
19. resuscitation
20. show photos of a neonatal intensive care nursery; explain equipment and care
21. listen; offer anticipatory guidance
22. 1. c
    2. a
    3. d
    4. b
    5. c
23. 1. b
    2. a
24. 1. a
    2. c

UNIT XIV

1. as an environment for birth that simulates a home environment but offers all the support systems of a hospital
2. emergencies may arise that require the support systems and interventions only hospitals are equipped to handle
3. out of an honest desire to have a memorable, safe, family-centered birth
4. a
5. b

APPENDIX A
Joint position statement on the development of family-centered maternity/newborn care in hospitals*

PREAMBLE

The Interprofessional Task Force on Health Care of Women and Children endorses the concept of family-centered maternity care as an acceptable approach to maternal/newborn care. The Task Force believes it would be beneficial to offer further comment and guidance to facilitate the implementation of such care. To this end, the organizations constituting the Task Force have participated in a multidisciplinary effort to develop a joint statement regarding the rationale behind and the practical implementation of family-centered maternity/newborn care. The effort has resulted in the development of this document, which the parent organizations believe can be helpful to those institutions considering or already implementing such programs. A description of potential components of family-centered maternity/newborn care is presented to assist implementation as judged appropriate at the local level.

DEFINITION: FAMILY-CENTERED MATERNITY/NEWBORN CARE

Family-centered maternity/newborn care can be defined as the delivery of safe, quality health care while recognizing, focusing on, and adapting to both the physical and psychosocial needs of the client-patient, the family, and the newly born. The emphasis is on the provision of maternity/newborn health care which fosters family unity while maintaining physical safety.

POSITION STATEMENT

The Task Force organizations, The American College of Obstetricians and Gynecologists, the American College of Nurse-Midwives, The Nurses Association of The American College of Obstetricians and Gynecologists, the American Academy of Pediatrics, and the American Nurses' Association, endorse the philosophy of family-centered maternity/newborn care. The development of this conviction is based upon a recognition that health includes not only physical dimensions, but social, economic and psychologic dimensions as well. Therefore, health care delivery, to be effective and satisfying for providers and

---

*Interprofessional Task Force on Health Care of Women and Children, June, 1978.

the community alike, does well to acknowledge all these dimensions by adhering to the following philosophy.

- That the family is the basic unit of society;
- That the family is viewed as a whole unit within which each member is an individual enjoying recognition and entitled to consideration;
- That childbearing and childrearing are unique and important functions of the family;
- That childbearing is an experience that is appropriate and beneficial for the family to share as a unit;
- That childbearing is a developmental opportunity and/or a situational crisis, during which the family members benefit from the supporting solidarity of the family unit.

To this end, the family-centered philosophy and delivery of maternal and newborn care is important in assisting families to cope with the childbearing experience and to achieve their own goals within the concept of a high level of wellness, and within the context of the cultural atmosphere of their choosing.

The implementation of family-centered care includes recognition that the provision of maternity/newborn care requires a team effort of the woman and her family, health care providers, and the community. The composition of the team may vary from setting to setting and include obstetricians, pediatricians, family physicians, certified nurse-midwives, nurse practitioners, and other nurses. While physicians are responsible for providing direction for medical management, other team members share appropriately in managing the health care of the family, and each team member must be individually accountable for the performance of his/her facet of care. The team concept includes the cooperative interrelationships of hospitals, health care providers, and the community in an organized system of care so as to provide for the total spectrum of maternity/newborn care within a particular geographic region.[1]

As programs are planned, it is the joint responsibility of all health professionals and their organizations involved with maternity/newborn care, through their assumptions and with input from the community, to establish guidelines for family-centered maternal and newborn care and to assure that such care will be made available to the community regardless of economic status. It is the joint concern and responsibility of the professional organizations to commit themselves to the delivery of maternal and newborn health care in settings where maximum physical safety and psychological well-being for mother and child can be assured. With these requirements met, the hospital setting provides the maximum opportunity for physical safety and for psychological well-being. The development of a family-centered philosophy and implementation of the full range of this family-centered care within innovative and safe hospital settings provides the community/family with the optimum services they desire, request and need.

In view of these insights and convictions, it is recommended that each hospital obstetric, pediatric, and family practice department choosing this approach designate a joint committee on family-centered maternity/newborn care encompassing all recognized and previously stated available team members, including the community. The mission of this committee would be to develop, implement, and regularly evaluate a positive and comprehensive plan for family-centered maternity/newborn care in that hospital.

In addition, it is recommended that all of this be accomplished in the context of joint support for:

- The published standards as presented by The American College of Obstetricians and Gynecologists, The American College of Nurse-Midwives, The Nurses Associ-

[1]Committee on Perinatal Health, The National Foundation–March of Dimes. *Toward Improving the Outcome of Pregnancy: Recommendations for the Regional Development of Maternal and Perinatal Health Services.* 1976.

ation of The American College of Obstetricians and Gynecologists, The American Academy of Pediatrics, and the American Nurses' Association.[2,3,4,5,6,7]

- The implementation of the recommendations for the regional planning of maternal and perinatal health services, as appropriate for each region.
- The availability of a family-centered maternity/newborn service at all levels of maternity care within the regional perinatal network.

POTENTIAL COMPONENTS OF FAMILY-CENTERED MATERNITY/NEWBORN CARE

No specific or detailed plan for implementation of family-centered maternity/newborn care is uniformly applicable, although general guidance as to the potential components of such care is commonly sought. The following description is intended to help those who seek such guidance and is not meant to be uniformly recommended for all maternity/newborn hospital units. The attitudes and needs of the community and the providers vary from geographic area to geographic area, and economic constraints may substantially modify the utilization of each component. The detailed implementation in each hospital unit should be left to that hospital's multidisciplinary committee established to deal with such development. In addition to the maternal/newborn health care team, community and hospital administrative input should be assured. In this manner, each hospital unit can best balance community needs within economic reality.

The major change in maternity/newborn units needed in order to make family-centered care work is attitudinal. Nevertheless, a description of the potential physical and functional components of family-centered care is useful. It remains for each hospital unit to implement those components judged feasible for that unit.

I. **Preparation of families:** The unit should provide preparation for childbirth classes taught by appropriately prepared health professionals. Whenever possible, physicians and hospital maternity nurses should participate in such programs so as to maximize cohesion of the team providing education and care. All class approaches should include a bibliography of reading materials. The objectives of these classes are as follows:
   A. To increase the community's awareness of their responsibility toward ensuring a healthy outcome for mother and child
   B. To serve as opportunities for the community and providers to match expectations and achieve mutual goals from the childbirth experience.
   C. To serve to assist the community to be eligible for participation in the full family-centered program.
   D. To include a tour of the hospital's maternity and newborn units. The tour should be offered as an integral part of the preparation for childbirth programs and be available to the community by appointment. The public should be informed of a mechanism for emergency communication with the maternity/newborn unit.

---

[2]The American College of Obstetricians and Gynecologists. *Standards for Obstetric-Gynecologic Services*, 1974.

[3]American College of Nurse-Midwives. *Functions, Standards, and Qualifications*, 1975.

[4]The Nurses Association of The American College of Obstetricians and Gynecologists. *Obstetric, Gynecologic and Neonatal Nursing Functions and Standards*, 1975.

[5]American Academy of Pediatrics. *Standards and Recommendations for Hospital Care of Newborn Infants*, 1977.

[6]American Nurses' Association. *Standards of Maternal-Child Health Nursing Practice*, 1973.

[7](a) The American College of Obstetricians and Gynecologists, the American College of Nurse-Midwives, and The Nurses Association of The American College of Obstetricians and Gynecologists. *Joint Statement on Maternity Care*, 1971. (b) The American College of Obstetricians and Gynecologists, The American College of Nurse-Midwives, and The Nurses Association of The American College of Obstetricians and Gynecologists. *Supplement to Joint Statement on Maternity Care*. 1975.

II. Preparation of hospital staff: A continuing education program should be conducted on an ongoing basis to educate *all levels* of hospital personnel who either directly or indirectly come in contact with the family-centered program. This education program may include:

- Content of local preparation for childbirth classes.
- Current trends in childbirth practices.
- Alternative childbirth practices: safe and unsafe, as they are being practiced.
- Needs of childbearing families to share the total experience.
- Ways to support those families experiencing less than optimal outcome of pregnancy.
- Explanation of term "family" so that it includes any "significant" or "supporting other" individual to the expectant mother.
- The advantages to families and to the larger society of establishing the parenting bond immediately after birth.
- The responsibilities of the patients toward ensuring a healthy outcome of the childbirth experience.
- The potential long-term economic advantage to the hospital for initiating the program and how this could benefit each employee.
- The satisfaction to be gained by each employee while assisting families to adjust to the new family member.
- How the family-centered program is to function and the role each employee is to perform to ensure its success.

III. Family-centered program within the maternity/newborn unit: The husband or "supporting other" can remain with the patient throughout the childbirth process as much as possible. Family-newborn interaction immediately after birth is encouraged.

A. *Family Waiting Room* and Early Labor Lounge, attractively painted and furnished, should be available in or near the obstetrical suite where:

1. Patients in early labor could walk and visit with children, husbands, and others.
2. The husband or "supporting other" person could go for a "rest break" if necessary.
3. Access to light nourishment should be available for the husband or "supporting other."
4. Reading materials are available.
5. Telephone/intercom connections with the labor area are available.

B. *A Diagnostic-Admitting Room* should be adjacent to or near the Family Waiting Room where:

1. Women could be examined to ascertain their status in labor without being formally admitted if they are in early labor.
2. Any woman patient past 20 weeks gestation could be evaluated for emergency health problems during pregnancy.

C. *"Birthing Room":*

1. A combination labor and delivery room for patient and the husband or "supporting other" during a normal labor and delivery.
2. A brightly and attractively decorated and furnished room designed to enhance a home-like atmosphere. A comfortable lounge chair is useful.
3. Stocked for medical emergencies for mother and infant with equipment concealed behind wall cabinets or drapes, but readily available when needed.
4. Wired for music or intercom as desired.

5. Equipped with a modern labor-delivery bed which can be:
   a. raised and lowered.
   b. adjustable to semi-sitting position.
   c. moved to the delivery room if the need arises.
6. Equipped with a cribbette with warmer and have the capacity for infant resuscitation.
7. Appropriately supplied for a normal spontaneous vaginal delivery and the immediate care of a normal newborn.
8. An environment in which breastfeeding and handling of the baby are encouraged immediately after delivery with due consideration given to maintaining the baby's normal temperature.

D. *Labor Rooms:*
   1. The husband or "supporting other" can be with a laboring patient whether progress in labor is normal or abnormal.
   2. Regulation hospital equipment is available.
   3. An emergency delivery can be performed.
   4. Attention is given to the surroundings which are attractively furnished and include a comfortable lounge chair.

E. *Delivery Rooms:* Should be properly equipped with standard items but, in addition, should have delivery tables with adjustable backrests. An overhead mirror should be available. The delivery rooms should accommodate breastfeeding and handling of the baby after delivery with due consideration to maintaining the baby's normal temperature.

F. *Recovery Room:* Patients may be returned from the delivery room to their original labor rooms, depending upon the demand, or to a recovery room. Such a recovery room should have all the standard equipment but also allow for the following options:
   1. The infant to be allowed to be with the mother and father or "supporting other" for a time period after delivery with due consideration given to the infant's physiologic adjustment to extrauterine life. Where feasible, post-caesarean section patients may be allowed the same option.
   2. The husband or "supporting other" to be allowed to visit with the new mother and baby with some provision for privacy.
   3. A "pass" to be given to the father or "supporting other" of the baby to allow for extended visiting privileges on the "new family unit."

G. The Postpartum *"new Family Unit"* should:
   1. Contain flexible rooming-in with a central nursery to allow:
      a. Optional "rooming-in."
      b. Babies to be returned to the central nursery for professional nursing care when desired by the mother.
      c. Maximum desired maternal/infant contact especially during the first 24 hours.
   2. Have extended visiting hours for the father or "supporting other" to provide the opportunity to assist with the care and feeding of the baby.
   3. Have limited visiting hours for friends since the emphasis of the family-centered approach is on the family.
   4. Contain a family room where:
      a. Children can visit with their mothers and fathers.
      b. Professional staff are available to answer questions about parenting and issues regarding adjustments to the enlarged family.
      c. Cafeteria-like meals can be served and eaten restaurant-style by the mothers.

5. Have group and individual instruction provided by appropriately prepared personnel on postpartum care, family planning, infant feeding, infant care, and parenting.
6. Allow visiting and feeding by the mothers in the special nurseries such as:
   a. Newborn, intensive care nursery.
   b. Isolation nursery.
7. Allow for breastfeeding/bottle feeding on demand with professional personnel available for assistance.

H. Discharge planning should include options for early discharge. If this option is desired, careful attention to continuing medical and/or nursing contact after discharge to ensure maternal and newborn health is important. Potential for utilization of appropriate referral systems should be available.

APPENDIX B
Preparation for childbirth organizations

American Academy of Husband-Coached Childbirth
P.O. Box 5224
Sherman Oaks, CA 91413

American Society for Psychoprophylaxis in Obstetrics, Inc.
1840 Wilson Blvd.
Suite 204
Arlington, Va. 22201

Childbirth without Pain Education Association
20134 Snowden
Detroit, MI 48235

Childbirth without Pain Education League
3940 Eleventh St.
Riverside, CA 92501

Council of Childbirth Education Specialists, Inc.
168 W. 86th St.
New York, NY 10024

c/sec, Inc., Cesearean/Support, Education and Concern
22 Forest Rd.
Framingham, MA 01701

International Childbirth Education Association
P.O. Box 20048
Minneapolis, MN 55420

LaLeche League International, Inc.
9616 Minneapolis Ave.
Box 1209
Franklin Park, IL 60131-8209

Maternity Center Association
48 West 92nd St.
New York, NY 10028

Midwest Parentcraft Center
627 Beaver Rd.
Glenview, IL 60025

Read Natural Childbirth Foundation, Inc.
1300 S. Eliseo Dr., Suite 102
Greenbrae, CA 94904

APPENDIX C
Preference profile

PREFERENCE PROFILE

Name ______________________________ Age ____________
Partner's name ______________________________ Age ____________
Grav. ____________ Para ____________ Age of children ____________
Due date ____________________ Physician ____________________
Other support person? ______________________________
Prenatal classes ______ Yes ______ No ______ What kind? ______ Where? ______
____
Baby care classes ______ Yes ______ No ______ What kind? ______ Where? ______
____
Desire to restrict visitors? ______________________________
Whom do you want with you in labor? ____________ For birth? ____________
Type of childbirth expected: ______________________________
____
____
Do you desire anesthesia for birth? ______________________________
____
Do you have any medical problems or allergies? ______________________________
____
Do you have any strong feelings about the following?

1. Episiotomy ______________________________
2. Breast-feeding ______________________________
3. Bottle feeding ______________________________
4. Circumcision ______________________________
5. Cutting of umbilical cord ______________________________
6. Lighting at birth ______________________________
7. Medications for mother or baby ______________________________
8. Fetal monitor—use of or type ______________________________
9. Intravenous fluids ______________________________
10. Partner's presence at cesarean birth ______________________________

Do you want the baby to go to a nursery or stay with you?
____
____
Is there something special you would like to learn or do while in the hospital? ____________
____
____
How can the medical and nursing staff help you to achieve your preferences for labor and delivery? ______________________________
____
____

APPENDIX D
Drugs in pregnancy and lactation

Potential problems from drugs known to be excreted in human milk

Drug	Effect
Analgesics	
Aspirin	Bleeding tendency in infant.
Heroin	Neonatal addiction.
Anti-infectives	
Ampicillin (Amcill, Omnipen, Penbritin, Polycillin)	Hypersensitivity upon repeated exposure.
Chloramphenicol (Chloromycetin)	Immature glucuronide conjugating system. May prevent adequate excretion and hence systemic toxicity.
Erythromycin (E-Mycin, Erythrocin, Ilosone)	Levels exceeding those in milk have been reported; potential neonatal jaundice.
Metronidazole (Flagyl)	Levels in milk equal those of plasma; may cause blood dyscrasia in infant.
Nalidixic acid (NegGram)	Hemolytic anemia in the absence of glucose-6-phosphate dehydrogenase.
Penicillin G and V	Hypersensitivity upon repeated exposure.
Sulfanilamide	Allergic skin rash; may cause hemolytic anemia in glucose-6-phosphase dehydrogenase deficiency.
Sulfapyridine	Allergic skin rash.
Sulfisoxazole (Gantrisin)	May cause kernicterus by displacing protein bound neonatal bilirubin.
Anticholinergics	
Atropine	May inhibit lactation and cause anticholinergic manifestations (that is, tachycardia) in infant.
Anticoagulants	
Phenindione (Hedulin)	Significant increase in prothrombin time and hence bleeding tendency of infant.
Bis-3:3-4 oxy-coumarinyl ethyl acetate	Hemorrhage of umbilical stump has been reported.
Cardiovascular drugs	
Reserpine (Serpasil)	Galactorrhea; nasal stuffiness and difficult breathing owing to enhanced production of bronchial mucus.
Thiazide diuretics (HydroDIURIL, Esidrix, Oretic, Thiuretic)	Maternal dehydration; manufacturers suggest discontinuance if nursing.
Central nervous system drugs	
Bromides	Have produced drowsiness; infant should be monitored for bromism.
Barbiturates	Barbital (Veronal) has produced sedation of infant; others may cause similar effect as well as induce neonatal microsomal enzyme activity. These or related anticonvulsants such as phenytoin may inhibit neonatal diaphorase and produce methemoglobinemia.

Continued.

Potential problems from drugs known to be excreted in human milk—cont'd

Drug	Effect
Caffeine	Irritability in infant after ingestion of large amounts of caffeine by mother.
Diazepam (Valium)	Parent compound or metabolite may accumulate and cause drowsiness, leading to reduced suckling and thus weight loss.
Lithium carbonate (Eskalith, Lithane)	Lithium can achieve levels in infant serum equal to that in mother's milk (0.3 milliequivalents per liter) and signs of lithium toxicity should be watched for.
Miscellaneous drugs	
Anthraquinone laxatives	If taken regularly by mother, infant may show signs of colic and diarrhea.
Carisoprodol (skeletal muscle relaxant) (Soma, Rela)	Levels equal to or greater than plasma levels are observed in milk; central nervous system depression and gastrointestinal upset may occur in the infant.
Dihydrotachysterol (Hytakerol)	Hypercalcemia may occur.
DDT	Poisoning can occur; levels as high as 5 mg% have been reached in milk.
Ergot (e.g., Cafergot)	Should be avoided; can cause changes in blood pressure as well as vomiting and diarrhea in the neonate.
Mercury	Central nervous system toxicity.
Oral contraceptive steroids	Combination estrogen-progestin products inhibit lactation if taken within first few weeks postpartum; proliferation of female infant's vaginal epithelium; gynecomastia in male infant; hyperbilirubinemia leading to kernicterus.
Phenylbutazone (Butazolidin, Azolid)	Levels in milk small, but if accumulation occurs, blood dyscrasias may occur in infant.
Potassium iodide	May alter infant's thyroid function; therefore should be avoided.
Thiouracil	M/P ratio < 1; may cause goiter or agranulocytosis.

Compiled from Knowles, J.A.: Pediatr. Currents (Ross Laboratories) **21**:28, 1972; O'Brien, T.E.: Am. J. Hosp. Pharm. **31**:844, 1974; Vorherr, H.: The breast, morphology, physiology and lactation, New York, 1974, Academic press; Ayd, F.J.: Int. Drug Therap. Newslett. **8**:9, 1973; Catz, C.S., and Giacola, G.P.: Ped. Clin. No. **19**:151, 1972; Takyi, B.E.: J. Hosp. Pharm. **28**:317, 1970; Illingsworth, R.S.: Practitioner **171**:533, 1953; Tyson, R.M., Shrader, E.A., and Perlman, H.H.: J. Pediatr. **11**:824, 1937. (From Gaginella, Timothy S.: U.S. Pharmacist **3**[3]: 40-50, 1978.)

How drugs given to a pregnant woman may harm her baby*

Drug	When given	Effect before birth	Effect at or following birth
Analgesic agents			
Narcotics: meperidine, morphine, propoxyphene, pentazocine, codeine (including codeine in cough medicines)	Throughout pregnancy	Poor intrauterine growth	Withdrawal symptoms; irritability, excessive crying, tremulousness, vomiting, diarrhea, hyperthermia, poor sleeping patterns, convulsions
Acetaminophen (large quantities)	Throughout pregnancy		Renal disease
Aspirin	Last few weeks of pregnancy		Lower albumin-binding capacity, platelet dysfunction, decrease in factor XII
Anesthetic agents			
General anesthetics	Any time during pregnancy	Temporary decrease in oxygen supply	
Local anesthetics, especially if given paracervically or as conduction anesthesia	Any time during pregnancy	Rapid absorption into fetal circulation causing bradycardia, acidosis, myocardial depression, convulsions, or death	Significant neurological impairment

How drugs given to a pregnant woman may harm her baby—cont'd

Drug	When given	Effect before birth	Effect at or following birth
Belladonna derivatives			
Atropine	Any time during pregnancy	Tachycardia	
Scopolamine	Third trimester	Second stage of labor prolonged, greater likelihood of need for cesarean birth	
Scopolamine interacting with methadone	Third trimester		Respiratory depression
Antihypertensives			
Diazoxide	Third trimester		Severe hypoglycemia, excess or absence of hair
Hexamethonium	Third trimester		Paralytic ileus, perforated intestine, death
Reserpine	Third trimester		Nasal congestion, bradycardia, hypothermia, abnormal neurological findings lasting 7 to 10 days and interfering with the infant's ability to feed
Intravenous therapy†			
Large volume of hypotonic fluids for diuretic therapy and pitocin	Preceding labor		Hyponatremic seizures reversible by rapid administration of sodium
Psychotropic agents			
Chloropyramine, imipramine, nortriptyline	First trimester		Some association with cranio-facial, skeletal, and central nervous system anomalies. Further verification needed.
Desipramine	Third trimester		Cyanosis, irritability, weight loss, excessive perspiration, respiratory distress
Nortriptyline	Third trimester		Urinary retention from bladder distention
Diazepam	Third trimester		Hypotonia lasting 6 to 9 months, poor suck reflex, hypothermia, low Apgar score, increased need for resuscitation
Meprobamate, amitriptyline	Throughout pregnancy		Coliclike syndrome lasting 6 to 9 months
Lithium	First and third trimesters		Lethargy, cyanosis, respiratory distress for the first week of life, often diagnosed as congenital heart disease
Phenothiazines	Third trimester		Extrapyramidal dysfunction lasting 9 months
Chlordiazepoxide	Throughout pregnancy		Withdrawal symptoms occurring up to 3 weeks following birth
Promethazine	Third trimester		Inhibition of platelet aggregation
Anticonvulsive agents			
Paramethadione, trimethadione	Throughout pregnancy		Congenital heart disease, microphthalmia, mental retardation

Continued.

How drugs given to a pregnant woman may harm her baby—cont'd

Drug	When given	Effect before birth	Effect at or following birth
Phenobarbital or phenytoin, possibly in unidentified interactions with other drugs	Various times and durations		Two to three times the normal incidence of birth defects, congenital heart disease, cleft lip and/or palate; less frequent incidence of deformed facial features, incomplete development of distal phalanges and nails, growth retardation, slow mental development
Anticoagulants			
Dicumarol	First trimester		Syndrome similar to Conradi-Hünermann's chondrodysplasia punctuate: eye anomalies, depressed nasal bridge, incompletely developed nose, stippled cartilaginous portions of the skeleton, respiratory distress, mental retardation, blindness
Anti-infective agents			
Sulfonamides (short-and long-acting)	Third trimester		Hemolytic anemia, jaundice, kernicterus at lower-than-expected bilirubin levels
Tetracycline	Second and third trimesters		Discoloration of teeth, enamel hypoplasia, increased incidence of dental caries
Nitrofurantoin	Third trimester		Hemolysis
Isoniazid	Throughout pregnancy		Pyridoxine (vitamin B_6) deficiency
Cholinesterase inhibitors			
	Throughout pregnancy		Symptoms resembling myasthenia gravis reportedly lasting 9 days, 10% to 20% incidence of muscle weakness
Hypoglycemic agents			
Chlorpropamide	Throughout pregnancy	Miscarriage	Prolonged hypoglycemia
Tolbutamide	Third trimester		Prolonged hypoglycemia
Sedatives			
Phenobarbital (as little as 1 gram daily)	Throughout pregnancy		Withdrawal symptoms beginning immediately or up to 2 weeks after birth and lasting 4 to 6 months
Bromides	Throughout pregnancy		Failure to grow, lethargy, dermatitis, hypotonia
Chloral hydrate (excessive amounts)	Throughout pregnancy	Miscarriage	
Magnesium sulfate (large amounts)	Third trimester		Respiratory depression, hypotonia, convulsions, death
Glutethimide	Third trimester		Withdrawal symptoms

How drugs given to a pregnant woman may harm her baby—cont'd

Drug	When given	Effect before birth	Effect at or following birth
Diagnostic procedures			
Radioiodine (^{131}I)	First trimester		Microcephaly, exophthalmos
Radioiodine (^{131}I)	Second and third trimesters		Hypothyroidism
Radiograph (low dose)	Any time during pregnancy		Increased incidence of leukemia
Radiograph with radiopaque media	Any time during pregnancy		Erroneous thyroid function studies months to years later; elevation of PBI (protein-bound iodine), decreased radioiodine (^{131}I) uptake
Thyroid medication			
Iodine, thioureas, cough medicines or bronchodilators containing iodine for patients with asthma	Throughout pregnancy		Trachea obstructed by large goiter, possible necessitating a tracheostomy and/or partial resection of the thyroid, hypo- or hyperthyroidism
Uterine stimulants			
Oxytocin	Throughout pregnancy	Decrease in blood supply	Stillbirth, marked depression
Ergot (large amounts in migraine-headache therapy)	Throughout pregnancy	Miscarriage	
Vitamins			
Menidione (water-soluble vitamin K)	Preceding delivery		Hemolytic anemia, jaundice, kernicterus
Excessive supplementation of pyridoxine (vitamin B_6)	Throughout pregnancy		Withdrawal seizures

*From Hill, R.M.: RN **40:**36-39, Aug. 1977.
†Fluid and electrolyte imbalance in the mother causes a similar imbalance in the fetus.

APPENDIX E
Audiovisual resources

Films, videocassettes, slide-tape packages

UNIT I

Five Women—Five Births (slide-tape)
Suzanne Arms Productions
151 Lytton Ave.
Palo Alto, CA 94301

The Bonding Birth Experience (16 mm film)
Parenting Pictures
121 N.W. Crystal St.
Crystal River, FL 32629

Hospital Maternity Care: Family Centered (16 mm film)
Mead Johnson Laboratories
Evansville, IN 47721

I'm Seventeen, Pregnant and Don't Know What to Do (16 mm film)
Children's Home Society of California
3100 W. Adams Blvd.
Los Angeles, CA 90018

Hunger in America, Parts I & II, CBS Reports Program (videotapes)
Carousel Films
1501 Broadway, Suite 1503
New York, NY 10036

Pregnant Fathers (16 mm film)
Joseph T. Anzalone Foundation
P.O. Box 5206
Santa Cruz, CA 95062

Working Pregnant to Working Mother (16 mm film)
Perennial Education, Inc.
930 Pitner Ave.
Evanston, IL 60202

A Sister for Stephanie (slide, color, audio cassette)
Bay Area Birth Education Supplies (BABES)
59 Berens Dr.
Kentfield, CA 94904

The Ties that Bind (16 mm film)
Ross Laboratories
585 Cleveland Ave.
Columbus, OH 43216

Pregnancy after 35 (16 mm film)
Polymorph Films
118 South St.
Boston, MA 02111

Single Parenting: Crisis and Challenge (16 mm film and videocassette)
Miller-Pickle Associates
211 E. 7th St., Suite 101
Austin, TX 78701

UNIT II

The Anatomy of the Female Pelvic and Reproductive Organs (slide/tape)
Medical Electronic Educational Services, Inc.
29423 W. Six Mile Rd.
Livonia, MI 48152

The Menstrual Cycle (16 mm film)
Eli Lilly Company
Audio-Visual Film Library, Dept. MC-340
Indianapolis, IN 46206

About Conception and Contraception (16 mm film)
Canadian Film Institute
303 Richmond Rd.
Ottawa, Ontario, Canada

Placental Circulation (16 mm, 8 mm, video)
Film Service ACOG
P.O. Box 299
Wheaton, IL 60187

Inner Woman (16 mm film)
Merrell Dow Pharmaceuticals, Inc.
Subsidiary of the Dow Chemical Co.
Cincinnati, OH 45215

The Beginning of Life (16 mm film)
Benchmark Films, Inc.
145 Scarborough Rd.
Briarcliff Manor, NY 10510

UNIT III

From Generation to Generation Genetic Counseling (slide/tape)
National Foundation—March of Dimes
Supply Division
Box 2000
White Plains, NY 10602

Life Before Birth (film strips)
Time Education Program
Time & Life Building
Rockefeller Center
New York, NY 10020

Genetic Defects: The Broken Code (16 mm film)
Indiana University Audio-Visual Center
Bloomington, IN 47401

Trying Times: Crisis in Fertility (16 mm film)
Fanlight Productions
P.O. Box 226
Cambridge, MA 02238

Alcohol: Crisis for the Unborn (16 mm film)
Film Distribution Division
The National Foundation—March of Dimes
1275 Mamaroneck Ave.
White Plains, NY 10605

Laparoscopy: The View Within (16 mm film)
Merrell Dow Pharmaceuticals, Inc.
Subsidiary of the Dow Chemical Co.
Cincinnati, OH 45215

Gynecologic Laparoscopy (16 mm film)
Upjohn Professional Film Library
7000 Portage Rd.
Kalamazoo, MI 49001

Born Drunk: The Fetal Alcohol Syndrome (16 mm film/videocassette)
ABC Learning Resources, Inc.
1330 Avenue of the Americas
New York, NY 10019

Gifts of Love (videocassette)
National Down's Syndrome Society
70 W. 40th St.
New York, NY 10018

Medicines Used during Pregnancy (videocassette)
National Audiovisual Center
National Archives Trust Fund Board
Washington, DC 20409

UNIT IV

Breast Feeding: Prenatal and Postpartum Preparation (16 mm film)
Health Sciences Communication Center
Case Western Reserve University
University Circle
Cleveland, OH 44106

The Biological Aspects of Sexuality (slide/tape)
Harper and Row
Media Department
10 E. 53rd St.
New York, NY 10022

The Case Against Rubella (16 mm film)
National Foundation—March of Dimes
Supply Division
Box 2000
White Plains, NY 10602

Facilitating Self-Disclosure (filmstrip/tape)
American Journal of Nursing Co.
Educational Services Division
10 Columbus Circle
New York, NY 10019

Nutrition in Pregnancy (16 mm film)
Jay Hathaway Productions, Inc.
4349 Tujunga Avenue
North Hollywood, CA 91604

Female Pelvic Exam (16 mm film)
Eli Lilly Company
Audio-Visual Film Library
Dept. MC-340
Indianapolis, IN 46206

A Study in Maternal Attitudes (16 mm film)
American Journal of Nursing
ANA-NLN Film Library
267 W. 25th St.
New York, NY 10001

Preparation of the Breast for Breast Feeding (16 mm film)
Mead Johnson Laboratories
Evansville, IN 47721

Nutritional Management of High-Risk Pregnancy (16 mm film, ¾" videocassette)
Films, Society for Nutrition Education
1736 Franklin St.
Oakland, CA 94612

Early Pregnancy (slide, cassette, sound, color)
Lifecircle
2378 Cornell Dr.
Costa Mesa, CA 92626

Feeding Your Baby—From Birth through the First Year (16 mm, ¾″ videotape, ½″ videocassette)
Fairview General Hospital
Audio Visual Communication
18101 Lorain Ave.
Cleveland, OH 44107

Teens Having Babies (16 mm, videocassette)
Polymorph Films, Inc.
118 South St.
Boston, MA 02111

Sex and Pregnancy (videos: ½″ beta, ½″ VHS, ¾″ U-matic)
Centre Films, Inc.
1103 North El Centro Ave.
Hollywood, CA 90038

Born Hooked (16 mm film)
Film Distribution Division
The National Foundation—March of Dimes
1275 Mamaroneck Ave.
White Plains, NY 10605

UNIT V

Right from the Start
Film Distribution Center
The New York Hospital
Cornell Medical Center
525 E. 68th St.
Box 581
New York, NY 10021

Modern Obstetrics: Fetal Evaluation
Wexler Film Productions
801 North Seward St.
Los Angeles, CA 90038

Diagnosis before Birth (16 mm film)
National Foundation—March of Dimes
Supply Division
Box 2000
White Plains, NY 10602

Hydatidiform Mole (slide/tape)
Oxford Tape-Slide Series in Obstetrics and Gynecology
Pretest Service, Inc.
71 South Turnpike
Wallingford, CT 06492

Modern Obstetrics: Pre-eclampsia (16 mm film)
ACOG Film and Video Service
P.O. Box 299
Wheaton, IL 60187

Intrauterine Fetal Transfusion (16 mm film)
Abbott Laboratories
Public Relations Department
Film Serive D-384
North Chicago, IL 60064

UNIT VI

Birth Experience (slides/tape)
Bay Area ASPO Slides
c/o Deanna Sollid, R.N.
59 Berens Dr.
Kentfield, CA 94904

Childbirth for the Joy of It
Jay Hathaway Productions
4349 Tujunga Ave.
N. Hollywood, CA 91604

That's Our Baby (16 mm film)
Lawren Productions, Inc.
P.O. Box 666
Mendocino, CA 95460

Saturday's Children
Parenting Pictures
121 N.W. Crystal St.
Crystal River, FL 32629

Labors of Love
Polymorph Films
118 South St.
Boston, MA 02111

Nicholas and the Baby
Centre Productions, Inc.
1327 Spruce St., #3
Boulder, CO 80302

Together with Love
Centre Films, Inc.
1103 North El Centro Ave.
Hollywood, CA 90038
Three films on childbirth education in a cultural context

Dar Pecho (breast-feeding)
Spanish (with Latino cast)
10-minute, color 16 mm film and ¾″ videocassette

Tamika's Birth
English with a black cast
11-minute, color 16 mm film, and ¾″ videocassette

Maternidad (Motherhood)
Spanish (with Latino cast)
10-minute, color 16 mm film and ¾″ videocassette
Childbirth Education Films
VIDEOGRAPH
2833 25th St.
San Francisco, CA 94110

UNIT VII

Birth Atlas Slide Series (with guide)
Maternity Center Association
48 E. 92nd St.
New York, NY 10028

UNIT VIII

Birth in the Squatting Position
Polymorph Films
118 South St.
Boston, MA 02111

All Together Now: A Birth Plan
Family Centered Childbirth Education Association
4635 N.W. 50th St.
Des Moines, IO 50323

Intrapartum Labor Monitoring (slide/booklet)
Corometrics Medical Systems, Inc.
Vic. American Home Products, Inc.
61 Barnes Park Rd. North
Wallingford, CT 06450

UNIT IX

Epidural Anesthesia for Vaginal Delivery (16 mm film)
Winthrop Laboratories
90 Park Ave.
New York, NY 10016

Family-Centered Cesareans (16 mm film)
Parenting Pictures
121 N.W. Crystal St.
Crystal River, FL 32629

Having a Section Is Having a Baby (slide/tape, videocassette)
Polymorph Films, Inc.
118 South St.
Boston, MA 02111

Deliverance: A Family's Cesarean Experience (16 mm film, videocassette)
Polymorph Films, Inc.
118 South St.
Boston, MA 02111

All the More Special (16 mm film)
Parenting Resources and Educational Programming
P.O. Box 36024
San Jose, CA 95158-6024

Abortion Clinic (videocassette)
Fanlight Productions
47 Halifax St.
Jamaica Plain, MA 02130

UNIT X

Adapting to Parenthood (16 mm film)
Polymorph Films
118 South St.
Boston, MA 02111

Are you Ready for the Postpartum Experience? (16 mm film)
Parenting Pictures
121 N.W. Crystal St.
Crystal River, FL 32629

Contraception: A Matter of Choice (filmstrips/cassette tapes)
Audio Visual Narrative Arts, Inc.
P.O. Box 398
Pleasantville, NY 10570

Family Planning (16 mm film)
Emko Co.
Div. of Schering, Inc.
411 E. Gano St.
St. Louis, MO 63147

Abortion (slide/tape)
Medical Electronic Educational Services, Inc.
29423 W. Six Mile Rd.
Livonia, MI 48152

2 A.M. Feeding (16 mm film)
New Day Films
P.O. Box 315
Franklin Lakes, NJ 07417

The Breast-Feeding Experience
Parenting Pictures
121 N.W. Crystal St.
Crystal River, FL 32629

Caring and Coping: The New Parent Experience (16 mm film and videocassette)
Parenting Pictures
121 N.W. Crystal St.
Crystal River, FL 32629

Breastfeeding: A Special Closeness (16 mm film, videocassette, super 8)
Motion, Inc.
203 3rd Street, N.E.
Washington, DC 20002

The First Two Weeks of Life (16 mm film)
Alert Letter Service
718 Main St.
Cincinnati, OH 45202

The Parenting Experience (16 mm film)
Alert Letter Service
718 Main St.
Cincinnati, OH 45202

UNIT XI

Modern Obstetrics: Postpartum Hemorrhage (16 mm film)
American Medical Association
535 N. Dearborn St.
Chicago, IL 60610

Death of a Newborn (16 mm film)
Ross Laboratories
585 Cleveland Ave.
Columbus, OH 43216

Death of a Wished-For Child
OGR Service Corporation
P.O. Box 3586
Springfield, IL 62708

To Pick Up the Pieces
Twenty-Twenty Media
Springfield, IL 62705

To Touch Today
Creative Marketing
P.O. Box 2432
Springfield, IL 62705

"We Were Sad, Remember"
IFDA
1045 Outer Park Dr., Suite 120
Springfield, IL 62704

To Have and Not to Hold (slide tape, videocassette)
Polymorph Films, Inc.
118 South St.
Boston, MA 02111

UNIT XII

The Amazing Newborn (16 mm film)
Ross Laboratories
585 Cleveland Ave.
Columbus, OH 43216

Newborn (16 mm film)
West Glen Films
West Glen Communications, Inc.
565 Fifth Ave.
New York, NY 10017

Nursery Sepsis (16 mm film)
American Hospital Association
840 North Lake Shore Dr.
Chicago, IL 60610

Changing Concepts: The Nursing Care of the Newborn (1) Introduction to Newborn Nursing (2) the First 12 Hours of Life
Health Media Corp.
P.O. Box 167
Tulsa, OK 74101

The Perinatal Assessment of Maturation (slide/tape)
National Medical Audiovisual Center
Washington, DC 20409

Jonah Has a Rainbow (16 mm film, videocassette)
Centre Productions, Inc.
1800 30th St., #207
Boulder, CO 80301

Prematurely Yours: Premature Infant Behavior and Personality (slide/tape, videocassette)
Polymorph Films, Inc.
118 South St.
Boston, MA 02111

The Sensational Baby (slide/tape, videocassette, 16 mm film)
Polymorph Films, Inc.
118 South St.
Boston, MA 02111

Falling in Love with Your Baby (16 mm film, ¾″ videocassette)
Johnson & Johnson Baby Products Co.
Grandview Rd.
Skillman, NJ 08558

UNIT XIII

PKU—Preventable Mental Retardation (16 mm film)
Mead Johnson Laboratories
Evansville, IN 47221

Hypoglycemia (slides/tape)
National Foundation—March of Dimes
Supply Division
Box 2000
White Plains, NY 10602

Resuscitation of the Newborn (16 mm film)
Mead Johnson Laboratories
Evansville, IN 47221

Thermal Regulation of the Neonate (16 mm film)
Mead Johnson Laboratories
Evansville, IN 47221

Born Dying (16 mm film, ¾″ beta or VHS videocassette)
Carle Medical Communications
510 W. Main, Department A
Urbana, IL 61801

Jaundice in the Newborn (slide/tape)
National Medical Audiovisual Center
Washington, DC 20409

Respiratory Distress Syndrome (16 mm film)
Mead Johnson Laboratories
Evansville, IL 47221

UNIT XIV

The Road (Frontier Nursing Service) (16 mm film)
ANA-NLN Film Library
267 W. 25th St.
New York, NY 10001

Birth without Violence (16 mm film)
New Yorker Films
43 W. 61st St.
New York, NY 10023

An Unremarkable Birth (16 mm film)
National Film Board of Canada
1251 Avenue of the Americas, 16th Floor
New York, NY 10020

Midwife: With Woman (16 mm film, videocassette)
Fanlight Productions
47 Halifax St.
Jamaica Plain, MA 02130

Homebirth? The Answer is Love (¾″ or ½″ VHS videocassette)
Educational Media
Route 1, Box 30
Winslow, AR 72959

Birth Reborn (16 mm film, videocassette)
The Texture Films Collection
P.O. Box 1337
Skokie, IL 60076

APPENDIX F
Organizations involved in maternity care

American Academy of Pediatrics
P.O. Box 1034
Evanston, IL 60204

American College of Home Obstetrics
2821 Rose St.
Franklin Park, IL 60131

American College of Nurse Midwives
1012 14th St., N.W., Suite 801
Washington, DC 20005

American College of Obstetricians and Gynecologists
600 Maryland Ave., S.W.
Suite 300 East
Washington, DC 20024

American National Red Cross
17th and D Sts., N.W.
Washington, DC 20006

American Nurses Association
2420 Pershing Rd.
Kansas City, MO 64108

Association for Childbirth at Home, International (ACHI)
P.O. Box 39498
Los Angeles, CA 90039

Healthy Mothers, Healthy Babies Coalition
721 Hubert Humphrey Building
200 Independence Ave., S.W.
Washington, DC 20201

Home Oriented Maternity Experience (HOME)
511 New York Ave.
Takoma Park, MD 20012

La Leche League International, Inc.
9616 Minneapolis Ave.
Franklin Park, IL 60131

Maternity Center Association
448 E. 92nd St.
New York, NY 10128

NAACOG: The Organization for Obstetric, Gynecologic, and Neonatal Nurses
600 Maryland Ave., SW
Suite 200 East
Washington, DC 20024

National Association of Parents and Professionals for Safe Alternatives in Childbirth (NAPSAC)
P.O. Box 267
Marble Hill, MO 63764

The National Committee for Prevention of Child Abuse (NCPCA)
332 South Michigan Ave., Suite 1250
Chicago, IL 60604

The National Foundation—March of Dimes
1275 Mamaroneck Ave.
White Plains, NY 10605

National League for Nursing
10 Columbus Circle
New York, NY 10019

National Organization of Mothers of Twins Club
5402 Amberwood Lane
Rockville, MD 20853

National Perinatal Association
1311-A Dolly Madison Suite 3A
McLean, VA 22101

National Sudden Infant Death Syndrome (SIDS) Foundation
2 Metro Plaza, Suite 205
8240 Professional Place
Landover, MD 20785

Planned Parenthood Federation of America
810 7th Ave.
New York, NY 10019

APPENDIX G
Groups for grief help

AMEND
c/o Maureen Connelly
4324 Berrywick Terrace
St. Louis, MO 63128
or
P.O. Box 30
Harbor City, CA 90710

Compassionate Friends
P.O. Box 1347
Oak Brook, IL 60521

HAND
P.O. Box 62
San Anselmo, CA 94960

National Sudden Infant Death Syndrome (SIDS) Foundation
310 S. Michigan Ave.
Chicago, IL 60604

SHARE
Sister Jane Marie Lamb, OSF
SHARE Chairperson
St. John's Hospital
Springfield, IL 62769

APPENDIX H

ICEA position paper: diagnostic ultrasound in obstetrics*

Since 1970, the use of ultrasound as a diagnostic tool in obstetrics has increased dramatically, accompanied by considerable debate concerning its appropriate use. In 1979, over 1 million pregnant women received at least one diagnostic ultrasound examination in the United States.[1] The United States Bureau of Radiological Health foresees that potentially all children born in this country after the early 1980's could be exposed in utero to ultrasound.[2] Routine early pregnancy scanning is done in Great Britain and increasingly in other countries.

Recently, new equipment and techniques have resulted in improved quality, reliability, convenience and quicker study time, adding impetus to the increased clinical use of ultrasound.[3] Nevertheless, most health professionals agree that risks are difficult to assess, and some questions of safety, especially on a long-term basis, remain unanswered.[1-11]

At the present time (1983) there are no performance regulations or standards for diagnostic ultrasound equipment nor standards for clinical use of the procedure in the United States or Canada. The Department of National Health and Welfare in Canada has published *Guidelines for the Safe Use of Ultrasound*.[5]

In 1979, A Notice of Intent to Propose Rules and Develop Recommendations for diagnostic ultrasound equipment in the United States was published, advising that the Commissioner of the United States Food and Drug Administration (FDA), "in accord with recommendations of the Obstetrical and Gynecological Device Classification Panel, believes it prudent to use the lowest practical exposure levels, consistent with obtaining needed diagnostic information, and to use diagnostic ultrasound only when there is a valid medical reason."[3]

In 1982, the FDA reaffirmed this position, stating that, "Until risks are better defined, a prudent public health policy dictates judicious use of diagnostic ultrasound. Ultrasound examinations should be used only when diagnostic benefits to patients are indicated, and the exposure duration and ultrasound intensity should be limited to that required to yield the necessary diagnostic information."[11]

A similarly conservative approach was recommended in 1981 by The American College of Obstetricians and Gynecologists, stating that, "At present, only indicated diagnostic studies should be ordered."[12]

In 1981 the International Childbirth Education Association published an *ICEA Position Statement on Electronic Fetal Monitoring*.[13] It should be read in conjunction with this statement on diagnostic ultrasound, since Doppler ultrasound is used in electronic fetal monitoring during labor and in Doptone monitoring during pregnancy. The use of ultrasound in these procedures is generally not understood by pregnant women. It is therefore essential that information be provided about the use, accuracy, complications, and costs of electronic fetal monitoring.[13]

---

*ICEA Position Paper: Diagnostic Ultrasound in Obstetrics, published by the International Childbirth Education Association (ICEA), P.O. Box 20048, Minneapolis, Minn. 55420 USA, Reprinted with permission from the ICEA.

ICEA'S POSITION

The International Childbirth Education Association (ICEA) takes the position that obstetrical intervention and technology should be used only in the presence of medically valid criteria.[16] Since "no well-controlled study has yet proved that routine scanning of all prenatal patients will improve the outcome of pregnancy,"[12] since professional consensus does not support use of ultrasound on all pregnant women,[3-8,12] and since studies on long-term effects are inconclusive,[3,6,8,11] ICEA makes the following recommendations with respect to the use of diagnostic ultrasound in obstetrics:

- Pregnant women should avoid ultrasound exposure unless there is a documented medical reason for its use and/or disease is suspected.
- Pregnancy is a normal physiological process which does not, by itself, constitute a medical reason for ultrasound exposure.
- Participation in an ultrasound examination must be voluntary.
- Pregnant women should be specifically informed that the Doptone and electronic fetal monitor are both ultrasound devices. Written informed consent should accompany the use of electronic fetal monitoring.
- Ultrasound examination should not be withheld when there are valid indications of potential psychological and physical benefit.
- The desire of a healthy pregnant woman to know the baby's sex or "see the baby move" should not, by itself, be considered a valid reason for exposure to ultrasound.
- Before an ultrasound examination, expectant parents should be given information about the procedure, its benefits and known risks, gaps in knowledge about biological effects, and alternative tests which might be done and their benefits and risks.
- The pregnant woman's partner (i.e., support person of her choice) should be offered the opportunity to accompany her during the scanning procedure to allay anxiety and promote family involvement.
- Pregnant women should be given the opportunity to view the ultrasound screen during the procedure.
- Pregnant women should not undergo an ultrasound examination for commercial demonstration of equipment.
- Ultrasound examinations should be conducted and interpreted only by skilled personnel trained in ultrasound use and interpretation. The pregnant woman has the right to inquire about the training in ultrasonography of her physician and operators of the equipment. Physicians should be able to verify qualifications on request.
- Public health agencies and medical and scientific organizations have an obligation to publicize information on the biological effects of ultrasound, known risks, areas of uncertainty, and availability of guidelines for ultrasound use.

Documentation in support of these positions follows.

INSTRUMENTATION

The ultrasound examination (scan) is a procedure that enables study of the inner organs of the body by means of sound waves. The use of this procedure in obstetrics is rapidly replacing the use of x-ray examinations. In the ultrasound scan, high-frequency sound waves are directed into the pregnant woman's abdomen, where they rebound from structures and surfaces, producing "echoes," which can then be measured and recorded on a video display screen. Ultrasound uses nonionizing energy in contrast with the ionizing energy of x-rays, which is potentially carcinogenic.

The major types of diagnostic equipment are the static B scan, real-time imaging, and Doppler unltrasound. The static B scan method emits pulsed sound waves that provide a two-dimensional or cross-sectional view of a body tissue or organ. Real-time imaging is very rapid pulsed scanning that provides a "moving picture" of body organs. Since its introduction in 1974, increasing numbers of obstetricians are installing this equipment in their offices.[11,14] The Doppler device uses continuous sound waves, in which "echoes returned from moving structures are recorded as audio signals."[12] Fetal heart tones can be measured by the Doppler principle using a Doptone device during pregnancy and an external fetal monitor during labor, in which the ultrasound beam may be focused on one spot for many hours. The duration of exposure to ultrasound varies with the equipment used.

The frequency of the sound waves in clinical ultrasound devices is in the range of 3.5 to 5 megahertz (MHz), which is above those heard by the human ear.[1]

The intensity of energy waves emitted from an ultrasound device is measured in watts or milliwatts per square centimeter (W/cm^2 or mW/cm^2) of tissue being exposed, that is, the power of sound divided by the area over which it is spread. The intensity of a sound beam is not constant throughout the beam at a given time, and for pulsed ultrasound it varies with time. As an ultrasound beam is transmitted through tissue, it undergoes a complex series of processes that absorb, scatter, and refract the beam from its initial path. These processes may reduce its intensity, but focusing the beam can increase the intensity more than tenfold.[15] It is known that an ultrasound beam of sufficiently high intensity for sufficient time and exposure can produce harmful effects in biological tissue.[11]

Most manufacturers do not currently provide information about ultrasound exposure levels with their equipment. However, intensity levels for obstetrical ultrasound have been reported as follows[11]: In pulsed or static (B) scan devices, the average intensity ranges from about 0.01 to 10 mW/cm^2 with peak intensity from 0.4 to 700 W/cm^2; in continuous wave devices (Doppler) the average intensity ranges from 0.26 to 25 mW/cm^2. The peak intensities associated with pulsed devices can go up to hundreds of watts per square centimeter, and it is possible that some biological effects may result.[11] No maximum intensity levels for medical ultrasound have been officially established.

INDICATIONS FOR USE

The American College of Obstetricians and Gynecologists does not support the routine use of ultrasound and recommends that only indicated scans be done.[12] It states that, "No well-controlled study has yet proved that routine scanning of all prenatal patients will improve the outcome of pregnancy."[12]

The following primary indications for the use of diagnostic ultrasound in obstetrics have been recommended by the National Institutes of Health and The American College of Obstetricians and Gynecologists[8,12]:

- To establish gestational age by measuring the gestational sac diameter (at 5-8 weeks), the crown-rump length of the fetus (at 8-14 weeks), and the biparietal diameter (BPD) of the fetal head (at 15-25 weeks).
- To detect abnormalities of early pregnancy, including ectopic pregnancy, hydatidiform mole, congenital malformations, and threatened abortions.
- To determine location of the placenta and ascertain fetal movement as an adjunct to diagnostic amniocentesis.
- To conduct fetal growth studies in the second trimester.
- To investigate vaginal bleeding.
- To confirm abnormal fetal presentation.
- To confirm multiple pregnancy.
- To ascertain fetal life.
- To detect pelvic masses (tumors).

It should be noted that the use of ultrasound solely as a screening tool for dating gestational age of the fetus, both in early pregnancy[17] and after 25 weeks' gestation, is controversial. **By listing these indications, ICEA does not imply endorsement in the absence of a high-risk indication.**

COSTS

New advances in ultrasound technology are constantly emerging, accompanied by increasing competition in the market for ultrasound equipment.[18] A 1981 update on real-time devices suitable for physician offices lists prices ranging from $16,500 to $30,000 and more elaborate systems up to $45,000.[19] In 1974, sales of ultrasound equipment were about $65 million in the United States; in 1983 it has been predicted they will be $490 million.[18]

In 1979 it was estimated that the total cost of ultrasonography for 100,000 scans could be as high as $10 million.[8] On the other hand, the use of ultrasound to determine fetal maturation offers a potential for cost savings by preventing premature births, and early detection of fetal abnormalities by ultrasound can avoid later medical and long-term costs.[8]

The actual cost of an ultrasound scan to the consumer varies depending on geographic location, facility, type of equipment, and type of scan. It ranged from $50 to $115 in the United States in 1982. Reimbursement for the procedure varies, but in 1981 it was noted that "third party payors have recently refused to pay for routine screening procedures."[12]

FACILITIES

Ultrasonography is performed in many settings—obstetrics and radiology departments, genetic counseling centers, separate ultrasound clinics and divisions in hospitals, and private physician offices. It has been recommended that diagnostic ultrasound be available on a 24-hour basis at all secondary and tertiary level hospitals.[12]

The National Institutes of Health observes that the use of pulsed diagnostic ultrasound alone to detect fetal abnormalities in midtrimester constitutes clinical research and should therefore be conducted in specialized medical centers with highly experienced ultrasonographers, counseling staff, and ongoing research.[8]

It was estimated in 1981 that about 20% of obstetricians' offices had a real-time ultrasound scanner[19] and that the purchase of this equipment for office use is expanding at an estimated rate of about 20% a year worldwide.[20] Currently, because Certificate of Need (i.e., regional and/or state approval) is not required for a private practitioner to buy ultrasound equipment in the United States but is a requirement for hospital purchase, expansion of ultrasonography into private physicians' offices is certain.[14]

The availability of ultrasound in private offices is more convenient for the pregnant woman and her physician, but it has been noted that the inexperience of some equipment operators (no training other than that provided by the physician-employer in 30% of offices in one survey[14]) increases the risk of inaccurate interpretation of scans and is cause for concern.[12]

OPERATORS

Questions have been raised about the adequacy of training and expertise of ultrasound operators (both physicians and technicians).[5,8,12,14] The American College of Obstetricians and Gynecologists observes that the use of ultrasound "without proper training could result in false diagnoses and reduced cost-effectiveness."[12] It has been recommended that ultrasound technologists complete an accredited ultrasound training program and qualify for certification and that physicians receive formal training.[12]

For physicians in the United States, 3 months' training in obstetrical and gynecological ultrasound followed by 2 months' practical experience is recommended for those who have not received special training in ultrasound during residency.[21] To obtain accreditation, the diagnostic medical sonographer, whose work should be under direct supervision of a physician experienced in ultrasound,[12] should receive 2 years' training in ultrasound if he or she is a high school graduate without postsecondary education, or 1 years' training if already qualified in an allied health profession.[22] Canadian guidelines for operator training have also been published that recommend 6 months or more of formal training and experience in the use of ultrasound.[5]

ACCURACY

Refinements in ultrasound technology offer continual improvements in resolution and accuracy, but it has been pointed out that "the quality and reliability of the images depend directly on the skill of the person operating the equipment."[18] In addition, several physical distortions (e.g., mottling) and factors directly affect image quality and the diagnostic capability of ultrasound devices.[23] The absence of routine testing and maintenance of equipment can also affect the quality of information provided, and output levels of ultrasound devices can vary widely without operator knowledge.[3]

The accuracy of ultrasound in establishing gestational age by measuring the biparietal diameter of the fetal head depends on when the procedure is done in pregnancy. The scan is most accurate between 15 and 25 weeks' gestation but is inaccurate after that time in predicting fetal age and maturity.[8,12]

Misleading information could result if prenatal scanning were done routinely at 20 to 24 weeks' gestation and showed conditions that usually resolve spontaneously by term.[12] The findings could indicate an incidence of abnormal fetal presentations (e.g., breech) that could be nine times the actual occurrence at term; similarly, the apparent incidence of placenta previa at 20 to 24 weeks could be 60 times the actual incidence at term.[12]

With electronic fetal monitoring (EFM) or Doppler ultrasound, inaccuracies in diagnosis can occur, interpretations of readings can vary, and EFM findings are therefore open to "both misinterpretation and erroneous clinical decisions" in labor and birth management.[8] Confirmation of EFM diagnoses by a fetal scalp blood test has been shown to improve diagnostic accuracy in the determination of fetal distress.[8] Additional information about EFM is provided in the *ICEA Position Statement on Electronic Fetal Monitoring.*[13]

SAFETY

The safety of diagnostic ultrasound in obstetrics has been extensively discussed and reviewed, and the consensus is that additional clinical, laboratory, and epidemiological research is necessary to evaluate its safety.[1-11,15] The biological mechanisms of the action of ultrasound are not fully understood, and the possibility of subtle or long-term health problems is not known. To date, harmful effects to human beings have not been reported, but since this technology has become widely used before all safey aspects and interactions with the human body have been determined, caution in its use is advised by public health and professional organizations[3,5,8,11,12] and by other health professionals.[4,15]

The effects of ultrasound on biological systems may result from the following actions[6,9]:

- Heating or thermal effects. The absorption of ultrasound wave energy causes heat production in tissue.
- Cavitation effects. Under certain conditions ultrasound can cause gaseous cavities or bubbles within the exposed tissue, in which the bubble's surface oscillates in response to pressure variations cased by the sound wave. To produce this effect, gas-filled bubbles, or micronuclei, must already be present in tissue.
- Mechanical effects. Vibrations of ultrasound waves can cause "direct" effects on particles and cells of living tissue, altering structure and function.

Recommended exposure levels for safety have not been determined, but the United States Bureau of Radiological Health[3] considers that the recommendations of the National Electrical Manufacturers Association provide reasonable guidelines: intensity levels of 10 mW/cm^2 for pulse-echo devices and 20 mW/cm^2 for Doppler (continuous) devices.[3,24] The American Institute of Ultrasound in Medicine has reported (1976,1978) no significant biological effects on mammalian tissue exposed to intensities below 100 mW/cm^2.[2,25]

In 1982 the United States Bureau of Radiological Health concluded, "Although the body of current evidence does not indicate that diagnostic ultrasound represents an acute risk to human health, it is insufficient to justify an unqualified acceptance of safety."[11]

LABORATORY STUDIES

The number of laboratory studies on the biological effects of ultrasound on cells, plants, and animals greatly exceeds those conducted with human beings. Recent extensive reviews of the literature demonstrate that the evidence on biological effects of ultrasound is inconclusive and difficult to compare, since (1) most experiments have not been verified by other studies, and (2) study methodology is often inadequate.[6,11] Other factors contibuting to the confusion include differences in experimental organisms, in stage of development at the time of exposure, in intensity levels, and in time and duration of exposure.[11] It is not known whether any effects of ultrasound on tissue are additive or cumulative, nor is it clear how the available data on biological effects of ultrasound can be related to possible effects on human beings.[11]

Recent reports of biological effects in animals (e.g., mice, rats) exposed to ultrasound have involved exposure at currently used diagnostic levels, both continuous wave (Doppler) and pulse-echo.[2,10] Studies have been cited that show delayed neuromuscular development, altered emotional behavior, fetal abnormalities, and rise in temperature in rodents exposed to clinical devices at intensity levels ranging from 10 to 40 mW/cm^2.[3,10,11] It has been suggested that these studies need to be repeated with improved experimental design.[1] Fetal weight reduction and smaller litter size among rodents exposed to high intensities of ultrasound have also been reported.[4,6,11] Low intensities of ultrasound can produce hematological and vascular alterations in some animals.[11]

Insect eggs and larvae, and plant and mammalian cells have been damaged by inducing cavitation (bubbles) by exposure to ultrasound.[4,6,11] It is not known, however, if the physical conditions necessary for cavitation are present in human tissue.

Another group of studies has examined ultrasound effects on cell function (i.e., genetic effects). One report indicated interaction of ultrasound at low intensities with DNA material in cells and changes in cell appearance and motility.[26] In attempts to reproduce these findings, some have succeeded and others have failed.[11] Other reports have not found evidence of chromosome damage in mammalian cells at intensities and frequencies used in diagnostic ultrasound.[6]

HUMAN STUDIES

Most studies have reported no adverse effects of ultrasound on human beings, except for one study showing a more than 90% increase in fetal activity with the Doppler (continuous wave) device.[27] Other investigators have not confirmed this increase in fetal activity,[28] and further study in this area is suggested.[6]

It has been concluded that an increase in chromosome abnormalities seems unlikely when the fetus is exposed during the second and third trimesters, but because of insufficient data, no conclusion can be reached on possible chromosome damage during the first trimester.[6]

The findings of human epidemiological studies to date have been judged inconclusive,[5] but two major epidemiological studies, one in the United States funded by the United States Food and Drug Administration and the other in Canada, are currently under way. The United States study, begun in 1975, is a long-term follow-up study that involves approximately 400 children exposed to ultrasound in utero and approximately 400 children matched for age and obstetrical complications who were not exposed. Results will be available soon. In a report on part of this study that examined birth records of 2,135 single births, an association between ultrasound exposure and low birth weight has been found,[29] which "raises concern about human exposure at diagnostic levels."[11] This association needs further study to determine if it is a random association or a cause-and-effect association.

The Canadian study, also begun in 1975, will involve 10,000 women and their children exposed to ultrasound and 2,000 controls.[4,11] Preliminary results from this study are reassuring, and the incidence of fetal death, congenital abnormalities, serious communicative disorders, and cancer was no greater than that expected for the size of the population studied.[4] Although a slight but significant increase occurred in the number of children who were underweight at birth, the weight difference had disappeared by 5 years of age, and the cause was attributed to the fact that most of the underweight children came from high-risk pregnancies.[4]

The question of safety of ultrasound with current human information is inconclusive, and although acute effects are unlikely, studies to detect "less obvious" effects have not been done.[11] General areas of concern include developmental (behavioral and neurological), hematological, immunological, and genetic effects.[11] The professional consensus at a 1981 symposium on ultrasound was that since the possibility of subtle or delayed harmful effects is unknown, the procedure should be used only when a valid medical indication exists.[4]

ADVANTAGES AND DISADVANTAGES

The following advantages for the use of ultrasound have been cited:

- More accurate pregnancy dating in midtrimester (16-25 weeks).[8,14]
- Parental reassurance by indicating absence of fetal abnormality.[8,14]
- Early diagnosis of twins.[8,14]
- Better detection of fetal abnormalities, enabling early decision making by parents.[8,14]
- Early diagnosis of small-for-gestational age children.[14]
- Little or no discomfort for the noninvasive procedure.[8]
- Reduced necessity for using x-ray procedures.[8]
- Early diagnosis of maternal disorders.[8]
- Possible enhancement of maternal- and paternal-fetal bonding through visualizing the fetus.[30]
- Increased likelihood of an uncomplicated amniocentesis and fetoscopy.[8]
- Avoidance of inappropriate amniocentesis if serious malformation is diagnosed by ultrasound.[8]

The following disadvantages for the use of ultrasound has been cited:

- Long-term safety unknown.[1-12]
- No evidence of benefit for early screening of low-risk pregnant women.[1,12]
- Increased anxiety for some parents by early detection of conditions that resolve themselves spontaneously by term without intervention (e.g., malpresentations, apparent placenta previa).[12,30]
- Timing (i.e., during pregnancy) and number of scans to be performed an issue of debate among professionals.[12]
- Scanning often performed by untrained personnel.[14]
- Potential for abuse in private physician practice[14] (e.g., personal gain, faulty interpretation) and at other pratice locations.
- Inaccuracy in predicting fetal age and maturity after 25 weeks' gestation.[12]
- Some technical equipment limitations.[6,23,31]
- Diagnostic inaccuracy (false-positives and false-negatives).[8,17]
- Prolonged maternal recumbent position and restriction of mobility for use of electronic fetal monitoring (Doppler ultrasound),[8,11] causing compression of maternal blood vessels and fetal distress.
- Increased health care costs.[14]

The foregoing advantages and disadvantages should be considered in the context of rapid developments in the field of diagnostic ultrasound. Changes in indications, methods, equipment, interpretation, training requirements, professional guidelines, and research findings occur constantly.

FAMILY-CENTERED ASPECTS

Obstetrical practice and care should be conducted within a family-centered atmosphere and environment, with (1) sensitivity to the psychological and social needs of parents, (2) provision of accurate and adequate information about all aspects of procedures or treatments, and (3) discussion of evidence for benefits and possible risks to mother and child.

To assist expectant parents in making well-informed decisions about the use of prenatal tests and increase understanding, they should be given the following information:

- Type of information the test can and cannot provide.[17,32]
- How the test results will determine the course of care, and how the course of care will be affected if the test is **not** done.[1]
- Accuracy of the test[17]; possibility and meaning of inaccurate diagnoses (falsely positive or falsely negative).[32]
- Cost and reimbursement information.[32]
- Considerations of options available, depending on the results of the test.[32]
- Information about diagnostic intervention that may be needed.[32]
- Explanation of the risks involved, as far as they are known[32]; gaps in knowledge about the effects of the test.
- Research purposes for the test, if any.[32]
- Assurance that the privacy of expectant parents will be "scrupulously protected," so that individuals cannot be identified through central registries and medical data banks.[32]
- Sources for additional information, e.g., for ultrasound use, effects, safety, etc. contact the American Institute of Ultrasound in Medicine, 4405 East-West Highway, Suite 504, Bethesda, Maryland 20814 U.S.A., or the Bureau of Radiological Health, Food and Drug Administration, Rockville, Maryland 20857 U.S.A.

When an ultrasound examination is medically indicated, factors that can enhance family-centered aspects of the test include the following[31]:

- Sensitive, relaxing, and reassuring atmosphere in scanning area.
- Attention to "human relation skills" by ultrasound operators, whereby the pregnant woman is "treated with courtesy, respect, and a kindness in word and action. . ."[31]
- Attention to individual needs, matching the technique to the situation, with appropriate position changes, flexibility, rest periods, and comfort measures.
- Opportunity for the woman's partner to accompany her throughout the scanning procedure to reduce anxiety and promote family involvement.
- Avoidance of overreading or underreading the images.
- Explanation of ultrasound procedures as they are occurring and what the parents are seeing on the video screen.

FUTURE DIRECTIONS AND NEEDS

It has been acknowledged that "Many deficiencies and gaps exist in the current data base for ultrasound induced bioeffects. The potential for acute adverse effects has been virtually ignored. Few of the experiments have been duplicated in other laboratories. More information is needed on the effects of low-intensity ultrasound, the biological impact of the high temporal intensities used in pulsed ultrasound, the possibility of cumulative effects, and the possibility of long-term effects."[11] Major fields for future ultrasound research include studies on molecules and cells, and developmental, hematological/cardiovascular, genetic, immunological, behavioral, and human effects.[11]

Additional research on ultrasound use and instrumentation is needed so that the health risk from exposure to ultrasound can be properly evaluated. Refinements of ultrasound devices are constantly occurring, yet very little information exists on the ultrasound exposure an individual receives during a scan.[6] Performance regulations for diagnostic ultrasound equipment and standards for clinical use are needed.

Research is necessary to determine possible subtle effects of ultrasound. It is especially important to determine effects of ultrasound on the developing ova of the female fetus.[11,33] The sensitivity of tissue and organs, including sensory organs, requires further study.[9] Cavitation induced by ultrasound is a complex activity, and whether the findings in insects and plant and animal cells have relevance for human biological systems is an important area for investigation.[6]

The National Research Council of Canada stresses that "long-term follow-up studies of both the mother and fetus exposed to ultrasound are desperately needed."[6] It has been suggested that children exposed to ultrasound in utero should receive "intensive developmental, behavioral, and functional assessment for a number of years."[9]

The field of ultrasound is progressing extremely rapidly, and medical applications continue to increase. Since the question of ultrasound safety is still unresolved, it is therefore essential that new information, guidelines, and research findings be made available to the public as they develop. With accurate information and a thorough understanding of the ultrasound examination and its implications, childbearing families will be better able to make informed decisions about the use of this diagnostic procedure.

REFERENCES

1. Hobbins, J.C., Berkowitz, R.L., and Hohler, C.W.: How safe is ultrasound in obstetrics? *Contemp Ob/Gyn* Special Issue 14:63-74, 1979.
2. Stratmeyer, M.E.: Research directions in ultrasound bio-effects—a public health view. In Symposium on biological effects and characterizations of ultrasound sources, Rockville, Md., Dec., 1977, U.S. Department of Health, Education, and Welfare, pp. 240-245.
3. Food and Drug Administration, U.S. Department of Health, Education, and Welfare: Diagnostic ultrasound equipment: Development of action program, *Fed Reg* 44(13):9542-9545, Feb. 13, 1979.
4. Bolsen, B.: Question of risk still hovers over routine prenatal use of ultrasound, *JAMA* 247:2195-2197, 1982.
5. Environmental Health Directorate, Health Protection Branch: Guidelines for the safe use of ultrasound. I. Medical and paramedical applications, Ottawa, 1980, Department of National Health and Welfare.
6. Repacholi, M.H.: Ultrasound: Characteristics and biological action, Ottawa, 1981, Publication no. NRCC 19244, National Research Council of Canada.
7. Kennedy, D.: Statement. In Obstetrical practices in the United States, 1978, Washington, D.C., April 17, 1978, Hearing before the Subcommittee on Human Resources, U.S. Senate, 95th Cong., 2nd sess., U.S. Government Printing Office.
8. Antenatal diagnosis, Bethesda, Md., 1979, National Institutes of Health Consensus Development Conference, NIH Publication no. 79-1973, U.S. Department of Health, Education, and Welfare.
9. Abdulla, U.: Biologic effects of ultrasound. In Sabbagha, R.E., editor: Diagnostic ultrasound applied to obstetrics and gynecology, New York, 1980, Harper & Row, Publishers.
10. Stratmeyer, M.E.: Research in ultrasound bioeffects: A public health view, *Birth Fam J* 7:92-100, Summer, 1980.
11. Stewart, H.F., and Stratmeyer, M.E.: An overview of ultrasound: Theory, measurement, medical applications, and biological effects, HHS Publication FDA 82-8190, July, 1982, Bureau of Radiological Health, Food and Drug Adminstration.
12. American College of Obstetricians and Gynecologists: Diagnostic ultrasound in obstetrics and gynecology, ACOG Technical Bulletin No. 63, Oct., 1981.
13. ICEA Position statement on electronic fetal monitoring, *ICEA News* 20:4-6, Nov., 1981.
14. Hohler, C.W.: Real-time ultrasound moves into the OB office, *Contemp Ob/Gyn* Special issue 16:75-80, 1980.
15. Waxham, R.D.: Ultrasound safety information, *Perinat Press* 3:67-68, May, 1979.
16. ICEA Position paper on planning comprehensive maternal and newborn services for the childbearing year, Minneapolis, 1979, International Childbirth Education Association.

17. Edwards, M., and Simkin, P.: Obstetric tests and technology: A consumer's guide, Seattle, 1980, the pennypress.
18. Office of Technology Assessment: Policy implications of the computed tomography (CT) scanner: An update, Appendix B, Research and development of CT and other diagnostic imaging technologies, Washington, D.C., Jan., 1981.
19. Hohler, C.W.: Update on real-time ultrasound equipment for the ob-gyn office, *Contemp Ob/Gyn* Special issue 18:13-26, 1981.
20. U.S. market forecast, 1980.
21. Joint Task Force Group on Training for Diagnosis in Obstetrical and Gynecological Ultrasound: Guidelines for minimum post-residency training on OB/GYN ultrasound, Washington, D.C., 1981, American Institute of Ultrasound in Medicine.
22. Joint Review Committee on Education in Diagnostic Medical Sonography: Essentials and guidelines of an accredited education program for the diagnostic medical sonographer, Philadelphia, 1979.
23. Popp, R.L., and Macovski, A.: Ultrasonic diagnostic instruments, *Science* 210:268-273, 1980.
24. Technical Committee of the Ultrasound Section of the Radiation Imaging Products Division, National Electrical Manufacturers Association: Recommendations of the Technical Committee proposed for consideration. Presented to the Ultrasound Subcommitee, Ob/Gyn Device Classification Panel, Bureau of Medical Devices, FDA, HEW, 1976, 1978.
25. American Institute of Ultrasound in Medicine Bioeffects Committee: Acoustical definitions; bioeffects safety, Oklahoma City, 1979.
26. Liebeskind, D., et al.: Diagnostic ultrasound: Effects on the DNA and growth patterns of animal cells, *Radiology* 131:177-184, 1979.
27. David, H., Weaver, J.B., and Pearson, J.F.: Doppler ultrasound and fetal activity, *Br Med J* 2:62-64, 1975.
28. Hertz, R.H., Timo-Tritsch, L.J., Chik, L., et al.: Continuous ultrasound and fetal movement, *Am J Obstet Gynecol* 135(1):152-154, 1979.
29. Moore, R.M., Barrick, M.K., and Hamilton, P.M.: Effects of sonic radiation on growth and development. Presented before the Society for Epidemiologic Research, Cincinnati, June 17, 1982.
30. Queenan, J.T.: In Ultrasound diagnosis: Update for the 1980's, *Contemp Ob/Gyn* 15:28-56, 1980.
31. Hughey, M.J.: The ultrasound scan. In Sabbagha, R.E., editor: Diagnostic ultrasound applied to obstetrics and gynecology, New York, 1980, Harper & Row, Publishers.
32. Powledge, T.M., and Fletcher, J.: Guidelines for the ethical, social and legal issues in prenatal diagnosis, *N Engl J Med* 300:168-172, 1979.
33. Haire, D.: How the FDA determines the "safety" of drugs—Just how safe is "safe"? Washington, D.C., 1980, National Women's Health Network.

Glossary

abortion Termination of pregnancy before the fetus is viable, that is, less than 20 to 24 weeks gestation.

abruptio placentae Premature separation of a normally implanted placenta.

acidosis A pathological condition resulting from accumulation of acid in, or loss of base from, the body.

acini cells Milk-producing cells in the breast.

acinus A small saclike dilation, particularly one found in various glands.

acme The highest point of a uterine contraction.

adolescent A teenager or young adult.

AGA Appropriately grown for gestational age.

alleles One or two or more alternative states of a gene.

amniocentesis Procedure to remove amniotic fluid from the uterine cavity by inserting a needle through the abdominal and uterine walls and into the amniotic sac.

amnion The inner of the two fetal membranes forming the sac that encloses the fetus in the uterus.

amnionitis Inflammation of the amnion.

amniotomy Articficial rupture of the amniotic sac (AROM).

analgesia Relief of pain without loss of consciousness.

anesthesia Loss of feeling or sensation, with or without loss of consciousness.

anteflexed The normal forward bending of the uterus.

antepartum The period of pregnancy before delivery.

anticipatory guidance Anticipating the needs of a family and thus providing teaching in advance of these needs.

Apgar score Numerical rating of an infant's condition at 1 and 5 minutes after birth, based on heart rate, respiratory effort, muscle tone, reflex irritability, and color. Developed by Dr. Virginia Apgar.

apnea Temporary cessation of respiration.

areola Pigmented ring aroung the nipple of the breast.

asphyxia A condition in which there is a deficiency of oxygen in the blood and an increase in carbon dioxide in the blood and tissues.

atelectasis Incomplete expansion or collapse of the lungs.

atony A lack of normal muscle tone or tension.

axis A line about which any revolving body turns.

ballottement A term used when, in examining the pregnant woman, the fetus can be pushed about in the uterus.

Bartholin's glands The vulvovaginal glands.

baseline fetal heart rate Fetal heart rate pattern between uterine contractions.

bicornate uterus Anomalous uterus that may be either a double or a single organ having two horns.

bilirubin Yellow or orange pigment produced by the breakdown of hemoglobin in cell elements and in the red blood cells.

blastoderm The germinal membrane of the ovum.

Braxton-Hicks contractions Light, irregular, painless contractions of the uterus during pregnancy.

breech The buttocks; in a breech presentation, the buttocks present for delivery instead of the head.

caput succedaneum Swelling produced on the presenting part of the fetal head during labor.

cephalic Pertaining to the head.

cephalopelvic disproportion (CPD) When the size of the fetal head is too large to pass through the maternal pelvis.

cephalhematoma An accumulation of blood under the periosteum of any one of the cranial bones.

cerclage Encircling an incompetent cervix with a ring or loop of suture.

cesarean birth Delivery of the fetus through a surgical incision into the abdominal and uterine walls.

Chadwick's sign Violet color of the vaginal mucous membrane during pregnancy.

chloasma A discoloration of the skin of the face occurring in yellowish-brown patches and spots, also known as the "mask of pregnancy."

chorion The outer of the two membranes forming the sac that encloses the fetus in the uterus.

chromosomes Structures in the nucleus of cells that carry the genes or hereditary factors.

cilia Minute hairlike processes.

circumcision The surgical removal of the end of the prepuce or foreskin of the penis.

cleavage The early successive splitting of a fertilized ovum into smaller cells (blastomere).

clitoris Structure of the female genitalia analogous to the penis in the male.

colostrum The first secretion from the breasts during pregnancy and before lactation.

congenital Existing at or before birth.

convoluted A tortuous irregularity caused by the unfolding of a structure upon itself.

Coomb's test Indirect: determination of Rh-positive antibodies in maternal blood; direct: determination of maternal Rh-positive antibodies in fetal cord blood.

cornu Horn; a hornlike projection.

corpus luteum The yellow mass found in the graafian follicle after the ovum has been expelled.

CPAP (continuous positive airway pressure) Often used in treating respiratory distress syndrome in the newborn.

crowning Stage in delivery when the widest part of the fetal head appears at the vulva.

cystitis Infection in the urinary bladder.

cytomegalovirus (CMV) A group of highly host-specific herpesviruses, causing cytomegalic inclusion disease in man.

deceleration A slowing down.

decidua The endometrium during pregnancy.

decidua basalis The portion of the decidua directly under the implanted zygote.

decrement Decrease in intrauterine pressure after the acme of a uterine contraction.

diabetogenic state Producing diabetes-like symptoms.

dilation and curettage (D & C) A surgical procedure involving dilation of the cervix and removal of uterine contents.

diuretics Drugs that cause an increased excretion of urine.

dizygotic Derived from two fertilized cells.

dominant Capable of expression when carried by only one of a pair of homologous chromosomes.

ductus arteriosus A communicating channel between the aorta and the pulmonary artery of the fetus.

ductus venosus A fetal vessel that establishes a direct communication between the umbilical veins, through the liver, to the inferior vena cava.

dura (dura mater) Outermost, toughest of the three meninges covering the brain and spinal cord.

dyspnea Difficult or labored breathing.

dystocia Difficult labor or delivery.

eclampsia Abnormal reaction of the body to pregnancy resulting in convulsions; preceded by pre-eclampsia.

ectopic pregnancy Implantation of the fertilized ovum outside the cavity of the uterus.

effacement A thinning and shortening of the cervix that occurs during late pregnancy and/or labor.

effleurage Gentle stroking of the abdomen used during labor in some childbirth preparation methods.

ejaculation A sudden expulsion of semen.

embolism The sudden blocking of an artery or vein by a clot or foreign material that has been brought to its site of lodgment by the blood current.

embryo Products of conception from the second to the eighth weeks of gestation.

endometritis Inflammation of the endometrium.

endometrium The membrane lining the cavity of the uterus.

endothelium The layer of epithelial cells that lines the cavities of the heart and of the blood and lymph vessels and the serous cavities of the body.

endotracheal tube A tube inserted within the trachea.

engagement In obstetrics engagement has occurred when the widest diameter of the fetal head has passed through the inlet of the pelvis.

engorgement Lymph and venous stasis occurring in the breasts prior to the flow of milk.

epidural External to the dura mater.

episiotomy Surgical incision of the perineum as the fetal head crowns, if necessary, to facilitate delivery.

erythema toxicum A rash of unknown cause occurring in the newborn. It goes away spontaneously without treatment.

erythroblastosis fetalis Blood disorder in the fetus or newborn in which maternal anti-Rh antibodies destroy fetal blood cells, causing jaundice and other symptoms.

estriol A relatively weak human estrogen that is the oxidized end product of estradiol and estrone.

estrogen Female sex hormone manufactured in the ovaries.

ethnic Pertaining to a social group who share cultural bonds or physical (racial) characteristics.

exchange transfusion Replacement of 75% to 85% of circulating blood by withdrawing the recipient's blood and injecting a donor's blood in equal amounts.

fallopian tubes The two oviducts extending from the sides of the uterine fundus.

fetal Pertaining to the fetus.

fetal advocate A person who recognizes the health and well-being of the fetus as top priority.

fetal bradycardia A slowing down of the fetal heart rate below 100 beats per minute.

fetal tachycardia Fetal heart rate over 160 beats per minute for 10 minutes or more.

fetoscope A scope used to visualize the fetus in its sac. A specially designed stethoscope for listening to fetal heart tones.

fetus Products of conception from the eighth week of gestation until birth.

fibrin An insoluble protein that is essential to

clotting of blood, formed from fibrinogen by action of thrombin.

fibrinogen A normal blood constituent necessary for the formation of clots.

flexion The act of bending, or the condition of being bent.

follicle Secretory cavity or sac.

follicle-stimulating hormone (FSH) Hormone that stimulates the maturation of the graafian follicle.

fontanel An unossified space or "soft spot" lying between the cranial bones of the skull of a fetus.

foramen ovale Opening between the right and left atria of the fetal heart.

gavage Feeding by a stomach tube.

genes The factors responsible for the transmission of hereditary characteristics to offspring.

gestation Length of time a pregnancy is carried.

Goodell's sign Softening of the cervix.

gravida The number of times a woman has been pregnant.

Hegar's sign Softening of the lower segment of the uterus that is classified as a probable sign of pregnancy.

hemangioma A benign tumor made up of newly formed blood vessels.

hematoma A collection of blood in tissue.

hemostasis The arrest of bleeding.

heterozygous Having different alleles in regard to a given characteristic on each gene of a pair.

homozygous Having identical alleles for a characteristic on each gene of a pair.

human chorionic gonadotropin (HCG) A hormone produced by the trophoblast.

hydrocephalus An excess of cerebrospinal fluid within the ventricular system.

hymen Membranous fold that partially closes the vaginal orifice.

hyperbilirubinemia Elevation of unconjugated serum bilirubin concentrations.

hyperplasia Increase in the number of normal cells in normal arrangement in an organ or tissue.

hypertonic Increased tonicity or tension.

hypoglycemia Low level of sugar (glucose) in the blood.

hypovolemic shock Shock caused by abnormally decreased volume of circulating fluid (plasma) in the body.

icterus neonatorum Jaundice in a newborn.

"incompetent" cervix A cervix that is prone to dilate before the normal period of gestation. Frequently this happens between the sixteenth and twenty-eighth weeks of gestation.

increment Increasing intrauterine pressure as a uterine contraction begins.

induction Labor brought on by artificial means.

inertia A sluggishness or inactivity of uterine contractions during labor

infant mortality rate (IMR) Number of deaths of live-born infants before the first year of life per 1000 live births.

innominate bone One of the two pelvic bones.

intubation The insertion of a tube.

inversion A turning inward, inside out, or upside down.

involution The return of the reproductive organs to the nonpregnant state when pregnancy is over.

ischium The lower part of the innominate bone.

isoimmunization Development of antibodies in response to isoantigens (e.g., development of anti-Rh antibodies in an Rh-negative person).

jaundice Yellow discoloration of the body tissues caused by the deposit of bile pigments (unconjugated bilirubin).

Kegel exercise An exercise to strengthen the perineal muscles, first described by Dr. Kegel.

kernicterus Erythroblastosis fetalis with brain damage.

ketoacidosis Acidosis resulting from accumulation of ketone bodies.

labia majora The large, outer lips of the vulva.

labia minora The folds of delicate skin inside the labia majora.

lactation The secretion of milk.

lactose Milk sugar.

lanugo Fine downy hair growing over the body of the fetus.

laryngoscope An endoscope for examining the larynx.

Leopold's maneuvers Abdominal inspection and palpation to determine how the fetus is postioned in utero.

"let-down" reflex A new mother's body's response to oxytocin that allows milk in the breast alveoli to flow into the milk ducts.

LGA (large for gestational age) An infant whose birth weight falls above the 90th percentile.

lie In obstetrics the relationship of the long axis of the fetus to the long axis of the mother.

lightening Descent of the uterus into the pelvic cavity before or during labor.

linea nigra A dark line appearing longitudinally on the abdomen of pregnant women.

lobule A small segment or lobe, especially one of the smaller divisions making up a lobe.

lochia The vaginal discharge during the puerperium, consisting of blood, mucus, and tissue.

lochia alba The final yellowish-white vaginal discharge after childbirth.

lochia rubra The red, sanguinous vaginal discharge of the first 2 to 4 days postpartum.

lochia serosa The serous vaginal discharge occurring 4 to 5 days after birth.

mastitis Inflammation or infection of the breast.

meconium The dark green or black, sticky, tarry substance in the large intestine of the fetus or newly born baby.

meningocele Congenital malformation of the spine in which the meninges protrude through a defect in the cranium or vertebral column.

milia Distended sebaceous glands commonly found over the bridge of the nose, chin, and cheeks of newborn infants; appear like tiny "whiteheads."

mongolian spots Areas of dark blue pigmentation over the lumbar, sacral, and gluteal regions.

moniliasis Infection of the mucous membranes of the skin caused by a yeastlike fungus.

monozygotic Derived from one fertilized cell, such as identical twins.

Montgomery's tubercles Sebaceous glands of the areola of the breast.

morbidity State of being sick or diseased.

mortality Death.

morula The solid mass of cells formed by the division and redivision of the fertilized ovum.

myometrium Muscle coat of the uterus.

Naegle's rule Method of estimating the expected date of confinement (EDC), or due date. Count back 3 months from the first day of the last menstrual period and add 1 year and 7 days.

neonatal From birth to 28 days of life.

occiput The back part of the head.

oscilloscope An instrument that displays a visual representation of electrical variations on the fluorescent screen of a cathode ray tube.

ovulation Rupture of the graafian follicle and discharge of the ovum.

oxytocin Pharmaceutical agent that stimulates uterine contractions. Also, a naturally-produced posterior pituitary hormone that causes contraction of uterine myometrial cells and myoepithelial cells of the breast.

para Past pregnancies continued to period of viability—referring to pregnancies and not fetuses.

pelvic floor The soft tissues closing the pelvic outlet.

perfusion The passage of a fluid through the vessels of a specific organ.

perimetrium The serous membrane enveloping the uterus.

perineum In obstetrics the area between the lower end of the vagina and the anus.

phenylketonuria (PKU) An inborn error in metabolism in which the infant lacks the enzyme necessary to metabolize phenylalanine (an essential amino acid).

placenta The organ attached to the wall of the uterus through which the fetus derives its nourishment and oxygen.

placenta accreta A placenta abnormally adherent to the uterine wall.

placenta previa A placenta that is implanted in the lower uterine segment so that it partially covers the internal os of the cervix.

posterior Behind, or back of.

pre-eclampsia A disorder that can be present during pregnancy or early in postpartum period, characterized by hyptertension, edema, and albuminuria.

preterm labor Labor that begins before 38 weeks gestation.

prepuce The fold of skin that covers the glans penis of the male and clitoris of the female.

presentation The part of the fetus that enters the pelvis first.

presumptive signs Manifestations that suggest pregnancy but that are not absolutely positive. These include the cessation of menses, Chadwick's sign, morning sickness, and quickening.

probable signs Manifestations or evidence which indicates that there is a definite likelihood of pregnancy. These include Goodell's sign, Hegar's sign, enlargement of the abdomen, and positive pregnancy tests.

prolactin Hormone that stimulates lactation.

prolapsed cord The umbilical cord presenting beside or ahead of the presenting part.

prostaglandins Biological substances naturally occurring in semen, menstrual fluid, and various tissues of the body; stimulate contractility of the uterine and other smooth muscle.

proteinuria Presence of protein (albumin) in the urine.

puerperal sepsis Infection during the puerperium (postpartum period).

recessive Inheritance requiring genes from both mother and father.

reflex Automatic response built into the nervous system.

regimen A strictly regulated scheme of diet, exercise, or other activity.

restitution Spontaneous turning of fetal head to right or left after it has extended through the vulva thus assuming a normal alignment with the baby's shoulders.

retrolental fibroplasia A formation of fibrous tissue behind the lens of the eye, resulting in blindness. One cause of this condition is administration of oxygen in too high concentrations to premature infants.

retroverted A condition in which the normally anteflexed uterus is tipped posteriorly.

rubella German measles.

sedative A drug that allays irritability or excitement.

septate Divided by a septum.

septicemia Severe generalized illness caused by bacteria in the blood stream.

SGA (small for gestational age) An infant who falls below the 10th percentile for weight.

sibling Any of two or more offspring of the same parents; a brother or sister.

Skene's glands Ducts found on each side of the urethral meatus.

spermatozoa The male generative cells.

spina bifida Defect in closure of the bony spinal canal.

station The location of the presenting part of the fetus in relation to the ischial spines of the pelvis.

striae gravidarum Reddish-purple, irregular depressions that appear in the skin of the abdomen, thighs, and buttocks of pregnant women.

subinvolution Failure of the uterus to return to its normal size following pregnancy.

surfactant A surface-active agent secreted by type II cells in the alveoli of the lungs. It reduces the surface tension of the pulmonary fluids and thus prevents the alveoli from collapsing.

symphysis pubis Thick mass of fibrocartilage formed at the union of the pubic bones.

tachypnea Rapid respiration.

testes The two glands contained in the male scrotum.

thermogenesis Heat production.

thrombophlebitis Inflammatory process along the walls of the blood vessels.

thrush A fungus infection of the oral membranes, usually caused by *Candida albicans*. White patches on a red, moist, inflamed surface are apparent in the mouth.

titer The quantity of a substance required to react with or to correspond to a given amount of another substance.

transition The last part of the active phase of labor (from 8- to 10-centimeter dilation).

trimester Three-month period

trisomy The presence of three chromosomes rather than the usual two.

trophoblast Cells that form outer layer of the blastula.

tuboplasty Plastic surgery to repair severed or damaged fallopian tubes.

ultrasonography A technique by which high-frequency sound waves are beamed into the body and then reflect back, enabling the deep structures of the body to be visualized on a screen.

umbilicus Navel.

urethra The passage through which urine is discharged from the bladder to outside the body.

uterus The womb; a hollow muscular organ in which the embryo and fetus develop.

vaginitis An infection in the vagina.

vernix A white cheeselike substance that covers the skin of the fetus.

version Manual turning of the fetus.

vertex The crown of the head.

vestibule The space below the clitoris and between the labia minora.

viable Able to live.

villi A small vascular process or protrusion on a membranous surface.

vulva The external genitals of the female.

zygote The fertilized ovum.

Index

N

O

P

S

T